ESSENTIALS of NUTRITION in MEDICINE and HEALTHCARE

A Practical Guide

ESSENTIALS of NUTRITION in MEDICINE and HEALTHCARE

A Practical Guide

Editors:

Sumantra (Shumone) Ray, MB BS, MPH, MD, DN (Health Education), RNutr (Public Health), FHEA, FIANE
Founding Chair, Chief Scientist & Executive Director
NNEdPro Global Institute for Food, Nutrition & Health
Cambridge, United Kingdom

Bye-Fellow in Human, Social & Political Sciences,
Fitzwilliam College at the University of Cambridge
Professor of Global Nutrition, Health & Disease at Ulster University
Visiting Professor of Public Health & Primary Care at Imperial College London
Lord Rana Foundation Honorary Professor of Strategy Development
Co-Chair, BMJ Nutrition, Prevention and Health

Mariana Markell, MD
Professor of Medicine
Division of Nephrology
SUNY Downstate Health Sciences University
Brooklyn, New York, USA

Associate Editors and Content Coordinators:

Jørgen Torgerstuen Johnsen, BSc Hons, MSc, MIANE
Visiting Academic Associate
NNEdPro Global Institute for Food, Nutrition and Health
Oslo, Norway

PhD Researcher
Ulster University
Coleraine, Northern Ireland

James Bradfield, BSc Hons, MSc, MIANE, RD, ANutr
Senior Dietitian
Department of Nutrition & Dietetics
Kings College NHS Foundation Trust
London, United Kingdom

Lead Global Innovation Panel & Visiting Senior Academic Associate
NNEdPro Global Institute for Food, Nutrition and Health
London, United Kingdom

NNEdPro Global Institute for Food, Nutrition and Health is an award-winning interdisciplinary think-tank, building upon over a decade of nutrition education, research and innovation. Anchored in Cambridge (UK), we develop adaptable and scalable educational models for nutrition capacity building in health systems. We also conduct a range of training courses, primary research studies, and syntheses to fill key evidence gaps.

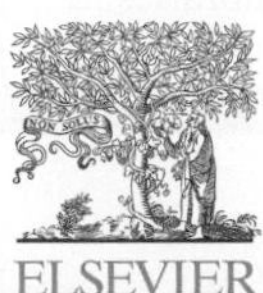

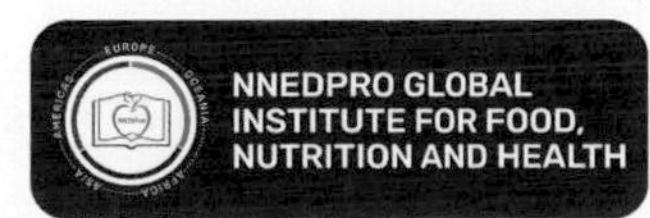

Social Enterprise | Independent Research Organisation
Education and Training Centre | Advisory Services

© 2024, Elsevier Limited. All rights reserved.

No part of this publication may be reproduced or transmitted in any form or by any means, electronic or mechanical, including photocopying, recording, or any information storage and retrieval system, without permission in writing from the publisher. Details on how to seek permission, further information about the Publisher's permissions policies and our arrangements with organizations such as the Copyright Clearance Center and the Copyright Licensing Agency, can be found at our website: www.elsevier.com/permissions

This book and the individual contributions contained in it are protected under copyright by the Publisher (other than as may be noted herein).

Notices

Practitioners and researchers must always rely on their own experience and knowledge in evaluating and using any information, methods, compounds or experiments described herein. Because of rapid advances in the medical sciences, in particular, independent verification of diagnoses and drug dosages should be made. To the fullest extent of the law, no responsibility is assumed by Elsevier, authors, editors or contributors for any injury and/or damage to persons or property as a matter of products liability, negligence or otherwise, or from any use or operation of any methods, products, instructions, or ideas contained in the material herein.

ISBN: 978-0-7020-8040-1

Senior Content Strategist: Alexandra Mortimer
Content Project Manager: Kritika Kaushik
Design: Patrick Ferguson
Art Buyer: Akshaya Mohan
Marketing Manager: Deborah Watkins

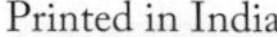

Printed in India

Last digit is the print number: 9 8 7 6 5 4 3 2 1

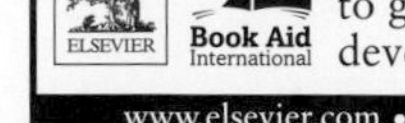

We, Sumantra (Shumone) Ray and Marianna (Marni) Markell, would like to dedicate this textbook to Shumone's daughter, Nikitah Rajput-Ray, as well as Marni's family, Jody, Miranda, Max, and Peter, for patiently listening to the travails of this book for years and cheering on to the finish line!

CONTENTS

The study of and clinical practice associated with nutrition has never been more important. The global COVID-19 pandemic has brought to the fore the importance of optimising nutrition to prevent and cure disease. Work in this area continues at pace at many levels from basic science to whole food systems and in the health policy and medical education arenas. This textbook represents a significant body of work, bringing together expert voices to produce a comprehensive outline of important nutrition concepts by body system, and is therefore an attractive publication for the qualified medical or health care professional and student alike.

Suboptimal nutrition management in health care systems is a leading cause of morbidity which at an individual level impacts on quality of life. In addition, for populations and health systems, it can result in economic catastrophe, with malnutrition costing the UK economy £13 billion annually as just one example. A way of tackling this growing problem is by working collaboratively across health care disciplines to address deficiencies in awareness, knowledge, and skills by providing appropriate education and training. Education schemes and medical or health care qualifications can use books like this one as a guide to ensure that core clinical nutrition competencies as applied to everyday practice can be implemented successfully.

A global crisis of the scale caused by COVID-19 has reduced incomes and disrupted vitally important supply chains, impacting the most vulnerable and exacerbating issues of food insecurity. As a result, health care professionals must also be equipped with the knowledge and skills to support efforts to address these widened health inequalities in the UK and internationally. That is why the nutrition and mental health section, with its chapter on public health, policy, prevention and implementation, is a welcome addition, widening the scope of this textbook and providing critical skills to support the broader responsibility that health care professionals have in society.

The demand for the information found in these pages does not just come from the need within society and our health systems, but also from practitioners themselves. There is a desire from them to learn more about the interface between nutrition and disease, as well as a need for greater clarity of a doctor's role working alongside established nutrition and dietetic professionals. Taking the steps outlined in this text will boost confidence and improve care for all patients as well as enhance public trust in medical and health care professionals.

Dr Harrison Carter
Chief of Staff, Vaccinations and Screening
at NHS England
NNEdPro senior collaborator

FOREWORD 2

Recently published research has demonstrated that there is a major gap within medical training in nutrition for both undergraduate and postgraduate students. This is a gap that we starkly experienced whilst studying at medical school and one that has been experienced by many other medical students in the United Kingdom and globally.

To address this gap, Nutritank (https://nutritank.com) was created in 2017 as an information and innovation hub for food, nutrition and lifestyle medicine. It is our firm belief that nutrition forms an essential component of every patient's management, with the food we eat impacting all bodily systems from the gastrointestinal system to the cardiovascular system to mental health. What's more, with the ongoing rise of lifestyle-related, noncommunicable disease, a fundamental understanding of nutrition will help doctors of the future to treat, as well as prevent, disease.

Nutrition education is vital to provide holistic, patient-centred care. The fact remains that at present, trainee doctors are ill prepared to talk about nutrition in practice, and they leave medical school without the knowledge or tools to navigate the nutritional space.

Our aim is to make a change to the current state of the health care system by ensuring that there is greater nutrition and lifestyle medicine education available to medical students and doctors throughout their training. We believe that this textbook provides an essential foundation of nutritional knowledge, which will prove invaluable for medical students and junior doctors alike, as well as other health care professionals not primarily trained in nutrition. This textbook will act as a reference guide to assist in clinical decision making and ensure patients are provided with evidence-based treatment and advice.

As medical students and junior doctors, we believe that this textbook provides a much-needed learning resource for current and future medical students. At present, there are few, if any, nutrition textbooks written specifically with medical students in mind, especially not one with a focus on how they can best support their patients through adequate nutrition provision alongside clinical dietitians and other members of the multidisciplinary team.

We are grateful to share our vision with the NNEdPro Global Centre for Nutrition and Health (https://www.nnedpro.org.uk/) and look forward to ongoing close collaborations with it to accomplish this mission. This textbook is a collaboration between leading voices in the reform of greater nutrition in medical training.

Nutritional education forms an essential role in the future of medicine, and this textbook is the ideal place to start, leading the way for a sea of change across the medical community and promoting a focus on patient-centred health care.

Dr Ally Jaffee and Dr Iain Broadley
Cofounders of Nutritank (Junior Doctors)
Juliet Burridge, Tally Abramovich and Esha Dandekar
Nutritank Core Team (Medical Students)

CONTRIBUTORS

The editor(s) would like to acknowledge and offer grateful thanks for the input of all contributors, without whom this new edition would not have been possible.

Contributors

Kirsty Alderton, MBChB, MRCPsych
Consultant Psychiatrist
Bristol Mental Health Services
Bristol, United Kingdom
Chapter 13

Sarah Armes, BSc (Hons), MSc, MIANE
Academic Officer
NNEdPro Global Institute for Food, Nutrition and Health
Cambridge, United Kingdom
Chapter 6

David Armstrong, MD, FRCP (Edin)
Consultant Rheumatologist, WHSCT
Clinical Lead for Fracture Liaison & Osteoporosis
Londonderry, United Kingdom

Visiting Professor
NICHE
Ulster University
Coleraine, United Kingdom
Chapter 10

Lauren Ball, BAppSc, MNutrDiet, PhD, Grad Dip Health Economics and Policy, Grad Cert Higher Education, FIANE
Professor of Community Health and Wellbeing
Centre for Community Health and Wellbeing
The University of Queensland
Brisbane, Queensland, Australia

Associate Director
NNEdPro Global Institute for Food, Nutrition and Health
Brisbane, Queensland, Australia
Chapters 3 and 14

Kaninika Basu, MBBS, MD
Clinical Fellow
Department of Medicine
Cambridge University Hospital NHS Foundation Trust
Cambridge, United Kingdom

Honorary Research Fellow
Brighton and Sussex Medical School
Brighton, United Kingdom
Chapter 12

Eleanor Beck, BSc Hons, Dip Nutr&Diet, PhD, FIANE
Professor and Head of School
Health Sciences
University of New South Wales
Kensington, New South Wales, Australia

Visiting Senior Academic Associate (Professorial)
NNEdPro Global Centre for Food, Nutrition and Health
Kensington, New South Wales, Australia
Chapter 2

Joanna Bond, RD
Advanced Renal Dietitian
Nutrition and dietetics
Brighton & Sussex University Hospital
United Kingdom
Chapter 9

James Bradfield, BSc Hons, MSc, MIANE, RD, ANutr
Senior Dietitian
Department of Nutrition & Dietetics
Kings College NHS Foundation Trust
London, United Kingdom

Lead Global Innovation Panel & Visiting Senior Academic Associate
NNEdPro Global Institute for Food, Nutrition and Health
London, United Kingdom
Chapter 9 and Appendix 3

Iain Broadley, BSc Hons, MBChB
Medical Doctor
General Medicine
Universities Hospitals Sussex
Sussex, United Kingdom

Nutritank C.I.C.
Appendix 2

Luke Buckner, BSc (Hons), BM BS, MSc, MIANE
Assistant Director
NNEdPro Global Institute for Food, Nutrition and Health
Cambridge, England
Chapter 6

Mei Yen Chan, BSc (Hons), PhD, FIANE
Associate Professor
School of Medicine
Nazarbayev University
Kazakhstan

Visiting Senior Academic Associate (Professorial)
NNEdPro Global Institute for Food, Nutrition and Health
Kazakhstan
Chapter 7

Dominic Crocombe, BSc Hons, MBBS, MSc, MRCP, MIANE
Gastroenterology Specialty Trainee and NIHR Academic Clinical Fellow in Hepatology
Sheila Sherlock Liver Centre & Institute of Liver and Digestive Health
Royal Free London NHS Foundation Trust & University College London
London, United Kingdom

NIHR Academic Clinical Fellow in Hepatology
Institute of Liver and Digestive Health
University College London
London, United Kingdom

Assistant Director
NNEdPro Global Institute for Food, Nutrition and Health
London, United Kingdom
Chapter 8

Pauline Douglas, BSc Hons, MBA, PgCHEP, RD, FBDA, FHEA, FIANE
Senior Dietetic Lecturer and Clinical Dietetics Facilitator
Department Nutrition Innovation Centre for Food and Health (NICHE)
Ulster University
Coleraine, United Kingdom

Lord Rana Foundation Honorary Professor of Leadership in Higher Education

Vice Chair & Operations Director
NNEdPro Global Institute for Food, Nutrition and Health
Coleraine, United Kingdom
Chapters 5 and 11

Tim Eden, BSc Hons (Dietetics), MB BS, MIANE, RD
GP Registrar and Freelance Dietitian
Berkshire Healthcare NHS FT
Berkshire, United Kingdom

Visiting Senior Academic Associate
NNEdPro Global Institute for Food, Nutrition and Health
Berkshire, United Kingdom
Chapter 2

Hala El-Agib El-Shafie, BSc Hons, RD
Consultant Dietitian, Clinical Speciality Eating Disorders and Bariatric Surgery
Nutrition and Dietetics
The Harley Nutrition Clinic
Nutrition Rocks LTD
London, United Kingdom
Appendix 2

Mary Feeney, MSc, RD
Paediatric Allergy Research Dietitian
Department of Women and Children's Health.
King's College London
London, United Kingdom
Chapter 12

Rajna Golubic, MD, MPhil PhD, DSc, MIANE, MRCP
NIHR Clinical Lecturer in Endocrinology and Diabetes
Oxford Centre for Diabetes, Endocrinology and Metabolism
University of Oxford
Oxford, United Kingdom

Associate Director
NNEdPro Global Institute for Food, Nutrition and Health
Oxford, United Kingdom
Chapter 7

Sandra Holasek, PhD
Associate Professor
Division of Immunology, Otto Loewi Research Center for Vascular Biology, Immunology and Inflammation
Medical University of Graz
Graz, Styria, Austria
Chapter 13

Ally Jaffee, BSc Hons, MBChB
Medical Doctor
General Medicine
NHS Luton & Dunstable Hospital
Luton, United Kingdom

Nutritank C.I.C.
Appendix 2

Jørgen Torgerstuen Johnsen, BSc Hons, MSc, MIANE
Visiting Academic Associate
NNEdPro Global Institute for Food, Nutrition and Health
Oslo, Norway

PhD Researcher
Ulster University
Coleraine, Northern Ireland
Chapter 14

Laura Keaver, MSc, RD
Lecturer in Human Nutrition and Dietetics
Health and Nutritional Science
Atlantic Technological University Sligo
Sligo, Ireland
Chapter 11

Ali Ahsan Khalid, MA (Cantab), MB BChir
Imperial College London
Faculty of Medicine
London, United Kingdom
Chapter 7

Sonja Lackner, PhD
Nutrition Scientist
Division of Immunology, Otto Loewi Research Center for Vascular Biology, Immunology and Inflammation
Medical University of Graz
Graz, Styria, Austria
Chapter 13

Celia Laur, BSc Hons, MSc, PhD, FIANE, RNutr
Associate Director
NNEdPro Global Institute for Food, Nutrition and Health
Toronto, Canada

Scientific Lead
Office of Spread & Scale, Implementation Science Team
Women's College Hospital Institute for Health System Solutions and Virtual Care (WIHV)
Toronto, Ontario, Canada

Assistant Professor
Institute of Health Policy, Management and Evaluation (IHPME)
University of Toronto
Toronto, Ontario, Canada
Chapters 3 and 14

Breanna Lepre, BNutrDiet (Hons), PhD, MIANE, APD
Research Fellow
Centre for Health System Reform and Integration
Mater Research Institute-University of Queensland (MRI-UQ)
Herston, Queensland, Australia

Assistant Director
NNEdPro Global Centre for Food, Nutrition and Health
Herston, Queensland, Australia
Chapters 1, 5, and 11

Elaine Macaninch, BSc Hons (nutrition & dietetics), PGDip (clinical education), PGCert (medical education), PGCert (diabetes & obesity), MIANE, RD
Research and Education Dietitian
University Hospitals Sussex
Brighton, East Sussex, United Kingdom

Visiting Senior Academic Associate
NNEdPro Global Centre for Food, Nutrition and Health
Brighton, United Kingdom
Chapter 9

Mariana Markell, MD
Professor of Medicine
Division of Nephrology
SUNY Downstate Health Sciences University
Brooklyn, New York, USA
Chapter 9

Kathy Martyn, BSc (Biological Sciences), BEd, MSc (Medical Nutrition), PhD, FIANE, RN, RNutr
Principal Lecturer Nutrition
School of Sport and Health Sciences
University of Brighton
Brighton, United Kingdom

Associate Director
NNEdPro Global Institute for Food, Nutrition and Health
Brighton, United Kingdom
Chapter 3

Shane McAuliffe, BSc Hons, MSc, MIANE, RD, APD, ANutr
Oncology Dietitian
Chris O'Brien Lifehouse
Sydney, New South Wales, Australia

Visiting Senior Academic Associate
NNEdPro Global Institute for Food, Nutrition and Health
Sydney, New South Wales, Australia
Chapter 5 and Appendix 3

Duane Mellor, BSc Hons, PhD, RD RNutr
Senior Lecturer and Associate Dean Public Engagement
Aston University
Birmingham, United Kingdom
Chapter 7 and Appendix 1

Claudia Gabriela Mitrofan, MB BChir, PhD, AFHEA
Junior Doctor
The National Health Service
Addenbrooke's Hospital, Cambridge
Cambridge, United Kingdom
Chapter 7

Sabrina Mörkl, MD, PhD
Consultant Psychiatrist
Division of Medical Psychology, Psychosomatics and Psychotherapeutic Medicine
Medical University of Graz,
Graz, Styria, Austria
Chapter 13

Minha Rajput-Ray, BSc Hons (Ost Med), MB ChB, DOccMed, DDAM, DIBLM, FIANE
Integrated & Lifestyle Medicine Physician and Medical Director
The Curaidh Clinic
East of Scotland

Non-Executive Director
NNEdPro Global Institute for Food, Nutrition and Health
Dundee, Scotland
Chapter 10

Sumantra (Shumone) Ray, MB BS, MPH, MD, DN (Health Education), RNutr (Public Health), FHEA, FIANE
Founding Chair, Chief Scientist & Executive Director
NNEdPro Global Institute for Food, Nutrition & Health
Cambridge, United Kingdom

Bye-Fellow in Human, Social & Political Sciences, Fitzwilliam College at the University of Cambridge
Professor of Global Nutrition, Health & Disease at Ulster University
Visiting Professor of Public Health & Primary Care at Imperial College London
Lord Rana Foundation Honorary Professor of Strategy Development
Co-Chair, BMJ Nutrition, Prevention and Health
Chapters 1 and 6

Lisa Sharkey, MA (Cantab), MB BChir, FRCP
Consultant
Department of Gastroenterology
Cambridge University Hospitals NHS Foundation Trust
Cambridge, United Kingdom
Chapters 4 and 8

Mercedes Zorrilla Tejeda, BSc (Hons), MSc, ANutr
Mexico Regional Network Co-Lead
NNEdPro Global Institute for Food, Nutrition and Health
Mexico City, Mexico
Chapter 14

Clare Wall, BSc Hons, MApplSci, PhD, RD, FIANE
Head of Department and Professor of Nutrition and Dietetics
Nutrition and Dietetics
University of Auckland
Auckland, New Zealand

Visiting Senior Academic Associate (Professorial)
NNEdPro Global Institute for Food, Nutrition and Health
Auckland, New Zealand
Chapter 6

Jeremy Woodward, MA (Cantab), MB BChir, PhD, FRCP
Consultant Gastroenterologist
Department of Gastroenterology and Clinical Nutrition
Addenbrooke's Hospital
Cambridge, United Kingdom
Chapter 4

ABBREVIATIONS

ACTH	adrenocorticotrophic hormone
AEC	Ambulatory Emergency Care
AKI	acute kidney injury
ALF	acute liver failure
anti-TTG	antitissue transglutaminase
APC	antigen-presenting cell
ARB	angiotensin receptor blocker
ARDS	acute respiratory distress syndrome
ASH	alcoholic steatohepatitis
B	Bacteroidetes
BCAA	branched-chain amino acid
BDA	British Dietetic Association
BFHI	Baby-Friendly Hospital Initiative
BIA	bioelectrical impedance analysis
BMD	bone mineral density
BMI	body mass index
BP	blood pressure
CF	cystic fibrosis
CFIR	Consolidated Framework for Implementation Research
CKD	chronic kidney disease
COPD	chronic obstructive pulmonary disease
CPAP	continuous positive airway pressure
CRBSI	catheter-related blood stream infections
CRP	C-reactive protein
CT	computed tomography
CVD	cardiovascular disease
D2	ergocalciferol
D3	cholecalciferol
DASH	Dietary Approaches to Stop Hypertension
DEXA	dual energy X-ray absorptiometry
DNL	de novo lipogenesis
DRV	dietary reference value
EE	energy expenditure
eGFR	estimated glomerular filtration rate
EOE	eosinophilic oesophagitis
EPA	eicosapentaenoic acid
ERAS	Enhanced Recovery After Surgery
ESKD	end-stage kidney disease
F	Firmicutes
FDEIA	food-dependent exercise-induced anaphylaxis
FRAIL	fatigue, resistance, ambulation, illnesses, and loss of weight
GDM	gestational diabetes mellitus
GI	gastrointestinal
GIT	gastrointestinal tract
GORD	gastro-oesophageal reflux disease
GP	general practitioner
HD	haemodialysis
HDU	high-dependency unit
HE	hepatic encephalopathy
HPN	long-term parenteral nutrition provided at home
IBS	irritable bowel syndrome
IBS-C	constipation-predominant IBS
IBW	ideal body weight
ICU	intensive care unit
IFALD	intestinal failure-associated liver disease
IgE	immunoglobulin E
IL	interleukin
ILCs	innate lymphoid cells
iNKT	invariant TCR+ CD1d-restricted natural killer T (cells)
INPAC	Integrated Nutrition Pathway for Acute Care
IPF	idiopathic pulmonary fibrosis
LDL	low-density lipoprotein
MAO	monoamine oxidase
MCV	mean corpuscular volume
MDD	major depressive disorder
MGBA	microbiota–gut–brain axis
MI	Motivational Interviewing
MNA	Mini Nutritional Assessment
MNA-SF	Mini Nutritional Assessment Short Form
MODY	maturity-onset diabetes in youth
MST	Malnutrition Screening Tool
MUFA	monounsaturated fatty acid
MUST	Malnutrition Universal Screening Tool
NAFLD	nonalcoholic fatty liver disease
NASH	nonalcoholic steatohepatitis
NEAP	net endogenous acid production

NEAT	nonexercise activity thermogenesis
NG	nasogastric
NICE	National Institute for Health and Clinical Excellence
NIV	noninvasive ventilation
NPY	neuropeptide Y
NRS	Nutrition Risk Screening 2002
NSAID	nonsteroidal anti-inflammatory drug
NST	nutrition support team
OGD	oeosphago-gastric duodenoscopy
ONS	oral nutritional supplements
OSA	obstructive sleep apnoea
PCOS	polycystic ovary syndrome
PD	peritoneal dialysis
PEG	percutaneous endoscopic gastrostomy
PEG-J	PEG with jejunal extension
PFS	pollen food syndrome
PG-SGA	patient-generated Subjective Global Assessment
PH	pulmonary hypertension
PN	parenteral nutrition
PPI	proton pump inhibitor
PTH	parathyroid hormone
PUD	peptic ulcer disease
PUFA	polyunsaturated fatty acid
RD	registered dietitian

RRT	renal replacement therapy
RTI	respiratory tract infection
SBS	short bowel syndrome
SCFA	short-chain fatty acid
SCREEN II	Seniors in the Community: Risk Evaluation for Eating and Nutrition, Version II
SDG	Sustainable Development Goals
SGA	Subjective Global Assessment
SIBO	small intestinal bacterial overgrowth
SIMPLE	Systematised, Interdisciplinary Malnutrition Pathway for Implementation and Evaluation in Hospitals
SMART	specific, measurable, accurate, reliable, timely
SPT	skin prick test
T1DM	type 1 diabetes mellitus
T2DM	type 2 diabetes mellitus
T3	triiodothyronine
T4	thyroxine
TB	tuberculosis
Th	T helper (Th1, Th2, etc.)
Treg	regulatory T cell
TSH	thyroid-stimulating hormone
UC	ulcerative colitis
WCRF	World Cancer Research Fund
WHO	World Health Organization

ACKNOWLEDGEMENTS

The editors and authors would like to specifically acknowledge Marjorie Lima Do Vale (NNEdPro Assistant Director) and Helena Trigueiro (NNEdPro Research Associate) for helpful inputs and comments as well as those colleagues who contributed to early conceptualisation of key chapters including Harrison Carter, Martin Kohlmeier, Melissa Adamski, Sharon Akabas, Marion Groetch, Sheepa Soni, Agnes Ayton, Dunecan Massey, Jenny Blythe, and Giuseppe Grosso.

Special thanks are due to operations colleagues within NNEdPro including Matheus Abrantes, Veronica Funk Petric, and several other members of our projects, operations, and strategy functions in their individual and collective efforts in supporting the production of this textbook.

Both editors would also have been lost without the unwavering support and skill of the associate editors, Jørgen Torgerstuen Johnsen and James Bradfield, in coproducing this text.

A huge debt of thanks goes to Elsevier colleagues including Alex Mortimer, Veronika Watkins, and Kritika Kaushik for their immense patience and guidance in steering this project through several challenges including the global pandemic.

All of the editorial team would like to pay tribute to their family members in standing by them throughout the challenging but rewarding journey of bringing this textbook together and in addition the 'NNEdPro global family' has been equally supportive at every step of this incredible adventure!

A final homage to Dame Professor Parveen Kumar CBE, for her encouragement at the time of the NNEdPro 10th Anniversary in 2018 and beyond, highlighting the clinical education needs that this textbook will meet as we look towards a better nutrition-trained health care workforce in the years to come.

PREFACE

From time immemorial, nutrition has been an integral part of the maintenance of health and the mitigation of disease. However, in recent times, there has been an uncoupling of nutrition from medicine, as well as health care practices. Although one contributing factor is the recognition that diet and disease requires its own field of study, multiple additional factors have driven this separation. One such factor is the advent of pharmacological and other interventional treatments driven by the growing burden of chronic diseases. Thanks to modern science and technology, we have new and better approaches to treatment, but with our growing (and in many regions aging) population and limited resources, we are grappling with increasing numbers of people affected by preventable disease. As a result, it is becoming ever more important to ensure that nutrition is reintegrated across all aspects of medical and health care practice. Whether in primary prevention, through the targeting of at risk populations, or as secondary prevention, where nutrition may slow disease progression or even prevent recurrence, nutrition is increasingly recognised as an integral part of care. Nutrition is also a key part of the interventional toolkit that we have at our disposal alongside pharmacological and other therapeutic approaches. Should we fail to consider the role of diet and nutrition in either prevention or intervention, we are underutilising a significant part of the evidence-informed machinery that modern medicine provides for effective health care. Hence the need for this textbook alongside others such as Clinical Medicine.

This textbook is organised by organ systems or specialties and is related back to medical practice through scenarios and case studies. In addition to the systems-based approach, there are several conceptual chapters that lay a solid foundation for the understanding of nutrition as a cognate scientific discipline and where it sits within health care pathways that straddle both primary and secondary care. This textbook also looks at population health, particularly through preventative approaches. There are several appendices, including information on the science behind key nutrition concepts, as well as the rapid application of nutrition knowledge to the recent COVID-19 pandemic. Other psychosocial aspects of nutrition in medical practice, for example weight stigma and how to recognise and sensitively handle it in clinical practice, are also covered.

We hope that this textbook will be suitable for both medical and other health care students as well as health care practitioners of all types who were not primarily trained in clinical nutrition. It is designed for those wishing to integrate nutrition knowledge and skills using a case based approach and serves as a practice ready toolkit.

SECTION A

Introduction to Nutrition and Health

SECTION OUTLINE

CHAPTER 1

Basic Principles of Nutrition

Sumantra Ray ■ Breanna Lepre

LEARNING POINTS

By the end of this chapter, you should be able to:

- Describe the relevance of nutriftion science discoveries in broad health and social systems over time
- Define nutrition, diet and malnutrition
- Demonstrate understanding of the biochemical demand for energy and nutrients
- Define nutrients, their physiological function and classification
- Identify dietary and other sources of major nutrients
- Gain awareness of food habits and the cultural and social importance of food
- Calculate available energy from food using the Atwater System
- Describe information available from food labels
- Describe the purpose of dietary reference values and dietary guidelines
- Describe indications for vitamin and mineral supplement use

DISCLAIMER

This chapter does not cover the mechanisms of lipid, carbohydrate and protein digestion, absorption and distribution which are well covered in standard human physiology texts

Historical Background

Nutrition is not a new discipline; food and nutrition have been studied for centuries. The historical perspective can be drawn back as far as Hippocrates and the well-known adage 'Let food be thy medicine and medicine be thy food'. However, in the 18th century a 'chemical revolution' took place and with it the development of methods of chemical analysis.

In the 1700s, Antoine Lavoisier, in collaboration with his assistant Armand Seguin, measured human respiratory output of carbonic acid (now known as carbon dioxide) at rest and during physical activity and demonstrated that the carbonic acid output increased with physical activity, thus providing important contribution for studies of energy balance and metabolism. In 1804, John Dalton proposed his atomic theory, an important advance in chemistry which underpins natural sciences even today.

Later in the 1800s, in his theory of mineral nutrients, Justus von Liebig identified the chemical elements of nitrogen as essential to plant growth, reporting that plants acquired carbon and hydrogen from the atmosphere and from water, and he later argued from experiments using muscle tissue that analyses failed to show the presence of fat or carbohydrate, the energy required for muscle contraction, and therefore this must be a result of a breakdown of the protein molecules themselves.

Throughout the 19th and 20th centuries, considerable advances in chemistry and our understanding of physiology took place. Kazimierz Funk, a Polish biochemist, was credited with the concept of vitamins in 1912, which he called vital amines. There was a focus on diseases of deprivation during this time, underpinned by new knowledge of the nature and function of nutrients. At that time, a pioneer of modern nutrition science, Dr. Elsie Widdowson, worked with Dr. Robert McCance to publish the first issue of *The Composition of Foods*. This was the first time that the nutrition intakes of individuals had been assessed and was the seminal work for nutritional databases around the world, which still today form the basis of dietary assessment.

Definitions

Nutrition is defined formally as the sum total of the processes involved in the taking in and the utilisation of food substances (nutrients) by which growth, repair and maintenance of the body are accomplished. It involves ingestion, digestion, absorption and assimilation. Nutrients are stored by the body in various forms and drawn upon when the food intake is not sufficient.

However, from a functional perspective, nutrition includes dietary intake (what you eat) which defines nutritional status (what you are) and, in turn, functional capacity (what you can do). There is also an overall goodness of fit (capacity to do) to individual requirements and circumstances, which defines your overall capacity based on nutrition available.

Diet refers to the food we eat rather than nutrients and encompasses the composition (quality and quantity) of food stuffs in meals and the way in which these meals are consumed (frequency and pattern). Exposure to dietary patterns determines nutritional status and, in turn, health outcomes.

Malnutrition is a related concept and is the consequence of prolonged inadequate dietary intake of one or more nutrients (undernutrition), excessive intake of one of more nutrients (overnutrition) or an imbalanced nutrient intake, such as those causing micronutrient deficiencies. Obesity is often considered a stand-alone problem but often represents one form of malnutrition. 'Hospital malnutrition' is another way we consider undernutrition in health care. Malnutrition manifests in multiple forms within individuals, households and populations and across the life course; it is often referred to as the double burden of malnutrition due to the coexistence of under- or overnutrition related to protein and energy, alongside micronutrient deficiencies.

Nutrients are chemical compounds that the human body requires for growth and metabolism. Nutrients can be organised as macronutrients, micronutrients and water.

Macronutrients are required in gram amounts in the diet and are major sources of energy for the body. They also provide essential nutrients, not synthesised in the body, such as amino acids and fatty acids, which are necessary for vital functions. The macronutrients are carbohydrate, proteins and fats.

Micronutrients are the nutrients the body needs in smaller amounts (milligrams or micrograms), namely, vitamins and minerals. Micronutrients are essential for health, cannot be made in the human body and are therefore obtained from the diet.

Carbohydrates

Carbohydrates are the most significant source of energy in the diet and can provide up to 85% of energy in the diet in developing countries and as little as 40% of energy in some developed countries. Our bodies convert carbohydrates into glucose, a type of sugar, which serves as the primary energy source in muscle, brain and other cells. Those carbohydrates which cannot be broken down are fermented by our gut bacteria or are egested. Carbohydrates also play an important role in the structure and function of cells, tissues and organs.

STRUCTURE AND CLASSIFICATION OF CARBOHYDRATES

Carbohydrates can be represented by the stoichiometric formula $(CH_2O)n$, where n represents the number of carbons in the molecule. Carbohydrates are classified as monosaccharides, oligosaccharides and polysaccharides, based on the number of sugar units, degree of polymerisation and how the sugar units are chemically bonded to each other. Oligosaccharides are further classified as disaccharide, trisaccharide and so forth depending on the number of monosaccharide units. They all provide a source of energy but differ in the way they are digested and absorbed. Carbohydrates come in two main forms, simple and complex, differing in chemical structure as well as how quickly they are digested and absorbed. Complex carbohydrates digest and raise blood sugar more slowly. Table 1.1 provides an overview of the carbohydrate family.

SOURCES OF CARBOHYDRATES

Carbohydrates are found in a variety of foods. Vegetables, fruits, whole grains, milk and milk products are major sources of carbohydrates. Grains, and some vegetables such as corn and potatoes, are generally rich in starch, whereas sweet potatoes are rich in sucrose. Other fruits and vegetables contain little to no starch, the polymeric form of glucose, but are a source of dietary fibre and contain other important micronutrients. The following section covers dietary sources of each subclass of carbohydrate.

Monosaccharides are simple sugars, whereby the number of carbons usually ranges from three to seven. As simple sugars, monosaccharides require the least effort by the body to break down, meaning they are available for energy more quickly than other types of carbohydrates. Monosaccharides include glucose, fructose and galactose. The most common monosaccharide is glucose, the body's main source of energy, which is found in foods such as dried fruit and fruit juice, sweetened beverages such as carbonated drinks, dairy and some vegetables. Fructose is found in foods such as fruit and honey, and it was previously found in fructose-rich corn syrup that the food industry used to sweeten soft drinks. Galactose, another monosaccharide, is a component of lactose and is found in dairy products as well as legumes and dried figs.

Oligosaccharides are formed when two or more monosaccharides are joined together by O-glycosidic bonds. Disaccharides contain two sugar units. Examples of disaccharides include sucrose, lactose and maltose. Sucrose is the most common disaccharide and is found in table sugar, the main dietary source of sucrose. Lactose is found in milk and milk products and is broken down into glucose and galactose. Maltose chemically consists of two glucose molecules and is present in malted wheat and barley products such as beer and melted candies. Other commonly occurring oligosaccharides include raffinose (trisaccharide), stachyose (tetrasaccharide) and verbacose (pentasaccharide), which can be found in legumes and seeds.

TABLE 1.1 ■ **An Overview of Carbohydrate Classification**

Simple Carbohydrates	Complex Carbohydrates
Monosaccharides: • Glucose • Fructose • Galactose Disaccharides: • Maltose • Sucrose • Lactose	Polysaccharides: • Glycogen • Starches • Fibres

Polysaccharides are complex carbohydrates, composed of 10 to up to several thousand monosaccharides arranged in chains by the same O-glycosidic bonds. Polysaccharides can be classified in different ways, including whether they are digestible or not digestible. Three main types of polysaccharides relevant to human nutrition include starch, glycogen and cellulose.

Starch is a digestible polysaccharide. It is an energy source obtained from plants and is the largest source of carbohydrate in the diet. Starch consists of two glucose polysaccharides: amylose and amylopectin. Starch is found in cereal grains (wheat, oats, barley, corn and rice) and products derived from these such as bread, pasta, pastries and cookies as well as potatoes.

Glycogen is the second type of polysaccharide; it is a storage form of glucose, found in the human liver and muscles. Glycogen functions as an energy reserve for short-term use as well as the triglyceride form stored in adipose tissue or body fat for long-term storage.

Cellulose and other nondigestible carbohydrates are structural polysaccharides found in plants. Cellulose can be found in whole grains, beans, peas and lentils. It is one type of nondigestible polysaccharide, which is also called fibre. Fibre, the edible portions of plant cell walls that are resistant to digestion, is an important component of a healthy diet. Dietary fibre can be classified based on water solubility as soluble or insoluble. Soluble fibre easily dissolves in water and slows the response of blood glucose to ingestion of simple carbohydrates. The reabsorption of bile acids is slowed by consumption of soluble fibre, leading to increased cholesterol losses in faeces. This in turn reduces blood cholesterol levels. Insoluble fibre consists mainly of cellulose and some hemicelluloses. Insoluble fibre binds to water in the colon and swells, adding bulk to stool and increasing transit time. This reduces the risk of constipation. The amount of soluble and insoluble fibre varies between foods. To receive the greatest health benefits from fibre, a wide variety of high-fibre foods should be consumed. Table 1.2 lists dietary sources of soluble and insoluble fibre.

GLYCAEMIC INDEX AND LOAD

Carbohydrates can also be classified based on glycaemic index or glycaemic load. Glycaemic index (GI) is a relative ranking out of 100 of carbohydrate content in foods according to how they affect

TABLE 1.2 ■ **Sources of Dietary Soluble and Insoluble Fibre**

Sources of Soluble Fibre	Actions in the Body	Health Benefits
Oats/oat bran Peas Beans Apples Citrus fruit Carrots Barley Rye Legumes Seeds and husks	• Lowers blood cholesterol by binding to bile • Slows glucose absorption • Slows transit of food through upper gastrointestinal tract • Retains water in stools, softening them	• May lower risk of heart disease • May lower risk of diabetes
Sources of Insoluble Fibre	**Actions in the Body**	**Health Benefits**
Whole grains Brown rice Wheat bran Nuts Beans and legumes Cauliflower Green beans Potatoes	• Increases weight of stool • Speeds up transit of stool through colon • Provide bulk to stool • Increases satiety (feelings of fullness)	• Prevent and alleviate constipation • Lowers risk of gastrointestinal-related issues such as diverticulitis, haemorrhoids and appendicitis • May assist in weight management

blood glucose levels. Carbohydrates with a GI value of 55 or less are considered low GI, meaning they are more slowly digested, absorbed and metabolised and create a more gradual rise in blood glucose. A GI value between 56 and 69 is considered medium GI, and 70+ is considered high GI. Fat and fibre content in foods relative to carbohydrate tends to lower GI.

Glycaemic load, on the other hand, considers both the quality and quantity of carbohydrate consumed. It can be used to compare the potential of different types and amounts of food to raise blood glucose levels by using the following formula:

Activity: Glycaemic Load

Glycaemic load = GI × carbohydrate (g) content per portion ÷ 100

Calculate the glycaemic load of a single apple with a GI of 38 and 13g carbohydrate.

Proteins

The human body contains an estimated 30,000 different kinds of proteins, many of which have not yet been studied. Proteins are large, complex molecules that have many critical functions. Proteins are essential primarily for growth and repair but have numerous structural and functional purposes including acting as transport carriers in the blood, as regulators of fluid balance and acid-base and as hormones and enzymes. Protein is also a source of energy and glucose during times of starvation or insufficient carbohydrate intake. In starvation, or when there is insufficient carbohydrate intake, the human body will break down tissue proteins to make amino acids available for energy or glucose production. Table 1.3 summarises some of the functions of protein in the human body and lists examples for each.

Protein is in a constant state of turnover in the body, which can be described using something known as 'nitrogen balance', which is calculated as the net difference between the intake of nitrogen in the diet (predominantly through protein) and its excretion, through urine as urea, ammonia and creatinine, or through faecal and miscellaneous losses.[1] In healthy adults, protein synthesis is in balance with protein degradation. When nitrogen intake equals nitrogen output, it is known as nitrogen equilibrium, or zero nitrogen balance. If the body synthesises more protein than is broken down, nitrogen status becomes positive. Nitrogen status is positive in growing infants, children, adolescents, pregnant women and people recovering from protein deficiency or illness. In states of growth and repair, protein is retained in new tissues as they build new blood, bone, skin and

TABLE 1.3 ■ **Functions of Protein**

Function in the Body	Description	Example(s)
Enzymes	Enzymes are proteins which carry out almost all of the chemical reactions that take place in cells	Phenylalanine hydroxylase
Hormones	Some hormones are proteins, which regulate body processes	Insulin, thyroxine
Transportation	Proteins bind and carry atoms and small molecules to and within cells and throughout the body	Ferritin, albumin, haemoglobin
Antibodies	Proteins bind to and inactivate specific foreign particles, such as viruses and bacteria, to help protect the body	Immunoglobulin G

muscle cells. Nitrogen status is negative in people who are in a state of starvation or suffering with burns, injuries, infections and fever. During these times, the body is breaking down muscle and other body protein for energy, which results in a nitrogen output which exceeds nitrogen intake (negative nitrogen status).

STRUCTURE AND CLASSIFICATION

Proteins are macronutrients consisting of chains of amino acids. All amino acids have the same basic chemical structure: a central carbon atom (C) with a hydrogen atom (H), an amino group (NH2) and an acid group (COOH). The fourth site distinguishes each amino acid from others. Reactive side groups of amino acids can combine to form other proteins.

Amino acids are joined together by peptide bonds and can form chains of various lengths, from two amino acids (dipeptide) up to more than 10 amino acids (polypeptides). There are approximately 20 amino acids, each with different properties. Many of the amino acids are nonessential, meaning that the body can synthesise them, given nitrogen is available to form the amino group and carbohydrate or fat to form the rest of the structure. Some amino acids cannot be synthesised by the body or only in sufficient quantities to meet its needs, and therefore must be supplied by the diet. These are known as essential amino acids (Table 1.4).

CONDITIONALLY ESSENTIAL AMINO ACIDS

In some cases, a nonessential amino acid can become essential. The body uses the essential amino acid phenylalanine to make tyrosine, a nonessential amino acid. If the diet does not supply adequate phenylalanine, or if the body cannot convert tyrosine to phenylalanine (such as in the inherited disease phenylketonuria), tyrosine becomes a conditionally essential amino acid.

SOURCES OF PROTEIN

Important sources of protein include meat, dairy, legumes, nuts, seafood and eggs. The amino acid content of a protein determines its biological value. A protein that contains all amino acids is sometimes referred to as a 'complete protein' and is considered to have high biological value. High

TABLE 1.4 ■ **Essential and Nonessential Amino Acids**

Essential Amino Acids	Nonessential Amino Acids
Histidine	Alanine
Isoleucine	Arginine
Leucine	Asparagine
Lysine	Aspartic acid
Methionine	Cysteine
Phenylalanine	Glutamic acid
Threonine	Glutamine
Tryptophan	Glycine
Valine	Proline Serine Tyrosine

biological value proteins include meat, eggs, soy and dairy products. Foods can be combined to create a meal that contains all essential amino acids.

LIPIDS

Lipids are substances poorly soluble or insoluble in water but soluble in organic solvents. Lipids are a good source of energy; aid the absorption of fat-soluble vitamins A, D, E and K; and improve the taste and appearance of food. Lipids are also a component of cell membranes, and cholesterol is converted to bile acids, which are important in digestion, as well as forming the backbone of steroid hormones. Lipids can be classified as triglycerides (triacylglycerols), cholesterol, phospholipids and sterols. Alternatively, lipids can also be classified as simple, complex, derived, and miscellaneous. Simple lipids are esters of fatty acids combined with different alcohols. Complex lipids are simple lipids combined with other groups. Derived lipids are products of simple or complex lipids.

Fatty Acids

Fatty acids are classified as derived lipids. They are organic acids composed of carbon (C), hydrogen (H), and oxygen (O). They generally consist of a straight chain with an even number of carbon and hydrogen atoms along the length of the chain at one end of the chain and a carboxyl group (-COOH) at the other end, which is what makes it an acid. They are the building blocks from which lipids are made and can be found in plants, animals and microorganisms. Fatty acids are a means of energy storage, provide energy for the body and are an essential component of stable cellular membranes.

Fatty acids can be saturated or unsaturated, depending on if the bonds are single (saturated) or double or triple (unsaturated). Whereas most saturated fatty acids are solid at room temperature, monounsaturated fatty acids may be solid or liquid. Table 1.5 summarises important definitions and dietary sources of different fatty acids.

TABLE 1.5 ■ **Key Definitions Related to Fatty Acids and Important Dietary Sources**

Term	Definition	Sources
Saturated fatty acid	A fatty acid in which the carbon chain has all or predominantly single bonds	Some sources of saturated fatty acid include meat fat, milk, butter, cheese, coconut oil and palm oil
Unsaturated fatty acid	A fatty acid in which the carbon chain possesses one or more double or triple bonds	Plant foods, such as nuts, seeds, vegetable oils (olive, peanut, safflower, sunflower, soybean and corn)
Monounsaturated fatty acid	A fatty acid with one double bond in the fatty acid chain and all remaining carbon atoms being single bonded	Sources of monounsaturated fatty acid include olive and rapeseed oils, avocado and nuts. Cod liver oil, vegetable oil (blended), margarine, and butter contain some monounsaturated fatty acid as well as polyunsaturated or saturated fatty acids
Polyunsaturated fatty acid	A fatty acid with more than one double bond in the fatty acid chain	Dietary sources of polyunsaturated fatty acids include a number of plant-based oils, including soybean oil, corn oil and sunflower oil, as well as some nuts and seeds, such as walnuts and sunflower seeds, tofu and soybeans

Saturated fatty acids. Some common examples of fatty acids include butyric acid (found in butter), lauric acid (found in coconut oil, palm kernel oil and breast milk), myristic acid (found in cow's milk and dairy), palmitic acid (found in palm oil and meat) and stearic acid (found in meat and cocoa butter). The expert consultation report of the World Health Organization and Food and Agriculture Organization concluded that the intake of saturated fatty acids is directly related to cardiovascular risk leading to a default target to restrict intake of saturated fatty acids to less than 10% of daily energy intake and less than 7% for high-risk groups. Foods rich in myristic and palmitic acids are associated with higher risk.

Unsaturated fatty acids. Some common examples include vegetable oils such as olive, peanut, safflower, sunflower, soybean and corn. Unsaturated fats are either monounsaturated, polyunsaturated or a combination of both and do not raise blood cholesterol or low-density lipoprotein (LDL) levels. Monounsaturated fats can reduce high blood cholesterol levels and potentially increase high-density lipoprotein ('good' cholesterol).

Monounsaturated fatty acids. Monounsaturated fatty acids include palmitic (C16:1), oleic (C18:1), elaidic (C18:1) and vacentic acids (C18:1). The most abundant monounsaturated fatty acid in the diet is oleic acid (C18:1 n-9). Diets rich in monounsaturated fatty acids have been shown to have favourable antiinflammatory and cardiovascular benefits and lower plasma total, LDL cholesterol and triglycerides.[2]

Polyunsaturated fatty acids. Polyunsaturated fatty acids are also differentiated by the position of the double bond nearest the methyl (CH3) end of the carbon chain, which is described by an omega number. An omega-3 fatty acid is a polyunsaturated fatty acid with its first double bond three carbons away from the methyl end. Similarly, an omega-6 fatty acid is a polyunsaturated fatty acid with its first double bond six carbons away from the methyl end. Arachidonic acid is an example of a polyunsaturated omega-6 fatty acid and is a precursor in the biosynthesis of prostaglandins, thromboxane and leukotrienes which are involved in cell signalling and the mediation of inflammation.

Essential fatty acids. There are only two fatty acids which cannot be synthesised by the body: linoleic acid (an omega-6 fatty acid) and alpha-linolenic acid (an omega-3 fatty acid). These fatty acids are considered *essential* fatty acids and must be supplied by the diet. Omega-3 and omega-6 fatty acids can be found in vegetable oils, seeds, nuts, oily fish and other marine foods. Omega-3 and omega-6 fatty acids are important components of cell membranes and are precursors to many other substances in the body, including prostaglandins and leukotrienes. Omega-3 fatty acids also have a role in neurotransmitter function.

Much of the research on essential fatty acids is focussed on omega-3 fatty acids in the context of cardiovascular disease risk. Eicosapentaenoic acid and docosahexaenoic acid are highly unsaturated omega-3 fatty acids. Omega-3 polyunsaturated fatty acids can reduce inflammation and may help to lower risk of chronic diseases such as heart disease, cancer and arthritis. Large trials of omega-3 fatty acids which assess the associations of omega-3 fatty acid supplements with the risk of fatal and nonfatal coronary heart disease and major vascular events have produced conflicting results. Table 1.6 lists sources of omega-3 and omega-6 fatty acids.

Omega-3:omega-6 ratio. Omega-3 and omega-6 fatty acids compete for the same enzymes and have opposite actions in the body. As a result, researchers have studied the impact of the ratio of these essential fatty acids on cardiovascular health. There is no scientific consensus on the ideal

TABLE 1.6 ■ **Sources of Omega-3 and Omega-6 Fatty Acids**

Omega-6 Fatty Acids	
Linoleic acid	Vegetable oils (corn, sunflower, safflower, soybean, cottonseed); fat from poultry; nuts and seeds
Arachidonic acid	Meats, poultry, eggs, can also be made from linoleic acid
Omega-3 Fatty Acids	
Alpha-linolenic acid	Oils (flaxseed, canola, walnut, soybean); nuts and seeds, particularly walnuts, almonds, flaxseeds, soybean kernels; soybeans
Eicosapentaenoic acid and docosahexaenoic acid	Human breast milk; pacific oysters and fish (blue-eye trevally, Atlantic salmon, blue mackerel, salmon, sardines, tuna); can also be made from alpha-linolenic acid; lean red meat

ratio, although suggested ratios range from 5:1 to 10:1. Increasing intake of omega-3 fatty acids in the diet has been suggested to be most effective in improving cardiovascular health.

***Trans*-fatty acids.** *Trans*-fatty acids are produced by hydrogenation of unsaturated oils or naturally by biohydrogenation in the stomach of ruminant animals. Hydrogenation increases the saturation of polyunsaturated fats. In the food industry, hydrogenation aims to protect fatty acids against oxidation (increase the shelf life) and to alter their texture (by making liquid vegetable oils more solid). Most often, a fat is partially hydrogenated, meaning that some of the double bonds that remain after processing change from *cis* to *trans*. Whereas in a *cis* configuration the hydrogens next to the double bonds are on the same side of the carbon chain, in a *trans* configuration, fatty acids where the hydrogen is next to the double bonds are on opposite sides of the carbon chain. This difference in structure affects function; *trans*-fatty acids derived from hydrogenation have been shown to behave more like saturated fats than unsaturated. Consumption of *trans*-fatty acids has shown to increase blood levels of triglycerides when compared with the intake of other fats and reduce the particle size of LDL cholesterol. Small LDL cholesterol has been associated with increased risk of coronary heart disease and has recently been included in guidelines for prevention of atherosclerosis.

Several studies have shown a relationship between *trans*-fatty acid consumption and increased risk of cardiovascular disease. Several countries have now committed to eliminate *trans*-fatty acids from their manufacturing process.

Triglycerides

Most of the fat from our diet is in the form of triglycerides, which are made up of three fatty acids esterified to glycerol. Triglycerides are classified as simple lipids. Most triglycerides contain a mixture of more than one type of fatty acid. Plasma triglycerides (found in the blood) are derived from dietary sources as well as from de novo triglyceride synthesis in a process called lipogenesis, which occurs in the liver.

Triglycerides are a major component of very-low-density lipoprotein and are the main source of lipid storage and energy in the human body. Serum triglyceride concentration is used to assess the presence of hypertriglyceridemia (elevated triglycerides in the blood), which can increase the risk of stroke, heart attack and heart disease.[6]

Phospholipids

Phospholipids are a class of lipids with a hydrophilic 'head' containing a phosphate group and two hydrophobic 'tails' derived from fatty acids and joined by an alcohol residue. They are classified as simple lipids. The nature of alcohol and the fatty acids varies from compound to compound. The fatty acids make phospholipids soluble in fat, and the phosphate group allows them to dissolve in water. Due to their unique chemical structure that allows them to be soluble in both water and fat, the food industry uses phospholipids as emulsifiers to mix fats with water (e.g., in mayonnaise). Phospholipids are also found naturally in foods such as eggs, liver, soybeans, wheat germ and peanuts.

Phospholipids are divided into two broad categories based on the alcohol residue present in their backbone: glycerophospholipids and sphingophospholipids.

Glycerophospholipids have a glycerol alcohol backbone and are the most abundant phospholipid. Sphingophospholipids have a backbone made of sphingosine alcohol. Both glycerophospholipids and sphingophospholipids perform important functions. For example, sphingomyelin, an important sphingophospholipid, is a component of the myelin sheath, an insulating layer that forms around the nerve axon in a spiral fashion. This myelin sheath allows electrical impulses to transmit quickly and efficiently along nerve cells.

Phospholipids are important constituents of cell membranes. As membrane components, phospholipids are selectively permeable (semipermeable), meaning only certain molecules can move in and out of the cell. Because phospholipids are soluble in both water and fat, lipids are able to move back and forth across the cell membrane into the watery fluids on both sides. Fat-soluble substances, including some vitamins and hormones, can pass in and out of cells without the need for transport proteins.

Sterols

Sterols are a subgroup of steroids with a multiple-ring structure. They are also classified as simple lipids. The most well-known sterol is cholesterol, formed of a steroid nucleus and branched hydrocarbon tail. Cholesterol is found in foods of animal origin (such as meats, eggs, fish, poultry and dairy products) in free form and esterified to fatty acids. Plant materials, such as vegetables, fruits, wheat germ, whole grains, beans and many vegetable oils, contain phytosterols, compounds chemically related to cholesterol but containing a different chemical side chain configuration and steroid ring-bonding pattern. Plant sterols interfere with cholesterol absorption in the intestine and in turn lower blood cholesterol levels. The food industry permits the use of plant sterols in foods such as margarine, low-fat milk, yoghurt, breakfast cereals and cheese. These 'functional' foods may help to reduce blood cholesterol when consumed as part of a healthy, balanced diet.

Vital body compounds, such as bile acids, sex hormones (e.g., oestrogen, testosterone), the adrenal hormones (e.g., cortisol) and vitamin D, are sterols synthesised from cholesterol in the body. Cholesterol also has a role as a structural component of cell membranes. The human body can synthesise cholesterol in the liver from fragments of carbohydrate, protein and fat.

Energy Turnover

Normal function of the human body requires a constant input and output (turnover) of energy to maintain life, allowing it to respond rapidly to changes in metabolic state (change synthesis and/or degradation). This concept can be applied at the cellular, tissue/organ or whole-body level, and can also relate to the conversion of one substrate/nutrient to another (i.e., movement between metabolic pathways).

The various chemical components of food provide energy to the human body. The chemical breakdown of carbohydrates, lipids and proteins provides the energy required for thousands of body functions that allow the human body to perform daily tasks such as breathing, reading, and exercising. Energy requirements can be affected by disease. For example, injury or acute stress can increase requirements for energy and protein.

ENERGY BALANCE AND THE HUMAN BODY

When the body uses carbohydrate, fat or protein for energy, the bonds between the nutrient's atoms break. As these bonds break, they release energy, some of which is released as heat and some of which is used as an energy source. The balance between energy intake and energy expenditure determines energy stores in the body. If the body does not use the energy from nutrients in food as fuel for its current activities, the human body rearranges nutrients into storage compounds (such as glycogen or body fat) for use between meals and overnight when energy supplies run low. If less energy is consumed than expended, the result is a decrease in energy stores and weight loss.

UNITS OF ENERGY

The international unit for measuring food energy is the joule, a measure of energy based on work accomplished (i.e., the energy required to produce a specific amount of force). In the United States, the kilocalorie (kcal), often referred to as the 'calorie', is the most used unit of energy. A kilocalorie is the amount of energy in the form of heat that is required to heat 1 kg of water 1°C. As calories and Joules are both units of energy, one can be converted to the other, where 1 kcal = 4.18 J.

NUTRIENT-ENERGY CONVERSION AND THE ATWATER SYSTEM

In the body, only macronutrients are energy yielding: carbohydrate, fat and protein. Each macronutrient provides a slightly different amount of energy per gram of food. The amount of energy a food provides depends on how much carbohydrate, fat and protein it contains. Most foods contain all three energy-yielding nutrients as well as water, vitamins, minerals and more. The Atwater system, named after Wilbur Olin Atwater, is used to calculate the available energy from foods. Lipids are a concentrated source of energy and provide almost double the amount of energy per gram than proteins and carbohydrates (Table 1.7.). Alcohol is not considered a nutrient but is a source of energy when metabolised in the body (29 kJ or 7 kcal per gram). When alcohol is consumed in excess of energy needs, it can be converted to body fat and stored.

ACTIVITY: THE ATWATER SYSTEM

Joel consumes 100 g chocolate, which contains 7.6 g protein, 30.4 g fat and 57.3 g carbohydrate. Calculate the total energy (kilocalories) available from the chocolate bar once consumed.

To calculate the available energy in a food or recipe, multiply the grams by the energy per gram.

TABLE 1.7 ■ **Average Kilojoule and Kilocalorie Values of Energy-Yielding Nutrients**

Nutrient	Energy (kJ/g)	Energy (kcal/g)
Carbohydrate	17	4
Protein	17	4
Fat	37	9

Micronutrients

VITAMINS

Vitamins are organic, essential compounds required in small amounts to serve a variety of functions in the human body that promote growth, reproduction, or the maintenance of health. The consequences of vitamin deficiencies are significant and attest to their central role in human physiology and health. Vitamins do not provide energy, but rather, they facilitate the release of energy from carbohydrate, fat and protein. They also have a variety of other roles, such as aiding in DNA synthesis and in blood clotting (Table 1.8).

There are 13 different vitamins, categorised as fat-soluble and water-soluble groups. The roles and sources of fat-soluble vitamins are different from that of water-soluble vitamins, yet they are all essential to life. Vitamins A, E, D and K are fat soluble and can be stored in the human body. Fat-soluble vitamins require bile for their absorption, and many of them require protein carriers for transport in the bloodstream. Because fat-soluble vitamins can accumulate in fat-storage sites in the body rather than being excreted, they are more likely than water-soluble vitamins to result in toxicity when consumed in excess. The B group vitamins (B1, B2, B3, B5, B6, B7, B9 and B12) and vitamin C are water-soluble vitamins. Due to these differences in solubility, the food matrix itself can affect vitamin absorption.

VITAMIN CONTENT AND RETENTION

As vitamins are complex organic molecules, they are vulnerable to destruction by heat, light and chemical agents. Therefore, the way one prepares, cooks and stores food can affect the vitamin content. To minimise nutrient loses, (most) fruits and vegetables should be refrigerated where possible; fruits and vegetables that have been cut should be stored in airtight wrappers or sealed containers; and fruits and vegetables should be rinsed before cutting them to avoid leeching of micronutrients. To minimise losses during cooking, vegetables should be microwaved or steamed in a small amount of water to reduce leaching of water-soluble vitamins C and B.

Table 1.8 summarises information on fat- and water-soluble vitamins.

ACTIVITY: VITAMIN B12 AND VEGANISM

1. Explain why B12 is important for human health.
2. Explain why it may be harder for vegans to reach their B12 requirements.
3. Identify three *plant-based* sources of B12.

A FOCUS ON FOLATE (VITAMIN B9) AND NEURAL TUBE DEFECTS

The brain and spinal cord develop from the neural tube, and defects in its formation during early weeks of pregnancy can result in central nervous system disorders and even death.

Folate supplements taken 1 month before conception and continued throughout the first trimester of pregnancy (the periconception period) can help prevent neural tube defects. As a preventive measure, all women of childbearing age who can become pregnant or who are planning a pregnancy should consume 400 mg of folate per day.

TABLE 1.8 ■ **Overview of Vitamins**

Vitamin	Other Names	Physiological Function(s)	Food Sources	Deficiency Disease and Presentation	Toxicity Disease and Symptoms
Vitamin A	Retinol, retinoic acid, retinal, carotenoid	Growth, maintenance of skin, bone development, maintenance of myelin, vision	Sources of retinoids: beef liver, eggs, fish, fortified milk, butter, cheese Sources of beta carotene: sweet potatoes, carrots, pumpkin, leafy, dark green vegetables	Lack of vitamin A or hypovitaminosis A; signs and symptoms include night blindness, corneal drying, triangular grey spots on eye (Bitot spots), softening of the cornea of the eye (keratomalacia), impaired immunity to infectious diseases	Vitamin A toxicity or hypervitaminosis A; signs and symptoms include blurred vision, nausea, vomiting, vertigo, increase of pressure inside skull, mimicking brain tumour, headaches, muscle uncoordination
Vitamin B1	Thiamine	Growth, appetite and digestion, nerve activity, part of coenzyme thiamine pyrophosphate used in energy metabolism	Pork, whole grain, fortified or enriched grain products, legumes, nuts, and seeds	Enlarged heart, cardiac failure, muscular weakness, apathy, confusion, poor short-term memory, irritability, weight loss Diseases related to vitamin B1 deficiency include beriberi (wet, with oedema; dry, with muscle wasting) and Wernicke-Korsakoff syndrome	Limited reports
Vitamin B2	Riboflavin	Growth and development, maintenance of mucosal, epithelial and eye tissues	Milk, milk products, leafy green vegetables, whole grain breads and cereals	Deficiency of vitamin B12 is called ariboflavinosis; signs and symptoms include sore throat; cracked corners of the mouth; smooth, red and painful tongue; inflammation characterised by skin lesions with a greasy appearance	Limited reports
Vitamin B3	Nicotinamide, niacinamide, nicotinic acid, niacin	Maintenance of NAD and NADP, coenzyme in lipid catabolism, oxidative deamination	Meat, poultry, fish, whole grain breads and cereals, mushrooms, asparagus, leafy green vegetables, peanut butter	Pellagra is the disease caused by lack of vitamin B3; signs and symptoms include diarrhoea; abdominal pain; vomiting; smooth, swollen, bright red tongue; depression; fatigue; apathy; loss of memory; headache; rash on areas exposed to sunlight	Painful flush, hives and rash, nausea and vomiting, liver damage, impaired glucose tolerance

TABLE 1.8 ■ **Overview of Vitamins—cont'd**

Vitamin	Other Names	Physiological Function(s)	Food Sources	Deficiency Disease and Presentation	Toxicity Disease and Symptoms
Vitamin B5	Pantothenic acid	Lipid and protein metabolism, part of coenzyme A in carbohydrate metabolism	Chicken, beef, potatoes, oats, tomatoes, liver, egg yolk, broccoli and whole grains	Vomiting, nausea, stomach cramps, insomnia, irritability, restlessness, apathy, hypoglycaemia, increased sensitivity to insulin, numbness, muscle cramps and inability to walk	Limited reports
Vitamin B6	Pyridoxine, pyridoxol, adermine	Growth, protein, carbohydrate and lipid metabolism, coenzyme in amino acid metabolism	Meat, fish, poultry, noncitrus fruits, fortified cereals, potatoes and other starchy vegetables	Scaly dermatitis, anaemia (small-cell types), depression, confusion, convulsions	Depression, fatigue, irritability, headaches, skin lesions and nerve damage resulting in numbness and muscle weakness, which may lead to an inability to walk and convulsions
Vitamin B7	Biotin, protective factor X	Growth, maintenance of skin, hair, bone marrow and sex glands, biosynthesis of aspartate and unsaturated fatty acids	Liver, egg yolks, soybeans, fish, whole grains; also produced by gastrointestinal bacteria	Depression, lethargy, hallucinations; a numb or tingling sensation in arms and legs; a red, scaly rash around the eyes, nose and mouth; hair loss	Limited reports
Vitamin B9	Folic acid, folacin, folinic acid	Synthesis of nucleic acid, differentiation of embryonic nervous system	Leafy green vegetables, fortified grains, legumes, seeds, orange juice, liver	Anaemia (large-cell types), smooth red tongue, mental confusion, weakness, fatigue, irritability, headaches, shortness of breath, elevated homocysteine	Masks symptoms of vitamin B12 deficiency
Vitamin B12	Cobalamin	Coenzyme in nucleic acid, protein and lipid synthesis, maintenance of epithelial cells and the nervous system	Animal products including meat, poultry, fish, seafood, eggs, milk and milk products	Megaloblastic anaemia is caused by lack of vitamin B12; signs and symptoms include anaemia (large-cell types), fatigue, degeneration of peripheral nerves progressing to paralysis, sore tongue, loss of appetite, constipation	None reported

(Continued)

TABLE 1.8 ■ **Overview of Vitamins—cont'd**

Vitamin	Other Names	Physiological Function(s)	Food Sources	Deficiency Disease and Presentation	Toxicity Disease and Symptoms
Vitamin C	Ascorbic acid	Absorption of iron, antioxidant activity, growth, wound healing, formation of cartilage, bone and teeth, maintenance of capillaries	Fruits and vegetables, especially citrus fruits, strawberries, tomatoes, potatoes, mangoes, lettuce and vegetables in the cabbage family	Lack of vitamin C causes scurvy; signs and symptoms include anaemia (small-cell type), atherosclerotic plaques, bone fragility, joint pain, poor wound healing, frequent infections, bleeding gums, loosened teeth, muscle degeneration and pain, hysteria, depression, rough skin, blotchy bruises	Nausea, abdominal cramps, diarrhoea, headache, fatigue, insomnia, hot flushes, rashes, aggravation of gout symptoms, urinary tract problems, kidney stones
Vitamin D	Calciferol, 1,25-dihydroxy vitamin D (calcitriol), vitamin D3 or cholecalciferol, vitamin D2 or ergocalciferol; the precursor is the body's own cholesterol	Normal growth, calcium and phosphorus absorption, maintenance of bone health, maintains serum calcium and phosphorous levels	Egg yolks, liver, fatty fish (herring, salmon, sardines and their oil), fortified milk, fortified margarine, synthesised in the body with the aid of sunlight	Rickets in children: inadequate calcification resulting in bowed legs, enlargement of ends of long bones, deformities of ribs, delayed closing of fontanelle (open space in the top of a baby's skull) resulting in rapid enlargement of head, lax muscles Osteomalacia or osteoporosis in adults: loss of calcium resulting in soft, flexible, brittle and deformed bones, progressive weakness, pain in pelvis, lower back and legs	Vitamin D toxicity or hypervitaminosis D is associated with elevated blood calcium, calcification of soft tissues (blood vessels, kidneys, heart, lungs, tissues around the joints)
Vitamin E	Alpha-tocopherol, tokopharm, tocotrienols	Antioxidant properties, growth maintenance, aids the absorption of unsaturated fatty acids, maintains muscular metabolism, vascular system, and central nervous system	Polyunsaturated plant oils (soybean, corn, cottonseed, safflower), leafy green vegetables, whole grain cereals and products, liver, egg yolk, nuts and seeds	Red blood cell breakage, nerve damage	Increases the effects of anticlotting medication
Vitamin K	Prothrombin factor, menaquinone, phylloquinone, menadione, naphthoquinone	Blood-clotting mechanisms, electron transport mechanisms, growth, prothrombin synthesis in the liver	Leafy green vegetables, broccoli, brussels sprouts, asparagus	Haemorrhaging	None reported

NAD, Nicotinamide adenine dinucleotide; *NADP*, nicotinamide adenine dinucleotide phosphate.
Source[7]: Fricker RA, Green E, Jenkins SI, et al. The influence of nicotinamide on health and disease in the central nervous system. *Int J Tryptophan Res*. 2018;11:1–11.

New Evidence on Vitamin D and COVID-19

MINERALS AND TRACE ELEMENTS

Minerals and trace elements are present in healthy human tissue. Minerals are inorganic substances required by the body in gram or milligram amounts, and trace elements are required in microgram amounts. Minerals have a variety of functions such as in the formation of bone and teeth, they are essential constituents of body fluids and tissues and components of enzymes, and they are involved in nerve function. The body requires different amounts of each mineral and people have different requirements, according to factors such as age, sex and physiological state (e.g., pregnancy). Table 1.9 provides an overview of the minerals and trace elements known to be essential to humans. Table 1.10 provides a summary of the function of minerals, dietary sources and deficiency or toxicity symptoms.

VITAMIN AND MINERAL SUPPLEMENTS

Most adults can normally meet their nutrient requirements by eating a varied diet consisting of nutrient-rich foods. Vitamins and mineral supplements are the most commonly used dietary supplements internationally.[8] In some cases, vitamin and mineral supplements are appropriate to correct or prevent deficiencies, to support increased nutrient needs during certain stages of life (e.g., pregnancy), to improve nutrition status where it is not possible to meet requirements with food (e.g., vegetarianism and veganism) and to reduce risk of disease (e.g., calcium supplement use in postmenopausal women to reduce bone degeneration of osteoporosis associated with age). Outside of these circumstances, the upper level of intake of the nutrient reference values provides a benchmark for the highest amount which appears safe for most healthy people.

In most cases supplement use is harmless, albeit costly. Supplement toxicity is a risk which often goes unrecognised. Toxic overdoses of vitamins and minerals can have significant adverse health effects and, in some cases, can result in coma or death. For example, large doses of fish oil can lead to decreased blood clotting. High-potency iron supplements are the leading cause of accidental ingestion fatalities among children. Even mild toxicity symptoms include gastrointestinal distress, nausea, and black diarrhoea.

TABLE 1.9 ■ **Minerals and Trace Elements Essential to Humans**

Major Minerals	Trace Minerals
Calcium	Copper
Chloride	Chromium
Magnesium	Iodine
Phosphorus	Iron
Potassium	Fluoride
Sodium	Manganese
Sulphate	Molybdenum Selenium Zinc

TABLE 1.10 ■ **Overview of Minerals and Trace Minerals**

Mineral	Physiological Function(s)	Food Sources	Deficiency Symptoms	Toxicity Symptoms
Calcium	Mineralisation of bones and teeth, muscle contraction and relaxation, nerve functioning, blood clotting and blood pressure	Milk and milk products, canned fish with bones (e.g., salmon, sardines), fortified tofu, fortified dairy alternatives (e.g., soy milk)	Stunted growth in children, bone loss (osteoporosis) in adults	Constipation, acute kidney injury, loss of appetite, nausea and vomiting, irregular heartbeat, seizure
Chloride	Fluid and electrolyte balance, assists in digestion (part of hydrochloric acid found in the stomach)	Soy sauce, table salt, processed foods, milk, meat, eggs	Rare	Vomiting
Chromium	Potentiating insulin action, potential role in carbohydrate, lipid and protein metabolism	Meats, whole grain products, fruits, vegetables, nuts, spices, brewer's yeast, beer and wine	Impaired glucose tolerance	None reported
Copper	Helps to form haemoglobin, cofactor for several enzymes which are involved in energy production, iron metabolism, neuropeptide activation connective tissue synthesis and neurotransmitter synthesis	Shellfish, nuts and seeds, organ meats, whole grains and whole grain products and chocolate	Anaemia, bone abnormalities	Liver damage
Fluoride	Maintains bone and teeth health, small amounts of fluoride help reduce tooth decay	Fluoridated drinking water, tea, seafood	Susceptibility to tooth decay	Fluorosis (characterised by hypomineralisation of tooth enamel caused by excessive ingestion of fluoride)
Iodine	Component of thyroid hormones which help to regulate growth, development and metabolism	Iodised salt, seaweed (e.g., kelp, nori, kombu, wakame), seafood, plants grown in iodine rich soil, dairy products (milk, yoghurt and cheese), fortified bread	Underactive thyroid gland, goitre, mental and physical retardation (cretinism)	Underactive thyroid gland, elevated thyroid stimulating hormone
Iron	Component of the protein haemoglobin which carries oxygen around the body in the blood, component of the protein myoglobin (found in muscles) which makes oxygen available for muscle contraction, energy metabolism	Red meat, fish, poultry, shellfish, eggs, legumes, dried fruits (e.g., apricots), iron-fortified breakfast cereals, cashews	Anaemia, fatigue, headaches, impaired productivity, impaired immunity, pale skin, nail beds, mucous membranes and palm creases, inability to regulate body temperature	Gastrointestinal distress, fatigue, joint pain, skin pigmentation, organ damage

Magnesium	Muscle contraction, nerve transmission, immune system health, bone mineralisation and teeth health	Nuts, seeds, whole grains, dark green vegetables (e.g., spinach), legumes	Weakness, confusion, convulsions, muscle spasms, hallucinations, difficulty swallowing	Diarrhoea, alkalosis, dehydration (from nonfood sources)
Manganese	Cofactor for several enzymes involved in amino acid, cholesterol, glucose and carbohydrate metabolism, bone formation, reproduction and immune response	Whole grains, seafood (clams, oysters, mussels), nuts, soybeans and other legumes, rice, leafy vegetables, tea	Rare	Nervous system disorders
Molybdenum	Structural constituent of molybdopterin, a cofactor synthesised by the body and required for the function of several enzymes	Legumes, whole grains, nuts and beef liver	Unknown	None reported
Phosphorus	Mineralisation of bones and teeth, component of every cell, component of phospholipids, energy transfer and acid-base balance	Animal products (meat, fish, poultry, eggs, milk, yoghurt)	Muscle weakness, bone pain	Symptoms may result from the effects of hypocalcaemia.
Potassium	Fluid and electrolyte balance, supports cell integrity, assists in nerve impulse transmission and muscle contractions	All whole foods (meat, milk, fruits, vegetables, grains, and legumes)	Muscle weakness, irregular heartbeat, glucose intolerance	Muscle weakness, cardiac arrest
Selenium	Component of an antioxidant enzymes which prevent oxidation (cell damage), regulates thyroid hormone	Brazil nuts, fish (tuna, halibut, sardines), meats, whole grains	Associated with Keshan disease (a cardiomyopathy), male infertility	Nail and hair brittleness, fatigue, irritability, nervous system disorders, skin rash
Sodium	Fluid and electrolyte balance, nerve impulse transmission and muscle contraction	Table salt, soy sauce, processed foods, moderate amounts found in meat, milk, bread and vegetables	Muscle cramps, loss of appetite, nausea and vomiting, headache, confusion, seizures	Dizziness, vomiting and diarrhoea, oedema, acute hypertension, confusion, coma
Sulfate	Stabilise protein structures, component of the hormone insulin and the B vitamins biotin and thiamine	All protein containing foods (meat, fish, poultry, eggs, milk, legumes, nuts)	None known	Only occurs in animals
Zinc	Component of the hormone insulin, wound healing, immune reactions, transport of vitamin A, taste perception, sperm production, normal foetal development, component of many enzymes involved in cell division and cell growth	Shellfish, meats, legumes, mushrooms, whole grains and fortified breakfast cereals	Growth retardation, delayed sexual maturation, hair loss, eye and skin lesions, loss of appetite, impaired immunity	Loss of appetite, impaired immunity, low high-density lipoprotein cholesterol, copper and iron deficiencies

Dietary Reference Values

Dietary reference values (DRVs) or nutrient reference values are a set of standards which define the amounts of energy, nutrients and other dietary components to promote health and prevent disease. DRVs are based on distribution within a particular population and are based on currently available scientific knowledge. Many countries internationally have their own DRVs, and international reference values have been published by organisations such as Food and Agriculture Organization and the World Health Organization. The definitions of DRVs will vary based on the country and organisation responsible for the recommendation. Table 1.11 lists key definitions and the uses of the various DRVs adapted from the from the Food and Nutrition Board Institutes of Medicine (2000) publication, *Dietary Reference Intakes: Applications in Dietary Assessment*.[10]

Reading Labels

Food labels appear on most packaged foods and can be confusing to the consumer. Fresh fruit, vegetables, nuts, lentils, beans, fresh meat and fish and foods with few nutrients, such as plain coffee, tea and spices, do not carry a nutrition label. Food labels contain many different types of information such as:

- Nutrition information panel
- Percentage labelling
- Information for people with food allergies or intolerances
- Date marking
- Ingredient list
- Food additives
- Directions for use and storage
- Nutrition and health claims

The nutrition information panel shows the average amount of energy, protein, fat, saturated fat, carbohydrate, sugars and sodium in a serving and in 100 g (or 100 mL) of the food. This can be used to compare the serving size with how much is eaten. For example, if the serving size is half a cup of dry rolled oats and you eat a cup, you will need to double the nutrient and kilojoule values per serving. Many products contain more than a single serving. The nutrient information panel can also be used to compare similar foods and to choose a product which provides less saturated fat, salt (sodium), added sugars and energy per 100 g. It is important to understand that when prescribing a diet for a patient, their ability to follow the prescription may be hampered by poor numeric skills or literacy. See Chapter 14, Public Health, Policy, Prevention, and Implementation for more.

Functional Foods

'Functional foods' are foods and food components that have physiological and psychological effects when consumed regularly as part of a varied diet and have recognised roles in protecting against disease, preventing deficiency of a nutrient or promoting growth and development. These may be whole foods, modified foods or fortified foods.

AN EXAMPLE OF FUNCTIONAL FOODS: OAT

Oat is a nutritious cereal which contains a high concentration of soluble fibre, a subclass of carbohydrate. Oat is a good source of the functional component, beta-glucan. Beta-glucan has been shown to have effects on the glycaemic, insulin and cholesterol responses to foods. Oats and whole-grain oat products have positive physiological benefits on blood cholesterol, blood glucose metabolism, satiety and gastrointestinal health.

TABLE 1.11 ■ **Summary of Dietary Reference Values and Their Application**

Term	Abbreviation	Definition	For individuals	For groups
Estimated average requirement (also referred to as recommended dietary allowance or RDI)	EAR	A daily nutrient level estimated to meet the requirements of half the healthy individuals in a particular life stage and gender group	Used to examine the probability that usual intake is inadequate	Used to estimate the prevalence of inadequate intakes within a group
Recommended dietary intake	RDI	The average dietary intake level that is sufficient to meet the nutrient requirements of nearly all (97%–98%) of healthy individuals in a particular life stage and gender group	Usual intake at or above this level has a low probability of inadequacy	Do not use to assess intakes of groups
Adequate intake	AI	Used when an RDI cannot be determined; the average daily nutrient intake level based on observed or experimentally determined approximations or estimates of nutrient intake by a group (or groups) of healthy people that are assumed to be adequate	Usual intake at or above this level has a low probability of inadequacy; when the AI is based on median intakes of healthy populations, this assessment is made with less confidence	Mean usual intake at or above this level implies a low prevalence of inadequate intakes
Estimated energy requirement	EER	The average dietary energy intake that is predicted to maintain energy balance in a healthy adult of defined age, gender, weight, height and level of physical activity, consistent with good health	Used to assess average dietary intake to maintain energy balance in a healthy adult	Do not use to assess requirements of groups
Upper level of intake	UL	The highest average daily nutrient intake level likely to pose no adverse health effects to almost all individuals in the general population; as intake increases above the UL, the potential risk of adverse effects increases	Usual intake above this level may place an individual at risk of adverse effects from excessive nutrient intake	Use to estimate the percentage of the population at potential risk of adverse effects from excessive nutrient intake

Source[10]: Institute of Medicine (US) Subcommittee on Interpretation and Uses of Dietary Reference Intakes; Institute of Medicine (US) Standing Committee on the Scientific Evaluation of Dietary Reference Intakes. *DRI Dietary Reference Intakes: Applications in Dietary Assessment*. Washington, DC: National Academies Press; 2000.

ACTIVITY: FUNCTIONAL FOODS

Identify three other functional foods and describe their uses in dietary advice.

Food Groups and Dietary Guidelines

Foods are categorised into what is known as 'food groups' based on their nutrient profile. Each of the food groups provides a range of important nutrients and are essential as part of a healthy, balanced diet. The food groups are typically as follows:

- Fruits
- Vegetables
- Whole grains and cereals
- Milk, yoghurt, cheese and/or alternatives
- Lean meat, fish, poultry, eggs, nuts, and legumes

Dietary guidelines are developed for use in practice at the level of the practitioner, the public or policy with the aim to promote health and well-being, reduce risk of diet-related conditions and chronic diseases. Dietary guidelines are often based on food groups classification and might include recommendations on the amount of each food group to be consumed daily (servings).

Dietary guidelines are based on the best available scientific evidence underlying food, diet and health relationships that improve public health outcomes and support improvements to the country's food environment. In recent years, the environmental impact of food choices and diet has become an important consideration of dietary guidelines, for example, Canada's Food Guide, which emphasises a diet rich in fruit and vegetables, plant-based protein foods and whole grain products. As we know, nutrition evidence is often changing, which poses a difficulty in the development of dietary guidelines that are up to date with the latest nutrition evidence.

A HEALTH PHILOSOPHY TOWARD FOOD

Good nutrition is important to human health and well-being. No food is necessarily 'good' or 'bad' per se. The concept of 'good' nutrition encompasses the need to consume adequate fuel (food) for growth and development, for the prevention of disease and to meet any social and cultural preferences. A healthy philosophy toward food recognises the social and cultural value of food, beyond composition of nutrients and energy consumption.

FACTORS THAT DRIVE FOOD CHOICE

Individuals choose whether to eat, what to eat and when to eat based on a number of motives. These motives might include biological determinants, such as hunger and appetite, personal preference, habit, ethnic heritage or tradition, convenience and economy, negative associations with food and body, and values. Skills such as the ability to cook and store food also drive food choice. Many consumers also make food choices based on the nutrition and perceived health benefits. The balance of foods selected over time can have an important influence on health status and outcomes.

References

1. Tessari P. (2006). Nitrogen Balance and Protein Requirements: Definition and Measurements. In: Mantovani G, et al. *Cachexia and Wasting: A Modern Approach*. Springer, Milano. https://doi.org/10.1007/978-88-470-0552-5_8.
2. Kris-Etherton P, Hecker K, Shaffer Taylor D, et al. *Nutrition in the Prevention and Treatment of Disease*. Cambridge, Massachusetts: Academic Press; 2001:279–290.

3. Wall R, Ross RP, Fitzgerald GF, et al. Fatty acids from fish: The anti-inflammatory potential of long chain omega-3 fatty acids. *Nutr Rev.* 2010;68:280–289.
4. Aung T, Halsey J, Kromhout D, et al. Associations of omega-3 fatty acid supplement use with cardiovascular disease risks: Meta-analysis of 10 trials involving 77 917 individuals. *JAMA Cardiol.* 2018;3(3):14–22.
5. Iqbal MP. Trans fatty acids—a risk factor for cardiovascular disease. *Pak J Med Sci.* 2014;30(1):194–197.
6. Bayly GR. *Clinical Biochemistry: Metabolic and Clinical Aspects.* 3rd ed. London, UK: Churchill Livingstone; 2014.
7. Fricker RA, Green E, Jenkins SI, et al. The influence of nicotinamide on health and disease in the central nervous system. *Int J Tryptophan Res.* 2018;11:1–11.
8. Zhang FF, Barr SI, McNulty H, Li D, Blumberg JB. Health effects of vitamin and mineral supplements. *BMJ.* 2020:369:m2511. https://doi.org/10.1136/bmj.m2511.
9. Carson TL, Desmond R, Hardy S, et al. A study of the relationship between food group recommendations and perceived stress: Findings from Black women in the deep south. *Journal of Obesity*, 2015; 203164. https://doi.org/10.1155/2015/203164.
10. Institute of Medicine (US) Subcommittee on Interpretation and Uses of Dietary Reference Intakes; Institute of Medicine (US) Standing Committee on the Scientific Evaluation of Dietary Reference Intakes. *DRI Dietary Reference Intakes: Applications in Dietary Assessment.* Washington, DC: National Academies Press; 2000.

CHAPTER 2

Basic Principles of Screening and Assessment

Tim Eden ■ Eleanor Beck

LEARNING POINTS

By the end of this chapter, you should be able to:

- Identify and describe measures of anthropometry, biochemistry, clinical and dietary and environmental assessment which can be used to assess nutritional status
- Describe the advantages and challenges of using different dietary assessment methods
- Understand the difference between nutrition screening and assessment and the relevance of these in modern health care to nutrition and nonnutrition professionals
- Recognise validated nutrition screening and assessment tools
- Apply nutrition screening tools suitable to the designated population/setting
- Understand the role of doctors/health professionals (e.g., nurses) and the role of the dietitian in nutrition screening and assessment and how assessment tools may be used in research and practice to measure change/progress
- Outline groups at risk of malnutrition

CASE STUDY 2.1 Nutrition Screening Examples

NUTRITION SCREENING EXAMPLE 1

Mr. Jones, aged 82 years, presents to hospital with unstable angina. On admission to hospital the nurse undertaking the routine admission procedures administers the Malnutrition Screening Tool (MST), recording the details in the electronic medical record. Mr. Jones is asked,

1. 'Have you lost weight recently without trying?'
2. 'Have you been eating poorly because of a decreased appetite?'

Mr. Jones states that he has lost weight recently without trying to, and the nurse asks how much weight. Mr. Jones believes he has lost 3–4 kg. He also states that he has not been eating all his meals as he has a poor appetite. Scoring (out of a total of 4) only 1 for question 1, but 2 for question 2 categorises Mr. Jones as at risk, and he is referred automatically to the dietitian for nutrition assessment.

NUTRITION SCREENING EXAMPLE 2

Molly is a nutrition student on a first-year observational placement in a primary care clinic. Molly will be undertaking the task of nutrition screening on individuals presenting for routine health care assessments with the primary care doctor. The individuals presenting are between 55 and 90 years of age. Molly chooses to use the Malnutrition Universal Screening Tool (MUST) over the Mini-Nutritional Assessment Short Form (MNA-SF), as some individuals are under 65 years of age. Molly's first patient is Mary, who was recently discharged from hospital after hip replacement surgery. Using chair scales today, Mary's weight was 58 kg and she reports a height of 166 cm. She has lost 5 kg in the lead-up to surgery over 3 months. Mary states this is primarily due to the pain she experienced presurgery. Mary is now undertaking all activities of daily living and states she feels very well and is eating all of her meals after discharge.

CASE STUDY 2.1 Nutrition Screening Examples—(Continued)

In application of the MUST:

1. Mary has a body mass index (BMI) of 21 km/m^2, scoring 0 on Step 1 of the MUST.
2. Mary has experienced weight loss of approximately 8% (5 kg from 63 kg starting weight), scoring 1 on Step 2 of the MUST.
3. Mary has recently been unwell but is now well and is not describing any ongoing symptoms, scoring 0 on Step 3 of the MUST.
4. Step 4 of MUST indicates that Mary is at medium risk of malnutrition, scoring a total of 1 on Steps 1–3 of the tool.
5. Step 5 indicates that Mary should be observed. Management may include highlighting to Mary that unintentional weight loss is not ideal, that she should be sure she is eating all of her meals and that she should weigh herself to ensure no ongoing decrease in body weight. Molly should flag that Mary is screened at all subsequent visits to ensure the situation (of significant weight loss recently) is resolved.
6. The importance of using the right tool. For example, using MUST on a patient with renal impairment or liver disease and how the fluid retention may lead to the patient's risk being underestimated.

NUTRITION ASSESSMENT EXAMPLE 1

Marjo, aged 45 years, attends clinic for advice on healthy eating. Her dietary recall includes the following information:

Breakfast:	2 slices of white toast, a thin scrape of olive-based margarine and jam, black tea
Morning tea:	apple or banana, a tub of low-fat yoghurt
Lunch:	2 slices of white bread with cheese and ham and margarine (made at home), cappuccino (about 300 mL), 2 chocolate biscuits
Afternoon tea:	30 g of mixed nuts, 1 slice of white bread with margarine and jam, black tea
Dinner:	180 g mince or ½ chicken breast or lean steak, cooked in a small amount of sunflower (polyunsaturated) oil, 2 potatoes with skin (microwaved) with sour cream and 1.5 cups of mixed vegetables (eats a variety each night), water to drink
Supper:	4–6 squares of chocolate

Simple dietary assessment against guidelines such as EatWell (UK) can compare Marjo's diet to review basic nutritional adequacy. Marjo is eating five servings of breads and cereals (five slices of bread/day) which alongside the potato portion makes up her total carbohydrate intake. The one piece of fruit (morning tea) and up to 2–3 servings of vegetables (dinner) gives a daily intake of 3–4 fruit and vegetable portions. She has 2–3 milk/alternatives (yoghurt, cheese, and milk in cappuccino). Marjo is eating two servings of meat/alternatives (equating to approximately 90 g of cooked meat per portion). Marjo is also consuming a serve of nuts, and discretionary (eat occasionally) foods, namely the chocolate biscuits, the chocolate, and the sour cream. Marjo's margarine and oil is predominantly high in monounsaturated (olives) and polyunsaturated (vegetable) oil, and her bread and cereal foods are not whole grain (they are refined).

The professional assessing Marjo's diet compares her intake against recommended guidelines and notes that she may have a diet low in fibre and whole grains as refined grains are consumed and Marjo has only one piece of fruit daily where two are recommended. Marjo consumes more meat/alternatives than would be recommended for her age group. At 45 years of age, the number of discretionary foods is excessive and may add to weight gain. Marjo is choosing several poly- and monounsaturated food items including nuts, margarine and oil, and this is positive.

Continued

CASE STUDY 2.1 Nutrition Screening Examples—(Continued)

This dietary assessment is based on dietary and nutrient quality and quantity. Consider how the assessment of Marjo's diet and suggestion on ways for Marjo to improve her diet may (or may not) change if (1) she was newly diagnosed with coeliac disease and was required to avoid all gluten, (2) she was unable to eat any hard or difficult to chew foods due to jaw surgery or (3) she previously had a BMI of 45 kg/m² and has lost 30 kg. She is now stuck at her current weight and seeking advice on further improvement.

NUTRITION ASSESSMENT EXAMPLE 2

Gerald is a 75-year-old man admitted to the hospital after a fall at home fracturing his right neck of femur. He lives alone and reports his clothes no longer fit as well as before, and he struggles at home with cooking and cleaning. He has recovered well on the ward after total hip arthroplasty and is receiving regular physiotherapy. He remains on the ward awaiting a new package of care for discharge but has been referred for nutritional support. On review of his drug chart, he is prescribed an ACE inhibitor, beta blocker and various analgesia and has recently been started on a diuretic (furosemide) indicating a diagnosis of heart failure. His recorded weight at review is 64 kg (136 lb), and he is 1.78 m (5 ft 10 in) tall. You notice oedema present affecting both legs which is documented as 'moderate, pitting oedema'. As part of the nutritional assessment, estimated energy and protein requirements are calculated as follows. Additional factors to consider are noted in Table 2.1.

Anthropometry

Weight: 64 kg (but likely less than this factoring bilateral moderate pitting oedema ~ 5 kg)

Adjusted for fluid/oedema present: 59 kg

BMI: 18.6 kg/m² (59 kg ÷ 1.78²)

Calculate Energy (Kilocalories)

Energy: resting energy expenditure 1180–1475 kcal/day (based on 59 kg using 20–25 kcal/kg)

Total energy: 1416–1770 kcal/day (using resting energy expenditure and adding a multiplier of 1.2 to account for physical activity and diet-induced thermogenesis)

*Consider additional 500 kcal/day in view of history of weight loss (1916 – 2270 kcal/day). (Note: the modulation of kcal will depend on weight goals.)

Calculate Protein (Grams)

Protein: 59–88.5 g/day (based on dry/actual body weight using 1.0–1.5 g/kg per day)

*Consider using upper limit in view of recent surgical intervention and likely weight loss.

TABLE 2.1 ■ **Highlighting Factors to Consider When Calculating Nutritional Requirements**

Factors to Consider When Calculating Requirements	
Anthropometry	Establish baseline measures (weight/body mass index/mid-upper arm circumference) and monitor, consider factors impacting weight measures, e.g., fluid retention, oedema, ascites, method of measure, accuracy.
Weight history	Use visual cues, verbal reporting from patient, check previous admissions or primary care notes.
Current/previous dietary intake	Conduct appropriate dietary assessment. Discuss with patient, family, friends. Monitor from ward records.
Refeeding syndrome	Assess risk based on recent nutritional intake. Monitor appropriate blood test and instigate preventative measures accordingly.
Disease factor	Establish clinical context of disease pathology and impact on metabolic state, e.g., presence of inflammation, sepsis, hypermetabolic states, deplete status.
Physical activity	Assess current activity levels and how this has changed and may change in the future.

Nutrition Screening and Assessment: Key Questions Example

Gary, aged 80 years, attends a routine visit to his primary care physician. He states that he recently had a fall at home and is feeling less steady on his feet than usual. Gary lives alone in his own home, but his son and daughter-in-law live nearby and he eats meals with them once or twice each week. Gary still does his own shopping but occasionally has shopping delivered. Gary states he is not motivated to cook and has noticed a decreased appetite. His doctor notices that his belt is on a tighter notch than usual. Gary's temples are hollowed with his clavicles well defined. He has significant fat on his biceps or triceps, and although his knee bones are well defined, he still has reasonably well-developed thighs and calf muscles. His interosseous muscle is slightly depressed but he has no oedema or ascites.

Today Gary weighs 78 kg but his weight 6 months ago was 83 kg. He is 177 cm tall. Gary states he has eaten all his meals but does not prepare large meals. He denies any nausea or other gastrointestinal symptoms.

Gary's medications include digoxin (Lanoxin) and atenolol (Tenormin). He has a past history of mild angina but no recent measurement of his lipid profile. All haematology results are normal.

Gary's favourite activity is his once per week chess game with an old friend. He used to walk daily but gave up after his wife died around 1 year ago.

Dietary Intake

Breakfast: black tea with sugar, large bowl of porridge made with milk with a banana

Lunch: sandwich with white bread and butter and processed meat and cheese and tomato OR sardines, another piece of fruit

Dinner: 3 beef sausages with oven fries and 1 sachet of frozen vegetables or 2 eggs on toast with fried tomato and mushrooms and baked beans OR meal with his son and daughter-in-law: a roast 1/week (beef 120 g, 1 roast potato, roast pumpkin, peas and broccoli and gravy); BBQ chicken 1/week (maybe a leg and a small amount of other meat with skin; with a green salad and some pasta salad with creamy sauce)

Snacks: occasional handful of nuts, pieces of fruit, a couple of nights each week a small bowl of ice cream, 1 can of beer when he is cooking at night; drinks water or black tea throughout the day

Key Clinical Questions

If you are in the role of Gary's primary care physician:

Is Gary at risk of malnutrition (consider the tools available for screening)?

What factors (anthropometry, biochemistry, clinical, dietary, social) might assist you in finalising a nutrition assessment for Gary?

Is Gary malnourished (consider the tools available for assessment)?

Overview and Introduction

It is difficult to discuss nutrition without some consideration of how poor nutrition may affect the health outcomes of an individual. Malnutrition may manifest as undernutrition in food-insecure individuals, in whom children present weight (wasted) or height (stunted) below typically healthy reference ranges and adults manifest underweight. However, it may also manifest as overnutrition due to excessive energy intake. In both under- and overnutrition, poor diet quality, including specific nutritional deficiencies (micronutrient deficiency) can manifest. In the context of health care, nutrition is recognised as an important factor in affecting both risk of disease and outcomes related to disease. For example, obesity, related to overnutrition, is associated with a range of diseases including diabetes, hypertension and cardiovascular disease.[1] In addition to the association of overnutrition with risk of chronic disease, undernutrition has been associated with consequences such as increased length of stay in hospital settings,[2] increased risk of complications[3] and greater likelihood of hospital readmission.[4] Consequently, malnutrition places a burden on individuals' health and health care systems.[5,6]

Prevalence of malnutrition in hospitals may be as high as 50%, although averaging a lower level in acute wards than rehabilitation settings.[7,8] These rates justify early identification of individuals who may be at risk of malnutrition or malnourished. If malnourished individuals are presenting to hospitals, or for health care in other settings, then the screening of community-dwelling individuals, who may be at particular risk, is also relevant. To identify poor nutrition, health professionals and researchers may undertake a process of nutrition screening and assessment to highlight risk and identify problems. Some tools used in nutrition screening are developed for the general public, for example, the Healthy Eating Index developed by the US Department of Agriculture[9] or the modified version for Australian Adults.[10] These are simplistic measures, which may allow an individual to make a basic assessment of their own diet, forming part of a broad nutrition assessment process. The tools and processes used by health care professionals are more complex and consider a range of measures including anthropometry, biochemistry, clinical signs and symptoms (especially those affecting dietary intake), dietary evaluation and the broad social context of an individual. Most validated tools are designed for screening or assessment of individuals who may be at risk, such as the elderly or those presenting to hospital for treatment.

Malnutrition screening is typically focused on identifying undernutrition, and it is a process that ideally errs on the side of false-positives. Namely, these tools are simple, designed to be administered by professionals with little or no training in nutrition, and will occasionally flag well-nourished individuals as at risk, to ensure those who are malnourished are not missed. While the screening process flags individuals who may be at risk, full nutrition assessment is required to provide a diagnosis of 'malnutrition'. Furthermore, tools designed to determine a formal diagnosis of malnutrition tend to require greater complexity, and generally professionals with further clinical education, including dietitians and medical practitioners, are most likely to administer these tools. In addition to tools designed to streamline the process, nutrition assessment is included in standards for professionals such as dietitians who may follow specific processes, such as the Nutrition Care Process, and utilise specific terminology in diagnosing a nutrition-related problem, based on a full nutrition assessment.[11] Examples of tools and processes are provided in this chapter.

This chapter focuses on nutrition screening and assessment of the individual and not population-level screening/assessment as undertaken in surveillance. Although there is a focus on undernutrition (hereafter malnutrition), the *process* of nutrition assessment does not change between individuals. On completion, the objective is to be able to define and understand the various methods of nutrition screening and assessment, to appreciate how this varies in different clinical and nonclinical settings and to understand the rationale for disease-specific tools to improve sensitivity and clinical management.

What Are Nutrition Screening and Nutrition Assessment?

Nutritional screening is the application of simple, rapid and validated nutrition screening tools, which are reproducible with minimal training. These tools feed into care pathways seeking to further assess and manage nutritional status as required. Screening tools are applied in varied health care settings including primary, secondary and tertiary care services and wider population cohorts. Many screening tools focus on weight loss, and thus emphasis is often placed on undernutrition, and others exist for specific populations and disease-states. It is important to appreciate that

TABLE 2.2 ■ **Comparison of Nutrition Screening and Assessment**

	Nutrition Screening	Nutrition Assessment
Goal	Typically focused on identifying undernutrition	Full nutrition assessment focused on providing a diagnosis of malnutrition in all its forms, undernutrition, overnutrition and micronutrient deficiencies
Process	Simple processes and tools, designed to be administered by professionals with little or no training in nutrition	Complex processes and tools, applied by professionals with further clinical education including dietitians and medical practitioners
Examples	Healthy Eating Index[9] or the modified version for Australian Adults[10]	Anthropometry, biochemistry/haematology, clinical examination, diet history and social assessment

overweight or obese status does not preclude the risk of malnutrition, and all individuals require screening in some settings (e.g., hospital) regardless of appearance.

Nutritional assessment is a clinical skill to identify specific issues related to potential poor nutrition. These can occur in the context of under- and overnutrition and include an understanding of how diet quality is relevant to nutritional status. Nutritional assessment is a more detailed, specific, and more in-depth evaluation of nutritional status by an expert. It enables identification of specific dietary and nutritional needs, which may be addressed via individualised care plans (devised by a trained health care professional, namely dietitian, nutritionist or doctor). Nutritional assessments require the specialist interpretation of quantitative and qualitative data incorporating elements of anthropometry, biochemistry, clinical and dietary factors (Table 2.2).

Methods of Nutrition Screening

A review of nutrition screening tools[12] identified 34 malnutrition screening tools for older adults and highlighted the number of tools that may exist across varied patient groups, but also where single tools are used across patient groups. To understand the general principles of screening, it is valuable to consider the common elements of screening tools (Table 2.3). The most common questions in malnutrition screening tools relate to appetite, dietary intake and weight. Unintentional weight loss has long been associated with increased mortality, with as little as 4%–5% weight loss over a year associated with poorer outcomes.[13] Investigations of unintentional weight loss show that even in individuals who are overweight or obese, weight loss increases the risk of both major cardiac events and all-cause mortality.[14] Therefore, it is particularly relevant that several screening tools specifically address unintentional weight loss.

The most simple of these tools is the Malnutrition Screening Tool (MST)[15] which consists of two simple questions on unintentional weight loss and poor dietary intake due to a decreased appetite. This tool was originally developed to screen for malnutrition in all adults in a hospital environment. Similarly to most tools, questions attract a score based on responses to these questions. Individuals who present large weight loss (more than 5 kg) as well as those who are unsure about weight loss or the amount of weight lost are identified as potentially at risk of malnutrition, and referral is made for further review, namely nutrition assessment by a health care professional such as a dietitian. Likewise, the Malnutrition Universal Screening Tool (MUST)[16] used commonly in the United Kingdom, Mini-Nutritional Assessment Short Form (MNA-SF) adopted relatively globally,[17,18] and Nutrition Risk Screening 2002 (NRS)[19] all address weight loss as a key factor in nutritional risk, regardless of initial body weight. Other tools developed to predict a more general decline in health status, such as the FRAIL (fatigue, resistance, ambulation, illnesses and

TABLE 2.3 ■ **Commonly Used Malnutrition Screening Tools**

Tool	Format	Weight History	Appetite	Dietary Intake	Medical History/ Current Situation
MST	Two questions; score directs further care	X	X		
MUST	5-step process; score directs to further care	X		X	X
MNA-SF	6 questions; score directs to continue assessment	X	X	X	X
NRS	4 initial questions; further assessments if flagged at risk	X	X	X	X[a]

[a]The initial four questions only include reference to intensive care unit status. Further questions include reference to medical conditions.
MST, Malnutrition Screening Tool; *MUST*, Malnutrition University Screening Tool; *MNA-SF*, Mini-Nutritional Assessment—Short Form; *NRS*, Nutrition Risk Screening.

loss of weight) tool, also ask the question regarding recent weight loss,[20] again highlighting the relevance of unintentional weight loss in overall health. Ultimately, there are a number of tools (for example MUST, NRS and MNA-SF) that classify individuals as at risk of malnutrition where body weight is very low in the first instance irrespective of recent weight loss.

There is also recognition that illness creates risk either adding to decreased appetite, changed environment (such as hospital admission) or increased nutritional requirements related to a clinical condition. The MST and MNA-SF ask about appetite, and some tools such as the NRS more specifically address intake over a recent time frame. The MNA-SF, MUST and NRS all describe illness of relevance or, in the case of NRS, initially screen for intensive care patients (who are all at some risk). Understanding the factors that contribute to malnutrition provides broad understanding of how to screen individuals and recognises that while acute illness and hospitalisation add risk, the fundamental factors of unintentional weight loss and poor appetite, and therefore poor dietary intake, can occur in any setting.

Internationally, many organisations (such as government health departments) provide automatic screening for malnutrition to individuals admitted to hospital, recording of this score by electronic medical record, and subsequent referral for further investigation if risk is identified. A key element of using malnutrition screening tools is the pathway of care that follows an individual's risk classification. The care pathways highlighted in the MST, MUST and NRS all suggest referral to dietitians or nutrition care teams or invoking specific nutrition-related policies if individuals are identified as at risk of malnutrition.

It is also important to recognise that individuals experiencing acute illness may quickly deteriorate, and hence repeat screening is recommended weekly in hospital settings, regardless of the tool in use. For community-dwelling individuals, the tools recommend reassessment of lower risk of malnutrition with varied time frames of 1 to 12 months. The MUST suggests the 1-month time frame for the elderly in care homes, highlighting their poorer health generally as a risk for decreased dietary intake and hence malnutrition.

A final consideration may be around which tool is relevant for a particular population group. Recent work has highlighted the feasibility of screening in primary care as part of preventative health care, with positive outcomes.[21] A meta-analysis examining a range of tools for hospital inpatients found no single tool was likely to meet the purposes of both nutrition screening and also predict longer-term health outcomes of individuals.[22] However, some tools have been developed for specific patient groups. For example, the MNA-SF is specific to the elderly over 65 years of age, whereas the MST and MUST have been designed as generic tools for all adults. A comparison of the MST, MUST and MNA-SF identified the usefulness of the MST and MUST for hospitalised adults,[23] and the MST has been validated in oncology outpatients.[24] In contrast, the MNA-SF presents as less useful in hospitalised individuals due to false-positives.[23]

For community-dwelling individuals, the prevalence of malnutrition and both the MUST and MNA-SF have been validated in outpatient settings against full nutritional assessment.[23] A recent study investigating community living adults[25] suggests the Seniors in the Community: Risk Evaluation for Eating and Nutrition, Version II (SCREEN II) tool[26] may also be useful in this setting. SCREEN II is similar to many nutrition screening tools, with some more specific questions related to diet quality (for example fruit and vegetable intake) and can be self-administered.

Nutrition Assessment

The role of a nutritional assessment seeks to identify specific dietary and nutrition related risks, issues or concerns which may impact an individual's health. As previously discussed, this differs from nutritional screening in that the purpose goes beyond identifying at-risk groups or individuals. The aim is to identify and establish an understanding of the specific dietary and nutritional concern and factors that may contribute to these concerns. This requires expert knowledge and an appreciation for the intricate interplay between nutrition and both normal physiological circumstance and that which may exist when a given disease process is present.

It is therefore the role of the health care professional to adopt a systematic approach when performing a thorough nutritional assessment. This involves the collection and interpretation of combined qualitative and quantitative data, which aims to provide the professional with the ability to apply a clinically relevant and appropriate nutritional intervention. Albeit a variety of methodologies have been developed to perform such a task, there is broadly a common process which aims to incorporate relevant factors, enabling appropriate clinical decision-making.[27,28]

Around the world the global nutrition community has adopted a variety of structured assessment models which have been validated in their respective countries.[11] Nutrition and dietetics professional bodies and organisations often provide country-specific methods and documentation preferences for nutritional assessment processes. These are typically incorporated into the education of nutrition specialists and dietetic students.[29,30] Common examples of this include the process and internationally used abbreviations first introduced by The Academy of Nutrition and Dietetics in the USA utilising the Nutrition Care Process Terminology and has been adopted by other influencing dietetic bodies such as the British Dietetic Association.[30] The processes are described as:

SOAP: Subjective, Objective, Assessment and Plan

ADIME: Assessment, Diagnosis, Intervention and Monitoring/Evaluation

A further commonality between the models is the use of the term 'nutrition or dietetic diagnosis' which is ultimately the outcome in which the health professional identifies a nutritional issue impacting physical, mental or social well-being. The diagnosis is specific to a problem which the nutritional health care professional will be directly involved in managing.[31] This may be a problem which is likely to impact medical management, for example, individually prescribed nutritional support products (e.g., high-energy, high-protein supplements) to prevent weight loss which influences a chemotherapy regimen. This may also be an existing nutritional issue such as an individual with known kidney disease and targeted nutritional advice is required to help manage electrolytes. The nutritional diagnosis is related to the nutritional intervention required, not the medical condition.

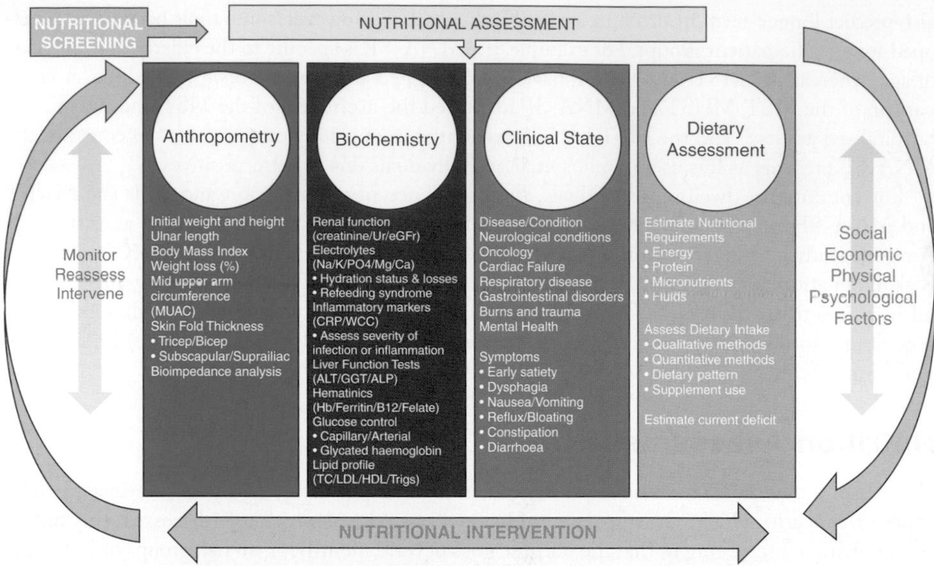

Fig. 2.1 The core components of the nutritional assessment process. *ALP*, alkaline phosphatase; *ALT*, alanine transaminase; *CRP*, C-reactive protein; *eGFR*, estimated glomerular filtration rate; *GGT*, gamma glutamyl transferase; *Hb*, haemoglobin; *HDL*, high-density lipoprotein; *LDL*, low-density lipoprotein; *TC*, total cholesterol; *Trigs*, triglyceride; *UR*, Urea; *WCC,* white cell count.

The aim of this section will be to highlight some of the core components used within the nutrition assessment process and is based around the commonly used frameworks in clinical practice (Fig. 2.1). While some aspects of specific assessment ideologies vary slightly, the basic principles are the same.

ANTHROPOMETRY

Anthropometry is the scientific study of the measurements and proportions of the human body. An initial part of the nutritional assessment is to identify current and previous anthropometric measures, which may be obtained using a variety of methods, from simple to complex. The most commonly used measures in clinical practice, primarily due to ease of collection, reproducibility and low cost, include weight, height, calculation of body mass index (BMI) (kg/m^2) and waist circumference measures. There is a wealth of literature associating high and low values of these measures with increased morbidity and mortality.[32] The World Health Organization (WHO) indicates crude nutritional status dependent on BMI value, whereas other organisations also factor for ethnic differences, adjusting for evidence that differing cutoffs associate with increased cardiometabolic risk (Table 2.4).[33,34]

In primary care, weight or other anthropometric measures can be conducted in the clinic environment using simple equipment. Other effective measures include the use of waist-to-hip ratio and waist-to-height ratio.[35] Both measures help to identify a degree of central adiposity, an established factor for obesity-related cardiometabolic disease, and can be used to assess disease risk with greater accuracy than a weight measure alone (Table 2.5).[36,37]

Clinicians and patients may replicate these measures at home to provide a trend and a record for the health professional. For example, waist-to-height ratio is calculated as waist measurement divided by height measurement (W ÷ H); therefore, a person with a waist of 71 cm (28 in) and height of 170 cm (5 ft 7 in) has a waist-to-height ratio of 0.42 (healthy category indicating no increased disease risk).[38] Weight history forms a significant part of assessment and monitoring

TABLE 2.4 ■ **Commonly Utilised BMI/Abdominal Circumference Cutoffs**

Variable	WHO International Criteria (kg/m²)	Consensus Guidelines for Asian Indians
Generalised descriptors and BMI cutoffs (kg/m²)	Underweight <18.5 Normal weight 18.5–24.9 Preobesity 25.0–29.9 Obesity ≥30.0	Underweight <18.0 Normal weight 18.0–22.9 Preobesity 23.0–24.9 Obesity ≥25.0
Abdominal obesity (waist circumference cutoffs in cm)	Male: ≥102 Female: ≥88	Male: ≥90 Female: ≥80

BMI, Body mass index; *WHO*, World Health Organization.
From WHO Expert Consultation. Appropriate body-mass index for Asian populations and its implications for policy and intervention strategies. *Lancet* 2004;363(9403):157–163.

TABLE 2.5 ■ **Gender-Specific Interpretation of Waist-to-Height Ratio**

Interpretation	Females	Males
Underweight	<0.35	<0.35
Slim	0.35–0.42	0.35–0.43
Healthy	0.42–0.49	0.43–0.53
Overweight	0.49–0.54	0.53–0.58
Obese	0.54–0.58	0.58–0.63
Highly obese	>0.58	>0.63

processes. This can be an invaluable determinant on assessing risk of nutritional issues such as malnutrition and obesity but also on assessing the effectiveness of a nutritional intervention.

In the secondary care setting, this may rely on health care assistants, nurses or other health workers to obtain weights and heights using additional equipment (e.g., hoisting, pad slides, chair scales) dependent on the individual's clinical condition and mobility. Other factors which will impact this measure may require additional physical examination, for example, assessing for fluid retention, oedema and ascites, which can be significant in individuals with end-stage renal disease, heart failure and decompensated liver disease. Correction of weight measures, if combined with physical examination, is also possible in these clinical conditions (Table 2.6).[39]

Other physical measures that are commonly utilised include mid-upper arm circumference or calf circumference and skinfold thickness, for example, measured at the tricep/bicep, whilst also looking closely to the individual to assess for loss of subcutaneous fat/muscle mass.[40] Skinfold thickness measurement is a specialised skill and not covered in detail here. More sophisticated measures of body composition can be used where available/appropriate such as bioelectrical impedance analysis (BIA). As technology has improved, such equipment has become more readily available as it is a noninvasive and relatively inexpensive method to assess for additional anthropometric measures.[41] BIA is based on the transmission of a low-voltage current through the body. Water is stored in muscle and lower impedance of the current will occur in individuals with higher muscle-to-fat ratios, providing measures of the various compartment such as fat mass, fat-free mass and skeletal muscle mass. However, it should be noted that BIA is not advised

TABLE 2.6 ■ **Estimations of Weight Contribution from Oedema and Ascites**

	Ascites	Pitting Oedema
Mild	2.2 kg (detectable on ultrasound scan examination only)	1.0 kg (barely visible, immediate rebound time)
Moderate	6.0 kg (causing moderate symmetrical abdominal distension)	5.0 kg (slight indentation, 10–20-second rebound time)
Severe	14.0 kg (marked abdominal distension and discomfort)	10.0 kg (very deep indentation, >20-second rebound time)

Based on from Mendenhall CL, Anderson S, Weesner RE, Goldberg SJ, Crolic KA. Protein-calorie malnutrition associated with alcoholic hepatitis: Veterans Administration cooperative study group on alcoholic hepatitis. *Am J Med*. 1984;76(2):211–222.

where an individual is at the extreme of weights (high and low) or in clinical cases where extreme fluid shifts occur (patients on dialysis or haemofiltration). An emerging alternative to address this has been the development of bioelectrical impedance vector analysis.[42] This is a type of bedside measure using bioelectrical impedance which adjusts using a theoretical model that differentiates hydration from cell mass, making this less susceptible to inaccuracies caused by fluid and hydration status.

A further bedside measure which is attracting use to assess muscle mass and quality in the context of sarcopenia is the use of cross-sectional ultrasound. Ultrasonography helps to differentiate between subcutaneous fat mass and muscle such that advancing techniques can help to establish changes in muscle groups, quantity and quality when taken as serial measures.[43] While in the vast majority of situations simple measurements of weight or waist circumference and changes in these will provide sufficient anthropometric information, the choice of measurements used is related to the situation of the individual and other clinical factors. Table 2.7 summarises clinical significance, advantages and disadvantages of anthropometric and physical measures commonly used in clinical practice.

BIOCHEMISTRY

An important aspect to the nutritional assessment process is being able to identify specific nutritional deficiencies, which may include specific blood tests and markers. Often in clinical practice the presenting symptomatology and physical assessment will help to identify potential deficiencies thus enabling a targeted approach when ordering specific nutrition-related blood tests. Equally, appreciating the clinical context, inclusive of the individual's past medical history and surgical history, will help to illicit further questioning or investigations.

A broad appreciation of the relevant and commonly ordered laboratory tests, which are either directly or indirectly impacted by nutritional status, is key. One of the most common panels reviewed in assessment of nutritional status is haematological bloods (haemoglobin, mean corpuscular volume, platelets), alongside haematinics (vitamin B12/folate) and iron studies to determine anaemias, either macrocytic or microcytic. Other commonly utilised tests include the use of serum 25-OHD (vitamin D) in conjunction with renal and bone profiles to assess for deficiencies and potential causality.

Measurement of specific vitamin markers may be warranted on the background of severe gastrointestinal symptoms and/or pathology which could influence digestion and absorption, thus increasing the risk of suboptimal levels and deficiency. For example, certain types of surgery, chiefly involving the gastrointestinal tract, will warrant specific monitoring and potential

TABLE 2.7 ■ **Anthropometric and Physical Measures Commonly Used in Clinical Practice**

Physical Measurement	Clinical Significance	Advantages	Disadvantages
BMI kg/m²	Crude marker for obesity-related cardiometabolic disease risk; used in primary/secondary care (individual/population comparisons easily made)	Simple, cheap, accessible, reproducible, involves minimal equipment and is noninvasive	Does not distinguish between excess fat, muscle or bone mass; influenced by factors such as age, sex, ethnicity
WHR Waist circumference divided by hip circumference **WHtR** Waist circumference divided by Height	Proxy for measuring subcutaneous fat and central adiposity; marker for obesity-related cardiometabolic disease with greater accuracy and sensitivity vs BMI alone	Simple calculation, cheap, accessible, reproducible, involves minimal equipment and is noninvasive; can adjust for sex, ethnicity	Interoperator differences in measures, less accurate at extremes of weight, especially when BMI >35.0 kg/m²; not advised for use in children
MUAC >23.5 cm likely to have a healthy BMI and is at low risk of malnutrition <23.5 cm likely to have a BMI <20 kg/m² and may be at high risk of malnutrition	Rapid assessment of over-/undernutrition; predominantly used for children and adolescents but can be used in adult population	Simple, quick, cheap, minimal training required, age dependent, comparisons can be made; high sensitivity, specificity for assessing over- and undernutrition when weight not available	Interoperator differences, significant variability if using as one-off measure; less reliable in elderly and when significant weight loss occurred (presence of skin folds)
Skinfold thickness	Proxy marker for fat mass and indicator of total fat mass; should be conducted at multiple body sites for most accurate interpretation	Quick, cheap, portable equipment, noninvasive	Interoperator differences, requires significant skill to perform reliably; influenced by fat distribution which varies across sex, ethnicity, body type and age
BIA **BIVA**	Measure of body composition differentiating between fat mass % (visceral and subcutaneous), skeletal muscle mass; more reliable than BMI and skinfold thickness measurements	Simple, inexpensive and noninvasive	Less accurate with abnormal hydration status, extremes of BMI or elderly; note BIVA not confounded by hydration (therefore not impacted by presence of ascites/oedema)

Continued

TABLE 2.7 ■ **Anthropometric and Physical Measures Commonly Used in Clinical Practice—cont'd**

Physical Measurement	Clinical Significance	Advantages	Disadvantages
Ultrasound scan of skeletal muscle	More accurate measure of skeletal muscle mass and used to assess sarcopenic changes; can also assess muscle quality via tissue characteristics which is more commonly performed at the quadriceps muscles	Noninvasive, rapid information, portable equipment available, no exposure to radiation	Highly skilled, expensive equipment and training needs required, interoperator differences

BIA, Bioelectrical impedance analysis; *BIVA*, bioelectrical impedance vector analysis; *BMI*, body mass index; *MUAC*, mid-upper arm circumference; *WHR*, waist-to-hip ratio; *WHtR*, waist-to-height ratio.

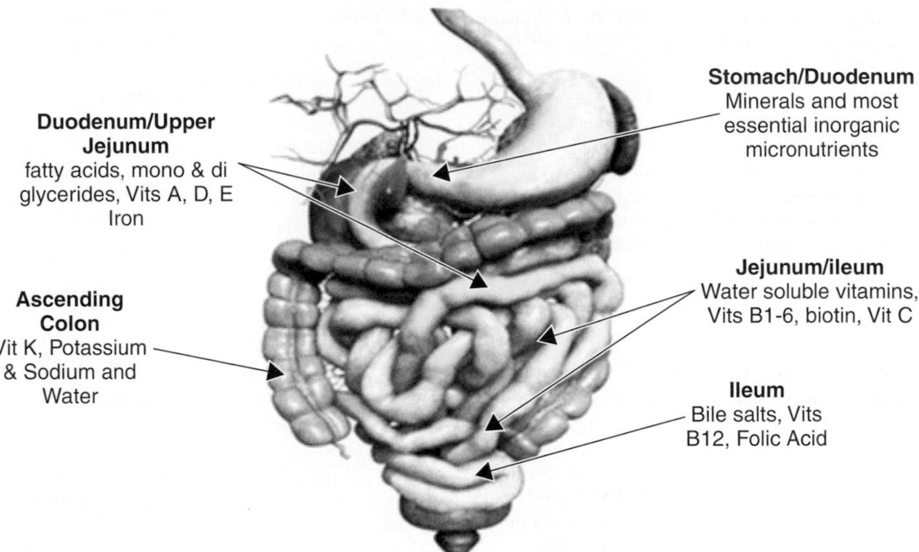

Fig. 2.2 Sites of absorption of nutrients. *Vit.*, Vitamin. (Adapted from Tappenden KA. Pathophysiology of short bowel syndrome: considerations of resected and residual anatomy. *JPEN J Parenteral Enteral Nutr*. 2014;38:14S–122S.)

supplementation. Commonly utilised weight loss procedures such as Roux-en-Y gastric bypass necessitate the need for supplementation of micronutrients absorbed in the duodenum and proximal part of the jejunum.[44] Another example is that of short bowel syndrome as a consequence of extensive bowel resections often requiring supplementation of micronutrients and electrolytes.[45] While it is beyond the scope of this chapter to discuss this in depth, having a familiarity with the site of absorption of vitamins and minerals (Fig. 2.2) will assist in understanding risk and therefore provide a basic appreciation of investigations which may be required.[46]

A further consideration is the role of infection and inflammation on nutritional markers. This can often influence the interpretation of various vitamin and minerals assessed for in clinical practice whereby it is recognised that levels of vitamin C, vitamin D, zinc and selenium are significantly impacted by increased inflammatory states. It is therefore important to recognise that laboratory testing can be very useful for interpreting disease state and severity but may be less useful for nutritional assessment. Table 2.8 outlines key parameters which may be relevant for general clinical assessment, particularly about nutritional assessment.

CLINICAL STATE

Understanding the current disease state and symptomatology is helpful to identify causes of why an individual may be at increased risk of malnutrition. This may relate to increased energy and/or protein requirements, reduced energy intake or increased nutritional losses. For example, an individual suffering from chronic obstructive pulmonary disease may have increased energy requirements related to the increased respiratory effort required to breathe.[47] However, they may also struggle to consume food due to the physical difficulties associated with breathlessness. Individuals with protein-losing nephropathies need to make up for protein losses through diet. Again, understanding the passage of food from ingestion to excretion may assist in understanding the relevant considerations in nutrition assessment. Each of these can then be considered in the context of a specific disease state which may impact one or more of the following:

Ingestion may be impaired by dysphagia (difficulty in swallowing), odynophagia (pain on swallowing) or not having the physical capacity to feed one's self. This may be a consequence of neurological conditions, trauma or surgical intervention directly affecting the upper gastrointestinal tract. It is also important to recognise psychological determinants, such as mood and mental health status. The influence of these psychological factors on appetite and food intake should always be considered in conjunction with physical factors.

Digestion may be compromised by pathology affecting the gastrointestinal tract, which may cause mechanical obstructions or reduced peristalsis, impacting the flow of food substances, gastric juices and chyme. Often this can be due to physical obstruction by malignancy, adhesions, fistulations, postoperative complications or compromised digestion, but may also be a result of medications that affect gastric motility.

Absorption may be compromised by various pathologies or disease states leading to malabsorption. These can be inherited or acquired and may vary in time, where some cases are transient and others more prolonged, all depending on the underlying cause.[48,49] Inherited conditions include cystic fibrosis where pancreatic insufficiency necessitates the need for artificial enzyme replacement therapy to ensure adequate nutrient absorption. Congenital conditions such as biliary atresia can impact bile duct development, impairing bile flow in infancy and causing long-term hepatic dysfunction and cirrhosis. Other more subtle conditions can impact absorption of nutrients, such as coeliac disease where inflammation causes flattening of the microvilli in the small intestine. This can cause malabsorption of nutrients specific to this part of the gastrointestinal tract such as iron, calcium and fat-soluble vitamins. Even less serious conditions, such as lactose intolerance, may add to gastric motility and affect absorption of other nutrients.

Other commonly encountered conditions include inflammatory bowel disease such as ulcerative colitis and Crohn disease. Diseases which involve the gallbladder, liver and pancreas can influence absorption via dysregulation to gastric juices, bile salts and pancreatic enzyme production. Equally, other iatrogenic causes should be considered such as medications damaging the gastric lining, including tetracyclines, colchicine or cholestyramine and even long-term antibiotic use influencing the microbiome. Common signs and symptoms of malabsorption (Table 2.9) can be either directly observed from physical examination or elicited from accurate and astute history taking.[50]

Metabolism is broadly described as the net result when combining complex biochemical processes and pathways that occur in living organisms to ensure normal cellular function. This involves substrate matter, which, in nutritional terms, can be categorised as energy (kilocalories/kilojoules)

TABLE 2.8 ■ **Laboratory Measures and Nutritional use with Added Reference Ranges (Available Tests and Reference Ranges Vary Across Health Systems)**

Measurement	Nutritional Rationale	Reference Ranges (lab/unit specific)
Haemoglobin (Hb)	Assess for iron status or indicate anaemia (differentiate between macro/microcytic; i.e., add in ferritin, B12, folate)	Women = 12.0 to 15.5 g/dL Men = 13.5 to 17.5 g/dL
Albumin	A negative acute phase protein; low levels may indicate presence of inflammation or infection, therefore an unreliable marker of protein/nutritional status; also significantly contributes to oncotic pressure and low levels can reflect fluid shifts causing oedema	35–50 g/L (3.5–5.0 g/dL)
CRP	A nonspecific marker of inflammation, raised when infection/inflammation is present; may indicate severity of inflammatory response; when excessively high can impact interpretation of certain vitamins and minerals (vitamins C, D and zinc and selenium)	Ideally <10 mg/L
White cell count	Immune system marker; is raised if infection is present	4–11 × 10^9/L
Glycated haemoglobin	Indicates an average blood sugar level over a period of months (2–3); cannot be used in the presence of certain haematological conditions (e.g., haemolytic anaemia, blood loss and conditions affecting Hb production such as iron deficiency, malaria, pregnancy)	Ideally <48 mmol/mol
Sodium	Indicator of hydration status and renal function; a raised sodium level may indicate dehydration, worsening renal function, iatrogenic causes (e.g., excessive intravenous fluids)	135–145 mmol/L
Urea	Used to assess renal function; high urea and other markers levels in combination may indicate dehydration and temporarily increased protein intake	2.5–7.1 mmol/L
Calcium and phosphate	Useful in context of refeeding syndrome (alongside potassium, magnesium); calcium is adjusted for albumin level (correct/adjusted levels); can be influenced by renal dysfunction which is responsible for calcium/phosphorus homeostasis	Adjusted Ca 2.0–2.6 mmol/L Phosphate 0.7–1.4 mmol/L
Magnesium	Likely to be low if there are large gastrointestinal losses and can be chronically low in type 2 diabetes and coeliac disease; role in refeeding syndrome whereby rapid depletion can result in cardiac instability	0.7–1.0 mmol/L
Micronutrients	Include vitamin and essential trace elements; these are affected by the acute phase response if inflammation or infection is present and should be measured when CRP is low (ideally < 20)	

CRP, C-reactive protein; *Hb*, haemoglobin.

TABLE 2.9 ■ **Signs and Symptoms Associated with Malabsorption**

Nutrient Component	Sign and Symptoms of Malabsorption
Fats/lipids	Light or 'clay'-coloured stools. Foul or off-smelling stools which are soft or runny. Stool may be difficult to flush or stick to side of the toilet pan (due to high lipid content).
Protein	Dry hair ± hair loss. Oedema caused by loss of proteins and subsequent reduction in maintaining oncotic pressures. Often can be pitting and tissue will form indent when compressed.
Certain sugars (FODMAPS)	Can cause symptoms often clustered as irritable bowel syndrome—abdominal bloating, excessive gas/flatus and diarrhoea.
Micronutrients	Anaemia (micro/macrocytic), malnutrition, skin breakdown, poor tissue/wound repair.

FODMAPS, fermentable oligo-, di-, mono-saccharides and polyols.
Based on from Nikaki K, Gupte GL. Assessment of intestinal malabsorption. *Best Pract Res Clin Gastroenterol.* 2016;30(2):225–235.

and its constituent macronutrients (fats, carbohydrates, proteins), appreciating that these can be further subcategorised (lipids, sugars and amino acids), but also its micronutrients inclusive of vitamins and minerals. Individual constituents can be influenced by the interaction along specific metabolic pathways involving enzymes and cofactors where the aim is to enable vital cellular function and processing to sustain life.

In health and disease there will be a large degree of variation, underpinned by the disease process itself and the host reaction, often termed the 'metabolic response' or 'stress response'.[51] This factors in the role of inflammation, cytokines and catabolic hormonal responses, to name a few, and the subsequent changes to energy expenditure and protein utilisation. It is therefore imperative to have an appreciation of how the 'disease effect' will influence nutritional requirements, enabling a tailored nutritional approach. For example, consider a patient with thermal/burns injuries, known to facilitate the highest metabolic response in critical care.[52] The role of this triggered hypermetabolic state is to support immune response, wound healing and tissue preservation and will therefore demand significantly higher energy (caloric), protein and micronutrient intake compared with baseline requirements. Compare this to a patient with low-grade inflammation often observed in individuals with cardiometabolic disease. Therefore, the nutritional and therapeutic target may aim to modulate the proinflammatory pathways but will not necessitate greater energy and/or protein demands.

When nutrition experts (such as clinical dietitians) determine the energy requirements of an individual, they will consider a wide range of factors in assessing individuals and incorporate this assessment into their nutritional intervention/management. It is beyond the scope of this chapter to explore this in further detail, but examples of dietary assessment in the context of methods used to calculate nutritional requirements are included herein.

Dietary Assessment

An integral part of the nutritional assessment process is to illicit an individual's current or recent dietary intake. This encompasses food sources and fluids consumed over a given period. Assessment of diet can be made against population dietary guidelines, measuring the intake of an individual against an 'ideal' diet which meets the macronutrient and micronutrient requirements of the general population.[53,54] Foods consumed are mapped against minimum servings from each food group recommended to achieve nutritional adequacy. This is a crude measure of dietary quality. The dietary assessment should also provide insights to overall dietary patterns inclusive of meal timings, portion sizing, snacking and other components. These include an awareness of the social setting and environment in which food is consumed, financial factors and any ethnic/cultural/religious dietary practices. Having an appreciation of the aforementioned considerations will help in the process of devising appropriate nutritional and dietary advice. That is, nutrition intervention, if required, can then be targeted toward the specific deficits, foods or eating patterns that may have deleterious effects. Dietary assessment may highlight deficiency or excess, which of course is also dependent on other pathological conditions.

The method of collection of dietary information will limit the ability to directly target specific aspects of dietary intake, where a differing methodology may be preferred in line with target audience or clinical question. There are various ways dietary assessment methods are classified, including categorisation as subjective or objective measures. Subjective measures are most utilised when assessing individual level dietary intake and rely on recall methods such as diet history, 24-hour dietary recalls, food frequency questionnaires and weighed food diaries. Alternative objective measures are less frequently used in clinical practice and sit within the realms of research. These include direct observation over a specified time/study period or duplicate diets whereby a duplicate portion of all food consumed is assessed for nutritional value and therefore mitigates reporting errors or respondent bias. Table 2.10 summarises the commonly recognised dietary assessment methods alongside advantages and disadvantages.[55]

TABLE 2.10 ■ **Applications of Dietary Assessment Outlining Advantages and Disadvantages**

Method of Assessment	Principal Use	Advantages	Disadvantages
Diet history	To identify meal patterns and choice of food groups alongside crude portions. Generalised assessment of dietary balance.	Easy, rapid and inexpensive to use. Can be used as face-to-face interview or phone. Literacy not required.	Limited by skill of interviewer. Requires ability to record, memorise and interpret food sources to meaningful nutritional measures.
24-hour dietary recall	Quick baseline assessment of specific food choices and quantity which can be used for specific analysis.	Easy, rapid and inexpensive to use. Will not influence responders' intake pattern. Literacy not required.	Only reflects past 24-hour, recall bias and is unable to establish dietary or habitual patterns of food intake.
Food frequency questionnaire	Identifies commonly consumed foods and establishes crude dietary patterns over a longer time period.	Easy and flexible to administer. Low respondent burden. Can assess food choices and relate to specific nutrient intake as part of risk assessment (e.g., detecting deficiencies or excessive consumption of particular food groups).	Limited by food contained on specific list. Reporter bias, high degree of literacy/numeracy skills for accurate reporting. Limited information about portion sizing and may not always include cultural/ethnic food choices.

Continued

TABLE 2.10 ■ **Applications of Dietary Assessment Outlining Advantages and Disadvantages—cont'd**

Method of Assessment	Principal Use	Advantages	Disadvantages
Weighed food diary	Detailed record of highlighted specific foods and ingredients with accurate portion representation.	Does not rely on individual recall. Accurate at the point of consumption and specific for weight and quantity.	Requires good compliance, motivation. Time-consuming and labour intensive. May alter eating habits for ease and omit foods eaten out.
Direct observation	Objective measure recording precise intake of food types indicating meal composition. Used to validate dietary assessment of subjective methods or when specific portions, brands and environmental influence are being assessed.	Observation provides objective measures minimising responder bias and reporting errors. Can identify physical and social influence in intake.	Extensive training for observers and highly intensive and expensive. Time limited and difficult to extrapolate whole dietary pattern.
Duplicate diets	Objective measure retaining a duplicate portion of all food and drinks consumed during a study period. Considered global standard method of assessing nutrient intakes in the research setting.	Accurate nutrient intake and portion recording minimising recording bias and reporter error. Does not rely on food composition estimates.	Expensive and intensive input required to collect and report data. High individual burden and reliant on all foods being duplicated.

Modified from Thompson FE, Subar AF. Dietary assessment methodology. Nutrition in the prevention and treatment of disease. Elsevier; 2017:5–48.

Many factors influence the choice of dietary assessment method used in practice, including the purpose of the assessment and the skill set of the observer or individual administering it. Another important consideration is the ability and expertise required to interpret the data collected.

International and national standards may help to guide this interpretation. Guidance is often country or region specific but commonality between recommendations can be observed.[56] Many of these commonly reference proportions of food groups and types to optimise health and specify food types to minimise intake of in view of their adverse health effects. Examples of this include the Eatwell guide in the UK,[53] the Australian Guide to Healthy Eating[57] and the MyPlate guidelines for the United States.[58] By providing a graphical representation, food guides aim to guide individuals in terms of balancing macro- and micronutrient indirectly via providing specific recommendation for each of the food groups. The outlined dietary guidelines help to provide a framework to enable comparisons when analysing a dietary assessment. However, these guidelines are devised to provide information to the general population and should not be used in isolation when interpreting assessments when a known disease pathology is present. Specific disease processes directly influencing nutritional requirements will therefore necessitate a different and more specialist form of analysis and should be undertaken by a health professional with appropriate expertise.

ESTIMATING NUTRITION REQUIREMENTS

As part of the nutritional assessment process, it is important to have an appreciation of an individual's specific energy and protein requirements. This will be influenced by the various clinical factors previously mentioned; notably, variations in energy and protein requirements will occur due to changing clinical status and will be influenced by metabolic stressors. Equally, baseline weight, age and gender will influence these requirements. The aim is that whether a patient is fed via oral, enteral or parenteral nutrition (elaborated in acute and chronic nutrition support), these needs can be met whilst avoiding the complications of over- or underfeeding individuals.[59]

Various methods are used in clinical practice to help establish estimates of energy requirements. In a healthy individual, comparing intake against generic guidelines and reviewing current weight and weight history may be sufficient to suggest that under- or overnutrition exists. However, in illness, the complexity of factors requires further estimation of factors affecting energy requirements.

Indirect calorimetry has been deemed the most accurate measure of energy expenditure[60] and is slowly becoming more readily available, most notably in the critical care setting. The individual is covered by a hood, with the technique measuring inspired and expired gas flows, volumes, and concentrations of O_2 and CO_2 and estimates substrate oxidation. This enables the calculation of an individualised respiratory quotient (CO_2 production/O_2 consumption) and therefore resting energy expenditure.[61] Resting energy expenditure includes any additional stressors the individual is experiencing, and so in this way, it accounts for illness. However, indirect calorimetry is not used routinely in clinical practice, due to the expense and the requirement for technical expertise to operate and maintain the equipment.

More commonly, other indirect methods are used in clinical practice and rely on equations deriving energy requirements through estimating basal metabolic rate (e.g., Henry Equations,[62] Harris-Benedict,[63] Schofield[64] and Mifflin St Jeor[65]equations). These predictive equations are based on regression models from population groups where indirect calorimetry (as a gold standard) was used. A calculated basal metabolic rate considers weight, age and gender and subsequently uses clinical judgement to determine if additional factors are required. These factors relate to metabolic stressors present, diet-induced thermogenesis and levels of physical activity, all of which will influence the total energy/caloric requirement. These predictive equations were developed on healthy populations and therefore, to adjust for illness, require significant clinical judgement. Alternative and more simplified numerical methods are also recommended to estimate resting energy expenditure for clinically stable patients (e.g., using 20–25 kcal/kg when BMI falls between 18.5 and 30 kg/m^2).[59,66] Consensus guidance advocating for the use of this simplified method of kcal/kg (using actual body weight) also requires an additional factor to allow for diet-induced thermogenesis and physical activity. This final value reflects the total energy expenditure and should be utilised in line with the health care professional's clinical judgement. Furthermore, disease-specific factors and guidance should also be considered alongside making appropriate adjustments in the extreme of BMI < 18.5 kg/m^2 and when BMI > 30.0 kg/m^2.

Estimating nutritional requirements also requires determining an appropriate guide to protein intake, thus necessitating the need to consider nitrogen balance. Similarly to energy, protein requirement estimates or calculations will be influenced by the clinical context, disease pathology and also premorbid status. For example, evidence of malnutrition or insufficient intake for a prolonged period may increase protein requirements. The overarching aim is to enable the body to achieve a neutral nitrogen balance, thus matching input for output and accounting for losses from faeces, urine, skin and other exudative losses such as burns, gastrointestinal losses and surgical drains. Individuals in hypermetabolic states will often have significantly higher requirements such that in the initial catabolic phase, it may be near impossible to achieve a positive nitrogen balance, for example, in burns, major trauma or severe sepsis.

In general, in clinical settings, individuals within a BMI range of 18.5–30.0 kg/m^2 will require approximately 1.0–1.5 g of protein/kg per day using actual body weight.[59,66] Protein requirements may be higher in the presence of pressures sores, cancer cachexia and liver disease. Disease-specific guidance will often be utilised by the nutritional specialist/team, and it should be noted that requirements should be adjusted at extremes of BMI < 18.5 kg/m^2 and >30.0 kg/m^2. For example, at the lower end of BMI (<18.5 kg/m^2), an element of depletion can be assumed and thus calculations should aim for the higher end of requirements, perhaps 1.5 g/kg (actual body weight) per day. Conversely, at the upper limits of BMI (>30.0 kg/m^2), utilising 65%–75% of calculated requirements is advocated to avoid excessive protein intake (based on British Dietetic Association guidelines, 2018).

NUTRITION DIAGNOSIS

After a thorough nutritional assessment has been conducted, health care professionals will be able to elicit the key nutritional problems and how these are linked with the global clinical issues. The final component of the assessment process is therefore to develop a nutrition diagnosis which helps to summarise the findings and enables the individual to establish targeted nutritional goals with the associated interventions. This has now become common practice amongst nutritional specialists and dietitians, adopted as a key part of the nutrition care process, and is incorporated in the structured assessments advocated by nutrition and dietetic professional associations worldwide.[28,30] Often this will take the form of a structured sentence describing the specific nutrition/dietetic problem that will be addressed as part of the proposed intervention. The three main components to the formulated 'nutrition diagnosis' can be referenced as the PASS (or PES) statement:

The problem (P): nutrition diagnosis

The aetiology (A): the root cause/s of the nutrition problem (nutrition diagnosis)

The signs and symptoms (SS): evidenced by signs and symptoms indicating that the nutrition problem (nutrition diagnosis) exists

The nutrition diagnosis enables the health care professionals involved in the individual's care to rapidly identify the core nutritional problems and understand what/which interventions have been proposed or implemented to address this. Follow-up and monitoring of the proposed intervention is a key part of the process and should allow for evaluation by utilising goals that are specific, measurable, accurate, reliable, timely (SMART).

SPECIFIC NUTRITION ASSESSMENT TOOLS

The extensive considerations of nutrition assessment described are important in managing the overall care of an individual. Similar to nutrition screening, researchers have developed specific and validated tools to quantify malnutrition and inform further management. Each of the tools use a range of measures, which may include anthropometry, collection of clinical symptoms including appetite and dietary intake, measures of physical capabilities and evidence of muscle wasting and fat loss. As these tools provide a score or ranking for malnutrition, they may also be used to manage progress or regression of nutritional status for an individual, or they may also be used in research as a measure of success of a particular intervention or to determine the association of malnutrition with conditions (medical or social). Tools commonly used across the globe are the Mini Nutritional Assessment (MNA),[67] Subjective Global Assessment (SGA)[68] or the patient-generated SGA (PG-SGA).[69]

The MNA was developed specifically for geriatric populations and therefore the questions are most relevant to ages over 65 years. The MNA provides a malnutrition indicator score where a higher score indicates normal nutritional status, slightly lower scores indicate risk of malnutrition and a lower score indicates that the individual is malnourished. The SGA was initially validated for use in hospital inpatients. The PG-SGA recognises that the health professional may have limited time to complete a full assessment but also that asking individuals to answer questions related to weight history, dietary intake and symptoms empowers them in their own care. This tool was initially developed for use in oncology patients.

WHY IS NUTRITION SCREENING AND ASSESSMENT RELEVANT?

As described, malnutrition is associated with increased morbidity and mortality. Therefore, identifying poor nutritional status allows timely intervention to positively influence health outcomes. The recognition of malnutrition is not new, but its prevalence remains high with various groups calling for continued recognition and action.[70] It is also important to consider the relevance of poor nutritional status on the resources of the health care system. Many countries have funding systems for health care based on the diagnosis of the individuals receiving care in that system. In the simplest example, a medical professional in a primary care setting who sees a patient for a longer appointment due to multiple medical conditions, may be reimbursed more for that visit than for a shorter visit. In the hospital setting, the funding system may be based around the concept of 'diagnostic-related group'. Research has identified that classification of an individual with a diagnosis of malnutrition is predictive of increased costs associated with the care of the patient.[4] It has been estimated that malnutrition costs the UK Health System billions of pounds each year and at least half of that is within the hospital system.[71] A similar European study also identified coding for malnutrition increased the severity of illness score for approximately 40% of patients in the funding model used in Portugal.[72] The additional funding received for each patient was significant and would add to the economic viability of individual centres. Critically, providing supplements to assist in amelioration of malnutrition may reduce costs in the first instance.[71]

References

1. Wilson PW, D'Agostino RB, Sullivan L, Parise H, Kannel WB. Overweight and obesity as determinants of cardiovascular risk: The Framingham experience. *Arch Intern Med.* 2002;162(16):1867–7182.
2. Kruizenga H, van Keeken S, Weijs P, et al. Undernutrition screening survey in 564,063 patients: Patients with a positive undernutrition screening score stay in hospital 1.4 d longer. *Am J Clin Nutr.* 2016;103(4):1026–1032.
3. Schneider SM, Veyres P, Pivot X, et al. Malnutrition is an independent factor associated with nosocomial infections. *Br J Nutr.* 2004;92(1):105–111.
4. Lim SL, Ong KCB, Chan YH, Loke WC, Ferguson M, Daniels L. Malnutrition and its impact on cost of hospitalization, length of stay, readmission and 3-year mortality. *Clin Nutr.* 2011;31(3):345–350.
5. Álvarez-Hernández J, Planas Vila M, León-Sanz M, et al. Prevalence and costs of malnutrition in hospitalized patients; the PREDyCES® Study. *Nutr Hosp.* 2012;27(4):1049–1059.
6. Australian Institute of Health and Welfare. *Impact of Overweight and Obesity as a Risk Factor for Chronic Conditions: Australian Burden of Disease Study.* Australian Burden of Disease Study series no 11. Canberra, Australia: AIHW; 2017.
7. Beck E, Patch C, Milosavljevic M, et al. Implementation of malnutrition screening and assessment by dietitians: malnutrition exists in acute and rehabilitation settings. *Australian Journal of Nutrition and Dietetics.* 2001;58(2):92–97.
8. Ray S, Laur C, Golubic R. Malnutrition in healthcare institutions: A review of the prevalence of undernutrition in hospitals and care homes since 1994 in England. *Clin Nutr.* 2014;33(5):829–835.
9. Guenther PM, Casavale KO, Reedy J, et al. Update of the Healthy Eating Index: HEI-2010. *J Acad Nutr Diet.* 2013;113(4):569–580.
10. Roy R, Hebden L, Rangan A, Allman-Farinelli M. The development, application, and validation of a Healthy Eating Index for Australian Adults (HEIFA-2013). *Nutrition.* 2016;32(4):432–440.
11. Swan WI, Vivanti A, Hakel-Smith NA, et al. Nutrition care process and model update: Toward realizing people-centered care and outcomes management. *J Acad Nutr Diet.* 2017;117(12):2003–2014.

12. Power L, Mullally D, Gibney ER, et al. A review of the validity of malnutrition screening tools used in older adults in community and healthcare settings—A MaNuEL study. *Clin Nutr ESPEN.* 2018;24:1–13.
13. Wallace JI, Schwartz RS, LaCroix AZ, Uhlmann RF, Pearlman RA. Involuntary weight loss in older outpatients: Incidence and clinical significance. *J Am Geriatr Soc.* 1995;43(4):329–337.
14. De Stefani FdC, Pietraroia PS, Fernandes-Silva MM, Faria-Neto J, Baena CP. Observational evidence for unintentional weight loss in all-cause mortality and major cardiovascular events: A systematic review and meta-analysis. *Sci Rep.* 2018;8:15447.
15. Ferguson M, Capra S, Bauer J, Banks M. Development of a valid and reliable malnutrition screening tool for adult acute hospital patients. *Nutrition.* 1999;15:458–464.
16. Elia M., Chairman and Editor. *Screening for Malnutrition: A Multidisciplinary Responsibility. Development and Use of the 'Malnutrition Universal Screening Tool' ('MUST') for Adults.* Malnutrition Advisory Group (MAG), a Standing Committee of BAPEN Redditch. Worcs: BAPEN; 2003.
17. Kaiser MJ, Bauer JM, Ramsch C, et al. Validation of the Mini Nutritional Assessment Short-Form (MNA-SF): A practical tool for identification of nutritional status. *J Nutr Health Aging.* 2009;13(9):782–788.
18. Rubenstein LZ, Harker JO, Salvà A, Guigoz Y, Vellas B. Screening for undernutrition in geriatric practice: developing the Short-Form Mini-Nutritional Assessment (MNA-SF). *J Gerontol A Biol Sci Med Sci.* 2001;56(6):M366–M372.
19. Kondrup J, Rasmussen HH, Hamberg O, Stanga Z. Nutritional risk screening (NRS 2002): A new method based on an analysis of controlled clinical trials. *Clin Nutr.* 2003;22(3):321–336.
20. Morley JE, Malmstrom TK, Miller DK. A simple frailty questionnaire (FRAIL) predicts outcomes in middle aged African Americans. *J Nutr Health Aging.* 2012;16(7):601–608.
21. Hamirudin A, Charlton K, Walton K, et al. Feasibility of implementing routine nutritional screening (MNA-SF) for older adults in Australian general practices: A mixed-methods study. *BMC Fam Pract.* 2014;15:186.
22. van Bokhorst-de van der Schueren MA, Guaitoli PR, Jansma EP, de Vet HC. Nutrition screening tools: does one size fit all? A systematic review of screening tools for the hospital setting. *Clin Nutr.* 2014 Feb;33(1):39-58. doi: 10.1016/j.clnu.2013.04.008. Epub 2013 Apr 19. PMID: 23688831.
23. Castro-Vegaa I, Veses-Martín S, Cantero-Llorca J, Barrios-Marta C, Banuls C, Hernández-Mijares A. Validity, efficacy and reliability of 3 nutritional screening tools regarding the nutritional assessment in different social and health areas. *Med Clin (Engl Ed).* 2018;150(5):185–187.
24. Isenring E, Cross G, Daniels L, Kellet E, Koczwara B. Validity of the malnutrition screening tool as an effective predictor of nutritional risk in oncology outpatients receiving chemotherapy. *Support Care Cancer.* 2006;14(11):1152–1156.
25. Dwyer JT, Gahche JJ, Weiler M, Arensberg M-B. Screening community-living older adults for protein energy malnutrition and frailty: Update and next steps. *J Community Health.* 2020;45(3):640–660.
26. Keller HH, Goy R, Kane S-L. Validity and reliability of SCREEN II (Seniors in the Community: Risk Evaluation for Eating and Nutrition, Version II). *Eur J Clin Nutr.* 2005;59(10):1149–1157.
27. ICDA. International competency standards for dietitian-nutritionists. 2016. Available at: https://www.internationaldietetics.org/Downloads/International-Competency-Standards-for-Dietitian-N.aspx.
28. Lövestam E, Vivanti A, Steiber A, et al. The international nutrition care process and terminology implementation survey: Towards a global evaluation tool to assess individual practitioner implementation in multiple countries and languages. *J Acad Nutr Diet.* 2019;119(2):242–260.
29. Noland D, Raj S. Revised 2019 Standards of practice and standards of professional performance for registered dietitian nutritionists (competent, proficient, and expert) in nutrition in integrative and functional medicine. *J Acad Nutr Diet.* 2019;118(6):1019–1036.
30. Lawrence J, Douglas P, Gandy J. *Model and Process for Nutrition and Dietetic Practice.* John Wiley & Sons, Ltd; 2016. Hoboken, New Jersey, USA.
31. Porter JM, Devine A, Vivanti A, Ferguson M, O'Sullivan TA. Development of a nutrition care process implementation package for hospital dietetic departments. *Nutr Diet.* 2015;72(3):205–212.
32. Aune D, Sen A, Prasad M, Norat T, Janszky I, Tonstad S et al. BMI and all cause mortality: systematic review and non-linear dose-response meta-analysis of 230 cohort studies with 3.74 million deaths among 30.3 million participants *BMJ* 2016; 353 :i2156 doi:10.1136/bmj.i2156

33. WHO Expert Consultation. Appropriate body-mass index for Asian populations and its implications for policy and intervention strategies. *Lancet*. 2004;363(9403):157–163.
34. WHO Expert Committee on Physical Status: the Use and Interpretation of Anthropometry (1993: Geneva, Switzerland) & World Health Organization. (1995).
35. Baioumi AYAA. Comparing measures of obesity: Waist circumference, waist-hip, and waist-height ratios. In: *Nutrition in the Prevention and Treatment of Abdominal Obesity*. 2nd Edn., Chapter 3, Academic Press, New York, USA., ISBN: 978-0-12-816093-0, pp: 29–40.
36. Ashwell M, Gibson S. Waist-to-height ratio as an indicator of early health risk: Simpler and more predictive than using a matrix based on BMI and waist circumference. *BMJ Open*. 2016;6(3).
37. Anwar SAB, Rashid HH, Moslhey GJ. Which is a better marker for overweight: Waist height ratio or waist circumference? *Int J Res Med Sci*. 2019;7(2):462.
38. Schneider HJ, Friedrich N, Klotsche J, et al. The predictive value of different measures of obesity for incident cardiovascular events and mortality. *J Clin Endocrinol Metab*. 2010;95(4):1777–1785.
39. Mendenhall CL, Anderson S, Weesner RE, Goldberg SJ, Crolic KA. Protein-calorie malnutrition associated with alcoholic hepatitis: Veterans Administration cooperative study group on alcoholic hepatitis. *Am J Med*. 1984;76(2):211–222.
40. Madden AM, Smith S. Body composition and morphological assessment of nutritional status in adults: A review of anthropometric variables. *J Hum Nutr Diet*. 2016;29(1):7–25.
41. Player EL, Morris P, Thomas T, et al. Bioelectrical impedance analysis (BIA)-derived phase angle (PA) is a practical aid to nutritional assessment in hospital in-patients. *Clin Nutr*. 2019;38(4):1700–1706.
42. Kyle UG, Soundar EP, Genton L, Pichard C. Can phase angle determined by bioelectrical impedance analysis assess nutritional risk? A comparison between healthy and hospitalized subjects. *Clin Nutr*. 2012;31(6):875–881.
43. Scott JM, Martin DS, Ploutz-Snyder R, et al. Panoramic ultrasound: a novel and valid tool for monitoring change in muscle mass. *J Cachexia Sarcopenia Muscle*. 2017;8(3):475–481.
44. Shankar P, Boylan M, Sriram K. Micronutrient deficiencies after bariatric surgery. *Nutrition*. 2010;26:1031–1037.
45. Matarese LE. Nutrition and fluid optimization for patients with short bowel syndrome. *JPEN J Parenteral Enteral Nutr*. 2013;37(2):161–170.
46. Tappenden KA. Pathophysiology of short bowel syndrome: considerations of resected and residual anatomy. *JPEN J Parenteral Enteral Nutr*. 2014;38:14S–122S.
47. Mete B, Pehlivan E, Gülbaş G, Günen H. Prevalence of malnutrition in COPD and its relationship with the parameters related to disease severit. *Int J COPD*. 2018;13:3307–3312.
48. Posovszky C. Congenital intestinal diarrhoeal diseases: A diagnostic and therapeutic challenge. *Baillieres Best Pract Res Clin Gastroenterol*. 2016;30(2):187–211.
49. Van der Heide F. Acquired causes of intestinal malabsorption. *Baillieres Best Pract Res Clin Gastroenterol*. 2016;30(2):213–224.
50. Nikaki K, Gupte GL. Assessment of intestinal malabsorption. *Baillieres Best Pract Res Clin Gastroenterol*. 2016;30(2):225–235.
51. Tappy LP. *The Stress Response of Critical Illness: Metabolic and Hormonal Aspects*. Springer International Publishing; 2016.
52. Porter C, Tompkins RG, Finnerty CC, Sidossis LS, Suman OE, Herndon DN. The metabolic stress response to burn trauma: Current understanding and therapies. *Lancet*. 2016;388(10052):1417–1426.
53. Public Health England. A Quick Guide to The Government's Healthy Eating Recommendations. 2018. Available at https://assets.publishing.service.gov.uk/government/uploads/system/uploads/attachment_data/file/742746/A_quick_guide_to_govt_healthy_eating_update.pdf.
54. Scientific Advisory Committee on Nutrition. Dietary Reference Values for Energy; 2011. ISBN: 9780108511370. Printed in the UK by The Stationery Office Limited. ID 2485597 04/12 15707 19585. Available at: https://www.gov.uk/government/publications/sacn-dietary-reference-values-for-energy.
55. Thompson FE, Subar AF. *Dietary Assessment Methodology. Nutrition in the Prevention and Treatment of Disease*. Elsevier; 2017:5–48. https://www.sciencedirect.com/book/9780128029282/nutrition-in-the-prevention-and-treatment-of-disease#book-info.
56. Herforth A, Arimond M, Álvarez-Sánchez C, Coates J, Christianson K, Muehlhoff E. Global review of food-based dietary guidelines. *Adv Nutr*. 2019;10(4):590–605.

57. National Health and Medical Research Council. Australian guide to healthy eating. 2015. Available at: https://www.eatforhealth.gov.au/guidelines/australian-guide-healthy-eating.
58. U.S. Department of Health and Human Services and U.S. Department of Agriculture. 2015–2020 Dietary Guidelines for Americans. 8th Edition. December 2015. Available at: https://health.gov/sites/default/files/2019-10/DGA_Recommendations-At-A-Glance.pdf.
59. National Collaborating Centre for Acute Care (UK). Nutrition Support for Adults: Oral Nutrition Support, Enteral Tube Feeding and Parenteral Nutrition. London: National Collaborating Centre for Acute Care (UK); 2006 Feb. PMID: 21309138.
60. Zusman O, Kagan I, Bendavid I, Theilla M, Cohen J, Singer P. Predictive equations versus measured energy expenditure by indirect calorimetry: A retrospective validation. *Clin Nutr.* 2019;38(3):1206–1210.
61. Oshima T, Berger MM, De Waele E, et al. Indirect calorimetry in nutritional therapy. A position paper by the ICALIC study group. *Clin Nutr.* 2017;36:651–662.
62. Henry C. Basal metabolic rate studies in humans: measurement and development of new equations. *Public Health Nutr.* 2005;8(7a):1133–1152.
63. Harris JA, Benedict FG. *A Biometric Study of Basal Metabolism in Man.* Washington, DC: 1919.
64. Schofield WN. Predicting basal metabolic rate, new standards and review of previous work. *Hum Nutr Clin Nutr.* 1985;39:5–41.
65. Mifflin MD, St Jeor ST, Hill LA, Scott BJ, Daugherty SA, Koh YO. A new predictive equation for resting energy expenditure in healthy individuals. *Am J Clin Nutr.* 1990;51(2):241–247.
66. McClave SA, Taylor BE, Martindale RG, et al. Guidelines for the provision and assessment of nutrition support therapy in the adult critically ill patient: Society of Critical Care Medicine (SCCM) and American Society for Parenteral and Enteral Nutrition (ASPEN). *JPEN J Parenter Enteral Nutr.* 2016;40(2):159–211.
67. Vellas B, Villars H, Abellan G, et al. Overview of the MNA—Its history and challenges. *Journal of Nutrition, Health and Aging.* 2006;10(6):456–465.
68. Detsky AS, McLaughlin JR, Baker JP, et al. What is subjective global assessment of nutritional status? *JPEN J Parenter Enteral Nutr.* 1987;11(1).8–13.
69. Ottery FD. Definition of standardized nutritional assessment and interventional pathways in oncology. *Nutrition.* 1996;12:S15–S19.
70. Tappenden KA, Quatrara B, Parkhurst ML, Malone AM, Fanjiang G, Ziegler TR. Critical role of nutrition in improving quality of care: An interdisciplinary call to action to address adult hospital malnutrition. *J Acad Nutr Diet.* 2013;113(9):1219–1237.
71. Russell CA. The impact of malnutrition on healthcare costs and economic considerations for the use of oral nutritional supplements. *Clinical Nutrition Supplements.* 2007;2(1):25–32.
72. Campos Fernandes A, Pessoa A, Antónia Vigário M, Jager-Wittenaar H, Pinho J. Does malnutrition influence hospital reimbursement? A call for malnutrition diagnosis and coding. *Nutrition.* 2020;74(6):110750, ISSN 0899-9007, https://doi.org/10.1016/j.nut.2020.110750.

CHAPTER 3

Basic Principles of Nutritional Care Pathways

Kathy Martyn ■ Celia Laur ■ Lauren Ball

LEARNING POINTS

By the end of this chapter, you should be able to:

- Identify and critique the principles and key components of nutrition care pathways
- Demonstrate awareness of the roles and responsibilities of multidisciplinary team members of nutrition care pathways
- Identify the optimal time for a nutrition care pathway to commence
- Describe how nutrition care pathways support appropriate care and clinical judgement, including consideration of the social determinants of health
- Demonstrate awareness of the benefits of pathways as guides to help in the transfer of care within and between primary, secondary and tertiary care.

CASE STUDY 3.1 Elderly Living in a Rural Community

Christine is 86 years of age, widowed and living alone in a rural community. She presented at her local community hospital having driven there with her 'heart that was racing'. An electrocardiogram revealed she had atrial fibrillation, and Christine was asked to attend the accident and emergency department at the local general hospital, about 45 minutes away.

Previous medical history: hysterectomy 1989; hypercholesterolaemia; bilateral knee replacements 2005; revision of right knee 2018

On admission, she was hypotensive, with blood pressure 98/67 and pulse 136, and dehydrated with bilateral swelling of both ankles up to the midcalf region. A social assessment indicated that she was a well-educated, articulate, 86-year-old widow, living alone with two dogs in a rural location. She has four children, but only two live nearby. She described her children as regularly seeing her, with her youngest son living less than a mile away. She had no additional care at home, managing to shop and cook her meals, and she was independent in her daily activities. On the Rockwood frailty index, she scored 4. Her treatment while in hospital focused on her admitting diagnosis of atrial fibrillation, and she was commenced on bisoprolol 2.5 mg BD (twice daily), rivaroxaban 20 mg, furosemide 20 mg and discharged home after 24 hours in the hospital, with a follow-up appointment for an echocardiogram. The nursing staff had noted that she appeared to be unkempt; she had admitted to finding it challenging to wash.

Three weeks later, Christine's family contacted her family doctor as they were concerned about Christine's physical well-being. They felt that she was increasingly drowsy, confused and disorientated. Both her legs were red, swollen and oozing fluid. The family members were taking turns sleeping at her house as they were concerned about her ability to care for herself and to ensure her safety. They had also arranged for carers to attend each day to ensure she had her medications and to help with personal hygiene.

Following an appointment with the doctor, furosemide was increased to 40 mg, and she was prescribed a 7-day course of erythromycin 250 mg QDS (four times daily) for cellulitis.

Drug doses as per British National Formulary

CASE STUDY 3.1 Elderly Living in a Rural Community—(Continued)

Seven weeks later, the family contacted the doctor, expressing their concerns that oedema had worsened. The general practitioner then referred her to the ambulatory emergency care (AEC) pathway, and she was admitted into the emergency department with bilateral oedema in the lower limbs extending to the sacrum and breathlessness. Her weight in the hospital was 71 kg, and the consultant considered that about 10 kg of this was fluid. In the hospital, she was given intravenous furosemide before being discharged 12 hours later. Her medications were adjusted to include spironolactone 2.5 mg BD and furosemide 80 mg BD. An appointment was made for the community frailty clinic for review 4 weeks later.

Later, Christine's condition further deteriorated, and she was confused and disorientated and falling asleep. The family were concerned that she was not eating or drinking enough. They had organised private care twice daily to ensure she had her medications and some help. They described their mother as being difficult to support as she was adamant that she could continue to care for herself independently. She was taken to her general practitioner, and following a blood test that revealed she had acute kidney failure due to severe dehydration, she was admitted to AEC for treatment.

On admission to AEC, she received 2 L Hartman's and her medications adjusted. Her furosemide was decreased to 40 mg BD. Her Rockwood frailty score was 5, and she was transferred to the frailty unit. On the frailty unit, she was screened using the Malnutrition Universal Screening Tool (MUST), scoring 1 (medium risk—observe). It was noted in the medical and nursing records that she had difficulties caring for herself and seemed forgetful of time and place. A dementia screen was completed and identified mild cognitive impairment. She showed little interest in caring for herself and needed prompting to wash and dress. Her appetite was good but only ate if food and fluids were presented to her.

She was discharged to her home with no referral for community services. The family remained concerned as their mother needed constant care to ensure she had her medications and was able to meet her hygiene needs, eat and drink regularly and remain safe. They contacted the general practitioner, and a visit by the district nursing team was arranged. Four days following her discharge, she was admitted into a long-term care facility for continuing care.

CASE STUDY 3.2 Younger Individual with Cystic Fibrosis and Transfer of Care

Cystic fibrosis (CF) is a genetic condition affecting more than 70,000 individuals worldwide, with approximately 1,000 new cases of CF diagnosed each year.[1] More than 75% of people with CF are diagnosed by age 2, and more than half of the CF population is age 18 or older.

Diet to support the treatment of CF is essential, and throughout the world, specialist dietitians are involved in supporting individuals and their families. Specialist dietetic support commences from diagnosis, and focuses on ensuring adequate dietary intake to support growth and promote positive outcomes, minimising exacerbations of the condition. Nutritional management is based on eating an energy-dense diet and optimising nutrient intake.[2] Many children will also be prescribed replacement pancreatic enzymes.

Theo has recently been transferred from paediatric to adult services. He had had routine 6-month appointments and had a close relationship with his paediatric dietitian whom he had known since he was 5 years of age. In recent years he had found the constant need to be thinking about his condition difficult and had missed the last appointment at the hospital. He was starting university in the autumn, moving to a town some distance from his home, and was looking forward to being 'normal'. He had received notification about his new consultant and had been requested to contact the clinic to arrange an appointment. He had not made contact, and every time his mother mentioned his condition, he had said he would do it later.

NOTE: Both case studies are referred to and discussed further in relation to principles covered over the course of this chapter.

Overview and Introduction

Nutrition is well recognised as a central component of healthy living, supporting healthy bodily functions such as moving and sleeping. Despite some diet fads changing over time, the scientific literature is clear that we need the right amounts of macronutrients and micronutrients to help us to live healthier and better.[3]

Drug doses as per British National Formulary

NUTRITION CARE IS EVERYONE'S RESPONSIBILITY

Health care works best when it is a collaborative process focused on patients' health. For nutrition, the optimum process would be that *everyone* involved in patients' care encourages *every person* they care for to eat well, *every time* they interact as described in 'Making Every Contact Count' by the National Institute of Health and Care Excellence in the UK.[76] As an example, family doctors are usually the first interaction patients have with the health care system. Imagine if *all* interactions between patients and family doctors included a check-in about whether or not patients are eating well, as well as reminders about how foods can affect health outcomes, ultimately referring to health professionals who can go into depth with our specific dietary needs (such as a registered dietitian). These actions may seem small, but they help reorient care systems to support optimum nutrition.

Now imagine nurses in a hospital who provide ongoing care to patients on their ward. If the nurses recognise the importance of diet and nutrition in the patients' care and recovery, they are more likely to help them order their meals, open food containers and inquire about their appetite and satisfaction. It is likely that patients would then be more likely to eat well and improve their physical and emotional health, aiding their recovery and eventual discharge. This support could also come from a dietitian, a health care assistant, or a registered volunteer. Making nutrition everyone's business and ensuring everyone works together makes a difference.

These are two simple examples, but they raise an important point. Regardless of our background or role, all health professionals, in fact, all people in the health system, have a role to play in supporting patients to eat well. In the nurse example, there would have been workers in the kitchen preparing the food, using a menu designed by a dietitian. The patient may be on a specialised diet supervised by a health care team. Thus, multiple people influence a person's dietary intake.

This is the fundamental basis of a nutrition care pathway—a range of people have input with a shared vision to promote good nutrition.

NUTRITION CARE PATHWAYS

Using standardised processes can help health professionals know when to provide additional or specialised support to individual patients. This standardisation is where nutrition care pathways have a role. Nutrition care pathways provide specific steps and processes with the aim to provide patients with optimal care based on the available resources, while allowing for clinical judgement.

Nutrition care pathways can take several forms. They can be general recommendations at all levels of care, or they can specify the ideal 'route' that individual patients are recommended to travel in that health care setting, based on their conditions and the options available in their context. These pathways advocate for efficiency, while still encouraging clinical judgement and flexibility to adapt to the local context and available resources.[4,5] For example, a pathway may need to be adapted based on the availability of a dietitian. In areas without access to a dietitian or nutrition professionals, pathways should provide potential directions, while still advocating for the inclusion of the specialised resource of a dietitian.

Nutrition care pathways can support effective nutrition management, minimising the impact of malnutrition and supporting recovery as care is transferred between care settings.[6] In the UK, guidance on nutritional screening in primary care, the first step in a nutritional care pathway, is linked to the 75 and over annual health check[7] and also in guidance on screening for malnutrition.[6] However, each of these is a stand-alone policy, and effectiveness is greatest when integrated into formalised nutrition care pathways.[8]

ROLES OF HEALTH PROFESSIONALS

The use of a nutrition care pathway can enable health care professionals to identify and monitor a patient's condition earlier to ensure that adequate, nourishing food and fluids are being provided. When used within a multiprofessional team, it can ensure that during the patients' journey between primary and secondary care, their nutritional needs are not forgotten.

Primary care professionals are often the first point of contact and thus the first opportunity to initiate a nutrition care pathway. This health care touch point is either part of the health facility or within the homes of the people they meet. In line with government recommendations, this point of contact provides opportunities for nutritional screening using a validated tool, as discussed in the previous chapter. Working in conjunction with the general practitioner[6,9] and commencing a nutritional care pathway will then alert other health and social professionals to the nutrition needs of the individual and may trigger onward referral.

As health care systems develop, an increasing number of other health care professionals can provide initial nutrition screening and presumptive assessment at that first point of contact. Frontline staff engaging in primary care assessments and consultations include, for example, pharmacists,[10] paramedic practitioners[11] and physiotherapists.[12] Although these assessments can occur in formal care settings or an individual's home, they can also occur in clinics, pharmacies, supermarkets, leisure centres, and other locations. Utilising a nutritional care pathway, with a validated nutrition screening tool integrated into the professional assessment, can identify early indicators of malnutrition. These health professionals can also play a role in other points within the pathway, such as watching for and flagging the nutrition risk factors mentioned herein.

EXAMPLES

One example of a nutrition care pathway is the Integrated Nutrition Pathway for Acute Care (INPAC) developed in Canada to address hospital malnutrition[13,14] (Fig. 3.1). INPAC was designed to facilitate appropriate nutrition care for all patients including screening, standardised assessment, monitoring of food intake and mealtime barriers, through to discharge planning.[13,14] Fig. 3.1 shows that all patients identified as being at risk of malnutrition during the nutrition screening at admission are recommended to be assessed by a dietitian or another designated health professional and then referred for advanced nutrition care or a comprehensive nutrition assessment before discharge. If this pathway is followed as suggested, no patient should miss out on support to eat well if they need it. All elements of the pathway support prevention, detection, monitoring and communication of malnutrition in hospitals.

A similar model for managing malnutrition is also used in Australia, called the Systematised, Interdisciplinary Malnutrition Pathway for Implementation and Evaluation in hospitals (SIMPLE).[15] Another, Enhanced Recovery After Surgery (ERAS), is designed to achieve early recovery for patients undergoing major surgery and includes a significant nutrition component. ERAS has been shown to decrease the amount of time needed to stay in hospital after surgery and to reduce complications.[16]

A hospital nutrition care pathway typically goes to the point of discharge when a patient returns to the community. At this point, other guides could be used, for example, the 'Guide to Managing Adult Malnutrition in the Community' developed by a multiprofessional consensus panel of UK organisations including the British Dietetics Association. This guide aims to support the implementation of National Institute for Health and Clinical Excellence guidelines and assist health care professionals in optimising patient outcomes through good nutritional care. It focuses on a few key areas, including a pathway for oral nutritional supplements.[17]

In the community, there are more potential options for health care touch points, making the pathways more diverse. Guidance from the UK recognises the importance of multiprofessional

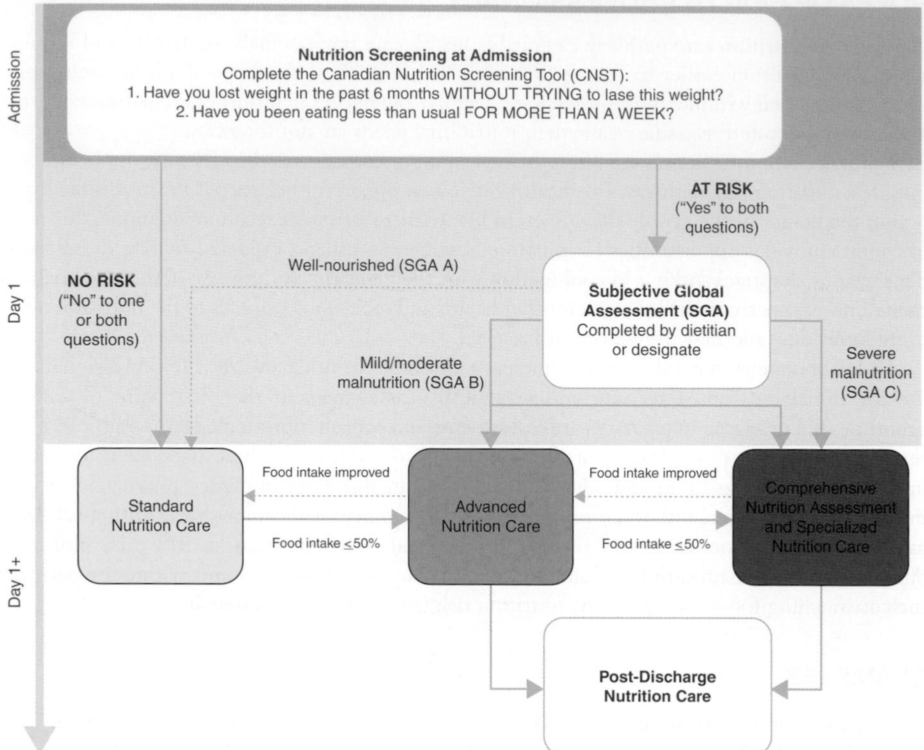

Fig. 3.1 From the Integrated Nutrition Pathway for Acute Care (INPAC). (Used with permission from the authors of Keller et al. 2018.

teams working across health and social care to develop integrated pathways. Within these pathways, it is important to recognise the needs of diverse populations, and using interprofessional working can ensure that those who are most vulnerable are identified. For example, older people present unique challenges due to the combination of ageing, comorbidities and polypharmacy, as mentioned in Case Study 3.1.

Pathways in Action

The effectiveness of nutritional care pathways is evident when viewed alongside the experiences of people in their journey between primary, secondary and tertiary care settings. A common feature at the beginning of a care pathway is the timing of the first nutritional screening or assessment process. In England, National Institute for Health and Clinical Excellence guidance states that a patient's initial nutrition assessment should be completed at the first point of contact in primary care and within 24 hours of admission in secondary care.[18] The earlier the assessment is completed, the more likely that planned nutritional care will be used.

Case Study 3.1 illustrates a typical trajectory for an older adult having multiple interactions with the health care system. This is a real case, and unfortunately, although there are many opportunities for nutrition care and major triggers, no nutritional care pathways were used. Read through the case and think of opportunities for nutrition care pathways and other interventions.

In the case, Christine had had little contact with her primary care service. She had received her annual flu vaccination and cholesterol testing but had not attended routine preventative health checks. Prior to the family's decision for Christine to leave her own home and move into a nursing home, there were several visits to her general practitioner and two admissions into hospital, each of which provide an opportunity for nutritional screening and the commencement of a nutritional care pathway.

As populations age, preventative health strategies, including screening for nutrition risk, frailty, and cognitive decline, continue to be beneficial. Governments across the world are considering how they can support their ageing population to age well and live independently.[19,20]

EARLY NUTRITION RISK SCREENING—HOSPITAL ADMISSION

Emergency departments are often fast-paced and busy. UK government standards for emergency treatment of older people recommend that ambulatory emergency care (AEC) is provided to avoid unnecessary admission into hospital.[21]AEC pathways are common across the world,[22] and in the UK, they form part of the acute care toolkit that includes short stays in a medical assessment unit with a focus on providing high-quality diagnostics and treatment with resource management. AEC includes diagnosis, observation, treatment and rehabilitation not provided within the traditional hospital bed base or within outpatient services.[23] These pathways are considered to be important in the assessment and management of frail, older patients as part of a pathway with links to services in primary care, the community, and local authorities. The aim is to offer a rapid assessment with coordinated access to services to avoid unnecessary admission into hospital.[24] Although there is some variation in how AEC is designed, the pathway provides an opportunity for nutritional screening, and if required, appropriate referral to community dietetic services.

In Case Study 3.1, Christine's first admission into the hospital was an opportunity for nutritional screening, using a validated screening tool, such as the Mini Nutritional Assessment-Short Form.[25] As approximately one in three patients are malnourished at admission to hospital,[26–29] screening at admission can trigger nutrition care pathways such as INPAC or SIMPLE that support patient care. This is particularly important in older adults, as identification of malnutrition at the earliest opportunity requires a coordinated, multiprofessional approach that brings together nutrition and geriatric screening tools with a good medical history, and both clinical and subjective evaluations.[30–32]

Ideally, nutrition risk screening and malnutrition assessments completed in the hospital should be shared with the primary care provider as part of an integrated care pathway.[33–35]

EARLY NUTRITION RISK SCREENING—PRIMARY CARE

In Case Study 3.1, Christine's visits to her family doctor were also opportunities for nutrition screening and to start nutrition care pathways designed to provide support in the community. Prevalence of nutrition risk in community-dwelling older people is also high, with estimates ranging from 30%–50%,[36] yet in Australia, less than one-third of patients ever recall speaking with a primary care provider about nutrition.[37] When detected early, the adverse effects can be avoided or improved by providing individualised nutrition care[38] or community food-based services[39] such as a community dietitian or third sector resources such as the 'Food for Life' project that supports older adults in the UK.[40] Malnutrition prevention needs to start early, and primary care is one option for this screening.[41,42]

NUTRITIONAL FACTORS TO CONSIDER

Recognising nutrition risk triggers is important and can be overlooked during acute admissions into the hospital where the focus is on treating the underlying disease, or during primary care, where visits typically focused on one symptom. It is at this stage that the multiprofessional team and interdisciplinary working can be most effective in identifying health and social care needs that could impact on recovery and reduce the readmission into secondary care. Exploring Christine's changing physical health, and the concerns raised by the family, provided opportunities to have conversations about care at home, including her ability to shop, cook and have regular meals. Some factors to consider in Case Study 3.1 include:

MUST score: Although a MUST score was taken for Christine, no actions were taken on the score of 1 (medium risk—observe). This score indicated the need to continue to monitor food and fluid intake, with a planned community review.[43]

Living situation: Those who live alone, are older, and have low social participation, disability, depression, or poor oral health have an increased likelihood of developing malnutrition.[36] Losing a partner and being alone can impact on nutritional status as everyday eating practice and dietary patterns change.[44]

Frailty: Frailty is a medical syndrome with multiple causes and contributors that is characterised by diminished strength and endurance and reduced physiological function that increases an individual's vulnerability, reflected in increasing dependency and/or death.[45] There is a strong connection between malnutrition and frailty,[46] indicating the importance of including frailty measures, such as the Rockwood Frailty tool (index).[47] Studies have identified how the inclusion of malnutrition screening and early dietetic involvement may reverse frailty and reduce readmission with more favourable long-term outcomes.[48]

Dehydration: Many older people in the community are underhydrated with diminished appetites.[49,50] Also, the intracellular water content in lean tissue has been related to muscle strength, functional capacity and frailty risk.[51] As such, recognising early signs of dehydration and planning support in community-dwelling older people, through the use of nutritional screening tools such as the Mini-Nutritional Assessment, is essential to reduce the risks of deteriorating independence and increased risk of admission into hospital.

Family concerns regarding eating and drinking: Family and carers are often best positioned to recognise changes to physical and mental well-being. Listening to their concerns, and those of the patient, can indicate subtle changes that, alongside a comprehensive assessment, can identify risk factors for developing malnutrition in the future.[52] Food and fluid consumption are closely linked, and with age, thirst and hunger signals can be lessened.

Noticing deterioration: Deteriorating physical health indicates that treatment and management of underlying conditions is not effective, necessitating a review of the treatment plan, and as in Christine's case, changes to medication. Older people admitted with cardiac conditions are at greater risk of functional decline following discharge, as often care is focused on the admitting condition with little consideration of functional needs.[53,54] Also, comorbidity and polypharmacy are common in older people and contribute to increased vulnerability and frailty. The high symptom burden, alongside medical complications, can lead to impaired physical function that impacts daily lives, including mobility, independence, self-sufficiency and social relations.[55] Comprehensive history taking, coupled with listening to the concerns of the family, can identify changes to dietary intake and self-care abilities that trigger a referral to primary care services. The World Health Organization recommends shifting from disease-driven attention models toward a personalised, integrated and continuous care aimed at the maintenance and enhancement of functional capacities.[56] Nutritional care as part of an integrated model of care can identify those most at risk of malnutrition and sarcopenia at an early stage to support individuals to maintain their independence and improve health outcomes.

Malnutrition is also a risk factor for cognitive frailty.[57] In Case Study 3.1, there was a gradual decline in cognitive function identified by both the family and health care professionals. Research has also indicated that nutrition can impact on vascular risk factors that are associated with dementia decline in those with cognitive frailty.[58]

Acute infection—cellulitis in the lower leg: Older people with long-term conditions and changing health status are at greater risk of infection when coupled with malnutrition and sarcopenia. Also, deficiency in micronutrients, such as vitamin D, is more common in older adults and is associated with impaired immune response.[59,60] Infections in older people often mark a deterioration in overall health as with age, there is a reduction in physiological, psychological and sociological resilience to acute events.[61,62] Infections are known to have a significant impact on nutritional needs through altered metabolism.[63] Cellulitis increases the risk of sepsis and as such is a trigger for further nutritional assessment.[64,65]

Other social demographic factors: Although we have limited sociodemographic information about Christine, it is known that diets low in energy and protein, the use of dentures and chewing difficulty and living alone are associated with increased risk of malnutrition in adults over 60 years.[66,67] Other sociodemographic characteristics associated with this increased risk include female sex, unmarried, low education level, food insecurity, unemployment, low income (<125% poverty), lifestyle choices including smoking and less physical activity.[66,68]

TRANSITION OF CARE BETWEEN SETTINGS AND MEDICAL SPECIALITIES

Transition in health care can occur many times, such as between treatment and rehabilitation, between therapeutic care and palliative care, and between medical specialities. In Case Study 3.2, the patient was moving from paediatric care to adult care, at a time when he was also demonstrating his emerging independence as a young adult. When transferring care, the importance of communication and collaborative working, ensuring people continue to be supported and to avoid repetition in assessment processes, is essential.[69] Instigating a nutritional care pathway can contribute to this smooth transition.

At times of transition, people can be more vulnerable, increasing the risk of not managing their health or worsening nutritional status. In the discharge and transfer of care between setting and medical specialities, individuals can become lost in the system or feel unable to participate in the decisions being made. Poor planning at this stage can lead to poor outcomes and increased risk of early readmission.[70–73] It is recommended that discharge planning from secondary to primary care begins at the point of admission.[74] Many people on discharge from secondary care will return to their normal lives and require little input from health or social care professionals. However, others will require complex care packages and input from many different professionals. When nutrition is part of the underlying therapeutic treatment, for example, as in diabetes mellitus, the appropriate referral to community diabetic teams is essential. For others undergoing rehabilitation or palliative care, the importance of nutrition as part of an integrated care pathway can improve outcomes.[75]

OPPORTUNITIES FOR INSTIGATING A NUTRITIONAL CARE PATHWAY

As people seek treatment and support, there are many opportunities for instigating a nutritional care pathway. At the differing touch points when people encounter health and social care professionals, recognising the role of food and nutrition in public health and social outcomes, alongside its role in addressing malnutrition and managing long-term conditions, can ensure a holistic approach to support.[76,77]

Conclusion

- Use of nutrition care pathways, when adapted to the local context and used along with clinical judgement, can lead to more appropriate care for patients, particularly for older adults.
- Using a multidisciplinary approach within nutrition care pathways can facilitate appropriate care.
- Nutrition care pathways are particularly important during transitions of care, when communication is often difficult and patients are also undergoing transitions in their own lives.

References

1. Cystic Fibrosis Foundation. About Cystic Fibrosis. 2020. Available at: https://www.cff.org/What-is-CF/About-Cystic-Fibrosis/. Accessed June 15, 2020.
2. National Institutes for Health and Care Excellence. Cystic fibrosis: diagnosis and management [NG78]. Guidelines. October 2017. Published by National Institutes for Health and Care Excellence (NICE) https://www.nice.org.uk/guidance/ng78
3. World Health Organization. Nutrition. 2019. Available at: https://www.who.int/westernpacific/about/how-we-work/programmes/nutrition. Accessed June 13, 2020.
4. Rotter T, Kinsman L, Machotta A, et al. Clinical pathways for primary care: Effects on professional practice, patient outcomes, and costs (protocol). *Cochrane Collab*. 2013(8).
5. Kinsman L, Rotter T, James E, Snow P, Willis J. What is a clinical pathway? Development of a definition to inform the debate. *BMC Med*. 2010:8.
6. National Institute for Health and Care Excellence. Nutrition support in adults. 2012. Published by National Institutes for Health and Care Excellence (NICE) https://www.nice.org.uk/guidance/qs24
7. Department of Health Social Services and Public Safety. *Service Framework for Older People*. Belfast; 2013. Social Care Institute for Excellence.
8. Bracher M, Steward K, Wallis K, May CR, Aburrow A, Murphy J. Implementing professional behaviour change in teams under pressure: Results from phase one of a prospective process evaluation (the Implementing Nutrition Screening in Community Care for Older People (INSCCOPe) project). *BMJ Open*. 2019;9(8).
9. Hamirudin AH, Charlton K, Walton K, et al. Feasibility of implementing routine nutritional screening for older adults in Australian general practices: A mixed-methods study. *BMC Fam Pract*. 2014;15(1).
10. Stuhec M, Gorenc K, Zelko E. Evaluation of a collaborative care approach between general practitioners and clinical pharmacists in primary care community settings in elderly patients on polypharmacy in Slovenia: A cohort retrospective study reveals positive evidence for implementation. *BMC Health Serv Res*. 2019;19(1):118.
11. McManamny T, Jennings PA, Boyd L, Sheen J, Lowthian JA. Paramedic involvement in health education within metropolitan, rural and remote Australia: A narrative review of the literature. *Aust Health Rev*. 2019;44(1):114–120.
12. Bornhöft L, Thorn J, Svensson M, Nordeman L, Eggertsen R, Larsson MEH. More cost-effective management of patients with musculoskeletal disorders in primary care after direct triaging to physiotherapists for initial assessment compared to initial general practitioner assessment. *BMC Musculoskelet Disord*. 2019;20(1).
13. Keller H, Laur C, Atkins M, et al. Update on the Integrated Nutrition Pathway for Acute Care (INPAC): Post implementation tailoring and toolkit to support practice improvements. *Nutr J*. 2018;17(1):2.
14. Keller H, McCullough J, Davidson B, et al. The Integrated Nutrition Pathway for Acute Care (INPAC): Building consensus with a modified Delphi. *Nutr J*. 2015;14(63).
15. Bell J, Young A, Hill J, et al. Rationale and developmental methodology for the SIMPLE approach: A systematised, interdisciplinary malnutrition pathway for implementation and evaluation in hospitals. *Nutr Diet*. 2018;75(2):226–234.
16. Greco M, Capretti G, Beretta L, Gemma M, Pecorelli N, Braga M. Enhanced recovery program in colorectal surgery: A meta-analysis of randomized controlled trials. *World J Surg*. 2014;38(6):1531–1541.
17. Holdoway A, Anderson L, McGregor I, et al. *A Guide to Managing Adult Malnutrition in the Community*. London; 2017. https://www.malnutritionpathway.co.uk/
18. National Institute for Health and Care Excellence. Nutrition support for adults: oral nutrition support, enteral tube feeding and parenteral nutrition. https://www.nice.org.uk/guidance/cg32. NICE Guide. 2017;CG32.
19. Government Office for Science. https://assets.publishing.service.gov.uk/government/uploads/system/uploads/attachment_data/file/816458/future-of-an-ageing-population.pdf *Future of an Ageing Population*. London; 2016.
20. United Nations Department of Economic and Social Affairs Population Division. World Population Ageing 2019: Highlights. 2019. United Nations. https://www.un.org/en/development/desa/population/publications/pdf/ageing/WorldPopulationAgeing2019-Report.pdf

21. Royal College of Physicians. Acute care toolkit 3: Acute medical care for frail older people. 2015. Available at: https://www.rcplondon.ac.uk/guidelines-policy/acute-care-toolkit-3-acute-medical-care-frail-older-people. Accessed June 15, 2020.
22. Conley J, O'Brien CW, Leff BA, Bolen S, Zulman D. Alternative strategies to inpatient hospitalization for acute medical conditions: A systematic review. *JAMA Intern Med.* 2016;176(11):1693–1702.
23. Ward D, Potter J, Ingham J, Percival F, Bell D. Acute medical care. The right person, in the right setting—first time: How does practice match the report recommendations? *Clin Med J R Coll Physicians London.* 2009;9(6):553–556.
24. Blunt I. Focus on preventable admissions: Trends in emergency admissions for ambulatory care sensitive conditions, 2001 to 2013. Research report. Nuffield Trust and Health Foundation; 2013. The Health Foundation and the Nuffield Trust. https://www.nuffieldtrust.org.uk/files/2018-10/qualitywatch-preventable-admissions.pdf
25. Power L, Mullally D, Gibney ER, et al. A review of the validity of malnutrition screening tools used in older adults in community and healthcare settings—a MaNuEL study. *Clin Nutr ESPEN.* 2018;24:1–13.
26. Schindler K, Pichard C, Sulz I, et al. nutritionDay: 10 years of growth. *Clin Nutr.* 2017;36(5):1207–1214.
27. Correia MITD, Perman MI, Waitzberg DL. Hospital malnutrition in Latin America: A systematic review. *Clin Nutr.* 2017;36(4):958-967. https://doi.org/10.1016/j.clnu.2016.06.025
28. Leij-Halfwerk S, Verwijs MH, van Houdt S, et al. Prevalence of protein-energy malnutrition risk in European older adults in community, residential and hospital settings, according to 22 malnutrition screening tools validated for use in adults ≥65 years: A systematic review and meta-analysis. *Maturitas.* 2019;126:80–89.
29. Allard J, Keller H, Jeejeebhoy K, et al. Malnutrition at hospital admission: contributors and effect on length of stay: A prospective cohort study from the Canadian Malnutrition Task Force. *JPEN J Parenter Enteral Nutr.* 2016;40(4):487–497.
30. Agarwal E, Miller M, Yaxley A, Isenring E. Malnutrition in the elderly: A narrative review. *Maturitas.* 2013;76:296–302.
31. National Institute for Health Care Excellence. Nutrition support in adults. Evidence update. 2013. NICE. https://www.nice.org.uk/guidance/cg32/evidence/evidence-update-194887261
32. Keller H. Promoting food intake in older adults living in the community: A review. *Appl Physiol Nutr Metab.* 2007;32(6):991–1000.
33. Braet A, Weltens C, Sermeus W. Effectiveness of discharge interventions from hospital to home on hospital readmissions: A systematic review. *JBI Database Syst Rev Implement Rep.* 2016;14(2):106–173.
34. Keller H, Laporte M, Payette H, et al. Prevalence and predictors of weight change post discharge from hospital: A study of the Canadian Malnutrition Task Force. *Eur J Clin Nutr.* 2017;71(6):766–772.
35. Young AM, Mudge AM, Banks MD, et al. From hospital to home: Limited nutritional and functional recovery for older adults. *J Frailty Aging.* 2015;4(2):69.
36. Ramage Morin P, Gilmour H, Rotermann M. Nutritional risk, hospitalization and mortality among community-dwelling Canadians aged 65 or older. *Health Rep.* 2017;28(9):17–27.
37. Harris MF, Fanaian M, Jayasinghe UW, et al. What predicts patient-reported GP management of smoking, nutrition, alcohol, physical activity and weight? *Aust J Prim Health.* 2012;18(2):123–128.
38. Munk T, Tolstrup U, Beck AM, et al. Individualised dietary counselling for nutritionally at-risk older patients following discharge from acute hospital to home: A systematic review and meta-analysis. *J Hum Nutr Diet.* 2015;29(2):196–208.
39. Wright L, Vance L, Sudduth C, Epps JB. The impact of a home-delivered meal program on nutritional risk, dietary intake, food security, loneliness, and social well-being. *J Nutr Gerontol Geriatr.* 2015;34(2):218–227.
40. Food for Life. Developing a good food culture to support health and wellbeing: Older people. 2020. Available at: https://www.foodforlife.org.uk/get-togethers/older-people. Accessed June 15, 2020.
41. Laur C, Keller H. Making the case for nutrition screening in older adults in primary care. *Nutr Today.* 2017;52(3):129.
42. Keller H, Brockest B, Haresign H. Building capacity for nutrition screening. *Nutr Today, Clin Community Trials.* 2006;41(4).
43. Todorovic V, Russell C, Elia M. The "MUST" Explanatory Booklet: A Guide to the "Malnutrition Universal Screening Tool" ('MUST') for Adults. 2011. British Association of Parenteral and Enteral Nutrition (BAPEN) https://www.bapen.org.uk/pdfs/must/must_explan.pdf

44. Whitelock E, Ensaff H. On your own: Older adults' food choice and dietary habits. *Nutrients*. 2018;10(4).
45. Doody P, Aunger J, Asamane E, Greig CA, Lord J, Whittaker A. Frailty Levels in Geriatric Hospital paTients (FLIGHT)—The prevalence of frailty among geriatric populations within hospital ward settings: A systematic review protocol. *BMJ Open*. 2019;9(8).
46. Laur C, McNicholl T, Valaitis R, Keller H. Malnutrition or frailty? Overlap and evidence gaps in the diagnosis and treatment of frailty and malnutrition. *Appl Physiol Nutr Metab*. 2017;42(5):449–458.
47. Rockwood K, Song X, MacKnight C, et al. A global clinical measure of fitness and frailty in elderly people. *CMAJ*. 2005;173(5):489–495.
48. Yang PH, Lin MC, Liu YY, Lee CL, Chang NJ. Effect of nutritional intervention programs on nutritional status and readmission rate in malnourished older adults with pneumonia: A randomized control trial. *Int J Environ Res Public Health*. 2019;16(23).
49. Abdallah L, Remington R, Houde S, Zhan L, Melillo KD. Dehydration reduction in community-dwelling older adults: Perspectives of community health care providers. *Res Gerontol Nurs*. 2009;2(1):49–57.
50. Keller M. Maintaining oral hydration in older adults living in residential aged care facilities. *Int J Evid Based Healthc*. 2006;4(1):68–73.
51. Lorenzo I, Serra-Prat M, Carlos Yébenes J. The role of water homeostasis in muscle function and frailty: A review. *Nutrients*. 2019;11(8).
52. Dickson M, Riddell H, Gilmour F, McCormack B. Delivering dignified care: A realist synthesis of evidence that promotes effective listening to and learning from older people's feedback in acute care settings. *J Clin Nurs*. 2017;26(23–24):4028–4038.
53. Van Grootven B, Jeuris A, Jonckers M, et al. Predicting hospitalisation-associated functional decline in older patients admitted to a cardiac care unit with cardiovascular disease: A prospective cohort study. *BMC Geriatr*. 2020;20(1):112.
54. Forman DE, Rich MW, Alexander KP, et al. Cardiac care for older adults: Time for a new paradigm. *J Am Coll Cardiol*. 2011;57(18):1801–1810.
55. Junius-Walker U, Schleef T, Vogelsang U, Dierks ML. How older patients prioritise their multiple health problems: A qualitative study. *BMC Geriatr*. 2019;19(1):362.
56. World Health Organization. World report on ageing and health. World Health Organization; 2015. https://www.who.int/
57. Gómez-Gómez ME, Zapico SC. Frailty, cognitive decline, neurodegenerative diseases and nutrition interventions. *Int J Mol Sci*. 2019;20(11):2842.
58. Panza F, Solfrizzi V, Seripa D, et al. Age-related hearing impairment and frailty in Alzheimer's disease: Interconnected associations and mechanisms. *Front Aging Neurosci*. 2015;7:113.
59. Kweder H, Eidi H. Vitamin D deficiency in elderly: Risk factors and drugs impact on vitamin D status. *Avicenna J Med*. 2018;8(4):139.
60. Calder PC. Nutrition, immunity and COVID-19. *BMJ Nutr Prev Health*. 2020 May 20;0: bmjnph-2020-000085. https://nutrition.bmj.com/content/bmjnph/3/1/74.full.pdf.
61. Richards C. Infections in residents of long-term care facilities: An agenda for research. Report of an expert panel. *J Am Geriatr Soc*. 2002;50(3):570–576.
62. Makam AN, Tran T, Miller ME, Xuan L, Nguyen OK, Halm EA. The clinical course after long-term acute care hospital admission among older Medicare beneficiaries. *J Am Geriatr Soc*. 2019;67(11):2282–2288.
63. Childs CE, Calder PC, Miles EA. Diet and immune function. *Nutrients*. 2019;11(8):1933.
64. Andersson M, Östholm-Balkhed Å, Fredrikson M, et al. Delay of appropriate antibiotic treatment is associated with high mortality in patients with community-onset sepsis in a Swedish setting. *Eur J Clin Microbiol Infect Dis*. 2019;38(7).
65. Van Niekerk G, Meaker C, Engelbrecht AM. Nutritional Support in Sepsis: When Less May Be More. Nutritional support in sepsis: when less may be more. *Crit Care*. 2020;24(1):53.
66. Wong MMH, So WKW, Choi KC, et al. Malnutrition risks and their associated factors among home-living older Chinese adults in Hong Kong: Hidden problems in an affluent Chinese community. *BMC Geriatr*. 2019;19(1).
67. Fanelli Kuczmarski M, Stave Shupe E, Pohlig RT, Rawal R, Zonderman AB, Evans MK. A longitudinal assessment of diet quality and risks associated with malnutrition in socioeconomic and racially diverse adults. *Nutrients*. 2019;11(9):2046.

68. Aliabadi M, Kimiagar M, Ghayour-Mobarhan M, et al. Prevalence of malnutrition in free living elderly people in Iran: a cross-sectional study. *Asia Pac J Clin Nutr*. 2008;17(2):285–289.
69. Loos S, Walia N, Becker T, Puschner B. Lost in transition? Professional perspectives on transitional mental health services for young people in Germany: A qualitative study. *BMC Health Serv Res*. 2018;18(1).
70. Coleman EA, Boult C. Improving the quality of transitional care for persons with complex care needs. *J Am Geriatr Soc*. 2003;51(4):556–557.
71. Zurlo A, Zuliani G. Management of care transition and hospital discharge. *Aging Clin Exp Res*. 2018;30(3):263–270.
72. Glette MK, Kringeland T, Røise O, Wiig S. Hospital physicians' views on discharge and readmission processes: A qualitative study from Norway. *BMJ Open*. 2019;9(8):31297.
73. Coffey A., Leahy-Warren P., Savage E., et al. Interventions to promote early discharge and avoid inappropriate hospital (Re)admission: A systematic review. *Int J Environ Res Public Health*. 2019;16(14):2457.
74. ACT Academy. Quality, Service Improvement and Redesign Tools: Discharge Planning. NHS England. Available at: https://www.england.nhs.uk/wp-content/uploads/2021/12/qsir-discharge-planning.pdf.
75. Oikonomou E, Chatburn E, Higham H, Murray J, Lawton R, Vincent C. Developing a measure to assess the quality of care transitions for older people. *BMC Health Serv Res*. 2019;19(1):505.
76. Darzi J. Be nutrition aware in primary care: Making every contact count. *British Journal of General Practice*. 2014;64(628):554–555.
77. Primary Care Workforce Commission. The future of primary care. Creating teams for tomorrow. 2015.

CHAPTER 4

Basic Principles of Acute and Chronic Nutrition Support

Lisa Sharkey ■ Jeremy Woodward

LEARNING POINTS

By the end of this chapter, you should be able to:

- Recognise a patient with undernutrition and take measures to safely initiate nutrition support
- Describe the indications for and ethical considerations around enteral tube feeding
- Know the indications for, and complications that can arise from, parenteral nutrition
- Know the definition and causes of intestinal failure
- Describe the different types of short bowel syndrome and the complications that can arise with each type
- Explain the composition and roles of a nutrition support team

CASE STUDY 4.1 Anorexia Nervosa

History

At the age of 20, Laura had just started her university course. When she returned home for the Easter holidays, her parents were concerned that she appeared to have lost a significant amount of weight and seemed very weak. Laura attributed this to a variety of factors including living on a student grant, the state in which her flatmates left the kitchen and not being organised enough to go out and buy food. However, when at home she ate very little at family mealtimes and complained of feeling sick and needing to vomit immediately afterward. She wore loose-fitting clothes that concealed the true extent of her loss of weight. One morning, her parents heard a loud thump from Laura's bedroom and dashed upstairs to find her collapsed on the floor. She was drowsy and confused, and they immediately called an ambulance which took her straight to the emergency department of the local hospital.

When she arrived, she was noted to be weak and speaking in a barely intelligible voice. Her body mass index (BMI) was 11 kg/m^2. Her temperature was 35.4°C, her blood pressure was 85/45 mm Hg, her pulse rate was 45 beats per minute and an electrocardiogram showed sinus bradycardia with a significantly prolonged QT interval of 476 ms. Blood tests showed a serum sodium concentration of 135 mmol/L, potassium of 3.0 mmol/L, blood glucose of 2.9 mmol/L, urea of 9 mmol/L and creatinine of 88 μmol/L. The alanine transaminase level was elevated as was the creatine kinase measurement. Her serum albumin was 35 g/L.

The medical team took her through to the resuscitation area and established intravenous access. They corrected her blood glucose with 50 mL of 50% dextrose given intravenously and her blood pressure with a 500-mL bag of intravenous colloid solution. However, her condition rapidly deteriorated and she became increasingly short of breath, requiring high-flow oxygen to maintain capillary oxygen saturation greater than 90%. Just as the junior doctor went to lunch, a cardiac arrest call was put out to the resuscitation area. Laura was unresponsive and had no palpable cardiac output. She was intubated and ventilated and given intravenous adrenaline before being transferred to the intensive care unit. Sadly, she required escalating amounts of inotropic support and died on the unit 4 hours later.

Discussion

Anorexia nervosa is an extremely dangerous condition and carries a high risk of mortality from suicide as well as from malnutrition. In Laura's case, the emergency medical team overlooked the fact that she

CASE STUDY 4.1 Anorexia Nervosa—(Continued)

was starving and that her physiological parameters were not those of a well-nourished individual. The bradycardia and hypotension are characteristic and should not be subject to rapid correction with fluid bolus, even though in this case there was biochemical evidence of relative renal impairment. The doctor interpreted the normal albumin level as being indicative of haemoconcentration; however, a normal serum albumin is usual in this setting. Whilst it was reasonable to consider correcting the serum glucose (due to the impaired conscious level on arrival), high-dose thiamine should have been given beforehand and a low dose of glucose—preferably orally or as 40% dextrose gel such as "hypostop" on the gums—would have been preferable to the excessive amount of intravenous dextrose delivered. The intravenous dextrose led to a rapid decline in blood levels of both phosphate and potassium, which would have precipitated a cardiac arrythmia and cardiac arrest. Wasting of the heart muscles through malnutrition and reduced contractility from low phosphate availability resulted in irreversible heart failure that could not be corrected by inotropic support.

This case demonstrates the critical importance of understanding the physiological derangements associated with malnutrition and the effects of attempting to correct them rapidly.

CASE STUDY 4.2 Cerebrovascular Accident

History

Manjeet was admitted into hospital having been found by his carer slumped in his chair with profound right-sided weakness and unintelligible speech. He was 78 years old and had a history of type 2 diabetes, obesity, hypertension and coronary artery bypass surgery following a non-ST elevation myocardial infarction the previous year. A CT scan showed a large infarct in the left middle cerebral artery territory. Thrombolytic therapy was initiated but there was no improvement in function. He was admitted to the stroke ward. The following day he failed a bedside swallow assessment and had a nasogastric (NG) feeding tube placed. The pH of the gastric aspirate was 6.1, and he therefore underwent a chest X-ray which confirmed that the tip of the NG tube was below the diaphragm and within the gastric air bubble. It was therefore deemed safe for use and he commenced NG feeding; the tube was also used for delivering oral medications.

Manjeet became disorientated on the ward and pulled at his NG tube overnight, dislodging it and making it unsafe for use. The following day a nutrition nurse specialist from the nutrition team replaced the NG tube and placed a 'nasal bridle'—a loop of tape around the nasal septum attached to the tube and preventing displacement. The dietitian prescribed an appropriate regimen for him based on his estimated nutritional requirements; however, his blood sugar level increased which required a sliding scale insulin infusion for control. Over the next few days Manjeet regained some cognitive function and was reviewed by the speech and language therapists who assessed his swallowing and found that he was unsafe to swallow at all consistencies from thin liquid to solid food. After 3 weeks he was referred to the feeding issues multidisciplinary team for consideration of placement of a percutaneous endoscopic gastrostomy (PEG) tube. On discussion it was ascertained that he was deemed to lack capacity to make this decision for himself under the terms of the Mental Capacity Act of 2005; his next of kin and close family felt that he would wish to pursue the slim chance of recovery and felt that a gastrostomy tube would allow him to be fed safely without the risk of aspiration pneumonia. The family were keen to learn how to manage the tube so that he could be looked after in his own home rather than a nursing home. The tube placement was scheduled for the following week and the home care nurse visited the family at home before Manjeet was discharged to train them how to manage the feed and medications through the tube. The palliative care team also visited Manjeet and his family on the ward prior to discharge to clarify advance decisions regarding his future care, for instance, if he should develop a pneumonia or consider further admission into hospital.

Discussion

The decision to place a gastrostomy tube for long-term feeding is complex and may require the patient to forego the pleasures of eating and drinking and mealtime social interactions to prevent the risk of developing aspiration pneumonia. When patients lack the mental capacity to make this decision for themselves, it has to be made in the patients' best interests by health care professionals, taking into consideration the views of family members as to what the patients might have wished for themselves had they the capacity to do so. A multiprofessional feeding issues team meeting permits the forum for these discussions to take place and also to decide the appropriate timing of PEG placement (should it be deemed appropriate), along with the involvement of the palliative care team and prior training of patient, family or carers in the management of PEG feeding prior to insertion to streamline discharge arrangements.

CASE STUDY 4.3 Mesenteric Ischaemia

History

Steve came into the sitting room just after breakfast to find his wife, Karen, ashen grey and clutching her abdomen in severe pain. She was 37 years old and they had been married for just 3 years. She had no medical history of any significance and took no regular medications, neither was there any family history of note. Steve immediately telephoned for an ambulance and Karen was taken to the hospital emergency department. The ambulance paramedic gave her an intramuscular injection of morphine for the pain and by the time she arrived in the emergency department the pain was considerably better. The doctor who examined her could find no evidence of any abdominal abnormality, and blood tests were normal apart from a mild elevation of the white cell count and platelet count. A diagnosis of gastritis was made and she was prescribed a proton pump inhibitor and discharged home. That night, Steve awoke to find his wife once again in agony but tried to settle her with paracetamol and a hot water bottle. After 2 hours he called an ambulance again and she returned to the hospital where a surgeon was called. Abdominal examination revealed peritonitis and an urgent CT scan was requested. This showed a blood clot within the superior mesenteric artery and bubbles of gas in the intestinal wall and portal vein. Karen was taken to the operating theatre and underwent a laparotomy where the intestine from just beyond the duodeno-jejunal flexure to the right colon was found to be ischaemic and nonviable and was therefore resected. Karen was left with a jejunostomy, and the midtransverse colon was stapled across. She was started on parenteral nutrition (PN), delivered via a central line in the intensive care unit where she stayed for 3 days before being moved to a ward. The output from her jejunostomy increased over the subsequent days as Karen started to eat and drink, and she found that however much she drank she still felt thirsty. When the output reached 8 L over a 24-hour period, the intestinal failure team were consulted and recommended fluid restriction to just 1 L of high sodium fluid (St. Mark solution) and twice daily administration of intravenous proton pump inhibitor. A tunnelled central line was placed into the right internal jugular vein for the administration of PN, and after 3 weeks Karen was discharged home, receiving a 4-L bag of PN overnight with connections and disconnections to the feed performed by visiting home care nurses. Karen became extremely depressed, and Steve gave up his job to care for her, learning how to manage the stoma and PN. When Karen was admitted into hospital with sepsis due to an infection on her line 9 months later, the intestinal failure team realised that the home situation was not sustainable and referred her to the national intestinal transplant service. During assessment, a liver biopsy was performed which showed evidence of intestinal failure-associated liver disease (IFALD) and mild fibrosis. She was listed for transplantation and suitable organs became available 3 months later. She received a small intestinal transplant with pancreas and right colon and spent 4 further weeks in hospital recovering from the operation. One year later, Karen is well, eating and drinking normally without a stoma, and visits the hospital twice a year for checkups with the transplant team. Steve has returned to full-time work and Karen now works as a volunteer in the local hospital.

Discussion

Although rare, mesenteric ischaemia can occur suddenly and without warning at any age. In Karen's case, a mutation of the *JAK2* gene led to a prothrombotic state and spontaneous arterial thrombosis, but other causes of ischaemia in otherwise well young adults include volvulus due to partial malrotation or congenital Ladd bands. With an ultra-short bowel IFALD can develop rapidly, and intestinal transplantation can significantly improve quality of life.

Overview and Introduction

Along with ever-rising levels of obesity in Westernised societies, the extent of undernutrition often goes unrecognised. Yet it affects over 10% of all adults over the age of 65 years in the community and more than 40% of all patients admitted into hospital. Undernutrition may have profound implications for the presentation of disease and recovery. It impacts physiological function and homeostatic reserves, immunity and susceptibility to infection, wound healing and factors such psychological motivation, mobility, mood and social interaction.

Weight is more easily lost than regained, and therefore prevention of undernutrition in the institutional setting is desirable, through provision of appropriate and palatable food at the correct times, quantity and temperature, in a conducive environment. For instance, eating with others can increase consumption by as much as 40% compared with eating alone. Such measures are

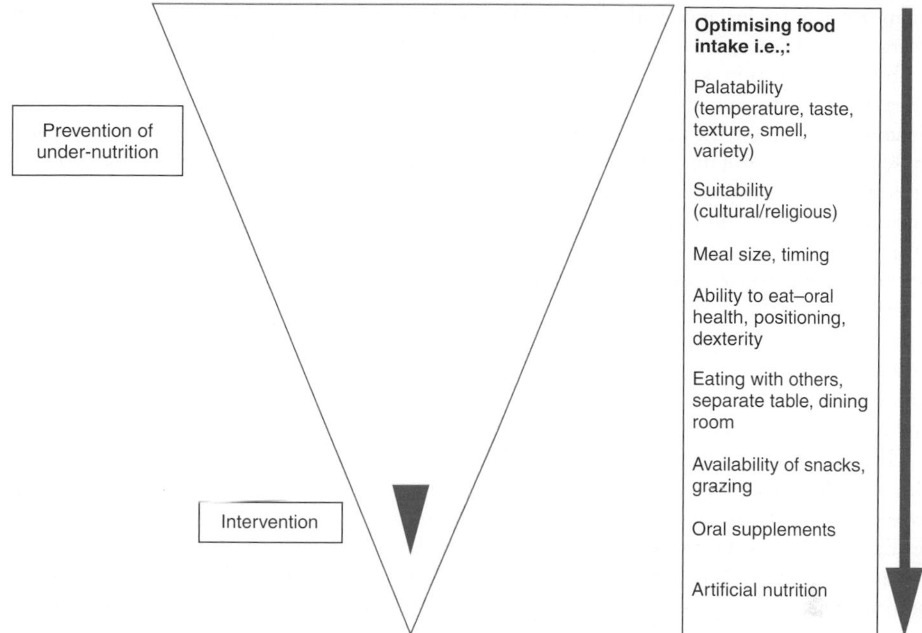

Fig. 4.1 The place of artificial nutrition in the institutional nutrition support pyramid.

frequently overlooked in hospitals where patients eat alone in their beds and are often poorly positioned and lack necessary assistance and mealtimes are treated by patients and staff alike as of secondary importance to ward rounds and investigations.

Nutrition support therefore necessarily comprises an inverted pyramid (Fig. 4.1). Prevention of undernutrition by appropriate measures is most effective for the largest number of individuals, with progressively smaller numbers requiring interventions through oral nutrition supplements (which have been shown to reduce hospital admissions by nearly 20% when used appropriately in certain settings) or tube feeding.

In this chapter, we will address the options for artificial nutrition in both the acute hospital setting and the community. However, in doing so, the greater good of prevention by optimising the consumption of a balanced diet ('food first') or the use of oral nutrition build-up sip feeds as supplements must not be forgotten.

Principles of Nutrition Support

RECOGNISING AND ASSESSING UNDERNUTRITION

Undernutrition is frequently overlooked until advanced stages, when complications have already developed and necessitate prolonged nutritional and physical rehabilitation. Its timely recognition is therefore of critical importance. Clues to weight loss may be apparent from a carefully taken history or physical examination, noting sunken cheeks (often an early sign, rapidly restored on weight gain), loose-fitting clothes or wedding rings and notches on belts. Blood tests are of little value in detecting undernutrition; serum albumin can fall precipitously in the acute phase through losses into third spaces rather than reduced synthesis, and a low full blood lymphocyte count, whilst more sensitive, also lacks specificity.

Weight is best assessed in proportion to height—using the BMI of weight (in kg) / height (in m)^2. However, care needs to be taken in interpreting BMI in particular instances of body dysmorphism (for instance, with severe kyphoscoliosis in individuals with cerebral palsy) or with alterations of body composition (for instance, with fluid overload and peripheral oedema).

Body composition is also affected by the rate and amount of weight lost and the underlying disease process. Lean body mass (muscle and protein) is critically important for all physiological functions, and unlike the case of carbohydrate and fat, there are no true stores of protein. Loss of muscle bulk leads to (amongst other issues) immobility, impaired swallowing function (and risk of pulmonary aspiration) and reduced ability to clear secretions. These combine to predispose to pneumonia, a common fatal complication of undernutrition. Muscle mass is preferentially lost during rapid weight loss and by cytokines released by inflammatory conditions such as infections or certain malignancies, leading to the condition of cachexia.

Body composition analysis complements BMI and can be undertaken using electrical impedance (current flows preferentially through lean rather than fat mass), or by using anthropometric measurements such as the mid-upper arm muscle circumference. The recently recognised condition of sarcopaenic obesity represents a situation of significant muscle loss despite a high BMI and can be quantified by algorithms applied to cross-sectional imaging modalities such as CT.

The rate of weight loss and the current BMI defined criteria for undernutrition are shown in Box 4.1. However, the risk of malnutrition for patients in an acute setting relies also on their projected trajectory, for instance, whether they are likely to continue with chronic inflammation or have restricted oral intake due to their underlying condition. These three indices—weight loss, current BMI and pending threats to nutritional intake—can be combined into a numerical score that quantifies nutritional risk. Scoring systems such as the Malnutrition Universal Screening Tool are now routinely incorporated into hospital and care home practice in the UK to identify patients at risk of malnutrition.

INITIATING NUTRITION SUPPORT

In hospitals and care homes, the malnutrition screening tool is used to stratify risk and steer appropriate intervention. For instance, measures may be implemented to augment and record oral food intake, a dietitian may be consulted to perform a formal nutritional assessment and advise on optimising food intake or the provision of oral nutrition supplements, or a form of artificial nutrition support may be initiated.

The timing of initiation of artificial nutrition support, through enteral or intravenous parenteral nutrition (PN) routes, depends on the current nutritional status of the patient and how likely the patient is to be able to recover oral intake in the near future. Such decisions therefore need to be made on an individual basis. Both routes of artificial nutrition are associated with a degree of risk (see discussion later in this chapter), and short-term benefits have been difficult to demonstrate in all but the most severely malnourished individuals.

BOX 4.1 ■ Indicators of Undernutrition in Adults

- BMI $< 18.5\,kg/m^2$

OR

- Weight loss of >10% over 6 months

OR

- BMI $< 20\,kg/m^2$

AND

- Weight loss of >5% over 6 months

From National Institute for Health and Clinical Excellence, Clinical Guideline 32. Clinical guideline [CG32]. Overview | Nutrition support for adults: oral nutrition support, enteral tube feeding and parenteral nutrition | Guidance | NICE. Published 22 February 2006. Last updated August 2017. Available at https://www.nice.org.uk/guidance/cg32

The chosen route for artificial nutrition depends primarily on the presence of a functioning gastrointestinal (GI) tract which can be utilised for enteral nutrition, without which PN is required. Artificial nutrition is frequently used to supplement oral intake rather than supplant it, especially where patients are unable to ingest 60% or more of their estimated nutritional requirements.

The calculation of estimated nutritional requirements takes place at the bedside using one of a number of different predictive equations based on gender, age and BMI. These can provide an approximation of resting energy expenditure that can then be modified by patient- and disease-related factors such as mobility, sepsis, area of burns or artificial ventilation to evaluate total requirements. Often the increased energy requirements of sepsis, burns or trauma are balanced by the lack of movement such that estimated requirements exceed calculated resting energy expenditure by as little as 10%–20%. Resting energy expenditure can also be measured using indirect calorimetry based on oxygen uptake and carbon dioxide measurement in exhaled gases, and reasonably accurate handheld devices are now available for this purpose.

Artificial feeds provided by the enteral route, and some parenteral feeds, are ready-made fixed formulations containing the necessary macro- and micronutrients in sufficient quantities to meet standard recommended daily allowances if given in the appropriate volume. However, PN also permits the modulation of separate components—within the limitations of chemical stability—and provides greater flexibility to match requirements to the individual. Table 4.1 shows baseline ranges of requirements for key nutrients.

REFEEDING SYNDROME

It is important to realise that prolonged starvation results in significant changes to body composition and metabolism. Following exhaustion of carbohydrate (glycogen) stores in the liver (usually within the first 24 hours), protein is initially broken down rapidly to provide the necessary three-carbon chains for glucose synthesis. To minimise loss of muscle, fat stores are then mobilised and metabolised through ketone body oxidation to provide energy. In the starved state, small amounts of glucose are still produced by the liver and kidney to supply cells that cannot adapt to ketone body oxidation—neurones and red blood cells. A process of reductive adaptation takes place that alters the physiological working parameters—the core temperature may drop, blood pressure and pulse are usually low, cortisol levels are elevated and thyroxine levels diminished. The ability to reset these parameters and reverse metabolic processes on refeeding is limited by the reduction in reserves due to prolonged fasting and therefore needs to take place gradually.

TABLE 4.1 ■ **Approximate Normal Nutrient Intake Requirements**

Energy	25–35 kcal/kg per day
Fluid	30–35 mL/kg per day (+ replacement of additional losses)
Protein	0.75–1.5 g/kg per day
Lipid	35%–50% of energy requirements (minimum of 4.5% energy intake required to provide essential fatty acids)
Carbohydrate	50%–65% of energy requirements <5 g/kg per day oxidised 5–15 g/kg per day stored as glycogen >15 g/kg per day results in lipogenesis/hepatic steatosis
Sodium	1 mmol/kg per day
Potassium	1 mmol/kg per day

Attempting to apply 'normal' physiological parameters to a starving patient can be catastrophic; the heart muscle is wasted and unable to tolerate intravenous fluid boluses which can result in irreversible heart failure, and the use of a warming blanket to increase core body temperature can result in vasodilatation and collapse of blood pressure. The rapid reintroduction of carbohydrates may lead to rapid consumption of cofactors such as thiamine that are critically required for glucose oxidation. Thiamine deficiency leads to cessation of glycolysis, paradoxically so in those cells that remain dependent on glucose, and can lead to a characteristic pattern of irreversible brain damage. This is known as Wernicke encephalopathy, and results in profound short-term memory loss, confusion and external ophthalmoplegia. In addition, the slowing of glycolysis reduces the availability of inorganic phosphate as it is bound to metabolic intermediates and limits energetic processes within cells including muscle fibre contraction. Finally, the stimulation of insulin secretion by glucose results in activation of the membrane sodium/potassium ATPase pump and rapid transmembrane flux of potassium into cells, which can dangerously destabilise cardiac muscle action potentials and result in fatal arrythmia. These adverse consequences of attempting to restore the individual to 'normal' physiological parameters are known as refeeding syndrome and must be prevented by the slow reintroduction of feed (as little as 5–10 kcal/kg per day to start with), prior intravenous administration of B vitamins (including high-dose thiamine), careful use of intravenous fluids and generous replacement of electrolytes (potassium, magnesium and phosphate) with regular monitoring of blood concentrations.

AIMS AND OUTCOMES OF NUTRITION SUPPORT

The principle aim of nutrition support is to preserve physiological function by retaining lean body mass (protein). Severe illnesses including trauma, sepsis and burns result in a significant catabolic state of protein breakdown. Provision of appropriate nutrition support in such states can attenuate protein loss but rarely is it reversible until the underlying drive to catabolism has resolved. Providing excess nutrients does not improve nitrogen balance nor result in net protein synthesis but merely increases metabolic side effects and is toxic. Unsurprisingly, therefore, studies have repeatedly shown the benefit of early intervention with appropriate nutrition support in a critical care setting but demonstrate increased mortality when given in excess to estimated requirements.

Weight gain on refeeding an undernourished patient is slow and initially comprises fluid and fat rather than lean muscle mass; the body composition and function may take a considerable period of time to reequilibrate after weight has regained to premorbid levels. Once again this demonstrates the importance of prevention of malnutrition and early recognition of those at nutritional risk.

Enteral Nutrition

INDICATIONS FOR ENTERAL FEEDING AND ETHICAL CONSIDERATIONS

Enteral feeding is used when oral feeding is unsafe or insufficient to meet demands and requires placement of a feeding tube into the GI tract. Hence, it is also called tube feeding or enteral tube feeding.[1] Table 4.2 shows some common indications for enteral feeding.

For longer-term feeding, the majority of patients have either a neurological or GI problem necessitating artificial nutrition (Table 4.3).

Clinically assisted nutrition and hydration are medical interventions, and the risks and benefits must be weighed for each individual patient, as for any other treatment. The General Medical Council provides guidance on this area for medical professionals. Often patients being considered for tube feeding lack the capacity to make decisions about their own health, in which case the treating team must make the decision they feel is in the patient's best interests. It is preferable

TABLE 4.2 ■ **Indications for Short-Term Enteral Tube Feeding**

Category	Examples
Acute neurological impairment	Stroke, head injury, ventilated patients
Acute gastrointestinal conditions	Oesophageal obstruction, delayed gastric emptying, optimisation for gastrointestinal surgery, inflammatory bowel disease
Increased nutritional requirements	Burns, intensive care unit patients, severe sepsis, postoperative patients, liver disease
Psychological	Anorexia nervosa, severe depression

TABLE 4.3 ■ **Indications for Longer-Term Enteral Tube Feeding**

Category	Examples
Neurological disorders	Stroke, multiple sclerosis, motor neuron disease, cerebral palsy, traumatic brain injury
Gastrointestinal	Dysmotility, pharyngeal or oesophageal obstruction, gastroparesis/gastric outlet obstruction (jejunal tube), malabsorption
Increased nutritional requirements	Cystic fibrosis, short bowel

TABLE 4.4 ■ **Types of Enteral Feeding Tube**

	Short Term (4–6 Weeks)	Long Term
Gastric feeding	Nasogastric tube	PEG tube RIG
Jejunal feeding	Nasojejunal tube	PEG-J Direct PEJ Surgical jejunostomy

PEG, Percutaneous endoscopically placed gastric tube; *PEG-J*, PEG with jejunal extension; *PEJ*, percutaneous endoscopically inserted jejunal tube; *RIG*, radiologically inserted gastric tube.

that this be discussed with the patient's family and decisions be made in a multidisciplinary team forum, a feeding multidisciplinary team.

TYPES OF ENTERAL FEEDING TUBE

The type of tube used depends on whether the anticipated duration of feeding is short or long term and whether feed can be delivered into the stomach or needs to be postpyloric (Table 4.4). Insertion methods can be at the bedside, for simple NG tubes, or require endoscopic, radiological or surgical placement.[2]

COMPLICATIONS OF TUBES AND ENTERAL FEEDING

NG tubes are generally inserted at the bedside. Misplacement into the lungs, or very occasionally intracranially, have been described. NG tubes should not be used in any patient with a suspected or confirmed base of skull fracture. Lung misplacement is unfortunately more common, and feeding must never commence without confirmation of intragastric placement with acidic aspirate or an X-ray. Pharyngeal pouches can be perforated during insertion and care should be taken in patients with known oesophageal varices, but placement of an NG tube is not contraindicated in such patients. Minor complications include nasal trauma, reactions to dressings and pharyngeal discomfort. Tubes can fall out or be accidentally or deliberately pulled out, which can cause feed to enter the lungs and cause a chemical pneumonitis, which can be fatal.

Nasojejunal tubes often displace back into the stomach. pH testing should be undertaken in all short-term tubes before any flushes, feed or medications are administered.

The risks of PEG tube insertion include pain, bleeding, peritonitis, site infection and non-target organ damage. Often a gastrocolic fistula is not recognised until many months after the PEG insertion and results from transfixing the colon onto the gastric wall during insertion. Risks can be minimised with adequate operator experience. A three-point approach to ensuring safe placement begins with checking position with finger indentation and transillumination from the endoscope light through the abdominal wall. Following this, a safe tract can be established using a small needle attached to a syringe and aspirating the syringe during withdrawal. If a patient complains of abdominal pain post-PEG insertion and has an X-ray or CT scan, it must be remembered that some degree of pneumoperitoneum may occur as a result of the procedure.

Longer-term PEG problems include overgranulation at the exit site, leakage, corrosion of the tube and buried bumper syndrome. The latter can be prevented by weekly insertion and rotation of the tube, to free it from the gastric wall. For PEG tubes with jejunal extensions, the additional problem of displacement of the jejunal tube is common, and repeat endoscopy to replace this is necessary.

The enteral feed itself can cause metabolic and GI problems. Gastro-oesophageal reflux can be reduced by correct positioning of the patient during feeding—at least 30 degrees during and for 30 minutes after feeding. Nausea and bloating may respond to slower rates of feeding. For inpatients experiencing diarrhoea, other causes such as infections, antibiotics or other medications and underlying GI conditions should be checked first, before a change of feed is considered. To ensure the patient is not being over- or underfed, a dietitian should prescribe and adjust the rate and type of feed given. At-risk patients should be monitored for refeeding syndrome and hyperglycaemia.[2]

CHOOSING THE TYPE OF FEED

A wide range of enteral feeds are available from a number of commercial suppliers. Polymeric feeds contain whole protein, carbohydrate as partially hydrolysed starch and long-chain triglycerides. Semielemental feeds are partially predigested and consist of short peptide chains, simple carbohydrates and medium-chain triglycerides. Elemental feeds are fully predigested and contain individual amino acids and medium-chain triglycerides. Both of these may be used in patients with malabsorption, but their high osmolality can result in diarrhoea.

Food allergies can be accommodated, with soya-based and gluten-free feeds. High-protein, high-fibre and energy-dense formulations can be used where appropriate. Involvement of a dietitian in prescribing the type and rate of feeding is essential to maximise tolerance and ensure nutritional requirements are being met.

MEDICATIONS AND TUBE FEEDING

Many medications are not licensed for use with enteral tubes and in the absence of evidence, best practice advice and/or guidelines are needed and input from a pharmacist is essential.

The main concerns are blocking the tube, reducing efficacy by crushing or otherwise manipulating medications, or interactions/precipitation. The site of absorption should be considered, especially for patients with jejunal tubes, as some medications are largely absorbed in the stomach or proximal duodenum. Drugs which cause particular problems include phenytoin, digoxin, some antibiotics and antacids. The British Association for Parenteral and Enteral Nutrition has useful and practical information on this on their website (https://www.bapen.org.uk).

Adequate flushes must be given between medications. Drug administration can become very time-consuming for a patient or carer, if lots of medications need to be crushed or liquids measured out, with flushes between each. On each clinical review, consideration should be given to whether some drugs can safely be stopped to ease the burden.

HOME ENTERAL FEEDING

Enteral tube feeding at home requires cooperation between the nutrition support team (NST) and the general practitioner, community dietitian, community nurses and the patient and carers. In many countries, home care companies take responsibility for provision of equipment and training. Patients need to be provided with written information on looking after their tube and contacts for problems.

Intestinal Failure and Parenteral Nutrition

DEFINITION AND CLASSIFICATION

The principal function of the GI tract is the digestion and absorption of micro- and macronutrients, salts and fluid. If it is unable to fulfil these functions, it can be said to have failed. Intestinal failure has been defined as follows: 'The reduction of gut function below the minimum necessary for the absorption of macronutrients and/or water and electrolytes, such that intravenous supplementation is required to maintain health and/or growth'.[3]

It is important to distinguish absorptive from digestive processes. Maldigestion—for instance, as a result of pancreatic exocrine insufficiency—may lead to malabsorption as nutrients are not appropriately reduced to their absorbable components.

Intestinal failure can be acute and self-limiting or chronic and long-lasting. These are respectively categorised as type 1 intestinal failure and type 3 intestinal failure. Type 2 intestinal failure is a classification used for a potentially remediable situation that may require complex surgery to restore GI continuity.

CAUSES OF INTESTINAL FAILURE

Intestinal failure can result from conditions that diminish the length or absorptive area of the intestine or its propulsive ability. These have been grouped into five pathophysiological groups as shown in Table 4.5.

SHORT BOWEL SYNDROME

Short bowel syndrome commonly results in intestinal failure through lack of adequate intestinal length for absorption. This is the commonest cause of type 3 intestinal failure, accounting for approximately one-third of cases in the UK. The effects of reduced intestinal length are frequently compounded by increased motility due to ileocolonic resection. This leads to a lack of secretion of the enteric hormones (peptide YY and glucagon-like peptide 1) that comprise the physiological 'ileal brake' mechanism.

As much as 8 L of fluid may enter the proximal jejunum in the human adult every day under normal circumstances due to ingested fluid augmented by the secretions of saliva, gastric juice, bile

TABLE 4.5 ■ **Classification and Causes of Intestinal Failure**

Pathophysiological Group	Mechanism of Intestinal Failure	Examples
Short bowel	Reduced absorptive surface area • Increased fluid losses • Secondary reduced oral intake to control losses • Rapid gastrointestinal transit	Type 2: 'Defunctioning' stoma formed in proximal intestine to protect a distal surgical anastomosis Type 3: Intestinal resection due to: • Mesenteric infarction arterial or venous), volvulus, Crohn disease, radiation enteritis, trauma (adults) • Congenital intestinal malformation, gastroschisis, atresia (children)
Intestinal fistula	Bypass of gastrointestinal absorptive mucosa • Increased fluid losses • Secondary reduced oral intake to control losses • Metabolic demands due to associated sepsis or inflammation	Type 2: Surgically remediable enterocutaneous fistula due to iatrogenic surgical injury to the intestine Type 3: Fistulation where further surgery is not possible in cases such as trauma or Crohn disease
Intestinal dysmotility	Intolerance of oral/enteral feeding due to symptoms • Small bowel bacterial overgrowth • Increased fluid secretion in obstructed segments • Increased gastrointestinal losses due to vomiting, diarrhoea or gastric drainage	Type 1: Self-limiting postoperative ileus Type 3: Chronic intestinal pseudo-obstruction either primary (visceral myopathy or neuropathy) or secondary to a wide variety of underlying medical conditions or medication use
Mechanical obstruction	Reduced oral intake due to symptoms and lack of absorption • Increased fluid secretion in obstructed segments • Increased gastrointestinal losses due to vomiting, diarrhoea or gastric drainage	Type 2: Obstructing tumour of the gastrointestinal tract remediable through surgery, chemo- or radiotherapy Type 3: Obstructing tumour of the gastrointestinal tract or caused by peritoneal metastatic disease, not remediable through surgery, chemo- or radiotherapy
Extensive intestinal mucosal disease	Inefficient nutrient absorption or nutrient and fluid loss from mucosal surface	Type 3: • Refractory coeliac disease, Crohn disease, common variable immunodeficiency with chronic noroviral infection (adults) • Tufting enteropathy, microvillous inclusion disease (children)

and pancreatic and duodenal secretions. All but 1–2 L of this fluid is absorbed in the ileum, which has greater absorptive capacity than the jejunum. The ileum is also specialised for the absorption of bile salts (for reclamation via the enterohepatic circulation) and vitamin B12.

The normal length of small intestine can vary in adults from 3 metres to over 8 metres. It is considered that a minimum of 2 metres of small intestine is required for adequate nutrient absorption if ending in a stoma. It is likely that if the small intestine is shorter than 1 metre in length, fluid losses will exceed fluid intake. A high-output stoma is often defined as producing more than

2 L of effluent per day, although a better definition may be where the output exceeds the ability to maintain hydration through oral intake.[4] Due to the permeability of jejunal mucosa, sodium concentrations tend to equilibrate across the epithelium, and the average electrolyte concentrations within the jejunal lumen are greater than 90 mmol sodium and 5 mmol potassium per litre. The absorptive capacity of the colon is such that if residual small intestine is surgically reconnected to it, then as little as 50 cm of small intestine may be adequate, especially if the ileo-caecal valve is present. However, the vulnerability of the ileo-caecal complex to diseases such as ischaemia and Crohn disease makes this an unusual configuration. Common types of short bowel configuration are shown in Table 4.6.

MANAGEMENT OF INTESTINAL FAILURE

By definition, the management of intestinal failure requires (intravenous) nutrition (PN). Specific management depends on the cause of intestinal failure. Excessive stomal outputs may make replacement of fluid and electrolytes challenging, and even when PN is required, efforts should be made to reduce losses and parenteral requirements for balance. In some instances, it may be possible to wean off intravenous requirements through appropriate medical management.[5]

Patients should be encouraged to eat and drink where it is possible and safe, for maintenance of psychosocial interactions and endogenous physiological regulation by enteric nutrient sensing (secretion of hormones such as cholecystokinin, insulin and regulation of motility. Stomal output can be reduced by decreasing GI secretions—proton pump inhibitors diminish gastric fluid production, octreotide injections may (in some cases) reduce biliopancreatic secretions. In those with a jejuno-colic anastomosis, diarrhoea may be reduced by sequestering bile salts (using a resin such as colestyramine) and taking a low-fat diet as colonic excess of both of these lead to fluid secretion. Motility slowing agents such as opiate receptor agonists (loperamide, codeine) may reduce intestinal transit and aid absorption.

The paradoxical increase of oxalic acid absorption through the colon in patients with a jejuno-colic anastomosis can lead to its precipitation in the kidneys as stones and avoidance of foods containing large amounts of oxalate is encouraged (such foods include chocolate, coffee, beer, rhubarb and strawberries). Patients with a high-output jejunostomy require careful fluid balance management. Hypotonic and hypertonic drinks need to be avoided, and a concentration of at least 100 mmol of sodium per litre of fluid is required to prevent additional salt and fluid losses. Standard World Health Organization rehydration salts contain 60 mmol per litre and are inadequate for this purpose when made up to standard strength. Sodium and fluid depletion leads to hyperaldosteronism and additional potassium and magnesium losses through the kidney, and therefore maintenance of hydration status is essential. Specific nutrient deficiencies (vitamin B12, magnesium, fat-soluble vitamins such as A and D) may require monitoring and replacement.

Peptide analogues of enteroendocrine trophic factors (such as glucagon-like peptide 2) can be injected to increase absorption and reduce stomal output and parenteral requirements. High cost and marginal benefits currently preclude this approach in the majority of cases. For type 1 intestinal failure, time and parenteral support may be all that is required until spontaneous recovery occurs. Specialist surgery may restore GI continuity and remove the requirement for intravenous support with type 2 intestinal failure. Intestinal lengthening operations can be undertaken in highly selected cases to increase absorption. Type 3 intestinal failure requires long-term support by PN (see next section) or intestinal transplantation to correct.

PARENTERAL NUTRITION

PN support is a means of providing supplementary nutrition intravenously when required. Total PN is when a patient's entire requirements are delivered intravenously. Long-term PN can be

TABLE 4.6 ■ **Common Types of Configuration of Short Bowel**

Configuration	Ileo-Colonic Anastomosis	Jejuno-Colic Anastomosis	End-Jejunostomy
Diagram	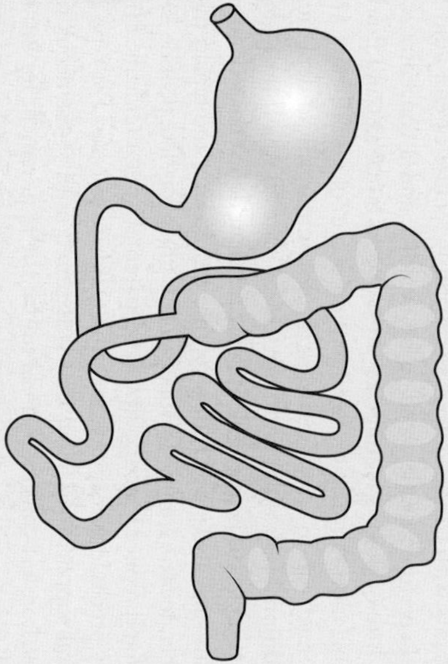	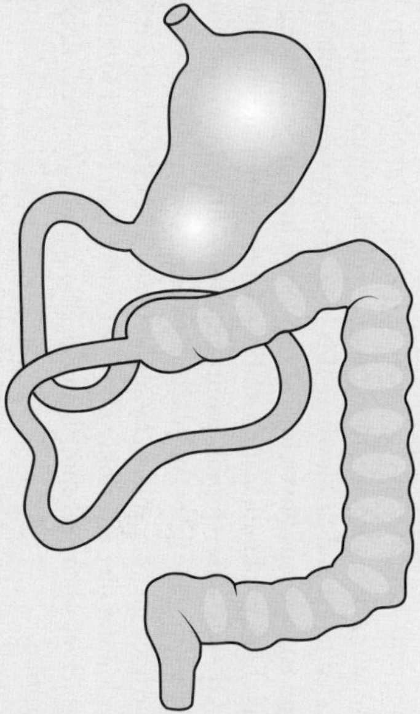	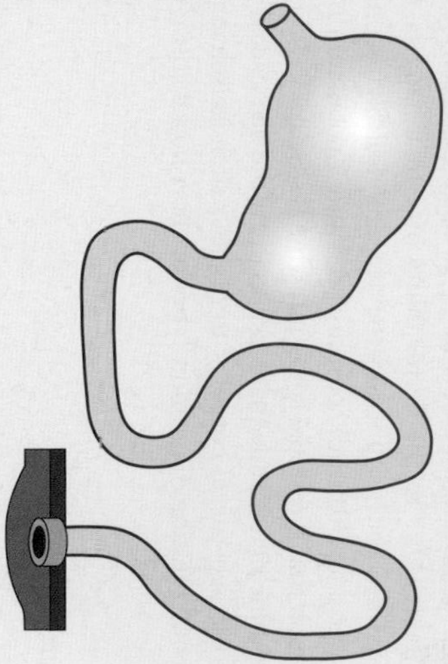
Malabsorption (depending on length of residual intestine)	Bile salts, vitamin B12, magnesium	Bile salts, vitamin B12, magnesium, macronutrients (0- to 50-cm residual intestine)	Fluid, electrolytes (sodium 90 mmol/L; potassium 5 mmol/L), micronutrients, macronutrients
Management	Bile salt sequestrant, low-fat diet, parenteral vitamin B12, oral magnesium replacement	Bile salt sequestrant, low-fat diet, low-oxalate diet, magnesium, vitamin B12 replacement, parenteral nutrition (0- to 50-cm intestine), oral nutrition (50- to 100-cm intestine)	Parenteral nutrition (0–100 cm), parenteral fluid ± magnesium (100- to 200-cm intestine)
Complications	Gallstones	Gallstones (45%), calcium oxalate kidney stones (25%)	Gallstones (45%), acute kidney injury

provided at home (HPN) for patients with type 2 intestinal failure (awaiting restorative surgery) or long-term (type 3) intestinal failure. In the UK, the requirement for HPN has increased from 10 per million population in 2000 to over 40 per million population in 2015. The use of HPN varies significantly between different health care systems in terms of numbers and indications for its use.

PN may contain all or some of the individuals' nutrient and fluid requirements depending on the amount that can be absorbed when taken orally or enterally. It is usually delivered in one bag and can be infused over varying amounts of time dictated by its volume and constituents. There are significant physico-chemical challenges in mixing the entire nutritional requirements together within one container and the amounts of individual components may be limited by their interactions (Table 4.7). To remain stable in solution without reaction or precipitation, ingredients can only be added within certain concentration ranges. The stability of different mixtures may be time or temperature dependent. PN emulsions can be specially formulated (compounded) on an individual patient basis or dispensed from a range of ready-made mixtures 'off the shelf'. These often contain separate aqueous, lipid and micronutrient partitions with breakable seals between them for mixing prior to administration as multichamber bags.

INDICATIONS AND USE OF PARENTERAL NUTRITION

PN is required to support individuals with intestinal failure, and for logistical and safety reasons it should not be used where oral or enteral alternatives are available. It may be required for a limited period of time only in hospital patients with type 1 intestinal failure or at home for patients with type 2 intestinal failure awaiting restorative surgery. However, long-term use may be required for patients with type 3 intestinal failure, and total PN has been used successfully in such individuals for periods of over 25 years.

The use of HPN in the palliative care setting is commonplace in some regions (United States, southern Europe) and is increasing in the UK due to increasing ease of use. The commonest palliative indication is for intestinal obstruction secondary to peritoneal metastatic disease arising from ovarian adenocarcinoma in which condition long-term survivors (more than 3 years) are reported. Short-term use of palliative HPN in terminally ill patients is contentious but in selected cases, benefits may outweigh burdens, particularly where a good performance status is maintained.

PN must be delivered into a large vein close to the heart where it is quickly diluted. Secure and long-term central venous access can be achieved through a line tunnelled under the skin or inserted peripherally and via the cephalic vein in the upper arm. There are only six major veins for normal access purposes: internal jugular, subclavian and femoral on each side. An injectable port attached to the line can be inserted under the skin and may be preferable to a protruding catheter for more active or younger patients, although it is not associated with fewer complications.

An infusion pump is used to deliver the PN at a variable rate. It is usually infused initially over 24 hours but for longer-term use it can be run over shorter periods of time (often overnight) to minimise lifestyle disruption.

For patients to manage PN at home, they require a medical-grade refrigerator unit and adequate storage space for feed and ancillaries. They also need to be trained how to maintain sterility in connection and disconnection of feed. Such training is usually carried out by home care company nurses in the home environment. Voluntary organisations such as Patients on Intravenous and Nasogastric Nutrition Therapy in the UK and the Oley Foundation in the United States provide support and advice for patients on HPN.

OUTCOMES AND COMPLICATIONS OF PARENTERAL NUTRITION

PN can be used safely over long periods of time, and it is the underlying disease process leading to intestinal failure that is responsible for the majority of associated morbidity and mortality. Only

TABLE 4.7 ■ **Components of Parenteral Nutrition Emulsions**

Component	Special Considerations
Fluid	• Volumes of over 3 L in one bag may be difficult to carry and manipulate. • High volumes with low solute concentrations may risk haemolysis. Low volumes with high solute content may risk precipitation and particulate formation or acute kidney injury. • Stability of the mixture may impose volume constraints. • Delivery into a central vein is essential.
Electrolytes	• Sodium requirements may be high when there are high obligatory losses body fluids. Measurement of urinary sodium concentration may be helpful to monitor balance (>20 mmol/L of urine for repletion). • High concentrations of potassium should be avoided when infusion times are short in view of potential for cardiac dysrhythmia. • Calcium and magnesium concentrations are limited by their ability to precipitate in solution with anions.
Amino acids	• Each amino acid requires administration in appropriate concentration—this may depend on disease state. Only a small number of mixed amino acid formulations are available for use. • Glutamine hydrolyses spontaneously to glutamic acid in solution and has hitherto been excluded from parenteral amino acid solutions but can be added separately as a dimer. • Some amino acids can precipitate with copper or zinc (reducing their availability).
Lipids	• Requires emulsification with phospholipids such as lecithin. A high ratio of phospholipids to triglyceride can accumulate and impair reticulo-endothelial cell function. • Phospholipids for emulsification sourced from egg yolk can be unsafe for egg-allergy sufferers. • A minimum amount of essential fatty acids (linoleic and a-linolenic acids) are required to be delivered to prevent deficiency states. • Lipid peroxidation (from sunlight) can lead to reactive oxygen species generation and requires emulsions to be kept in the dark. Excess vitamin E is added as an antioxidant to counteract this effect. • Hepatic and endothelial toxicity depends on optimal long-/medium-chain triglyceride and w-3-to-w-6 fatty acid ratios. • Separation of the lipid and aqueous components of the emulsion is called 'cracking' and renders the PN unsafe for use.
Carbohydrates	• Glucose is used as the carbohydrate source. • Too much or too rapid glucose infusion can exceed uptake and oxidation ability (especially as enteric incretin secretion is bypassed by parenteral use) and lead to hyperglycaemia or de novo lipogenesis and fatty liver.
Micronutrients	• Micronutrients may be required in small quantities but are essential for a range of enzyme functions. • Some—such as manganese, which is accumulated in the basal ganglia and can lead to movement disorders—are toxic in excess.
Vitamins	• Water-soluble vitamins are rapidly depleted due to lack of stores. • Vitamin D may be lost through interruption of the enterohepatic cycle and be required in high quantities. • Vitamin K is usually omitted from parenteral nutrition in order not to circumvent therapeutic anticoagulation with coumarin derivatives.

around 20% of deaths of patients receiving long-term HPN are attributable to complications of the PN delivery, approximately equally due to liver disease and catheter-related blood stream infections (CRBSIs).

CRBSIs occur at a rate of 0.35–2.27 per 1000 days of PN use and can usually be successfully treated with intravenous antibiotics, often salvaging the line for future use. Line-associated fungaemia carries a particularly high fatality rate. Thrombosis or stenosis of central veins can lead to impaired venous drainage of the limbs or head and create significant challenges for successful line replacement but occurs less frequently than CRBSI.

IFALD may be predominantly cholestatic, steatohepatitic or mixed. The aetiology is multifactorial and relates to the nonphysiological route of delivery and the components of the PN itself. Soy lipid-based emulsions contain phytosterols that lead to cholestasis, whereas glucose excess can lead to de novo lipogenesis and hepatic steatosis. Patients with ultra-short small intestine (less than 20 cm from duodeno-jejunal flexure to stoma) can rapidly progress to liver cirrhosis in as little as 3 years.[6]

Quality of life can be maintained in some cases on HPN; however, it is often impaired through the restrictions imposed on travel, the overnight volume load causing disturbed sleep, as well as the effects of a high stoma output and the psychosocial consequences of reduced meal-related interactions.

FAILURE OF PARENTERAL NUTRITION

PN can be said to have failed when it is unable to maintain fluid or nutrient balance, when intravenous access is no longer possible or safe (as a result of venous thromboses or recurrent infections) or due to the development of liver disease. Under such circumstances, intestinal transplantation should be considered. Postoperative survival rates match those of any solid organ with greater than 80% 5-year survival reported for isolated intestinal grafts (usually transplanted with pancreas, and some colon for fluid absorption). Outcomes are not as good for multivisceral transplant operations (containing stomach and liver in addition), and it is preferable to identify progressive IFALD at an early enough stage to transplant intestine without the additional requirement for a liver graft, as this can result in regression of liver fibrosis and resolution of IFALD.[6] Intestinal transplantation can also improve quality of life where it is significantly impaired as a result of intestinal failure and HPN.

Multiprofessional Working in Nutrition Support

THE NUTRITION SUPPORT TEAM

Patients requiring artificial nutrition support in a hospital setting require the coordinated input of physicians, dietitians and specialist nursing staff. The optimal way to achieve this is with a dedicated NST working together as recommended by the National Institute for Health and Clinical Excellence in its guidance on nutrition support in adults (Clinical Guideline 32).[2]

Introducing an NST has proven benefits in reducing unnecessary nutritional interventions, metabolic and infective complications of nutrition therapy and length of stay. NSTs can reduce inappropriate use of PN and ensure patients with indications for PN are not missed, but also improve individual patient's attainment of adequate energy and protein requirements.

COMPOSITION AND PURPOSE OF THE NUTRITION SUPPORT TEAM

The exact composition of an NST is flexible but must, as a minimum, have a senior clinician with an interest in nutrition (which may be a gastroenterologist, a surgeon, a clinical biochemist or an intensivist), a nutrition support nurse(s), pharmacist and dietitian. Many other specialities and allied health professionals contribute on a more intermittent basis with specific patient groups. Intestinal failure centres must also have good support from surgeons, stoma care nurses, vascular access units, interventional radiologists, microbiologists and psychologists. Details of the individual roles of team members can be found in Table 4.8.

The scope of practice of the NST varies from hospital to hospital; in some they operate in an advisory capacity, with the patients remaining under the primary care of their medical or surgical team.

TABLE 4.8 ■ **Roles and Responsibilities of the Members of the Nutrition Support Team**

Team Member	Clinical Roles	Nonclinical Roles
Nutrition nurse specialist	• Expertise in managing complications related to enteral feeding tubes and venous catheters • Conducts/participates in outpatient care of patients receiving HEN or HPN • Maintains clinical records • Participates in clinical audits • Develops nursing protocols and practice guidelines	• Training of ward nurses in the care of feeding tubes and venous catheters, including aseptic technique • Educating patients in self-care of tubes and lines • Education of all health professionals in good nutrition care • Contributes to decisions regarding procurement
Dietitian	• Carries out a thorough dietary assessment on all patients • Gives individualised advice on diet, supplements, EN or PN, as appropriate • Liaises with housekeepers, catering and procurement to ensure availability of appropriate food and supplements • Conducts/participates in outpatient care	• Contributes to education and training of dietetic students, nursing and medical colleagues
Pharmacist	• Advises on suitability/stability of PN prescriptions • Responsibility for compounding procedures • Makes safe amendments to PN mixtures using aseptic technique • Advises on drug or drug-nutrient interactions, or drug changes for feeding tube administration	• Involved in contracts for PN and EN supplies • Contributes to audit and education
Nutrition consultant (or registrar)	• Assesses the nutritional needs of patients in the context of their comorbid medical/surgical conditions • Assesses patients' suitability for PEG placement • Prescribing responsibility for PN (therefore must be able to review and agree prescriptions)	• Participates in nutrition-based research • Maintains and develops the NST in the context of the Trusts planning and development strategies • Maintains links with endoscopy, vascular access and IR teams
Ward nurses	• Responsible for safe administration of EN and PN for all patients • Promotes good nutritional care for all patients • Communicates nutritional aims and care plans with patient and families	• Ward-based audits of nutrition screening, delivery and complications • Education of junior staff in safe and effective nutrition care

EN, Enteral nutrition; *HEN*, home enteral nutrition; *HPN*, home parenteral nutrition; *IR*, interventional radiology; *NST*, nutrition support team; *PEG*, percutaneous endoscopic gastrostomy; *PN*, parenteral nutrition.

This is suitable in many circumstances, particularly for haemato-oncology patients, trauma patients and others. However, for most surgical and gastroenterology patients receiving PN, it is preferable if the NST forms part of that primary team where they can be responsible for fluid balance, drug prescribing and coordinating discharge of patients. Post discharge, the NST often remains the first contact point for patient queries and will follow up some patients in dedicated clinics.

Members of the NST have a key role in educating others about optimal nutritional care, particularly ward nurses, who provide the majority of inpatient care, and junior doctors about screening, assessment and monitoring. Much of this education is carried out on the ward, at the bedside, but the team often host dedicated study sessions or study days within the hospital.

Nutrition nurses will often train both ward nurses and patients receiving PN in aseptic technique and line care and in the care of gastrostomy and other tubes for patients receiving enteral nutrition. Dietitians have a very important role to play in educating junior doctors regarding nutritional assessment, calculating requirements, monitoring of patients and options of nutritional supplements and enteral feeds available, as these areas are particularly overlooked during medical training.

All members of the NST should educate others and promote excellence in nutritional care, especially screening and assessment, interventions available and monitoring of patients receiving nutritional therapy. Teams can empower other members of staff to take responsibility promoting nutritional awareness in their own clinical area or ward.

MONITORING AND GOVERNANCE

How does the NST demonstrate effectiveness? The team must determine outcome measures which will be monitored and reported to the NHS Foundation Trusts. Such measures may include PEG site infection rates, mortality after PEG insertion, total number of PN days, catheter-associated infections and thromboses, complications of line insertion and metabolic complications including refeeding syndrome.

Regular audits should be carried out, both locally and as part of national initiatives such as the British Association for Parenteral and Enteral Nutrition nutritional care tool.[7] Teams should also actively participate in and promote events to raise awareness of nutritional care, for example, malnutrition awareness week and nutrition screening week.

NUTRITION STEERING COMMITTEE

Members of the NST may sit on the Hospital's Nutrition Steering Committee, but it is critical that this committee also has representation from senior medical and nursing management and catering. The committee has oversight of all aspects of hospital nutrition, including policies and protocols. The majority of patients within a hospital receive oral nutrition, so attention to catering facilities, hygiene, quality control and financial considerations of catering, as well as ensuring access to a wide range of different meals which are nutritionally balanced, are key priorities for the steering committee. Ensuring adherence to national legal requirements, such as the 'Meeting Nutritional and Hydration Needs' regulation of the Health and Social Care Act 2008 in the UK, fall under the remit of the steering committee.

References

1. Stroud M, Duncan H, Nightingale J. Guidelines for enteral feeding in adult hospital patients. *Gut*. 2003;52(Suppl 7):vii1–vii12.
2. NICE clinical guideline 32. Nutrition support for adults: oral nutrition support, enteral tube feeding and parenteral nutrition. 2017. Available at: https://www.nice.org.uk/Guidance/CG32.
3. Pironi L, Arends J, Baxter J, et al. ESPEN endorsed recommendations. Definition and classification of intestinal failure in adults. *Clin Nutr*. 2015;34(2):171–180.

4. Mountford CG, Manas DM, Thompson NP. A practical approach to the management of high-output stoma. *Frontline Gastroenterol.* 2014;5(3):203–207.
5. Nightingale J, Woodward JM, Small B. Nutrition Committee of the British Society of Gastroenterology. Guidelines for management of patients with a short bowel. *Gut.* 2006;55(Suppl 4):iv1–iv12.
6. Woodward JM, Massey D, Sharkey L. The long and short of IT: Intestinal failure-associated liver disease (IFALD) in adults—recommendations for early diagnosis and intestinal transplantation. *Frontline Gastroenterol.* 2020;11(1):34–39.
7. BAPEN (British Association of Parenteral and Enteral Nutrition). Organisation of Nutrition Support in Hospitals. 2018. Available at: https://www.bapen.org.uk/resources-and-education/tools/ofnosh.

SECTION B

Nutrition in Health Care Practice with Case Studies

SECTION OUTLINE

CHAPTER 5

Nutrition in Respiratory Medicine

Pauline Douglas ■ Breanna Lepre ■ Shane McAuliffe

LEARNING POINTS

By the end of this chapter, you should be able to:

- Describe the aetiology and pathogenesis of common chronic and acute respiratory diseases
- Identify clinical features of common chronic and acute respiratory diseases
- Demonstrate awareness of the relationship between diet and nutrition and the development of respiratory diseases
- Describe how respiratory diseases can affect nutritional status
- Describe the role of nutrition in treatment of chronic and acute respiratory diseases
- Describe dietary management strategies for chronic and acute respiratory diseases

CASE STUDY 5.1 Nutrition Support in Noninvasive Ventilation

On day 6 of hospital admission, Terry, a 56-year-old man, was transferred to the high-dependency unit (HDU) at a tertiary centre after a 24-hour period of persistently reduced oxygen saturations (<84%), pH < 7.35 and pCO2 > 6.5 kPa despite optimal medical therapy at ward-level care. The presentation was consistent with acute on chronic type 2 respiratory failure, secondary to an infectious exacerbation of chronic obstructive pulmonary disease (COPD). Admission blood levels indicated elevated inflammatory markers, including a raised C-Reactive Protein (320 mg/L), and White Cell Count of 17.5×10^9/L.

Nutritional assessment was completed on admission to hospital. Initial anthropometric data estimated weight/height (60 kg/1.75 m) provided a body mass index (BMI) of 19.6 kg/m^2. Despite persistence with ward-level nutrition support and oral nutritional supplements (ONS), nutritional intakes were significantly limited for 3 days due to increasing breathlessness and the need for supplemental oxygen. Early dietetic intervention was sought, which estimated that Terry was currently meeting <50% of his nutritional requirements (approximately 1450–1800 kcal/day) orally and as a result had lost 3 kg (4.7% body weight) in the week since his admission. On admission to the HDU, a nutrition specialist nurse facilitated early insertion of fine-bore 8Fr nasogastric (NG) feeding tube which allowed for enteral feeding to commence. This was initiated in a progressive fashion, gradually increasing in volume to meet 25%–50%–75% of nutritional requirements alongside regular use of metoclopramide (10 mg TDS Thrice daily) to reduce the risk of gastric distention and promote gastric emptying. No issues of air leakage, gastrointestinal (GI) disturbance/distention or concerns about the risk of aspiration were encountered during this period.

Time on noninvasive ventilation (NIV) was maximised in the first 24 hours due to persisting hypoxaemia and remained high during the first 2–3 days, allowing little or no time for self-ventilation and in turn limited opportunity for oral nutritional intakes. As per conventional practice, time on NIV was gradually reduced over the following 3–5 days, with increasingly prolonged periods off during the day, while continuing with NIV overnight. As self-ventilation times increased into the second week on HDU, oral intakes were encouraged through the use of low-volume nutritional supplements (approximately 125 mL/300 kcal each) and energy dense snacks, enabling Terry to meet >50% of his nutritional requirements through oral feeding, meaning provision of nutrition via the NG tube was reduced accordingly.

NIV was discontinued completely on day 9 of HDU stay, with normalisation of pH and pCO2 and a general improvement in Terry's condition. He was discharged back to ward-based care with NG still in

Drug doses are as per the British National Formulary.

CASE STUDY 5.1 Nutrition Support in Noninvasive Ventilation—(Continued)

situ but only providing 25% of nutritional requirements via this route. His weight on ward stepdown was 58 kg (BMI 18.9 kg/m^2), where his physical and nutritional rehabilitation was continued with the therapy teams. Overall improvement in his condition and intensive rehab at ward level resulted in discharge 2 weeks later weighing 62 kg, with further follow-up organised for continued nutrition and physical rehabilitation in the community.

Discussion

Malnutrition in respiratory disease is a significant clinical problem leading to increased mortality risk and longer length of hospital stay, meaning consideration of the risk of malnutrition in this patient group should be routine practice. Early Multidisciplinary team (MDT) (dietitian/nutrition specialist nurse) involvement and/or commencement of nutrition support is recommended for patients identified as at nutritional risk.

Patients on NIV often struggle to meet nutritional requirements orally. High levels of systemic inflammation, particularly during acute episodes of disease, are known to contribute to increased energy expenditure, reduced nutritional intakes and weight loss. This ultimately leads to reductions in both functional and physical status.

When nutritional intakes are suboptimal for more than 2 days, artificial nutrition support should be considered with NG feeding being the most readily available option. In most cases, NIV patients who are enterally fed receive significantly more energy and protein than those who receive oral nutrition only. Regular assessment of nutritional adequacy is key to guide such intervention.

Hesitancy to implement NG feeding for those requiring NIV/continuous positive airway pressure (CPAP) exists due to fear of complications such as air leakage, poor GI tolerance and aspiration. Many of these risks can be mitigated through proactive measures including the use of fine-bore feeding tubes and prescription of regular prokinetics. Early intervention with these measures can ensure safety and minimise both respiratory and nutritional compromise in patients requiring multilevel support. These interventions have the potential to be used in a complementary fashion to optimise treatment from both a medical and nutritional standpoint.

Talking Point

Early NG tube placement was a pivotal factor in supporting Terry's nutritional status in this case example. Had early assessment for NG feeding not been considered, it is very possible that tube placement may have been more difficult during a period of high NIV requirements during the first number of days due to the risk of desaturation during self-ventilation. Consequently, few opportunities for oral nutrition support would have been made possible during this period, following an already poor baseline and weight loss before HDU admission, placing Terry at further risk for nutritional and physical deconditioning. Conversely, early assessment, MDT involvement and action meant that this risk was mitigated, and instead, weight was stabilised during the acute phase of illness. This helped to facilitate early rehabilitation upon ward stepdown and ultimately improvement in physical condition on discharge back to the community.

Overview and Introduction

THE RESPIRATORY SYSTEM

The structure of the respiratory system includes the nose, pharynx, larynx, trachea and lungs, which contain bronchi, bronchioles and alveoli. These are supported by the skeleton, diaphragm and abdominal and intercostal muscles.

The primary function of the respiratory system is gas exchange. This ensures adequate provision of oxygen to all body tissues, which is vital for metabolic function. This also requires the removal of waste products produced as a result of these processes, such as carbon dioxide. These functions work in tandem to maintain blood acid-alkaline balance (pH).

The respiratory system also plays a role in immune function. Inspired air contains microorganisms and other particles which are potentially harmful to both the respiratory system and the body at large. Protective mechanisms include elements physical (mucous, cilia), chemical (surfactant), innate and adaptive immunity (phagocytosis).

WHAT IS RESPIRATORY DISEASE?

Respiratory disease can generally be classified as *acute*, for example, acute respiratory distress syndrome (ARDS) and anaphylaxis, or *chronic*. Chronic respiratory disease encompasses a number of subclasses including:

- *Obstructive lung disease*, characterized by airway obstruction, for example, chronic obstructive pulmonary disease (COPD) and asthma
- *Restrictive lung disease*, characterized by reduced lung volumes, for example, sarcoidosis and pulmonary fibrosis
- *Pulmonary vascular disease*, affecting the blood vessels leading to or from the lungs, characterised by shortness of breath, for example, pulmonary hypertension (PH)
- *Infectious respiratory disease*, disease caused by germs (i.e., viruses, bacteria or other pathogenic microbes), for example, tuberculosis (TB)
- *Genetic lung disease*, inherited disease, for example, cystic fibrosis (CF)
- *Lung cancer*, the uncontrolled growth of abnormal cells in one or both lungs (see Chapter 11: 'Nutrition in Haematology and Oncology'.)

SYMPTOMS AND DIAGNOSTIC MARKERS OF RESPIRATORY DISEASE

As clinical presentation can be highly variable, a comprehensive approach to history taking, including time course, nature and severity of individual symptoms and analysis of diagnostic markers, is an important factor in determining the cause, prognosis and appropriate treatment of respiratory disease. Clinical features of respiratory disease include dyspnoea, chest pain, wheeze, cough and associated sputum production and colour.[1]

NUTRITION AND RISK OF RESPIRATORY DISEASE

Adequate nutrition is required for optimal development and function of the lungs and respiratory system.[2] Nutritional status has an effect on the formation of lung structure, respiratory muscle mass and immune function. Diet and nutrition can be considered important modifiable risk factors for the development, progression and management of respiratory diseases such as asthma and COPD.[2] Although pharmacological management remains the mainstay for the treatment of respiratory diseases, dietary intervention could be an important adjuvant therapy for disease management, as well as a consideration for the prevention of disease.[2] Conversely, respiratory disease places strain on nutritional status.[2] Key to this relationship is an increase in energy expenditure and therefore increased energy and protein requirements. The combined effects of breathing difficulty, inflammation and related medications are also likely to negatively impact on nutritional intakes.[2,3] These factors combined often contribute to the depletion of body mass, which is correlated with disease progression and worse prognosis.[3,4]

The Mediterranean diet, a dietary pattern typically characterised by a high consumption of fruits, vegetables, nuts, grains and olive oil and moderate consumption of fish, seafood and dairy and low to moderate alcohol intake, has been shown to have a protective effect for allergic respiratory diseases.[2,5] Adequate fruit and vegetable intake has been shown to exert beneficial effects in association with risk of respiratory disease due to their favourable nutrient profile, consisting of antioxidants, vitamins, minerals, dietary fibre and phytochemicals.[2,6–8] Conversely, a 'Western' dietary pattern, characterised by high intake of refined grains, processed and red meat, desserts and sweets and high-fat dairy products, has been associated with increased risk of asthma exacerbation and COPD.[9–11] Overnutrition and resulting overweight and obesity are associated with an increased risk of respiratory disease, in particular asthma.[12–14]

Acute Respiratory Disease

AETIOLOGY, PATHOGENESIS AND CLINICAL FEATURES OF ACUTE RESPIRATORY DISEASE

Acute respiratory failure can be considered as an 'acute impairment in gas exchange between the lungs and the blood causing hypoxia with or without hypercapnia'.[15] This can be caused by both acute illness, such as infectious respiratory conditions, and/or an acute decompensation of chronic respiratory diseases (such as COPD). Hypoxic respiratory failure (type 1 respiratory failure) is hypoxia without hypercapnia and results from an inability of the respiratory system to provide sufficient alveolar ventilation to maintain a normal arterial partial pressure of oxygen.[16] Hypercapnic respiratory failure (type 2 respiratory failure) results from an inability of the respiratory system to provide sufficient alveolar ventilation to maintain a normal arterial pressure of carbon dioxide (pCO_2).[16] This can often coexist alongside hypoxia.

Management of acute respiratory failure involves first ensuring that the upper airway is patent and clear of obstructions. Supplemental oxygenation and ventilatory support are likely to be required, with immediate attention to the underlying cause or causes for respiratory failure.[15] Noninvasive ventilation (NIV) in the management of patients with respiratory failure reduces the work of breathing and may prevent further deterioration of the respiratory status, reducing the need for sedation and conventional mechanical ventilation.[17] When further compromise of respiratory function results, this often requires ventilatory support and admission to the intensive care unit (ICU).

NUTRITIONAL MANAGEMENT OF ACUTE RESPIRATORY DISEASE

During exacerbations of respiratory disease, pulmonary function can be impaired to a level that negatively impacts an individual's ability to achieve their nutritional requirements.[18] Patients requiring NIV often struggle to meet their nutritional requirements orally.[19] Poor nutritional status is associated with increased hospital length of stay, higher need for invasive ventilation and increased mortality in patients undergoing NIV.[20] In patients requiring ventilatory support in the ICU, malnutrition is characterised by weight loss, muscle wasting, sarcopenia and metabolic dysregulation, all of which are known to worsen clinical outcomes and result in physical debilitation and decreased quality of life.[21]

Early multidisciplinary team involvement and/or commencement of nutrition support is recommended for patients identified at nutritional risk. Food and oral nutritional supplements (ONS) should always be used initially in an aim to meet nutritional requirements.

In the case of patients on NIV, the risk of rapid desaturation increases, and nutritional requirements become more difficult to meet orally. When intakes are suboptimal for more than 2 days, early artificial nutrition support via nasogastric (NG) feeding should be considered. These issues have become increasingly prudent during the course of the COVID-19 pandemic.[22] Early involvement of a registered dietitian for regular assessment of nutritional status and calculation of feeding requirements and formulation is advised. NG feeding for patient's requiring NIV/continuous positive airway pressure (CPAP) can be perceived as unsafe due to possible risks, including air leakage (breaking the seal) and gastrointestinal (GI) disturbance/distention and concerns about the risk of aspiration.[23] This results in high levels of underfeeding in this patient group.[23] In such cases, a number of measures can be taken to minimise risk in these patients, including the use of fine-bore (8Fr) feeding tubes, early use of prokinetics (metoclopramide, erythromycin) and measurement of gastric aspirates to indicate feed tolerance.[22] In cases of poor tolerance, post pyloric feeding or parenteral nutrition may be considered.

In ARDS requiring ICU admission, nutritional goals aim to ensure adequate provision to counteract the detrimental effects (increased energy deficit, catabolism and sarcopenia) of critical illness on nutritional status. According to the recommendations of the European Society of

Intensive Care Medicine, early enteral nutrition should be initiated within 48 hours in patients in whom oral intake is not possible.[24] Early enteral nutrition is associated with benefits including maintenance of GI function and modulation of immune response. Enteral feeding in critical illness is subject to a number of challenges, which can be secondary to the impact of polypharmacy.

Proning refers to the adjustment of a patient from a supine (lying back down) into the prone (lying face/chest down), as a means of improving ventilation in patients with ARDS.[25] There is limited evidence evaluating the safety and tolerability of enteral nutrition delivered to patients in a prone position. Existing literature suggests that enteral nutrition provided to patients does not appear to increase the risk for aspiration, vomiting or additional GI symptoms. Feed tolerance can be monitored through measurement of gastric residual volumes and persistent intolerance of feed may require postpyloric feeding.[24] Parenteral nutrition should be considered when enteral and oral feeding are unsuccessful, especially in those with preexisting malnutrition.

NUTRITION AND PREVENTION OF ACUTE RESPIRATORY DISEASE

Emerging Therapies (Micronutrients)

Emerging evidence suggests a role for micronutrients in maintaining and improving immune function through a number of mechanisms.[26,27] Deficiency of these nutrients suppresses immune function and increases our susceptibility to infection, where key nutrients of concern have previously been associated with infectious and respiratory diseases.[26,27] Strongest evidence of effect is demonstrated through correction of suboptimal status in individual micronutrients, demonstrating the importance of screening and treating insufficiency and/or deficiency in routine practice:

- Vitamin C has demonstrated effectiveness in both prevention and treatment of respiratory tract infections, reducing incidence and duration of upper respiratory tract infection and common cold and severity of pneumonia in hospitalised older adults.[28,29] High-dose vitamin C has been suggested as an adjunctive therapy to support the immune system during ARDS; however, this has not been confirmed by recent trial evidence.[30]
- Observational data have suggested a long-standing association between vitamin D status and the incidence of respiratory tract infections.[31] The role of vitamin D in mediating viral inflammation of the respiratory tract is particularly relevant in acute respiratory infection leading to critical illness,[32] and its relevance in viral susceptibility has also been questioned.[33]
- Fish oils rich in omega-3 fatty acids possess antiinflammatory properties.[26] This has led to interest in a potential role for mediating the severe inflammatory response to acute respiratory disease and critical illness, having previously been associated with favourable outcomes in ARDS.[34]
- Particular interest in a potential role for vitamin D in mediating risk of COVID-19 infection has been evident across health care practice, public health policy and science research during the course of the pandemic.[33,35,36] Consideration of the role of micronutrient status in COVID-19 risk and recovery may also warrant further investigation.[26,27,37]

Chronic Obstructive Respiratory Diseases

CHRONIC OBSTRUCTIVE PULMONARY DISEASE

Aetiology, Pathogenesis and Clinical Features of Chronic Obstructive Respiratory Disease

The Global Burden of Disease Study reported a prevalence of 251 million cases of COPD globally in 2016.[38] COPD is a common condition which is frequently associated with malnutrition.[3,4,39]

COPD is characterised by airflow obstruction and an abnormal inflammatory response in the lungs.[40] The aetiology of COPD therefore requires an inflammatory insult to the lung, often long-term exposure to noxious particles and gases, particularly cigarette smoke. Cigarette smokers who develop COPD have an enhanced or abnormal response to inhaling toxic agents, which may result in mucous hypersecretion (chronic bronchitis), tissue destruction (emphysema) and disruption of normal repair and defence mechanisms resulting in small airway inflammation and fibrosis (bronchiolitis).[40] These pathological changes result in the characteristic features of COPD, such as an increased resistance to airflow in the small conducting airways, increased compliance of the lungs, air trapping and progressive airflow obstruction. Other processes involved in the pathogenesis of COPD are an imbalance between proteases and antiproteases and an imbalance between oxidants and antioxidants (oxidative stress) in the lungs.[40]

Nutritional Management of Chronic Obstructive Respiratory Disease

Weight loss, low body weight and muscle wasting are common in patients with COPD and are associated with reduced functional capacity, increased risk of exacerbation and mortality.[3,39] Risk of malnutrition is highest among those in the most severe stage of COPD.[3] The causes of undernutrition and resulting malnutrition in COPD are multifactorial including reduced energy intake due to poor appetite and dyspnoea while eating, inactivity and systemic inflammation.[3,39] Resting energy expenditure is also significantly higher in patients with COPD due to increased work of breathing and systemic inflammation, a hallmark of the disease.[3] For malnutrition to be successfully managed in COPD, each of these factors should be considered.[3]

Many patients with COPD are unlikely to meet their daily requirements for energy and nutrients.[41] Routine nutritional risk screening with a validated screening tool should be performed for all COPD patients across all settings. Nutrition screening tools, such as the Malnutrition Universal Screening Tool (see Chapter 2), which considers BMI as well as unintentional weight loss, have been validated in a COPD context. In light of the high mortality risk associated in malnourished patients with COPD, nutritional supplementation is indicated when BMI is below 20 kg/m^2 but may also be considered in patients with a BMI above this when involuntary weight loss (>5%) is progressive in the preceding 6 months (high risk of malnutrition). Nutritional support, by means of ONS, or enteral tube feeding has been shown to promote weight gain and increase fat free mass, grip strength and exercise tolerance and overall improve quality of life for patients with COPD.[41–43] All of these may be goals of intervention, although goals need to be adjusted according to phase of disease and be patient centred and realistic, for example, in palliative care or advanced illness, goals may include slowing rate of weight loss and improving quality of life. ONS can be prescribed as divided doses throughout the day to prevent early satiety, abdominal distension and a reduction in exercise tolerance, associated with a large supplemental load in patients with COPD.[42] If goals are not met or there is limited progress, check ONS compliance and amend the prescription as necessary (e.g., preference of flavours prescribed), consider goals of intervention and monitor thereafter every 3 months or sooner if there is clinical concern.

A combination of ONS and exercise or anabolic stimulus has been shown to achieve significant functional improvement and decreased mortality.[43] A multimodal approach, such as ONS as an integrated component of a pulmonary rehabilitation programme that includes exercise, is likely to be more effective than individual interventions in the accrual of lean tissue and subsequent improvements in functional capacity and health-related quality of life.[43] Branched chain amino acid supplementation in COPD has also been associated with increases in whole-body protein synthesis, body weight, fat-free mass and arterial blood oxygen levels.[44–46]

Nutrition and Prevention of Chronic Obstructive Respiratory Disease

Tobacco smoke, as well as environmental pollutants, infections, physical activity and nutritional status, play a role in the development and progression of COPD.[47] Diet is a modifiable risk factor for the development and progression of COPD and other chronic respiratory diseases.[2] A good diet can help to maintain good health and a healthy BMI, while visceral adiposity and poor dietary quality may increase risk of developing COPD.[47] Consumption of fruits and vegetables is associated with reduced COPD incidence in both current and ex-smokers, but not in individuals who have never smoked.[48] A recent systematic review and meta-analysis suggests that healthy dietary patterns, defined as those with high consumption of fruit, vegetables, beans and green vegetables, whole grains, dairy, seafood and plant proteins and fatty acids, coupled with low consumption of refined grains and sodium are associated with a lower prevalence of COPD, while unhealthy dietary patterns are not.[49]

ASTHMA

Aetiology, Pathogenesis and Clinical Features of Asthma

Asthma is the most common chronic disease among children worldwide. Worldwide, more than 339 million people are living with asthma.[50] The pathophysiology of asthma as a chronic respiratory disease involves airway inflammation, airflow obstruction and bronchial hyperresponsiveness. Asthma comprises a range of heterogeneous phenotypes that differ in presentation, aetiology and pathophysiology.[51] While clinical presentation may vary between patients with asthma, it is generally marked by recurrent episodes of wheezing, cough, dyspnea and chest tightness.[50,51] Risk factors for the development of asthma include genetic, environmental and host factors. Inhaled allergens, smoke exposure, indoor and outdoor air pollution are common triggers of asthma symptoms.[51]

Nutritional Management of Asthma

Chronic inflammation of the airways is a key characteristic of asthma and may be modulated by dietary intake. Higher fat intake and low fibre intake, characteristic of the Western diet, has been associated with increased eosinophilic airway inflammation.[52] Conversely, a reduction of dietary saturated fat intake was associated with a reduction in neutrophilic airway inflammation in overweight and obese asthmatics.[53] Fruits and vegetables and their antioxidants may lower airway inflammation and intake of fruits and vegetables was inversely associated with interleukin-8 protein in nasal lavage of asthmatic children.[54] In asthmatic adults, intake of tomato juice, which is rich in the antioxidant lycopene, reduced airway neutrophil influx and sputum neutrophil elastase activity after 1 week of supplementation.[55] Furthermore, in a randomised controlled trial with adults with asthma, a high fruit and vegetable intake (defined as greater than five servings of vegetables and two servings of fruit daily for 14 weeks) led to improvements in lung function, namely FEV_1 Forced Expiratory Volume and FVC Forced Vital Capacity.[7] The Global Initiative for Asthma recommends a healthy diet rich in fruits and vegetables for general health and weight management and as a nonpharmacological asthma intervention.[56]

Obesity in asthmatic patients has a relationship with symptom control, pulmonary function and quality of life.[57] Obese asthmatics have a distinct phenotype with a unique pathophysiology characterised by low eosinophilic inflammation and low allergen sensitisation.[58] Weight loss can improve respiratory symptoms in overweight asthmatic patients.[59] Conversely, an observational study in Japan reported that underweight subjects with asthma had poorer asthma control than subjects who were a normal weight.[60]

Nutrition and Prevention of Asthma

The influence of diet on asthma outcomes has emerged relatively recently, with dietary factors showing the potential to be directly involved in asthma pathogenesis. The literature examines the effect of both individual nutrients and whole dietary patterns on asthma risk and progression. Two commonly investigated dietary patterns are the Mediterranean diet and the Western diet.[52]

Prevention of Asthma During Pregnancy

Asthma susceptibility is likely determined early in life for many patients, and in utero exposures including maternal obesity can influence childhood respiratory disease risk.[61,62] The World

Health Organization emphasises the value of breastfeeding for infant health generally, and any duration of breastfeeding was inversely associated with asthma in children when compared with no breastfeeding.[63] Cross-sectional studies have shown a protective effect of the Mediterranean diet during pregnancy on infant wheeze in the first year of life and asthma development in childhood.[64,65] However, in two prospective cohort studies, the Mediterranean diet was not associated with a reduced risk of wheeze in the first year of life, at 1.5 years or at 4 years of age.[66,67] Intake of vitamins D and E during pregnancy has been associated with a reduction in childhood wheeze, although no effect of vitamin D or E on risk of childhood asthma has been found.[68–71] Fish oil supplementation during pregnancy has been shown to decrease wheeze or asthma in childhood, and this protection appears to be maintained into adulthood.[72–74] In contrast, in cross-sectional studies, fast-food consumption at least three times a week during pregnancy increased the odds of childhood wheeze when compared with a consumption of fast food less than once a week.[65,75]

Prevention of Asthma in Children

The Mediterranean diet, which emphasises a high intake of fruit, vegetables, whole grains and seafood, has been associated with a reduced risk of asthma in children.[76] Furthermore, intake of polyunsaturated fatty acids, particularly long-chain n-3 fatty acids, found primarily in seafood is inversely associated with asthma and/or recurrent wheeze and atopy in preschool children.[77] A Western dietary pattern, typically high in fat and processed foods, has been shown to increase the risk of asthma or wheeze in childhood.[78,79] Two studies have found an association between sugar-containing beverages (fruit drinks and soda), often consumed as part of the typical Western diet, and asthma.[80,81]

Prevention of Asthma in Adults

While evidence is low, fruit and vegetable consumption appears to decrease asthma risk in adults.[82,83] Evidence suggests that a higher intake of vitamin D and dietary antioxidants, such as those found in fruits and vegetables, also have a protective effect against asthma risk,[84] while sugar-sweetened beverage intake at least two times per day was associated with adult asthma.[85–87]

OBSTRUCTIVE SLEEP APNOEA

Aetiology, Pathogenesis and Clinical Features of Obstructive Sleep Apnoea

Obstructive sleep apnoea (OSA) is a clinical respiratory disorder marked by repeated episodes of partial or complete obstruction of the upper airway (pharynx) during sleep, typically accompanied by loud snoring and resulting in intermittent hypoxia. Close to 1 billion are affected by OSA globally,[88] and it is increasingly being recognised as a cause of cardiovascular mortality.[89,90]

Nutritional Management of Obstructive Sleep Apnoea

CPAP treatment is typically first line, is safe and effective, reduces sleepiness and improves quality of life; however, diet is also vital in clinical management of OSA. Dietary manipulation of macronutrient distribution, particularly low-carbohydrate dietary approaches, and a reduction in energy (calorie) intake have demonstrated effectiveness in decreasing the severity of OSA.[91] The Mediterranean diet, rich in fruits, vegetables and whole grains, can assist with weight reduction and has been shown to be beneficial in OSA.[90] Conversely, high fat intake is associated with daytime sleepiness and apnea-hyponea index and high alcohol intake is related to severity of OSA.[92,93] Dietary sodium restriction may be beneficial in the management of OSA in patients with comorbidities that result in fluid retention, for example, resistant hypertension.[91]

Nutrition and Prevention of Obstructive Sleep Apnoea

Obesity is the major risk factor for OSA and many bidirectional comorbidities of OSA, such as type 2 diabetes and hyperlipidaemia, have nutrition-related aetiology.[94] General advice around healthy eating and increased physical activity may assist in weight regulation, important for the prevention of OSA.

Chronic Restrictive Respiratory Diseases

PULMONARY FIBROSIS

Aetiology, Pathogenesis and Clinical Features of Pulmonary Fibrosis

Pulmonary fibrosis is a rare progressive lung disease that causes the tissue surrounding the air sacs or alveoli in the lungs to become thickened and scarred, known as fibrosis. This scarring makes it increasingly difficult to breath and halts the efficient delivery of oxygen into the bloodstream, leading to respiratory insufficiency. The most common form of pulmonary fibrosis is idiopathic pulmonary fibrosis (IPF), characterised symptomatically by exertional dyspnoea.[95] Other clinical features of pulmonary fibrosis include a dry cough, fatigue and unintentional weight loss.[95] Despite the advent of new antifibrotic treatments, such as nintedanib and pirfenidone, the prognosis of IPF remains poor.

Nutritional Management of Pulmonary Fibrosis

In pulmonary fibrosis, increased respiratory muscles load, release of inflammation mediators, GI adverse events induced by antifibrotic drugs, the coexistence of hypoxemia and physical inactivity may have an adverse impact on nutrition intake and subsequent nutritional status.[96] Malnutrition is common in patients with IPF, and body weight loss, lower BMI and vitamin D deficiency have a negative prognostic significance.[95–97] Fat-free mass is also a significant independent predictor of survival in patients with IPF.[98] Nutritional status and risk of malnutrition should be assessed by evaluating nutrient intake, energy expenditure and body functions and through anthropometric parameters and assessment of body composition, such as BMI, Malnutrition Universal Screening Tool, and/or hand grip strength accompanied with biochemical and micronutrient levels, in particular vitamin D status. A recent study showed that patients with IPF exhibited low serum vitamin D concentrations, and vitamin D deficiency correlated with all-cause mortality.[99]

Goals for nutrition intervention in pulmonary fibrosis may include to attain a healthy body weight, maintain lean body mass and manage nutrition-related symptoms of antifibrotic drugs. To meet increased energy and protein requirements associated with pulmonary fibrosis, nutrition support, such as ONS, is indicated for malnourished patients with pulmonary fibrosis. Nutrition support can favourably impact the development of complications and modulations of the immune response and result in improved clinical outcomes for IPF.[100–102] Adequate clinical management of GI complications induced by antifibrotic drugs, such as diarrhoea, makes drug treatments more feasible. Management of antifibrotic drug-induced diarrhoea may involve dietary recommendations to reduce intake of foods that are high in fat and fibre, milk and other dairy products (as lactase deficiency may be induced by mucosal injury) and gut irritants such as spicy foods, alcohol and caffeine-containing products, while ensuring adequate hydration status.[103]

Nutrition and the Prevention of Pulmonary Fibrosis

Risk factors associated with pulmonary fibrosis might include smoking, environmental exposures, gastroesophageal reflux disease, commonly prescribed drugs, diabetes mellitus, infectious agents and genetic factors.

Cardiovascular comorbidities, particularly coronary artery disease and arrhythmias, have been frequently observed in patients with IPF and may increase mortality risk.[104] Risk factors for cardiovascular diseases in IPF patients may include unhealthy lifestyles and a poor diet, such as low physical activity level, dyslipidaemia, metabolic syndrome, systemic hypertension and a history of smoking.[105] In Japan, consumption of fruit has been associated with a reduced risk of IPF, while intake of meat and saturated fatty acids was associated with an increased risk.[106,107] A recent study found that vitamin D prevents experimental lung fibrosis and predicts survival in patients with IPF.[99]

PULMONARY SARCOIDOSIS

Aetiology, Pathogenesis and Clinical Features of Pulmonary Sarcoidosis

Pulmonary sarcoidosis is a multisystem granulomatous disease of unknown aetiology. Pulmonary sarcoidosis is characterised by the growth of collections of inflammatory cells (granulomas) in the lungs. Generally, there are three different classes of clinical presentation: asymptomatic sarcoidosis, nonspecific constitutional symptoms and symptoms related to specific organ involvement.[108]

Management of Pulmonary Sarcoidosis

Treatment of sarcoidosis is dependent on stage and severity of disease and is generally limited to the symptomatic patient. Glucocorticosteroids are used in pulmonary sarcoidosis to reduce symptoms and minimise long-term damage. For some patients, topical therapy, such as fluorinated steroid creams, corticosteroid injections for skin lesions or steroid-containing eye drops, are sufficient to control the disease. For pulmonary patients who present with a cough, inhaled corticosteroids may be sufficient for symptom control. A variety of chemokines and cytokines have been associated with the granulomatous response in sarcoidosis, including tumour necrosis factor α.[108] Biologic agents capable of blocking tumuor necrosis factor are effective in treating some patients as third-line treatment for pulmonary sarcoidosis.[108]

Nutritional Management of Pulmonary Sarcoidosis

Osteoporosis is a potential complication in patients who are treated with corticosteroids. Sarcoidosis is known to induce hypercalciuria and hypercalcaemia due to increased endogenous vitamin D production. UK guidelines on the management of glucocorticoid-induced osteoporosis advise measurement of bone mineral density to assess fracture risk in patients with a history of exposure to, or intention to treat with, oral corticosteroids for 3 months or more.[109] The American College of Rheumatology recommends calcium and vitamin D supplementation (1500 mg/d and 800 IU/d, respectively), along with bisphosphonates, which has demonstrated potential to reverse steroid-induced osteoporosis in patients with sarcoidosis.[108,110] Management may be accompanied by general advice around healthy eating, physical activity and smoking cessation.

Chronic Vascular Respiratory Diseases

PULMONARY HYPERTENSION

Aetiology, Pathogenesis and Clinical Features of Pulmonary Hypertension

PH is a chronic vascular respiratory disease defined as an elevated mean pulmonary artery pressure of $\geq$25 mm Hg at rest, resulting in progressive right heart failure and eventually death. Patients with PH typically present with exertional dyspnea and fatigue that progresses over time. Irrespective of cause, the presence of PH is associated with poor prognosis. PH is classified into five groups according to their pathophysiological mechanisms, clinical presentation, haemodynamic characteristics and treatment:

- Pulmonary arterial hypertension, further classified into idiopathic, familial, associated with other disorders or infections, or resulting from drug or toxin exposure
- PH as a result of left-sided heart disease
- PH as a result of lung disease
- PH as a result of chronic blood clots
- PH as a result of other health conditions, such as inflammatory conditions (e.g., sarcoidosis), metabolic disorders (e.g., glycogen storage disease), blood disorders (e.g., thrombocythemia) or kidney disease.

Nutritional Management of Pulmonary Hypertension

The initial approach to treatment might include physical activity within symptom limits and supervised rehabilitation.[111] Goals of nutrition therapy in patients with PH might include to attain a healthy weight and maintain lean body mass. Nutritional management of PH might include sodium, fluid and alcohol restriction and dietary recommendations to increase consumption of vegetables and fruits, whole grains, fibre, fish, nuts and olive oil and reduce consumption of red meat and low-fat dairy products.[111,112]

With regard to micronutrient status, vitamin D deficiency is frequently seen in patients diagnosed with PH, and low serum levels of 25(OH)D are associated with severity of PH.[113] Vitamin D supplementation in rats with PH improved survival, suggesting that vitamin D deficiency might accelerate right ventricular hypertrophy.[113] Iron deficiency and anaemia have also been linked to the clinical course of PH.[114,115] Current treatment guidelines suggest regular assessment of iron status and iron supplementation for patients with iron deficiency.[114,115] Some studies suggest that oral iron absorption may be impaired in patients with PH, so intravenous iron administration may be preferable; however, controlled trials are lacking.[114,115]

Chronic Infective Respiratory Diseases

TUBERCULOSIS

Aetiology, Pathogenesis and Clinical Features of Tuberculosis

TB is an infectious, contagious respiratory disease caused by *Mycobacterium tuberculosis* and spreads through air. TB is one of the top 10 causes of death and the leading cause from a single infectious agent. Globally, a total of 1.4 million people died from TB in 2019.[116] There are two types of TB: latent and active TB. Patients with latent TB (meaning they do not have the active TB disease) can be treated using preventive therapy, which usually involves a daily dose of the antibiotic isoniazid (isonicotinic acid hydrazide) for 6 to 9 months.[116] Clinical features of active pulmonary TB include cough with sputum and blood at times, chest pains, weakness, weight loss, fever and night sweats. The use of rapid molecular diagnostic tests, such as Xpert MTB/RIF, Xpert Ultra and Truenat assays, are recommended as the initial diagnostic test in all persons who present with signs and symptoms of TB.[116] Treatment of active, drug-susceptible pulmonary TB is highly effective. The most common treatment for active TB is isoniazid (isonicotinic acid hydrazide or isonicotinic acid hydrazide) in combination with rifampin, pyrazinamide and ethambutol. However, despite microbiologic cure, up to half of TB survivors have some form of persistent pulmonary dysfunction, which can increase the risk of death from respiratory causes.[116]

Nutritional Management of Tuberculosis

All individuals with active TB should receive an assessment of their nutritional status and appropriate nutrition counselling at diagnosis and throughout treatment, based on their nutritional status. Many individuals with active TB present in a catabolic state and may show signs of weight loss and vitamin and mineral deficiencies at diagnosis.[117,118] Low BMI (less than 18.5 kg/m^2) and lack of adequate weight gain with TB treatment are associated with an increased risk of mortality and TB relapse.[117,118] Goals of nutritional management of TB include meeting increased energy requirements, attaining an appropriate weight (or weight-for-height in children) and ensuring adequate micronutrient status. Nutrition support, such as fortified foods and/or oral nutrition supplements, may assist in meeting increased energy requirements and improve outcome in TB patients.[118] One randomized controlled trial found that a combination of nutrition counselling and the provision of nutrition supplements in the initial phase of TB treatment produced a significant increase in body weight, total lean mass and physical functions after 6 weeks.[119] Low circulating concentrations of micronutrients, such as vitamins A, E and D and the minerals iron, zinc and selenium, have been reported from cohorts of patients with recently diagnosed active TB. Efforts should be made to ensure that patients with TB receive the recommended intake of micronutrients, preferably through food or fortified foods. If it is not possible to meet requirements through diet alone, micronutrient supplementation at 1× the recommended nutrient intake is indicated.[117] In accordance with World Health Organization's recommendations, all pregnant and lactating women with active TB should take micronutrient supplements that contain iron, folic acid and other vitamins and minerals to complement maternal micronutrient needs.[117] For pregnant women with active TB in settings where calcium intake is typically low, calcium supplementation is recommended for the prevention of preeclampsia.[117]

Nutrition and the Prevention of Tuberculosis

There is a bidirectional causal association between active TB and malnutrition.[120] TB can lead to malnutrition due to increased metabolic demands, reduced food intake and nutrient losses from vomiting and diarrhoea, and malnutrition weakens immunity, increasing the risk of developing active TB by 6 to 10 times.[117,118,121] Furthermore, poverty and food insecurity contribute to the prevalence of TB, and those involved in TB care must recognise and attempt to address these wider socioeconomic issues.[117]

Chronic Genetic Respiratory Diseases

CYSTIC FIBROSIS

Aetiology, Pathogenesis and Clinical Features of Cystic Fibrosis

CF is a genetic respiratory disease, caused by a mutation in the CF transmembrane conductance regulator *(CFTR)* gene. The CFTR protein produced by this gene regulates the movement of chloride and sodium ions across the epithelial cell membranes. When mutations occur in one or both copies of the *CFTR* gene, ion transport is defective, and results in a build-up of thick mucus through the body, leading to respiratory insufficiency.[122] CF is characterised by a progressive decline in pulmonary function secondary to chronic lung infections, exocrine pancreatic insufficiency, liver disease and growth impairment.[122]

Nutritional Management of Cystic Fibrosis

In CF, the destruction of acinar pancreatic tissue, pancreatic ductular obstruction and lack of enzymatic activity lead to malabsorption (particularly of fats), diarrhoea and failure to thrive.[123] Other factors, such as pancreatic insufficiency, chronic malabsorption, recurrent sinopulmonary infections, chronic inflammation, increased energy expenditure and suboptimal intake, contribute to impaired nutritional status in CF patients.[123] Conversely, nutritional status plays a key role in the progression of CF.[123] Effort must be made to ensure an adequate energy intake in patients with CF.

Nutrition management for CF includes the use of pancreatic enzyme replacement therapy and aggressive nutrition support to meet increased requirements for energy and protein.[124] All patients who demonstrate pancreatic insufficiency, by fat balance studies and/or indirect pancreatic function tests such as faecal elastase or chymotrypsin, require pancreatic enzyme supplements.[124] While pancreatic enzyme replacement therapy (PERT) is indicated in the management of CF, there are physiological and pathological variables which may make PERT inefficient, from variation in gastric emptying to variation in the enzyme content of supplements between batches and with time in storage. The amount needed may depend on the contents of the meal, and therefore patient education around PERT is suggested.

Energy requirements in people with CF are estimated to be between 120% and 150% of normal requirements.[123] Nutrition support may be oral, enteral or, rarely, parenteral. Oral nutrition supplements are most effective when administered at earliest presentation of nutritional decline and can assist with meeting increased energy needs, particularly when appetite is poor. In the case of newly diagnosed infants, whereby maintenance of growth velocity is a priority, continuation of breast feeding is strongly recommended.[125] Human breast milk provides key amino acids and essential fatty acids and contains lipase and amylase, which may mitigate diminished pancreatic secretion. Furthermore, immunoglobulins, lactoferrin, epidermal growth factor and lysozyme protect against infection and taurine in human breast milk is necessary for bile acid synthesis and may enhance fat absorption.[125]

A deficiency of specific nutrients including fat-soluble vitamins (particularly A, E and K), essential fatty acids and some minerals may occur in patients with CF.[124] Liver disease increases the likelihood of vitamin D deficiency, and vitamin E requirements are increased by oxidative stress which is a hallmark of chronic respiratory infection. Low vitamin E levels may reflect impaired secretion of the antioxidant glutathione due to a defective *CFTR* channel. As a result, free oxygen radicals are not quenched, and lipid peroxidation of the long-chain fatty acids in the cell membrane occurs, leading to fatty acid imbalances. A high-energy diet with unrestricted fat and supplementation with fat-soluble vitamins can help to optimise growth in infants and children and prevent nutrition deficiencies in patients with CF with pancreatic insufficiency.[126] Nutritional status should be regularly reviewed and monitored closely to anticipate and swiftly address any issues that may arise.

References

1. Leach RM. Symptoms and signs of respiratory disease. *Medicine*. 2008;36(3):P119–P125. https://doi.org/10.1016/j.mpmed.2007.12.003.
2. Berthon BS, Wood LG. Nutrition and respiratory health—feature review. *Nutrients*. 2015;7(3):1618–1643. https://doi.org/10.3390/nu7031618.
3. Mete B, Pehlivan E, Gulbas G, et al. Prevalence of malnutrition in COPD and its relationship with the parameters related to disease severity. *Int J Chron Obstruct Pulmon Dis*. 2018;13:3307–3312. https://doi.org/10.2147/COPD.S179609.
4. Yilmaz D, Capan N, Canbakan S, et al. Dietary intake of patients with moderate to severe COPD in relation to fat-free mass index: A cross-sectional study. *Nutr J*. 2015;10(14):35. https://doi.org/10.1186/s12937-015-0020-5.
5. Willett WC, Sacks F, Trichopoulou A, et al. Mediterranean diet pyramid: A cultural model for healthy eating. *Am J Clin Nutr*. 1995;61:1402S–1406S.
6. Saadeh D, Salameh P, Baldi I, et al. Diet and allergic diseases among population aged 0 to 18 years: Myth or reality? *Nutrients*. 2013;5:3399–3432.
7. Wood LG, Garg ML, Smart JM, et al. Manipulating antioxidant intake in asthma: A randomized controlled trial. *Am J Clin Nutr*. 2012;96:534–543.
8. Hosseini B, Berthon BS, Wark P, et al. Effects of fruit and vegetable consumption on risk of asthma, wheezing and immune responses: A systematic review and meta-analysis. *Nutrients*. 2017;9(4):341. https://doi.org/10.3390/nu9040341.

9. Varraso R, Kauffmann F, Leynaert B, et al. Dietary patterns and asthma in the E3N study. *Eur Respir J.* 2009;33(1).
10. Varraso R, Fung TT, Barr RG, et al. Prospective study of dietary patterns and chronic obstructive pulmonary disease among US women. *Am J Clin Nutr.* 2007;86(2):488–495.
11. Varraso R, Fung TT, Hu FB, et al. Prospective study of dietary patterns and chronic obstructive pulmonary disease among US men. *Thorax.* 2007;62:786–791.
12. Periyalil HA, Gibson PG, Wood LG. Immunometabolism in obese asthmatics: Are we there yet? *Nutrients.* 2013;5(9):3506–3530.
13. Zammit C, Liddicoat H, Moonsie I, et al. Obesity and respiratory diseases. *Int J Gen Med.* 2010;3:335–343. https://doi.org/10.2147/IJGM.S11926.
14. Murugan AT, Sharma G. Obesity and respiratory diseases. *Chron Respir Dis.* 2008;5:233–242.
15. Acute respiratory failure—Symptoms, diagnosis and treatment. *BMJ Best Pract* 2020.
16. Davidson A, Banham S, Elliot M, et al. BTS/ICS guideline for the ventilatory management of acute hypercapnic respiratory failure in adults. *Thorax.* 2016;71:ii1–ii35. https://doi.org/10.1136/thoraxjnl-2015-208209.
17. Hess D. Non-invasive ventilation for acute respiratory failure. *Respir Care.* 2013;58(6):950–972. https://doi.org/10.4187/respcare.02319. PMID: 23709194.
18. Reeves A, Tran K, Collins P. Nutrition during noninvasive ventilation: Clinical determinants and key practical recommendations. In: Esquinas AM, ed. *Noninvasive Mechanical Ventilation.* Cham, Switzerland: Springer; 2016.
19. Reeves A, White H, Sosnowski K, Tran K, Jones M, Palmer M. Energy and protein intakes of hospitalised patients with acute respiratory failure receiving non-invasive ventilation. *Clin Nutr.* 2014;33(6):1068–1073. https://doi.org/10.1016/j.clnu.2013.11.012.
20. Terzi N, Darmon M, Reignier J, et al. Initial nutritional management during noninvasive ventilation and outcomes: A retrospective cohort study. *Crit Care.* 2017;21(1):293. https://doi.org/10.1186/s13054-017-1867-y.
21. van Zanten ARH, De Waele E, Wischmeyer PE. Nutrition therapy and critical illness: Practical guidance for the ICU, post-ICU, and long term convalescence phases. *Crit Care.* 2019;23(368). https://doi.org/10.1186/s13054-019-2657-5.
22. Turner P, et al. Route of nutrition support in patients requiring NIV & CPAP during the COVID-19 response. 2020. Available at: https://www.bapen.org.uk/pdfs/covid-19/nutrition-in-niv-21-04-20.pdf. Intensive Care Society
23. Singer P, Rattanachaiwong S. To eat or to breathe? The answer is both! Nutritional management during noninvasive ventilation. *Crit Care.* 2018;22(1):27. https://doi.org/10.1186/s13054-018-1947-7.
24. Blaser A, Starkopf J, Alhazzani W, et al. Early enteral nutrition in critically ill patients: ESICM clinical practice guidelines. *Intensive Care Med.* 2017;43(3):380–398. https://doi.org/10.1007/s00134-016-4665-0. Intensive Care Medicine
25. Intensive Care Society & Faculty of Intensive Care Medicine. Guidance for prone positioning in adult critical care. 2019. Available at: https://www.wyccn.org/uploads/6/5/1/9/65199375/icsficm_proning_guidance_final_2019.pdf.
26. Calder P. Nutrition, immunity and COVID-19. *BMJ Nutr Prev Health.* 2020:0. https://doi.org/10.1136/bmjnph-2020-000085.
27. McAuliffe S, Ray S, Fallon E, Bradfield J, Eden T, Kohlmeier M. Dietary micronutrients in the wake of COVID-19: An appraisal of evidence with a focus on high-risk groups and preventative healthcare. *BMJ Nutr Prev Health.* 2020:0. https://doi.org/10.1136/bmjnph-2020-000100.
28. Hemilä H, Chalker E. Vitamin C for preventing and treating the common cold. *Cochrane Database Syst Rev.* 2013:CD000980.
29. Hemilä H, Louhiala P. Vitamin C for preventing and treating pneumonia. *Cochrane Database Syst Rev.* 2013:CD005532.
30. Fowler AA, Truwit J, Hite RD, et al. Effect of vitamin C infusion on organ failure and biomarkers of inflammation and vascular injury in patients with sepsis and severe acute respiratory failure: The CITRIS-ALI randomized clinical trial. *JAMA.* 2019;322:1261.
31. Martineau AR, Jolliffe D, Hooper RL, et al. Vitamin D supplementation to prevent acute respiratory tract infections: Systematic review and meta-analysis of individual participant data. *BMJ.* 2017:356.
32. Amrein K, Papinutti A, Mathew E, et al. Vitamin D and critical illness: What endocrinology can learn from intensive care and vice versa. *Endocr Connect.* 2018;7:R304–R315.

33. Kohlmeier M. Avoidance of vitamin D deficiency to slow the COVID-19 pandemic. *BMJ Nutr Prev Health*. 2020:0. https://doi.org/10.1136/bmjnph-2020-000096.
34. Dushianthan A, Cusack R, Burgess VA, Grocott MP, Calder PC. Immunonutrition for acute respiratory distress syndrome (ARDS) in adults. *Cochrane Database Syst Rev*. 2019;1(1):CD012041. https://doi.org/10.1002/14651858.CD012041.
35. Lanham-New SA, Webb A, Cashman KD, et al. Vitamin D and SARS-CoV-2 virus/COVID-19 disease. *BMJ Nutr Prev Health*. 2020:0. https://doi.org/10.1136/bmjnph-2020-000089.
36. Griffin G, Hewison M, Hopkin J, et al. Vitamin D and COVID-19: Evidence and recommendations for supplementation. *R Soc Open Sci*. 2020;7:201912. https://doi.org/10.1098/rsos.201912.
37. Minnelli N, Gibbs L, Larrivee J, Sahu KK. Challenges of maintaining optimal nutrition status in COVID-19 patients in intensive care settings. *JPEN J Parenter Enteral Nutr*. 2020;44:1439–1446. https://doi.org/10.1002/jpen.1996.
38. Mathers CD, Loncar D. Projections of global mortality and burden of disease from 2002 to 2030. *PLOS Med*. 2006;3(11):e442. https://doi.org/10.1371/journal.pmed.0030442.
39. Chambaneau A, Filaire M, Jubert L, et al. Nutritional intake, physical activity and quality of life in COPD patients. *Int J Sports Med*. 2016;37(9):730–737. https://doi.org/10.1055/s-0035-1569368.
40. MacNee W. ABC of chronic obstructive pulmonary disease: Pathology, pathogenesis and pathophysiology. *BMJ*. 2006;332(7551):1202–1204.
41. Planas M, Alvarez J, Garcia-Peris PA, et al. Nutritional support and quality of life in stable chronic obstructive pulmonary disease (COPD) patients. *Clin Nutr*. 2005;24(3):433–441. https://doi.org/10.1016/j.clnu.2005.01.005.
42. Sugawara K, Takahashi H, Kasai C, et al. Effects of nutritional supplementation combined with low-intensity exercise in malnourished patients with COPD. *Respir Med*. 2010;104(12):1883–1889. https://doi.org/10.1016/j.rmed.2010.05.008.
43. Collins PF, Yang IA, Chang YC, et al. Nutritional support in chronic obstructive pulmonary disease (COPD): An evidence update. *J Thorac Dis*. 2019;11:S2230–S2237. https://doi.org/10.21037/jtd.2019.10.41.
44. Dal Negro RW, Aquilani R, Bertacco S, et al. Comprehensive effects of supplemented essential amino acids in patients with severe COPD and sarcopenia. *Monaldi Arch Chest Dis*. 2010;73:25–33.
45. Engelen MP, Rutten EP, de Castro CL, et al. Supplementation of soy protein with branched-chain amino acids alters protein metabolism in healthy elderly and even more in patients with chronic respiratory pulmonary disease. *Am J Clin Nutr*. 2007;85:431–439.
46. Jonker R, Deutz NEP, Erbland ML, et al. Effectiveness of essential amino acid supplementation in stimulating whole body net protein anabolism is comparable between COPD patients and healthy older adults. *Metabolism*. 2017;69:120–129. https://doi.org/10.1016/j.metabol.2016.12.010.
47. Scoditti E, Massaro M, Garbarino S, et al. Role of diet in chronic obstructive pulmonary disease prevention and treatment. *Nutrients*. 2019;11(6):1357. https://doi.org/10.3390/nu11061357.
48. Kaluza J, Larsson S, Orsini N, et al. Fruit and vegetable consumption and risk of COPD: A prospective cohort study of men. *Thorax*. 2017;72(6):500–509.
49. Parvizian M, Dhaliwal M, Li J, et al. Relationship between dietary patterns and COPD: A systematic review and meta-analysis. *ERJ Open Res*. 2020:6. https://doi.org/10.1183/23120541.00168-2019.
50. World Health Organization. Chronic respiratory diseases: Asthma. 2020. Available at: https://www.who.int/news-room/q-a-detail/chronic-respiratory-diseases-asthma. Accessed January 28, 2021.
51. Holgate ST. Pathogenesis of asthma. In: Kay AB, Kaplan AB, Bousquet J, eds. *Allergy and Allergic Diseases*. 2nd ed. UK: Blackwell Publishing Ltd; 2008.
52. Guilleminault L, Williams EJ, Scott HA, et al. Diet and asthma: Is it time to adapt our message? *Nutrients*. 2017;9(11):1127. https://doi.org/10.3390/nu9111227.
53. Scott HA, Gibson PG, Garg ML, et al. Dietary restriction and exercise improve airway inflammation and clinical outcomes in overweight and obese asthma: A randomized trial. *Clin Exp Allergy*. 2013;43:36–49.
54. Romieu I, Barraza-Villarreal A, Escamilla-Nunez C, et al. Dietary intake, lung function and airway inflammation in Mexico City school children exposed to air pollutants. *Respir Res*. 2009;10(1):122. https://doi.org/10.1186/1465-9921-10-122.
55. Wood LG, Garg ML, Powell H, et al. Lycopene-rich treatments modify noneosinophilic airway inflammation in asthma: Proof of concept. *Free Radic Res*. 2008;42(1):94–102. https://doi.org/10.1080/10715760701767307.

56. Global strategy for asthma management and prevention: Global Initiative for Asthma https://ginasthma.org/gina-reports/. 2020.
57. Forte G, da Silva DR, Hennemann ML, et al. Diet effects in the asthma treatment: A systematic review. *Crit Rev Food Sci Nutr*. 2017;58(1). https://doi.org/10.1080/10408398.2017.1289893.
58. Haldar P, Pavord ID, Shaw DE, et al. Cluster analysis and clinical asthma phenotypes. *Am J Respir Crit Care Med*. 2008;178(3):218–224.
59. Forno E, Celedon JC. The effect of obesity, weight gain, and weight loss on asthma inception and control. *Curr Opin Allergy Clin Immunol*. 2017;17:123–130.
60. Furukawa T, Hasegawa T, Suzuki K, et al. Influence of underweight on asthma control. *Allergol Int*. 2012:61.
61. Kumar R. Prenatal factors and the development of asthma. *Curr Opin Pediatr*. 2008:682–687.
62. Forno E, Young OM, Kumar R, et al. Maternal obesity in pregnancy, gestational weight gain, and risk of childhood asthma. *Pediatrics*. 2014;134:e535–e546.
63. Dogaru CM, Nyffenegger D, Pescatore AM, et al. Breastfeeding and childhood asthma: Systematic review and meta-analysis. *Am J Epidemiol*. 2014;179:1153–1167.
64. Castro-Rodriguez JA, Garcia-Marcos L, Alfonseda Rojas JD, et al. Mediterranean diet as a protective factor for wheezing in preschool children. *J Paediatr*. 2008;152:823–828.
65. Pellegrini-Belinchón J, Lorente-Toledano F, Galindo-Villardón P, et al. Factors associated to recurrent wheezing in infants under one year of age in the province of Salamanca, Spain: Is intervention possible? A predictive model. *Allergol Immunopathol (Madr)*. 2016;44:393–399.
66. Chatzi L, Garcia R, Roumeliotaki T, et al. Mediterranean diet adherence during pregnancy and risk of wheeze and eczema in the first year of life: INMA (Spain) and RHEA (Greece) mother-child cohort studies. *Br J Nutr*. 2013;110(11):2058–2068. https://doi.org/10.1017/S0007114513001426.
67. Castro-Rodriguez JA, Ramirez-Hernandez M, Padilla O, et al. Effect of foods and Mediterranean diet during pregnancy and first years of life on wheezing, rhinitis and dermatitis in preschoolers. *Allergol Immunopathol (Madr)*. 2016;44:400–409.
68. Beckhaus AA, Garcia-Marcos L, Forno E, et al. Maternal nutrition during pregnancy and risk of asthma, wheeze, and atopic diseases during childhood: A systematic review and meta analysis. *Allergy*. 2015;70:1588–1604.
69. Vahdaninia M, Mackenzie H, Helps S, et al. Prenatal intake of vitamins and allergic outcomes in the offspring: A systematic review and meta-analysis. *J Allergy Clin Immunol Pract*. 2017;5:771–778.
70. Martindale S, McNeill G, Devereux G, Campbell D, Russell G, Seaton A. Antioxidant intake in pregnancy in relation to wheeze and eczema in the first two years of life. *Am J Respir Crit Care Med*. 2005;171:121–128.
71. Devereux GT, Stephen W, Craig LC, et al. Low maternal vitamin E intake during pregnancy is associated with asthma in 5-year-old children. *Am J Respir Crit Care Med*. 2006;174:499–507.
72. Hansen S, Strøm M, Maslova E, et al. Fish oil supplementation during pregnancy and allergic respiratory disease in the adult offspring. *J Allergy Clin Immunol*. 2017;139(1):104–111. https://doi.org/10.1016/j.jaci.2016.02.042.
73. Bisgaard H, Stokholm J, Chawes BL, et al. Fish oil-derived fatty acids in pregnancy and wheeze and asthma in offspring. *N Engl J Med*. 2016;375(26):2530–2539. https://doi.org/10.1056/NEJMoa1503734.
74. Olsen SF, Osterdal ML, Salvig JD, et al. Fish oil intake compared with olive oil intake in late pregnancy and asthma in the offspring: 16 y of registry-based follow-up from a randomized controlled trial. *Am J Clin Nutr*. 2008;88:167–175.
75. Ehrenstein O, Aralis H, Flores M, Ritz B. Fast food consumption in pregnancy and subsequent asthma symptoms in young children. *Pediatr Allergy Immunol*. 2015;26:571–577.
76. Lv N, Xiao L, Ma J. Dietary pattern and asthma: A systematic review and meta-analysis. *J Asthma Allergy*. 2014;7:105–121. https://doi.org/10.2147/JAA.S49960.
77. Adams S, Lopata A, Smuts C, et al. Relationship between serum omega-3 fatty acid and asthma endpoints. *Int J Environ Res Public Health*. 2019;16(1):43. https://doi.org/10.3390/ijerph16010043.
78. Patel S, Custovic A, Smith JA, Simpson A, Kerry G, Murray CS. Cross-sectional association of dietary patterns with asthma and atopic sensitization in childhood—in a cohort study. *Pediatr Allergy Immunol*. 2014;25:565–571.
79. Tromp IIK-dJ JC, de Vries JH, Jaddoe VW, et al. Dietary patterns and respiratory symptoms in preschool children: The Generation R Study. *Eur Respir J*. 2012;40:681–689.

80. DeChristopher LR, Uribarri J, Tucker KL. Intakes of apple juice, fruit drinks and soda are associated with prevalent asthma in US children aged 2–9 years. *Public Health Nutr.* 2016;19:123–130.
81. Berentzen NEvS VL, Gehring U, Koppelman GH, et al. Associations of sugar-containing beverages with asthma prevalence in 11-year-old children: The PIAMA birth cohort. *Eur J Clin Nutr.* 2015;69:303–308.
82. Uddenfeldt M, Janson C, Lampa E, et al. High BMI is related to higher incidence of asthma, while a fish and fruit diet is related to a lower—results from a long-term follow-up study of three age groups in Sweden. *Respir Med.* 2010;104:972–980.
83. Knekt P, Kumpulainen J, Jarvinen R, et al. Flavonoid intake and risk of chronic diseases. *Am J Clin Nutr.* 2002;76:560–568.
84. Garcia-Larsen V, Del Giacco S, Moreira A, et al. Asthma and dietary intake: An overview of systematic reviews. *Allergy.* 2016;71(4):433–442. https://doi.org/10.1111/all.12800.
85. Shi ZD, Grande E, Taylor AW, Gill TK, Adams R, Wittert GA. Association between soft drink consumption and asthma and chronic obstructive pulmonary disease among adults in Australia. *Respirology.* 2012;17:363–369.
86. Park S, Blanck HM, Sherry B, Jones SE, Pan LJ. Regular-soda intake independent of weight status is associated with asthma among US high school students. *Acad Nutr Diet.* 2013;113:106–111.
87. Park S, Akinbami LJ, McGuire LC, Blanck HM. Association of sugar-sweetened beverage intake frequency and asthma among U.S. adults. *Prev Med.* 2013;91:58–61.
88. Benjafield A, Ayas N, Eastwood P, et al. Estimation of the global prevalence and burden of obstructive sleep apnoea: A literature-based analysis. *Lancet Respir Med.* 2019;7(8):P687–P698. https://doi.org/10.1016/S2213-2600(19)30198-5.
89. Punjabi NM, Caffo B, Goodwin JL, et al. Sleep-disordered breathing and mortality: A prospective cohort study. *PLOS Med.* 2009;6(8):e1000132.
90. Dobrosielski D, Papandreou C, Patil S, et al. Diet and exercise in the management of obstructive sleep apnoea and cardiovascular disease risk. *Eur Respir Rev.* 2017;26:160110. https://doi.org/10.1183/16000617.0110-2016.
91. Morrow E. Medical nutritional therapy in the management of obstructive sleep apnea. *J Nutr Diet Pract.* 2020;4(3).
92. Cao Y, Wittert G, Taylor AW, Adams R, Shi Z. Associations between macronutrient intake and obstructive sleep apnoea as well as self-reported sleep symptoms: Results from a cohort of community dwelling Australian men. *Nutrients.* 2016;8:207.
93. Stelmach-Mardas M, Mardas M, Iqbal K, Kostrzewska M, Piorunek T. Dietary and cardio-metabolic risk factors in patients with obstructive sleep apnea: Cross-sectional study. *PeerJ.* 2017;5:e3259.
94. Peppard P, Young T, Palta M, et al. Longitudinal study of moderate weight change and sleep-disordered breathing. *JAMA.* 2000;284(23):3015–3021.
95. Gea J, Badenes D, Balcells E. Nutritional status in patients with idiopathic pulmonary fibrosis. *Pulm Crit Care Med.* 2018:3. https://doi.org/10.15761/PCCM.1000147.
96. Faverio P, Bocchino M, Caminati A, et al. Nutrition in patients with idiopathic pulmonary fibrosis: Critical issues analysis and future research directions. *Nutrients.* 2020;12(4):1131. https://doi.org/10.3390/nu12041131.
97. Alakhras M, Decker P, Nadrous H, et al. Body mass index and mortality in patients with idiopathic pulmonary fibrosis. *Chest.* 2007;131(5):1448–1453. https://doi.org/10.1378/chest.06-2784.
98. Nishiyama O, Yamazaki R, Sano H, et al. Fat-free mass index predicts survival in patients with idiopathic pulmonary fibrosis. *Respirology.* 2017;22:480–485.
99. Tzilas V, Bouros E, Barbayianni I, et al. Vitamin D prevents experimental lung fibrosis and predicts survival in patients with idiopathic pulmonary fibrosis. *Pulm Pharmacol Ther.* 2019;55:17–24.
100. Thomas JM, Isenring E, Kellett E. Nutritional status and length of stay in patients admitted to an acute assessment unit. *J Hum Nutr Diet.* 2007;20:320–832..
101. Jolliet P, Pichard C, Biolo G, et al. Enteral nutrition in intensive care patients: A practical approach. *Clin Nutr.* 1999;18(1):47–56. https://doi.org/10.1054/clnu.1998.0001.
102. Huang YC, Yen CE, Cheng CH, Jih KS, Kan MN. Nutritional status of mechanically ventilated critically ill patients: Comparison of different types of nutritional support. *Clin Nutr.* 2000;19:101–107.

103. Wadler S, Benson A, Engelking C, et al. Recommended guidelines for the treatment of chemotherapy-induced diarrhea. *J Clin Oncol*. 1998;16(9):3169–3178. https://doi.org/10.1200/JCO.1998.16.9.3169.
104. Oldham J, Collard H. Comorbid conditions in idiopathic pulmonary fibrosis: Recognition and management. *Front Med (Lausane)*. 2017;4:123.
105. Wernig G, Chen SY, Cui L, et al. Unifying mechanism for different fibrotic diseases. *Proc Natl Acad Sci U S A*. 2017;114(18):4757–4762.
106. Miyake Y, Sasaki S, Yokoyama T, et al. Vegetable, fruit and cereal intake and risk of idiopathic pulmonary fibrosis in Japan. *Ann Nutr Metab*. 2004;48(6):390–397.
107. Miyake Y, Sasaki S, Yokoyama T, et al. Dietary fat and meat intake and idiopathic pulmonary fibrosis: A case-control study in Japan. *Int J Tuberc Lung Dis*. 2006;10(3):333–339.
108. Costabel U. Sarcoidosis: Clinical update. *Eur Respir J*. 2001;18:56s–68s.
109. Payer J, Brazdilova K, Jàckuliak P. Management of glucocorticoid-induced osteoporosis: Prevalence, and emerging treatment options. *Drug Healthc Patient Saf*. 2010;2:49–59. https://doi.org/10.2147/dhps.s7197.
110. Osteoporosis. ACoRAHCoG-I Recommendations for the prevention and treatment of glucocorticoid-induced osteoporosis: 2001 update. *Arthritis Rheum*. 2001;44(7):1469–1503.
111. Galiè N, Humbert M, Vachiery J, et al. 2015 ESC/ERS Guidelines for the diagnosis and treatment of pulmonary hypertension. *Eur Respir J*. 2015;46:903–975. https://doi.org/10.1183/13993003.01032-2015.
112. Cuspidi C, Tadic M, Grassi G, Mancia G. Treatment of hypertension: The ESH/ESC guidelines recommendations. *Pharmacol Res*. 2018;128:315–321. https://doi.org/10.1016/j.phrs.2017.10.003.
113. Tanaka H, Kataoka M, Isobe S, et al. Therapeutic impact of dietary vitamin D supplementation for preventing right ventricular remodeling and improving survival in pulmonary hypertension. *PLoS ONE*. 2017;12(7):e0180615. https://doi.org/10.1371/journal.pone.0180615.
114. Ruiter G, Lankhorst S, Boonstra A, et al. Iron deficiency is common in idiopathic pulmonary arterial hypertension. *Eur Respir J*. 2011;37:1386–1391.
115. Ruiter G, Lanser I, de Man FS, et al. Iron deficiency in systemic sclerosis patients with and without pulmonary hypertension. *Rheumatology (Oxford)*. 2014;53:2852–2892.
116. World Health Organization. Tuberculosis. 2020. Available at: https://www.who.int/news-room/fact-sheets/detail/tuberculosis. Accessed February 2, 2021.
117. World Health Organization. *Guideline: Nutritional Care and Support for Patients With Tuberculosis*. Geneva: World Health Organization; 2013.
118. Gupta K, Gupta R, Atreja A, et al. Tuberculosis and nutrition. *Lung India*. 2009;26(1):9–16. https://doi.org/10.4103/0970-2113.45198.
119. Paton N, Chua Y, Earnest A, et al. Randomized controlled trial of nutritional supplementation in patients with newly diagnosed tuberculosis and wasting. *Am J Clin Nutr*. 2004;80:460–465.
120. Cegielski J, McMurray D. The relationship between malnutrition and tuberculosis: Evidence from studies in humans and experimental animals. *Int J Tuberc Lung Dis*. 2004;8(3):286–298.
121. Schaible U, Kaufmann S. Malnutrition and infection: Complex mechanisms and global impacts. *PLOS Medicine*. 2007;4:e115.
122. Elborn J. Cystic fibrosis. *Lancet*. 2016;388(10059):2519–2531.
123. Matel J, Milla C. Nutrition in cystic fibrosis. *Semin Respir Crit Care Med*. 2009;30(5):579.
124. Dodge J, Turck D. Cystic fibrosis: Nutritional consequences and management. *Best Pract Res Clin Gastroenterol*. 2006;20(3):531–546. https://doi.org/10.1016/j.bpg.2005.11.006.
125. Green M, Buchanan E, Weaver L. Nutritional management of the infant with cystic fibrosis. *Arch Dis Child*. 1995;72:452–456.
126. Sankararaman S, Schindler T, Sferra T. Management of exocrine pancreatic insufficiency in children. *Nutr Clin Pract*. 2019;34(S1). https://doi.org/10.1002/ncp.10388.

CHAPTER 6

Nutrition in Cardiovascular and Cerebrovascular Medicine

Luke Buckner ■ Sarah Armes ■ Sumantra Ray ■ Clare Wall

LEARNING POINTS

By the end of this chapter, you should be able to:

- Understand the different populations which exist when discussing cardiovascular disease and which level of prevention is targeted at them (mainly primary and secondary prevention)
- Recognise how to account for various lifestyle factors in cardiovascular disease risk assessment of an individual patient
- Be able to advocate for dietary patterns or specific nutrients which prevent atherosclerotic cardiovascular disease
- Know that for patients with chronic cardiovascular disease (stroke and heart failure), nutrition advice must be tailored and will therefore be different to the advice for acute cardiovascular events such as myocardial infarction

CASE STUDY 6.1 Coronary Heart Disease Risk

Background

A 30-year-old South Asian male presented to his general practitioner (GP) with concerns about his weight. He has gained 10 kg in weight over the last 5 years and his body mass index (BMI) is 35 kg/m^2. His father died of a myocardial infarction (MI) at 55 years of age, and he expresses concern about his risk of coronary heart disease (CHD). His mother is well. He is married with two children, 5 and 3 years of age.

He has no significant past medical history, has not seen a doctor in over 5 years and takes no regular medications or over-the-counter dietary or herbal supplements. He works as an accountant in a large company and is generally inactive but does try to go for an occasional walk. He is a nonsmoker and drinks 8 units of alcohol, typically lager, per week.

He describes his diet as 'healthy' and his wife does most of the food shopping and preparation. At home they often eat traditional northern Indian cuisine. He buys his lunch when he is at work and regularly takes clients out for lunch.

Findings

On physical examination his cardiovascular and respiratory systems are unremarkable.

The GP arranges the following investigations:

- Full blood count
- Fasting lipid profile

These test results are shown in Table 6.1.

Intervention

His GP prescribes a lifestyle management approach to treatment with the primary goal of reducing his weight through a tailored healthy diet and physical activity approach. He refers the patient to a dietitian who completes a full dietary assessment with the patient and his wife and commences a stepwise approach to supporting him to make positive changes to his lifestyle behaviours.

CASE STUDY 6.1 Coronary Heart Disease Risk—(Continued)

TABLE 6.1 ■ **Blood Lipid Results and Classification**

Result	Case Study (mmol/L)	Healthy Level (mmol/L)
Total cholesterol	5.5	<5
HDL cholesterol	0.9	>1
LDL cholesterol	3.5	<3
Triglycerides	2	<2.3
Cholesterol/HDL ratio	6.1	<6

HDL, High-density lipoprotein; *LDL*, low-density lipoprotein.

Discussion

Overweight and obesity are recognised as a major risk factor for CHD. A hypocaloric diet, which supports weight loss, can improve his lipid profile along with recommending monounsaturated fatty acids and omega-3 fatty acids in place of saturated and omega-6 fatty acids in his diet. Increasing his intake of soluble dietary fibre would also assist with reducing his cholesterol absorption. Supporting him to explore sustainable ways to change his lunchtime eating behaviour would be an important consideration, as well as the cultural significance of foods which may have to be limited due to their high energy and saturated fat content.

Take-Home Points

- An approach to integrate lifestyle-based healthy habits into the course of a person's daily routine is the mainstay of primary and secondary prevention.
- Lifestyle changes are not a one-size-fits-all intervention and require individualised adaptation to patients and their habits, culture and preferences.
- Supporting people to make sustained changes to their weight requires education, support and empathy of the numerous factors feeding into their lifestyle and biological risk of developing obesity.

CASE STUDY 6.2 Cardiovascular Disease—Hypertension

Background

A 45 -year-old women presents to her GP with concerns about headaches. On a previous visit she was diagnosed with prehypertension and her GP recommended a 24-hour ambulatory blood pressure monitor which showed a 24-hour mean blood pressure 138/87 mm Hg.

See Table 6.2 for a general guide.

Her BMI is 22 kg/m^2. Her mother had a stroke at age 70 years, and her paternal grandfather had an MI at 60 years of age. She is married and lives with her husband and one child, who is 15 years of age. She is a shift worker in a local factory.

TABLE 6.2 ■ **Blood Pressure Classification**

Risk	Result
Ideal blood pressure	Between 90/60 mm Hg and 120/80 mm Hg
Pre–high blood pressure	Between 120/80 mm Hg and 140/90 mm Hg
High blood pressure	140/90 mm Hg or higher
Low blood pressure	90/60 mm Hg or lower

Continued

CASE STUDY 6.2 Cardiovascular Disease—Hypertension—(Continued)

She has no significant past medical history and takes no regular medications or over-the-counter preparations or vitamin and mineral supplements. She tries to walk regularly but this is challenging with her hours of work. She smokes 10 to 20 cigarettes per day and drinks alcohol very occasionally.

She describes her diet as sporadic and due to her shift work, she tends to eat quite a lot of ready-made meals and takeaways.

Findings

A general physical examination was unremarkable.

Intervention

Her GP prescribes a lifestyle management approach to treatment with the primary goal of reducing her blood pressure through a tailored dietary intervention, cessation of smoking and increasing physical activity. He refers the patient to a dietitian who completes a full dietary assessment with her and commences a stepwise approach to supporting her to make positive changes to her lifestyle behaviours. The dietitian recommends to the patient a modified Dietary Approaches to Stop Hypertension (DASH) diet with the goal of reducing her dietary sodium intake and increasing her fruit and vegetable intake.

Discussion

Recognising the difficulties of adopting these changes due to her current work schedule is essential to ensure compliance to the recommended changes to her diet.

Take-Home Points

- Reducing cardiovascular disease (CVD) risk is not solely about diet; it should incorporate and emphasise the benefits of stopping smoking, increasing exercise and other factors as well.
- Individualised advice will again be vital to success; this patient is unlikely to want complex recipes, but simple easy-to-follow advice given her busy schedule.

CASE STUDY 6.3 Heart Failure and Cachexia

Background

A 70-year-old man is admitted to hospital with progressive increase in breathlessness and ankle oedema over the previous month. He has heart disease and had an MI 5 years ago.

Findings

After suitable intervention his oedema resolves, and his BMI is calculated as 17 kg/m^2.

He lives with his wife who commented on admission that his appetite has been poor for a couple of months. He was subsequently diagnosed with cachexia.

The cardiologist advises a low-sodium diet and refers the patient to a dietitian.

A full dietary assessment reveals that this patient is only meeting 70% of his daily energy and protein requirements and that his dietary sodium intake is approximately 2000 mg a day which is within the recommended range for patients with heart failure. However, this may only be in range because of low energy intake.

Intervention

The dietitian formulates a dietary care plan with the patient, which aims to provide adequate energy and protein intakes to reduce the risk of further weight loss and promote weight gain. This is to be achieved by providing small frequent meals and concentrated oral nutritional supplements which are energy and protein dense, low in volume and low in sodium.

Discussion

Cachexia is a complex, multifactorial wasting syndrome characterised by involuntary weight loss with ongoing loss of skeletal muscle mass with or without loss of fat mass. It occurs in many conditions, perhaps most prominently in cancer. At present, there is no standard effective treatment of cancer-related cachexia, or any other type of cachexia, available. Strategies to address cachexia should therefore target the issues of anorexia, poor oral intakes and treatment side effects, using food-based interventions, oral nutritional supplements or artificial nutrition as appropriate.

CASE STUDY 6.3 Heart Failure and Cachexia—(Continued)

Take-Home Points

- This case highlights how CVD prevention is not just about weight loss and reducing risk factors; in this case, unfortunately the patient had a CVD event. The intervention is now in optimising the person's function and quality of life within the context of his chronic heart failure.
- Cardiac cachexia is a serious prognostic marker, and intervention to optimise a patient's medical treatment as well as nutritional status can improve quality of life and, potentially, prognosis.

Definition and Impact of Cardiovascular Disease

CARDIOVASCULAR DISEASE

Cardiovascular disease (CVD) is a group of common conditions affecting the heart and blood vessels[1] including, but not exclusively, hypertension, coronary heart disease (CHD), stroke, peripheral vascular disease (PVD) and heart failure. They remain the leading cause of death worldwide, with the World Health Organization reporting 17.9 million deaths, 32% of total deaths, worldwide in 2019. A large proportion (over 75%) occur in low- to middle-income countries; however, MI and stroke are still leading causes of death in high-income countries, primarily through the increasing rates of its noncommunicable risk factors and metabolic syndrome.

METABOLIC SYNDROME

'Metabolic syndrome' is a term used to describe a cluster of conditions which places a person at higher risk of developing CVD. These conditions include abdominal obesity, dyslipidaemia, hypertension and hyperglycaemia. Incidence of metabolic syndrome puts individuals at double the risk of CVD and increases the risk for type 2 diabetes approximately fivefold.

Factors associated with the development of metabolic syndrome include polycystic ovary syndrome, lipodystrophy, fatty liver disease, low birth weight and macrosomia (a birth weight defined as >4 kg).

According to the National Cholesterol Education Program Adult Treatment Panel III definition, at least three of the five following criteria must be met to diagnose a person with metabolic syndrome:

- **Abdominal obesity:** waist circumference of ≥102 cm in men and ≥88 cm in women
- **Hypertriglyceridemia:** ≥150 mg/dL (1.695 mmol/L)
- **Low high-density lipoprotein (HDL) cholesterol:** <40 mg/dL (1.04 mmol/dL) in men and <50 mg/dL (1.30 mmol/dL) in women
- **High blood pressure:** >130/85 mm Hg
- **High fasting glucose:** >110 mg/dL (6.1 mmol/L)

Primary and Secondary Prevention in CVD

Patients at risk of CVD should be advised to make lifestyle modifications including dietary changes (increasing the consumption of fruits and vegetables and reducing saturated fat to <11% of food energy intake and dietary salt intake to <6 g/day), reducing alcohol consumption, increasing physical activity, achieving or maintaining a healthy weight and cessation of smoking.

Further preventative measures with drug treatment should be taken to attenuate risk in those patients at highest risk who have not yet established the disease (primary prevention) and to reduce recurrence of events in patients with established CVD (secondary prevention).

Drug therapy includes:

- Antiplatelet therapy
- Antihypertensive therapy
- Lipid-lowering therapy

AETIOLOGY AND RISK FACTORS FOR CVD

A huge amount of research has evaluated risk factors for CVD, but to be clinically relevant they must be practical to test for and have enough evidence to support inclusion. Table 6.3 demonstrates some of these risk factors and defines them as either modifiable or nonmodifiable. Risk stratification scores such as QRISK3 have made their way into clinical care to identify high-risk patients who could benefit from early intervention to their lifestyle and, potentially, medication by summarising the cumulative effect of risk factors into a risk of a cardiovascular event.

Atherosclerosis is a process of fat deposition in the intima of the arterial wall, which can occur slowly over decades before a patient notices any symptoms. Fatty streak deposition occurs following damage to the artery wall, due to factors such as oxidative stress from smoking or increased pressure from hypertension. This subsequently leads to an increase in endothelial permeability. The 'response to retention' hypothesis proposes that low-density lipoprotein (LDL) particles interact with matrix proteins, resulting in their subsequent retention and greater risk of oxidative modification. This then provides a target for immune cells such as macrophages to infiltrate the intima in an attempt to begin clearing the fat; however, in uncontrolled phagocytosis these cells fill their cytoplasm with oxidised LDL cholesterol triggering conversion to foam cells.[3] It is this dysfunction when foam cells are formed, which leads to plaque formation with a fat core and plaque wall, stopping fat exposure to the blood stream.

At this point it is the plaque wall stability which controls progression of disease. Using the example of the coronary arteries, if the plaque is stable, it continues to grow, eventually causing stenosis to a point of symptoms during exercise (angina). If the plaque is unstable and ruptures,

TABLE 6.3 ■ **Modifiable and Nonmodifiable Risk Factors for Cardiovascular Disease**

Modifiable	Nonmodifiable
Lipid dysfunction (high total cholesterol, raised LDLc/low HDLc, raised triglycerides)	Gender
Hypertension	Age
Smoking	Family history
Physical inactivity	Ethnicity
Overweight and obesity	Genetic disorders of lipid metabolism
Alcohol intake	Foetal and childhood factors*
Oxidative stress[a]	
Coagulation[a]	
Endothelial function[a]	
Inflammation (IL-6, CRP, TNF-alpha[2])[a]	

[a]Emerging risk factors.
CRP, C-reactive protein; *HDLc*, high-density lipoprotein cholesterol; *IL-6*, interleukin-6; *LDLc*, low-density lipoprotein cholesterol; *TNF-alpha*, tumour necrosis factor alpha.

causing the contents of the atherosclerotic plaque to be exposed to the blood stream, then a clot will form acutely, obscuring the vessel and leading to major changes in blood supply to the myocardium (acute coronary syndrome)[4] (Figs. 6.1 and 6.2).

BENEFITS OF LIFESTYLE MODIFICATION ALONGSIDE MEDICATION IN CVD

CVD is a good example of a condition where the additive benefits of diet and lifestyle changes alongside medication are evident (Fig. 6.3). Good evidence exists that both lifestyle change and medication should be utilised in a complementary fashion, particularly with evidence demonstrating benefit to outcomes of CVD with multidisciplinary team input.[6–8] Examples of this in action include a prospective cohort study of approximately 10,000 dyslipidaemic patients comparing levels of physical fitness from an exercise test, as well as statin use, to mortality. Results demonstrated increased survival in both fit patients and those using statins, but a higher survival rate in those fit and using a statin.[9] Typically lifestyle modification is the mainstay for prevention of CVD until a threshold of risk is met. In the UK this level is 10% through the scoring system QRISK,[10] which predicts risk of a CVD event in the next 10 years with initial recommendation of statin prescription.[11]

Lifestyle changes such as increasing exercise, improving diet or reductions in smoking and alcohol intake can be difficult to achieve and so understandably time pressure becomes a barrier to clinicians engaging with advising patients. However, the same can be said for medical therapy; just because a medicine is prescribed does not mean it is being taken. Clinicians must recognise the importance of these aspects to patient care and work within a multidisciplinary group to provide advice on both medication and lifestyle changes and then support patients in implementing this.

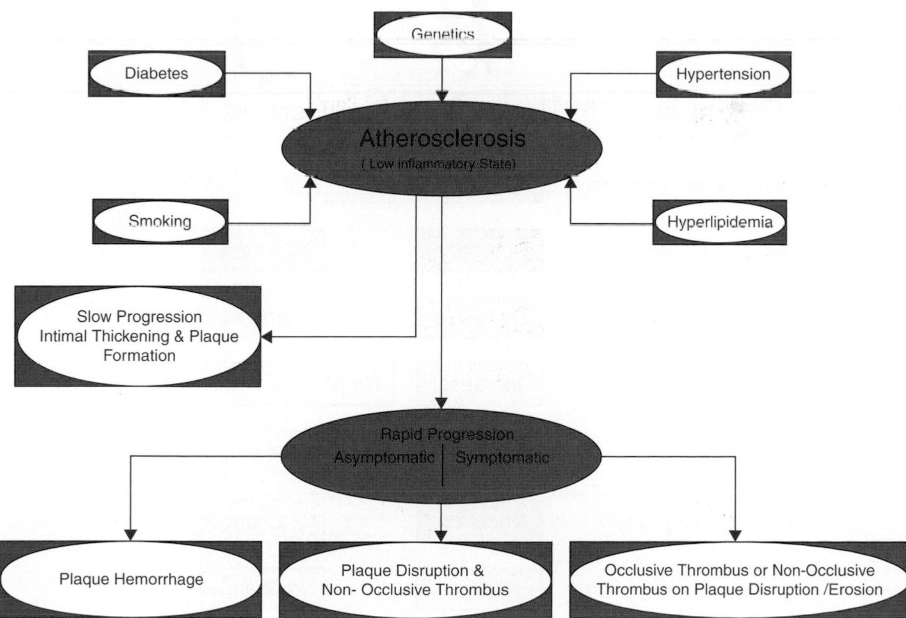

Fig. 6.1 Interactions of risk factors leading to atherosclerosis and acute coronary syndrome. (Adapted from Ambrose and Singh (2015).[4])

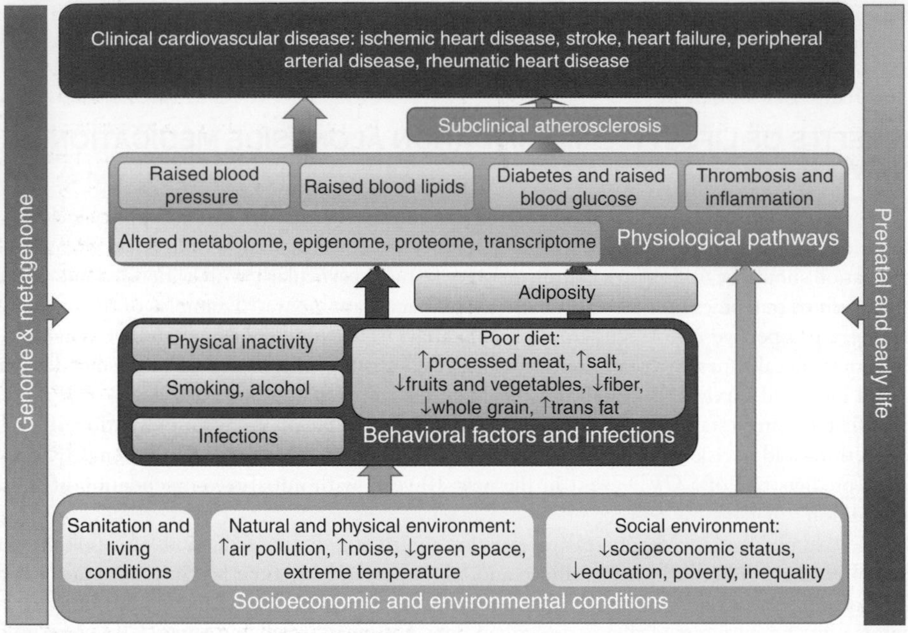

Fig. 6.2 Wider determinants of risk for CVD. (Adapted from Tzoulaki et al. (2016).[5])

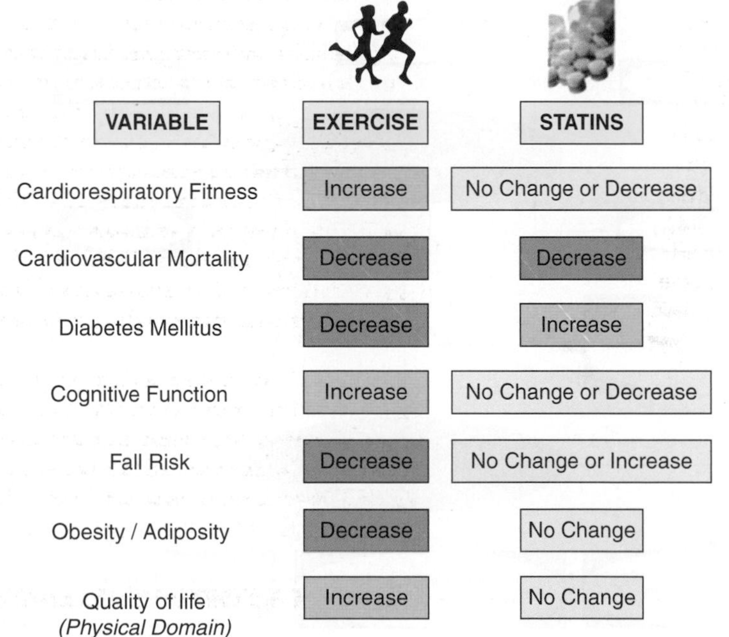

Fig. 6.3. How medication and exercise can work together. (Adapted from Brinks et al. (2017).[6])

Mediterranean, DASH and Low-Carb Diets

MEDITERRANEAN DIET

The Mediterranean diet has been heavily researched and is based on the principles detailed in Table 6.4, largely focussing on increasing mono/polyunsaturated fats, vegetables and fruit, legumes, fish and white meat instead of red meats.

TABLE 6.4 ■ **Dietary Components of the Mediterranean Diet Intervention in PREDIMED Trial**[12]

Food	Goal
Mediterranean diet	
Recommended	
Olive oil	≥4 tbsp/day
Tree nuts and peanuts	≥3 servings/wk
Fresh fruits	≥3 servings/day
Vegetables	≥2 servings/day
Fish (especially fatty fish), seafood	≥3 servings/wk
Legumes	≥3 servings/wk
Sofrito	≥2 servings/wk
White meat	Instead of red meat
Wine with meals (optionally, only for habitual drinkers)	≥7 glasses/wk
Discouraged	
Soda drinks	<1 drink/day
Commercial bakery goods, sweets and pastries	<2 servings/wk
Spread fats	<1 serving/day
Red and processed meats	<1 serving/day
Low-fat diet (control)	
Recommended	
Low-fat dairy products	≥3 servings/day
Bread, potatoes, pasta, rice	≥3 servings/day
Fresh fruits	≥3 servings/day
Vegetables	≥2 servings/day
Lean fish and seafood	≥3 servings/wk
Discouraged	
Vegetable oils (including olive oil)	≤2 tbsp/day
Commercial bakery goods, sweets and pastries	≤1 serving/wk
Nuts and fried snacks	≤1 serving/wk
Red and processed fatty meats	≤1 serving/wk
Visible fat in meats and soups‖	Always remove
Fatty fish, seafood canned in oil	≤1 serving/wk
Spread fats	≤1 serving/wk
Sofrito	≤2 servings/wk

Robust evidence supports an association between the Mediterranean diet with many health benefits, in particular with improvements in cardiovascular risk factors and the development of CVD itself, alongside reduction in mortality.

This has been shown through observational data, as well as in trials such as the PREDIMED trial, where 7447 participants with high risk of developing CVD were allocated to one of three diets (control diet—reduce dietary fat, Mediterranean diet with olive oil, Mediterranean diet with nuts). The participants received quarterly education sessions, and, depending on their group, free provision of extra-virgin olive oil, mixed nuts or small food gifts. They found that at 4.8 years' median follow up, the incidence of CVD was lower in the Mediterranean diet both with olive oil (hazard ratio 0.69 [95% confidence interval 0.53–0.91]) and nuts (0.72 [95% confidence interval 0.54–0.95]) compared with control advice.[12]

DASH DIET

The DASH diet has also gathered a good evidence base that adherence can reduce cardiovascular risk factors.

The principles of the DASH diet include a reduction in salt and saturated fat intake and an increase in the consumption of fruit and vegetables. Adherence to the DASH diet has been associated with improved health outcomes including hypertension, as well as outcomes like CVD events.[13]

LOW-CARB DIETS

The low-carbohydrate diet has been shown to result in moderate weight loss. Meta-analysis has shown that a low-carbohydrate diet resulted in improved blood pressure and lipid profiles. However, the long-term effects of this diet are uncertain when reviewing CVD itself. Whereas DASH and Mediterranean diets have evidence on end point improvements, the low-carb diet is yet to have reliable evidence for its effects on CVD end points.[14] However, if it works to improve a patient's CVD risk factors, it remains a clinical option and can be particularly useful in reducing blood glucose for patients with type 2 diabetes (Table 6.5).

Diet and Heart Disease

PRIMARY PREVENTION OF CORONARY ARTERY DISEASE

Coronary artery disease (CAD) is a condition whereby the coronary arteries supplying blood to the myocardium become narrowed or blocked, thereby reducing nutrient and oxygen supply to metabolically active muscle.

Primary prevention can be defined as the prevention of first events of CAD, whereas secondary prevention is working on similar principles but to reduce disease in those who already have disease. The mainstay of management focusses on treating the risk factors described previously, but primarily hypertension, dyslipidaemia, weight management, inactivity, smoking, alcohol intake and diabetes. Individual dietary recommendations will be described below, but cumulative benefit is seen in the management of each risk factor.

DYSLIPIDAEMIA

As previously described, cholesterol deposition into the intima of the coronary artery wall is the pathogenesis of atherosclerosis. Research has demonstrated that through manipulation of blood lipids, we can reduce the incidence and mortality from CAD. To understand the different interventions, we must first understand that it is the composition of the cholesterol and lipids, rather

TABLE 6.5 ■ **Overview of Key Dietary Patterns and Their Impact on Cardiovascular Disease**

Dietary Pattern	Author (Date)	Type of Study (Number of Studies)	Key Findings
Mediterranean diet	Rosato et al. (2019)[15]	Meta-analysis; observational studies (n = 29)	Exerts a protective effect on the risk of CVD, including CHD and ischemic stroke, but not haemorrhagic stroke.
	Sofi et al. (2014)[16]	Meta-analysis; cohort studies (n = 18)	A 2-point increase in adherence score was reported to determine an 8% reduction of overall mortality, a 10% reduced risk of CVD.
DASH diet	Siervo et al. (2015)[17]	Meta-analysis; RCTs (n = 20)	Decreases in SBP, DBP, total cholesterol and LDL cholesterol and a reduction of ~13% in the 10-year Framingham risk score for CVD.
	Filippou, et al. (2020)[18]	Meta-analysis; RCTs (n = 30)	Reductions in both SBP and DBP. Additionally, higher daily sodium intake and younger age enhanced the blood pressure–lowering effect.
Low-carbohydrate diet	Dong et al. (2020)[14]	Meta-analysis; RCTs (n = 12)	Decreases in SBP, DBP and triglyceride levels. Additionally, it was shown to increase plasma HDL cholesterol, serum total cholesterol and plasma LDL.
	Noto et al. (2012)[19]	Meta-analysis; observational studies (n = 9)	Significantly higher risk of all-cause mortality, and no significant association with risk of CVD mortality and incidence.

CHD, Coronary heart disease; *CVD*, cardiovascular disease; *DASH*, Dietary Approaches to Stop Hypertension; *DBP*, diastolic blood pressure; *HDL*, high-density lipoprotein; *LDL*, low-density lipoprotein; *SBP*, systolic blood pressure; *RCT*, randomised controlled trial.

than total amount, which has been associated with CAD. LDL cholesterol and triglycerides, for example, have numerous cohort studies linking raised levels with CAD, whereas there is good association demonstrated that high HDL cholesterol levels are associated with lower CAD risk. Whilst intervention trials demonstrating reductions in LDL and triglycerides levels lead to a reduction in CAD events and mortality, this cannot be said for interventions that raise HDL cholesterol (Table 6.6).

HYPERTENSION

Hypertension is a chronic elevation of blood pressure and a major risk factor for CVD. In the long term, high blood pressure causes end-organ damage and results in increased morbidity and mortality.

TABLE 6.6 ■ **The Impact of Nutrients on Cardiovascular Disease**

Nutrient	Evidence
Saturated fat	• There is clear evidence that dietary reduction in saturated fat leads to a decrease in LDL cholesterol. • Evidence is less clear about what we should replace this with, i.e., monounsaturated fat, polyunsaturated fat or carbohydrate.
Mono/polyunsaturated fat	• Replacement of saturated fat with polyunsaturated fat has been shown to decrease total, LDL and HDL cholesterol. • It is recommended to increase intake of monounsaturated fats with olive oil, rapeseed oil or spreads based on these oils and to use them in food preparation.
Omega-3	• Research has shown that intake of omega-3 fatty acids can reduce triglycerides and reduce small dense while increasing large buoyant LDL and increasing HDL cholesterol.
Carbohydrates[20]	• Evidence has shown that replacing fats with carbohydrates may increase fasting triacylglycerol concentrations, and isoenergetic replacement of SFAs with carbohydrates does not improve the serum total:HDL cholesterol.
Fibre	• Consistent evidence shows that soluble fibre moderately reduces total cholesterol and LDL cholesterol levels. • Current dietary guidelines recommend a total daily fibre intake of at least 20 to 30 g for adults.

HDL, High-density lipoprotein; *LDL*, low-density lipoprotein; *SFAs*, saturated fatty acids.

Consequences of hypertension include left ventricular hypertrophy and CAD, and it is a major risk factor for stroke. Left ventricular hypertrophy is an increase in muscle mass and wall thickness but not ventricular volume. It promotes a decrease of 'coronary reserve' and increases myocardial oxygen demand, both mechanisms contributing to myocardial ischaemia. CAD is associated with, and accelerated by, chronic arterial hypertension, leading to myocardial ischaemia and MI. Additionally, hypertension induces endothelial dysfunction, exacerbates atherogenesis and contributes to atherosclerotic plaque instability (Table 6.7).

In accordance with National Institute for Health and Clinical Excellence guidelines, do not offer calcium, magnesium or potassium supplements as a method for reducing blood pressure.

ALCOHOL

A reduction in excess consumption of alcohol is associated with a 3 to 4 mm Hg reduction in systolic and diastolic blood pressure. Small amounts (1–2 units per day) are perhaps protective with regards to CHD (weaker evidence for stroke); however, larger amounts are detrimental to health.

Given the other health effects related to alcohol, it is not best to advise patients to start drinking for their heart, but if they are drinking in moderation, it appears not to harm their risk of CVD (also the type of alcohol is worth considering, as there may be benefits from polyphenols in wine versus other drinks, for example).

DIETARY APPROACHES TO STOP HYPERTENSION

The DASH diet was originally tested in 1997 in the United States; it was a randomised control trial comparing a new dietary approach with a control diet. First the populations were all given 3

TABLE 6.7 ■ **The Impact of Nutrients on Hypertension**

Nutrient	Evidence
Salt	• Reduce total salt intake to 6 g/day (2.4 g sodium) including salt within foods and addition of salt to meals. • Strong and consistent evidence suggests that dietary sodium and blood pressure are positively linked.
Potassium	• Some evidence to demonstrate that low potassium intakes are linked with higher blood pressure, but less convincing evidence that raising intakes above sufficient levels has a dose response to blood pressure. In fact higher doses in this review were shown to lead to increase in BP (U-shaped curve).[21]
Calcium	• High dose supplementation (1000–1500 mg/day) has high evidence of some reduction in blood pressure, but these reductions are not hugely significant for an individual, more of a population advice reduction. • The quality of evidence is moderate for lower or higher doses of calcium.[22]
Magnesium[23]	• Poor quality of evidence to suggest that magnesium supplementation can reduce possible consequences of high blood pressure.
Caffeine	• Low-quality evidence did not show any significant effects of coffee consumption on blood pressure or the risk of hypertension.

BP, Blood pressure.

weeks of a control diet low in fruit, vegetables and dairy, with a fat content typical for Americans at the time. They were then randomised to continue the control diet or consume the DASH diet or a fruit- and vegetable-rich diet for 8 weeks. The fruit- and vegetable-rich diet solely focussed on increased intake of fruit and vegetable, whereas others were randomised to the DASH diet where the additional aspects were inclusion of low-fat dairy products, low-saturated-fat products and low-salt products.

Overall, the fruit and vegetable diet did reduce blood pressure significantly compared with the control diet, by 2.8 mm Hg systolic and 1.1 mm Hg diastolic, whereas the DASH diet reduced it further by 5.5 mm Hg systolic and 3.0 mm Hg diastolic. This was even more pronounced in those participants with hypertension, with the DASH diet reducing blood pressure by 11.4 and 5.5 mm Hg more than control for systolic and diastolic, respectively[13] (Table 6.8).

From this, further research has continued, highlighting its effectiveness in reducing CVD overall, not solely hypertension.

Secondary Prevention and Treatment of Heart Disease

CORONARY ARTERY DISEASE

The secondary prevention of CAD follows the same general principles as primary prevention. However, individuals will also have started several cardioprotective medications to prevent cardiac remodelling by their cardiologist usually including angiotensin-converting enzyme inhibitors, beta blockers, antiplatelets and a statin, as well as potentially a mineralocorticoid receptor antagonist (MRA) and sodium–glucose cotransporter-2 (SGLT-2) inhibitor depending on if their left

TABLE 6.8 ■ **The Effects of Macronutrients and Nutraceuticals on Cardiovascular Disease**

Nutrient	Evidence
Saturated fat, *trans*-fat and cholesterol	• Patients with metabolic syndrome obtain a favourable outcome from a diet low in saturated fats and high in unsaturated fats. • Fats should constitute 20% to 35% of the total calorie intake and, of these, saturated fats must be reduced to <7%, *trans*-fatty acids to <1% and cholesterol to <200 mg/day.
Fibre	• A diet high in complex unrefined carbohydrates and fibre (10–25 g/day) is beneficial and should be achieved through the diet, for example, emphasis on the consumption of beans, legumes, oats, flax seeds, fruit and vegetables. • Increased fibre intake is associated with reductions in total and LDL cholesterol and diastolic blood pressure.
Plant sterols	• Intakes of 2–3 g of plant stanol/sterol esters per day have been reported to decrease total and LDL cholesterol levels by 9% to 20%. • Intakes of plant sterols >3 g/day confer no additional benefit with respect to total or LDL cholesterol lowering. • However, there is substantial variability in response among individuals and little effect on HDL cholesterol or triglyceride levels has been reported. The evidence overall for plant sterols is weak, and they are not routinely advised in guidelines.[24]
Soy consumption	• Observational data linking replacing meat with soy protein leads to improvements in cholesterol profile and subsequently CVD risk. This may well be seen differently for different soy products. • Currently intervention trials using soy as a replacement have demonstrated unconvincing results or have too few trials to confirm any supposed effects on blood pressure, glycaemic control, weight loss or inflammation—therefore, no convincing effect.[25]
Nutraceuticals[26]	• Nutraceuticals and dietary supplements are not routinely recommended for the prevention or treatment of metabolic syndrome. However, this is a field with a wide range of compounds with mechanistic pathways which could influence metabolic syndrome and consequently CVD. • Foods rich in polyphenols and phenolic compounds, in addition to vitamin D, fruits and vegetables, have demonstrated a reduction in pro-inflammatory cytokines found in metabolic syndrome. • In addition, the presence of phenolic compounds and catechins reduced body weight in adults and they are a potential adjuvant treatment for obesity. • The inclusion of fish oil in the diet, especially with EPA and DHA, improved the lipid profile, inflammatory markers and endothelial function. • However, to date, changes in lifestyle, such as diet, play a fundamental role in these results.

CVD, Cardiovascular disease; *DHA*, docosahexanoic acid; *EPA*, eicosapentaenoic acid.

ventricular ejection fraction is reduced. Dietary advice should acknowledge these and they should be introduced alongside other key components, such as cardiac rehabilitation.

NUTRITION IN HEART FAILURE

Heart failure is a chronic disease, which carries a high burden of malnutrition. In heart failure, this is primarily due to cachexia (weight loss and muscle wasting), which has been associated with poor prognosis.[27] It also proves relatively difficult to screen for, as markers such as BMI, which are often used for undernutrition screening in acute care, rely on weight, which can significantly fluctuate in a patient in acute heart failure due to fluid retention.

A primary consideration in heart failure is acute versus chronic management. In acute decompensation, the focus is around fluid offloading, with diuresis and fluid restriction. Alongside this, medication can be reviewed to prevent further heart remodelling. In preserving this balance, patients may be advised to follow long-term fluid restriction to maintain a state of euvolemia.

Nutrition interventions are required both to aid symptoms of heart failure itself but also to prevent the adverse outcomes on prognosis and quality of life associated with cachexia.

FLUID RESTRICTION

In severe heart failure, patients are advised to restrict their fluid intake to 1.5 to 2.0 L/day. In moderate or mild heart failure, patients are unlikely to benefit from fluid restriction.

SODIUM

Sodium reduction is one such approach to symptom relief in heart failure, and the consensus is that this is likely to be helpful but will need to be tailored to the patient and their disease severity.

Patient knowledge of sodium reduction is a risk factor for hospital admission from heart failure. However, no significant difference is seen in studies evaluating the effects of sodium restriction, largely because patients do not recall the advice given. There are other factors complicating the evaluation of sodium restriction, including the changes in medication for optimisation of symptom control.[28]

CALORIES[29]

Patients can have difficulty eating enough calories, particularly when suffering from severe heart failure due to shortness of breath whilst eating or early satiety from ascitic/liver congestion. As such, an approach should start with slowly increasing calories, as sharp increases in intake may stimulate insulin levels to increase, which in return induces renal sodium and water absorption leading to risk of decompensation. Small frequent meals and energy fortification can be helpful if the patient is becoming full without finishing their food.

PROTEIN

Protein content should also be a focus to ensure adequate intake (1.0 g/kg/day), but there are no current recommendations for higher intakes than normal. The most effective way to maintain muscle mass is to include resistance exercise with adequate protein intake.

VITAMINS

- Thiamine deficiency has been observed in 13% to 30% of heart failure patients, and supplements are recommended. Patients with thiamine deficiency may have reduced cardiac function although causation for heart failure has not been established.[30]
- Supplementation of vitamins A, D, E and K may also be required because of reduced intestinal absorption.

Diet and Cerebrovascular Disease

Risk factors for cerebrovascular disease (stroke) may be similar to that of CAD, due to shared pathophysiology. As such, prevention is targeted around weight loss, moderating alcohol intake, quitting smoking, exercising, reducing blood pressure, maintaining normoglycaemia and modulating lipid profiles, as with other cardiovascular disorders. Lifestyle changes including diet and accessibility to healthy foods have also been highlighted to reduce stroke risk.

However, there are factors for cerebrovascular disease which need to be considered in a slightly different manner, both in prevention and then subsequent management of symptoms associated with the disease itself.

Primary Prevention of Cerebrovascular Disease

HYPERHOMOCYSTEINAEMIA, ENDOTHELIAL FUNCTION AND OXIDATIVE STRESS

Homocysteine is a metabolic compound which has been associated with risk of ischaemic stroke when elevated. There are several postulated mechanisms for this, including increased free radical damage and oxidative stress. However, over time it has largely been accepted that homocysteine is a marker, rather than target for prevention. Even then including homocysteine with traditional risk scores adds very little.

On the other hand, endothelial function and oxidative stress are still thought to play an important role in the development of atheroma, with evidence linking smoking, oxidised LDL cholesterol, HDL cholesterol and hyperglycaemia with changes in vascular functioning.[31]

OMEGA-3 (N-3) FATTY ACIDS

Omega-3 fatty acids, particularly through oily fish, have been demonstrated to have cardioprotective effects, and whilst the exact mechanisms are not well known, they exert desirable effects on endothelial function which could explain its mechanism.

However, there is little evidence to show that supplementation with omega-3 fatty acids reduces the risk of stroke in a healthy population, and so the advice continues to be where possible, obtain omega-3 from the diet through oily fish.

VITAMIN E

Vitamin E has been linked through cohort studies showing inverse association between intake and risk of CVD and stroke, potentially through reduction of oxidative stress. However, when this was translated to supplements of vitamin E, the results have been less conclusive. For the general population, many trials have demonstrated no benefit in supplementation for primary or secondary CVD prevention. However, there remains some interest in the use of vitamin E in more of a nutraceutical sense for patients with high oxidative stress burdens, although the evidence is still not strong enough for a clinical recommendation.

MEDITERRANEAN DIET

Fruit and vegetables, fish, olive oil and white meat have been associated with reduced risk of stroke, whereas red meat, processed meat and alcohol are associated with increased risk. As such, many of the components of a Mediterranean diet can help reduce risk of stroke in a healthy population.

Secondary Prevention and Treatment of Cerebrovascular Disease

After a stroke, depending on the subtype, dysphagia can be a major impact to the patient themselves and the managing medical team. Following diagnosis of a stroke with dysphagia, patients require assessment of their swallow to ensure it is safe, before taking food, liquids or medications through the oral route.

Whilst numerous key medical decisions are made with regards to imaging, medications, further investigations and rehabilitation, feeding must not be forgotten. In these patients, it is important to have multidisciplinary team focus on ensuring monitorings of food and fluid are documented, reviewed and acted on to ensure reduction in acute complications.[32]

Evidence demonstrates that early enteral feeding may improve survival in patients who fail a swallow assessment at baseline, but the clinician is uncertain whether to initiate nasogastric feeding at the start or monitor progress. However, in these patients it has been demonstrated that their level of disability and reduction in quality of life is subsequently higher, so it does raise an ethical question of whether this is prolonging the survival of patients severely disabled by stroke who would otherwise have died and whether this is the correct approach.[33] Ultimately as is the case with many aspects of medicine, it is important to have honest conversations with the family, and if possible, the patient, to establish what they would want to focus on in their treatment.

Patients should undergo screening for malnutrition on admission; additionally, hydration status should be assessed on admission and reviewed regularly. It is also worth noting that energy and protein requirements can be increased in the first 2 months after a stroke due to hypermetabolism.

MODIFIED TEXTURE FOODS/FLUID

If a patient is able to take food orally, the speech and language therapist team may advocate adjusting the consistency to facilitate a safer swallow. Modified texture foods/fluids may facilitate safe oral intake. It is worth remembering that by adding fluid to modify the texture of a food, the nutritional density can be diluted if you fill the same volume. However, it can be a useful way of hydrating a patient with poor oral intake, as the moisture content of food can be a leading source of water for individuals with dysphagia.

On the other hand, the modification of the texture of food, visual appeal and loss of vibrancy in colour may affect palatability. As such the long-term care of stroke patients, particularly those with dysphagia, carries high risk of undernourishment, and appropriate nutrition support should be provided, in the shape of food fortification, oral nutritional supplements or enteral feeding (e.g., via gastrostomy tube).

If a patient's swallow has not been affected and they are not at risk of undernutrition, their secondary prevention for stroke focusses on reduction of the impact of their risk factors through medications and lifestyle change.

Diet and Peripheral Vascular Disease

PVD shares very similar pathogenesis to ischaemic stroke due to atheromatous disease, as well as CAD. As such several risk factors are the same, and the lifestyle advice is the same as described previously. However, as with stroke, there are specific factors to consider in the management of PVD as shown next.

PRIMARY PREVENTION OF PVD

A large body of cohort data has looked at dietary patterns associated with the development of PVD and found that diets high in saturated fat, meat and meat products have the highest risk, whilst diets high in fibre, antioxidants (vitamins A, C and E) and polyunsaturated fat carried the least risk.[34] To date, there is a lack of evidence to suggest that supplementation of these nutrients has beneficial effects, but instead intake should be encouraged through the diet (Table 6.9).

Cardioprotective Diet and Lifestyle Recommendations

Overall, dietary patterns can improve overall health whilst preventing CVD. The best dietary advice for CAD, stroke, and PVD tends to follow many of the same core principles in what would be best described as a cardioprotective dietary pattern. Key features of a cardioprotective diet include increased consumption of fruits, vegetables, legumes and beans, nuts and oils with high unsaturated fat contents (e.g., olive oil), whole grains and fish, and limited intake of red or processed meats, refined carbohydrates and other ultraprocessed foods. These should be incorporated alongside other lifestyle factors such as exercise, moderating alcohol and stopping smoking, as well as potentially initiating medications.

CARDIOPROTECTIVE DIET

See Table 6.10 for food groups recommended to reduce cardiovascular risk.

OTHER LIFESTYLE RECOMMENDATIONS

See Table 6.11 for facts beyond diet that reduce risk of cardiovascular disease.

Conclusion

Following this chapter, we hope that you feel more confident in the breadth of research looking at diet, lifestyle and CVD and also recognise its place as both a primary presentation perspective,

TABLE 6.9 ■ **Primary prevention of PVD**

Nutrient	Evidence
Folate	• As described previously for stroke, there is an association between PAD and elevated levels of plasma homocysteine; this is associated with low folate intake. • However, there is insufficient evidence to suggest that supplementation has a beneficial effect.
Vitamin D	• Prevalence of PAD is associated with low serum vitamin D level, where supplementation helps overall bone and muscle health clearly with possible benefits to other systems.
Niacin	• Further avenues explored for treatment of PAD include the use of niacin to modulate increased levels of HDL cholesterol. • Whilst some effect has been shown, this is usually matched by placebo and put down to other factors, such as exercise.

HDL, high-density lipoprotein; *PAD*, peripheral artery disease.

TABLE 6.10 ■ **Food Groups Recommended to Reduce Cardiovascular Disease Risk**

Foods[a]	Comment
Fruit and vegetables	• Eat 5 or more portions a day.
Fish	• Eat 2 portions per week, including one of oily fish.
Nuts, seeds and legumes	• Eat 4 or more portions per week. • Consume unsalted nuts.
Fat	• Replace saturated fats with monounsaturated and polyunsaturated fats. • Decrease consumption of fried food, high fat products and foods containing *trans*-fats.
Oils and spreads	• Choose plant-based oils and spreads, such as olive, rapeseed or sunflower oil, that are high in mono/polyunsaturated fatty acids and lower in saturated fats.
Salt	• Reduce salt consumption, including salt within foods and addition of salt to meals.
Carbohydrates	• Choose foods high in fibre, for example, wholemeal bread and pasta instead of refined versions.
Sugar	• Limit intake of sugar and foods containing refined sugars.
Alcohol	• Limit intake to below 14 units per week spread out over >3 days.
Energy intake	• Limit energy intake if overweight or obesity are present.

Modified from Webster-Gandy J, Madden A, Holdsworth M, eds. 2020. *Oxford Handbook of Nutrition and Dietetics*. Oxford University Press.[35]
[a]These focus on key aspects of a cardioprotective diet and are not a comprehensive list of all foods

TABLE 6.11 ■ **Factors Beyond Diet That Reduce Risk of Cardiovascular Disease**

Recommendation	Comment
Body weight	• Reduce excess body weight. • Aim for BMI of 18.5–24.9 kg/m^2.
Physical activity/exercise	• Participate in >150 minutes of moderate intensity aerobic activity a week or 75 minutes of vigorous intensity aerobic activity (or mix of moderate and vigorous) and muscle-strengthening activity >2 days a week.
Smoking	• Cease smoking.

but also as a factor which works alongside long-term medical management of heart disease, stroke and peripheral vascular disease.

It should be noted that a large body of evidence in CVD comes from large-scale cohort data demonstrating associations, some weak and some strong. Many have been followed with interventional trials and subsequent meta-analysis/reviews. The ways shown to reduce CVD risk from these trials tend to be through adjusting to a dietary pattern with low saturated/*trans*-fat, increased mono-/polyunsaturated fatty acids, reduced salt content, whole grains/legumes, high fibre and high intakes of fruits and vegetables which are rich in vitamins, antioxidants and polyphenols.

Typically, this is captured through a Mediterranean diet; however, it has to be noted that this approach will only work for a proportion of patients, and other cultural factors and availability of foods need to be considered. Other diets such as the DASH diet demonstrate similar impact on CVD risk factors but have their own challenges, placing importance on a clinician to begin educating and supporting an individual to trial and adjust lifestyle to the approach that works for the patient.

Whilst other factors may prove significant additions to risk reduction in future research with regards to nutraceutical approaches, it is reasonable to suggest that if we were able to focus on changes to food environment and availability, with successful focus and support in clinical care on the lifestyle factors and dietary changes outlined in this chapter, major reductions in CVD would be seen.

Further Reading

Dong T, Guo M, Zhang P, Sun G, Chen B. The effects of low-carbohydrate diets on cardiovascular risk factors: a meta-analysis. *PLoS One*. 2020;15(1):e0225348.

Filippou CD, Tsioufis CP, Thomopoulos CG, et al. Dietary Approaches to Stop Hypertension (DASH) diet and blood pressure reduction in adults with and without hypertension: a systematic review and meta-analysis of randomized controlled trials. *Adv Nutr*. 2020;11(5):1150–1160.

Guo R, Li N, Yang R, Liao XY, et al. Effects of the modified DASH diet on adults with elevated blood pressure or hypertension: a systematic review and meta-analysis. *Front Nutr*. 2021;7:621.

Noto H, Goto A, Tsujimoto T, Noda M. Low-carbohydrate diets and all-cause mortality: a systematic review and meta-analysis of observational studies. *PLoS One*. 2013;8(1):e55030.

Rosato V, Temple NJ, La Vecchia C, Castellan G, Tavani A, Guercio V. Mediterranean diet and cardiovascular disease: a systematic review and meta-analysis of observational studies. *Eur J Nutr*. 2019;58(1):173–191.

Siervo M, Lara J, Chowdhury S, Ashor A, Oggioni C, Mathers JC. Effects of the Dietary Approach to Stop Hypertension (DASH) diet on cardiovascular risk factors: a systematic review and meta-analysis. *Br J Nutr*. 2015;113(1):1–5.

Sofi F, Macchi C, Abbate R, Gensini GF, Casini A. Mediterranean diet and health status: an updated meta-analysis and a proposal for a literature-based adherence score. *Public Health Nutr*. 2014;17(12):2769–2882.

References

1. World Health Organization. Cardiovascular disease (CVDs). Available at: https://www.who.int/newsroom/fact-sheets/detail/cardiovascular-diseases-(cvds). Published 11 June 2021.
2. Li J, Lee DH, Hu J, et al. Dietary inflammatory potential and risk of cardiovascular disease among men and women in the U.S. *J Am Coll Cardiol*. 2020;76(19):2181–2193.
3. Yu X-H, Fu Y-C, Zhang D-W, Yin K, Tang C-K. Foam cells in atherosclerosis. *Clin Chim Acta*. 2013;424:245–252.
4. Ambrose JA, Singh M. Pathophysiology of coronary artery disease leading to acute coronary syndromes. *F1000Prime Rep*. 2015;7:08.
5. Tzoulaki I., Elliott P., Kontis V., Ezzati M. Worldwide exposures to cardiovascular risk factors and associated health effects: current knowledge and data gaps. Available at: https://spiral.imperial.ac.uk/bitstream/10044/1/33984/2/Tzoulaki Ezzati Circulation review accepted 29 04 2016.pdf. Cited November 15, 2020.
6. Brinks J, Fowler A, Franklin BA, Dulai J. Lifestyle modification in secondary prevention: beyond pharmacotherapy. *Am J Lifestyle Med*. 2017;11(2):137–152.
7. Welty FK, Stuart E, O'Meara M, Huddleston J. Effect of addition of exercise to therapeutic lifestyle changes diet in enabling women and men with coronary heart disease to reach Adult Treatment Panel III low-density lipoprotein cholesterol goal without lowering high-density lipoprotein cholesterol. *Am J Cardiol*. 2002;89(10):1201–1204.
8. Wood D, Kotseva K, Connolly S, et al. Nurse-coordinated multidisciplinary, family-based cardiovascular disease prevention programme (EUROACTION) for patients with coronary heart disease and asymptomatic individuals at high risk of cardiovascular disease: a paired, cluster-randomised controlled trial. *Lancet*. 2008;371(9629):1999–2012.

9. Kokkinos PF, Faselis C, Myers J, Panagiotakos D, Doumas M. Interactive effects of fitness and statin treatment on mortality risk in veterans with dyslipidaemia: a cohort study. *Lancet.* 2013;381(9864):394–399.
10. ClinRisk. QRISK3. Available at: https://qrisk.org/three/. Published 2018. Cited January 5, 2021.
11. National Institute for Health and Care Excellence. CVD risk assessment and management. Available at: https://cks.nice.org.uk/topics/cvd-risk-assessment-management/. Published 2020. Cited February 2, 2021.
12. Estruch R, Ros E, Salas-Salvadó J, et al. Primary prevention of cardiovascular disease with a Mediterranean diet supplemented with extra-virgin olive oil or nuts. *N Engl J Med.* 2018;378(25):e34.
13. Chiavaroli L, Viguiliouk E, Nishi SK, et al. DASH dietary pattern and cardiometabolic outcomes: an umbrella review of systematic reviews and meta-analyses. *Nutrients.* 2019;11(2):338.
14. Dong T, Guo M, Zhang P, Sun G, Chen B. The effects of low-carbohydrate diets on cardiovascular risk factors: a meta-analysis. *PLoS One.* 2020;15(1):e0225348.
15. Rosato V, Temple NJ, La Vecchia C, Castellan G, Tavani A, Guercio V. Mediterranean diet and cardiovascular disease: a systematic review and meta-analysis of observational studies. *Eur J Nutr.* 2019;58(1):173–191.
16. Sofi F, Macchi C, Abbate R, Gensini GF, Casini A. Mediterranean diet and health status: an updated meta-analysis and a proposal for a literature-based adherence score. *Public Health Nutr.* 2014;17(12):2769–2782.
17. Siervo M, Lara J, Chowdhury S, Ashor A, Oggioni C, Mathers JC. Effects of the Dietary Approach to Stop Hypertension (DASH) diet on cardiovascular risk factors: a systematic review and meta-analysis. *Br J Nutr.* 2015;113(1):1–5.
18. Filippou CD, Tsioufis CP, Thomopoulos CG, et al. Dietary Approaches to Stop Hypertension (DASH) diet and blood pressure reduction in adults with and without hypertension: a systematic review and meta-analysis of randomized controlled trials. *Adv Nutr.* 2020;11(5):1150–1160.
19. Noto H, Goto A, Tsujimoto T, Noda M. Low-carbohydrate diets and all-cause mortality: a systematic review and meta-analysis of observational studies. *PLoS One.* 2013;8(1):e55030.
20. Mensink RP, Zock PL, Kester AD, Katan MB. Effects of dietary fatty acids and carbohydrates on the ratio of serum total to HDL cholesterol and on serum lipids and apolipoproteins: a meta-analysis of 60 controlled trials. *Am J Clin Nutr.* 2003;77(5):1146–1155.
21. Filippini T, Naska A, Kasdagli M-I, et al. Potassium intake and blood pressure: a dose-response meta-analysis of randomized controlled trials. *J Am Heart Assoc.* 2020;9(12):e015719.
22. Cormick G, Ciapponi A, Cafferata ML, Cormick MS, Belizán JM. Calcium supplementation for prevention of primary hypertension. Cochrane Database Syst Rev. 2021 Aug 10;8(8):CD010037. doi: 10.1002/14651858.CD010037.pub3. Update in: Cochrane Database Syst Rev. 2022 Jan 11;1:CD010037. PMID: 34693985; PMCID: PMC8543682.
23. Dickinson HO, Nicolson D, Campbell F, et al. Magnesium supplementation for the management of primary hypertension in adults. *Cochrane Database Syst Rev.* 2006(3):CD004640.
24. National Institute for Health and Clinical Excellence. Cardiovascular disease: risk assessment and reduction, including lipid modification. Clinical guideline. Available at: www.nice.org.uk/guidance/cg181. Published 2014. Cited November 8, 2020.
25. Ramdath DD, Padhi EMT, Sarfaraz S, Renwick S, Duncan AM. Beyond the cholesterol-lowering effect of soy protein: a review of the effects of dietary soy and its constituents on risk factors for cardiovascular disease. *Nutrients.* 2017;9(4):324.
26. Silva Figueiredo P, Inada AC, Ribeiro Fernandes M, et al. An overview of novel dietary supplements and food ingredients in patients with metabolic syndrome and non-alcoholic fatty liver disease. *Molecules.* 2018;23(4):877.
27. Sze S, Pellicori P, Kazmi S, et al. Prevalence and prognostic significance of malnutrition using 3 scoring systems among outpatients with heart failure: a comparison with body mass index. *JACC Hear Fail.* 2018;6(6):476–486.
28. Konerman MC, Hummel SL. Sodium restriction in heart failure: benefit or harm? *Curr Treat Options Cardiovasc Med.* 2014;16(2):286.
29. Okoshi MP, Capalbo RV, Romeiro FG, Okoshi K. Cardiac cachexia: perspectives for prevention and treatment. *Arq Bras Cardiol.* 2017;108(1):74–80.
30. Krim SR, Campbell P, Lavie CJ, Ventura H. Micronutrients in chronic heart failure. *Curr Heart Fail Rep.* 2013;10(1):46–53.

31. Brown AA, Hu FB. Dietary modulation of endothelial function: implications for cardiovascular disease. *Am J Clin Nutr*. 2001;73(4):673–686.
32. Buoite Stella A, Gaio M, Furlanis G, Douglas P, Naccarato M, Manganotti P. Fluid and energy intake in stroke patients during acute hospitalization in a stroke unit. *J Clin Neurosci*. 2019;62:27–32.
33. The FOOD Trial Collaboration. Effect of timing and method of enteral tube feeding for dysphagic stroke patients (FOOD): a multicentre randomised controlled trial. *Lancet*. 2005;365(9461):764–772.
34. Brostow DP, Hirsch AT, Collins TC, Kurzer MS. The role of nutrition and body composition in peripheral arterial disease. *Nat Rev Cardiol*. 2012;9(11):634–643.
35. Webster-Gandy J, Madden A, Holdsworth M, eds. *Oxford Handbook of Nutrition and Dietetics*. Oxford University Press; 2020.

CHAPTER 7

Nutrition in Endocrine (Obesity/ Diabetes) and Reproductive Medicine

Ali Ahsan Khalid ■ Rajna Golubic ■ Duane Mellor ■ Mei Yen Chan ■ Claudia Mitrofan

LEARNING POINTS

By the end of this chapter you should be able to:

- Understand the interplay between endocrinology and nutrition and how this can influence human health
- Describe the criteria used to define obesity and assess weight using various measurements
- Explain the relationship between energy requirements and expenditure
- Understand the role of hormones in controlling feeding behaviours (both hunger and satiation)
- Describe the medical conditions associated with obesity as well as their management and treatment
- Explain the pathophysiology of diabetes mellitus and understand its multifactorial aetiology
- Describe dietary approaches to managing type 2 diabetes
- Understand the role of thyroid in metabolism and ways of managing thyroid disease
- Explain the role of glucocorticoids in metabolism
- Describe the interplay between endocrinology and reproductive health
- Describe key nutritional and hormonal changes in pregnancy and lactation
- Define gestational diabetes
- Apply key principles of nutrition in endocrinology to clinical scenarios

CASE STUDY 7.1 Weight gain and its implications

A 20-year-old male university student is otherwise healthy with no other clinical conditions. He played sports at high school, but since starting university, he has reduced his physical activity level and started to drink alcohol, and his diet has become more based on convenience foods. On returning home it was noted that his body mass index (BMI) had increased in the last year from 22 kg/m^2 to 28 kg/m^2.

What is the classification of his initial and current BMI?

If he continued this type of lifestyle, what diseases might he be at risk of developing?

What would be the primary focus of any intervention in this case?

CASE STUDY 7.2 Diagnosing metabolic syndrome

A 46-year-old female business professional attends her family physician. She reports increased sleep disturbance and thinks she should have a general health review. Her blood pressure is 136/82 mm Hg, HbA1c 42 mmol/L, total cholesterol 4.6 mmol/L, high-density lipoprotein cholesterol 1.4 mmol/L and triglycerides 1.4 mmol/L. Her current weight is 89 kg, her height is 1.68 metres and her waist circumference is 112 cm.

What is her BMI and how would she be classified?

What are the implications of her waist circumference?

Does this patient currently have metabolic syndrome?

What might your initial advice be in this case?

CASE STUDY 7.3 Evaluation of the patient with elevated glucose

A 39-year-old man with a BMI of 37 kg/m^2 visits his family physician after reporting feeling somewhat tired over the past 6 months. His blood pressure is currently 146/90 mm Hg, his lipid profile suggested no significant findings, and his HbA1c was 45 mmol/mol which prompted his physician to arrange a glucose tolerance test. Fasting glucose was noted to be 5.9 mmol/L and 2-hour reading of 9.6 mmol/L.

What are the initial impressions of this case?

What are the most likely diagnoses?

What would the initial lifestyle recommendations and targets be?

CASE STUDY 7.4 Remission in diabetes

A 43-year-old woman who has recently been diagnosed with type 2 diabetes attends diabetes education. Her BMI is 36 kg/m^2 and her HbA1c was 53 mmol/mol when she was diagnosed 4 months ago. Currently she reports feeling well and her blood pressure and lipid results are unremarkable. She is currently not taking any medication. She wants to know if she can bring her diabetes into remission.

What lifestyle or health change is most likely to help bring her diabetes into remission?

Which dietary approaches could be discussed to help improve this patient's diabetes control?

CASE STUDY 7.5 Nutritional recommendations in Type 1 diabetes

A 23-year-old man with type 1 diabetes mellitus (T1DM) is managed using an insulin pump and supported using a continuous glucose monitor which provides glucose readings every few minutes. He is interested in improving his diet and is unsure about what next steps to take. His BMI is 22 kg/m^2, and his blood pressure and lipid profile are within recommended targets. He would like to engage in more exercise but is not clear how to do this. Consider how diet affects his glycaemic control compared with the need to match insulin dose to food (especially carbohydrate eaten).

What might happen to his carbohydrate and insulin requirements if he increases his exercise levels?

If he starts having more hypoglycaemic episodes, how might he manage these, and how could he reduce the risks of these happening in the future?

CASE STUDY 7.6 Primary infertility

A 26-year-old woman is referred to the gynaecology clinic by her general practitioner for investigation of primary infertility. Her partner is a 30-year-old man with no medical history and an offspring from a previous relationship. They stopped using contraception 2 years ago and have had regular intercourse since then. They both drink occasionally and have never smoked. She has previously been diagnosed with migraine but does not take any medications for it. She suffers from oligomenorrhea with periods occurring

CASE STUDY 7.6 Primary infertility—(Continued)

every 33 to 45 days. She does not suffer from menorrhagia or dysmenorrhoea. She does not have any intermenstrual or postcoital bleeding. Her cervical smears have been unremarkable, and she has never had a sexually transmitted disease.

EXAMINATION

Her BMI is 31 kg/m^2. She has slight hirsutism. Rest of the skin examination is normal.
She has a normal speculum and bimanual examination.

Investigations of Significance

follicle stimulating hormone 6.0 mIU/mL
Testosterone 5.0 nmol/L (elevated)
luteinizing hormone 6.1 IU/L
Transvaginal US report: left ovary 7 antral follicles and right ovary 13 antral follicles
What are the initial impressions of this case?
What is the most likely diagnosis and why?
Why would screening for type 2 diabetes be recommended in this case?
What would be the primary medical and lifestyle management interventions in this case?

FSH, Follicle stimulating hormone; *LH*, luteinising hormone, *US*, ultrasound

CASE STUDY 7.7 Osteoporosis

A 40-year-old woman visits her general practitioner. She underwent menopause when she was 37 years old due to premature ovarian failure of unknown aetiology. Similarly, her mother underwent menopause in her late thirties. Her mother had a fragility fracture of the head of the femur last month, which was fixed surgically. The patient has been reading on the subject and is terrified of getting a fracture herself later in life. She would like to know the risks associated with premature menopause to her health. Currently, she is not taking any medications. On inquiring, she reports preferring 'natural treatments' over drugs. However, she is open to pharmacological treatments if 'that is what's required to prevent a fracture'.
Why might this woman feel that she has an increased risk of developing osteoporosis?
What nutritional and medical interventions might be indicated in this case?
What modes of exercise are indicated in this case?

CASE STUDY 7.8 Gestational diabetes

A 31-year-old woman who is 24 weeks pregnant attends the antenatal clinic. It is her third pregnancy, and her last baby was born at term following an emergency caesarean and weighed 4.5 kg. Her pre-pregnancy BMI was 33 kg/m^2 and both her parents have type 2 diabetes mellitus (T2DM).
What are this woman's risk factors for having gestational diabetes mellitus (GDM)?
How and when might she be screened for GDM?
What might be the initial management and dietary advice given to this woman if she were diagnosed with GDM?

Overview of Endocrinology With Respect to Nutrition

The consumption of food results in a change in our body's internal environment that needs to be regulated so that the physiological processes are not impeded. Regulation is in part undertaken via the liver and first-pass metabolism via portal circulation; however, as the liver has limited storage capacity, other homeostatic mechanisms are required. This illustrates the underlying principle of endocrinology, the regulation and control of changes in metabolite levels following a meal.

The key principle of homeostasis and milieu interieur is defined as the ability of the extracellular fluid to regulate its composition and in turn maintain a protective stability for the intracellular environment. This is achieved via several key endocrinological principles:

1. Principle of negative feedback
2. Principle of positive feedback
3. Control of hormone levels by stimulating hormones and prohormones

How nutritional intake influences and changes extracellular/plasma levels of a metabolite is influenced by a number of factors summarised in Fig. 7.1. Hormones and their associated feedback mechanisms can potentially act on all of the referenced metabolic processes. In the case of iron metabolism, there is no active mechanism for excretion, but absorption can be moderated via a feedback mechanism. With respect to calcium metabolism, hormonal control can influence absorption, storage (bone deposition and resorption) and excretion (reabsorption in the kidney). With respect to metabolism, a number of enzymes in glucose and fat metabolism are insulin sensitive so metabolic processes are also influenced by hormones.

The ingestion of nutrients results in either direct or indirect changes to the extracellular levels of specific substrates. Metabolic processes vary between nutrients, and pathways to store and recycle nutrients or excrete waste substances are diverse. Some nutrients can be recycled but not excreted (e.g., iron), whereas other nutrients are metabolised and excreted. Homeostasis of macronutrients is subtly different, as there is a degree of interconversion between nutrients (e.g., deamination of amino acids prior to either gluconeogenesis, lipogenesis or ketogenesis).

The studying of the core principles influencing how endocrinology can respond to the challenges of the external environment is essential for the understanding of both system and whole-body physiology. In addition, when homeostasis is challenged beyond its capacity to maintain the internal environment within normal limits, disease occurs. In endocrinology, several pathologies that result from genetic, epigenetic or environmental factors, especially dietary factors and physical activity, have nutritional factors implicated in their causality as well as their management. This chapter considers the role of nutrition in the risk of developing, the potential causality and the management of common endocrine disease and related risk factors including obesity, diabetes,

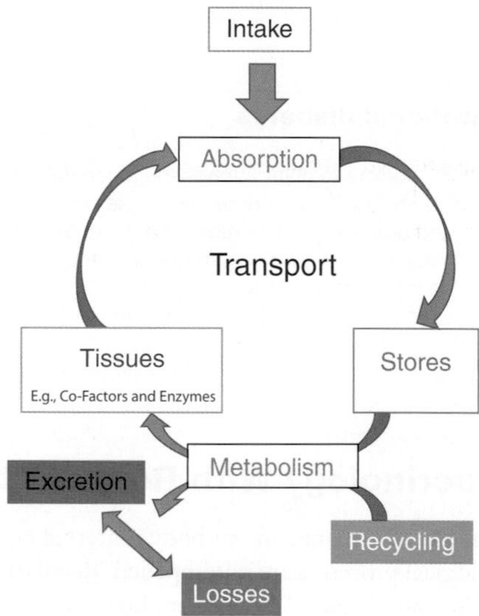

Fig. 7.1 Overview of metabolic processes. This can apply to most nutrients as well as xenobiotics including pharmaceutical agents.

thyroid dysfunction and adrenal function. Additionally, pregnancy and reproductive health will be considered as the hormonal regulation of menstruation and fertility can be influenced by nutrition as well as by other endocrine-related conditions.

Obesity

Many countries are currently seeing obesity rates of more than 20%. Over the last 30 years, obesity prevalence has tripled. Globally, about 40% of adults were overweight or obese in 2020.[1] Obesity is one of the world's greatest public health challenges—one that has shifted from being a problem in predominantly wealthy countries to one that spans all countries at all income levels and has been affecting developing countries, which are now faced with the double burden of malnutrition increasing the pathogen burden and extrinsic mortality risk.[2]

Obese individuals are at higher risks for adverse health outcomes; this includes increased risk of developing cardiovascular diseases, type 2 diabetes mellitus (T2DM) and at least 13 different cancers, including breast, colon and prostate.[3] Not only is the treatment of obesity and its related diseases extremely costly to society, but also the social and psychological burden on individuals is significant. In the United States, direct medical costs alone total about 100–200 billion dollars per year. The World Health Organization estimates that the percentage of children who are overweight or obese has risen from 4% in 1975 to around 18% in 2020.[1] If left unmanaged, childhood obesity is a significant predictor of obesity in adulthood, making it harder to manage and predisposing the individual to increased risk of earlier development of obesity-related chronic diseases. The recent coronavirus pandemic has been difficult for so many, restricting physical activity and altering food choices and habits, together with the associated psychological stress. A systematic review showed that obesity is an independent risk factor for poor COVID-19 disease outcome, and it increases the risks of individuals with COVID-19 having to seek advanced medical treatment.[4] Additionally, obesity was shown to increase the death risk in patients with COVID-19 younger than 50. This association with increased risk of an adverse outcome in people suffering from COVID-19 serves as a wake-up call to many that our general health, particularly lifestyle and body weight, can influence the outcome of disease.

ASSESSING BODY WEIGHT

As discussed in more detail in Chapter 2, in routine clinical settings, BMI is commonly used to help clinicians to identify patients who are underweight, in the healthy range, overweight or obese, and it gives an estimate of total body fat. This is a relatively simple measurement and calculation; however, it is in part limited as it is based on a Northern European population, and therefore may not reflect differences in muscle mass between different ethnic groups. This observation has led to the proposal that for individuals of Asian origin, alternative lower cutoff values should be considered. BMI is calculated by dividing body weight (in kilograms) by height (in metres) squared. Weight and height should be measured in bare feet, with the individual wearing light clothing. Measurements should be taken using calibrated equipment, and in the case of height checking, the head must be in the correct position (Frankfurt plane) and the person's heels must be against the measuring board.

With the advent of technology, it is much easier to measure the percentage of body fat, so researchers have argued that BMI is of decreasing utility and potentially should be replaced. There are limitations to the use of BMI. For instance, it should not be used for athletes who are very muscular or for pregnant women. BMI cutoffs should be ethnically specific and may not be applicable to all populations. Some have also argued that body fat distribution is a better predictor of the health hazards of obesity than is the absolute amount of body fat.

Research has shown that individuals with an upper body fat pattern (i.e., apple body shape or android pattern obesity), reflecting an excess of intra-abdominal or visceral fat, have significantly greater risk of T2DM, hypertension, and hyperlipidaemia as compared with individuals with a lower body fat accumulation pattern (pear shape or gynoid pattern obesity with the accumulation of excess fat in the hips and thigh region). The effect of visceral fat distribution appears to be separate from that of total body fat. Waist circumference can be a practical method for assessing body fat pattern, although measurements can be subject to greater error, both in defining the waist position and measuring over clothing. A BMI of 18.5–24.9 kg/m^2, indicating a normal weight, corresponds to a waist circumference of 88 cm in women and 102 cm in men. A waist circumference higher than 105 cm in women and 110 cm in men is connected to high risk of future coronary events and developing diabetes. As with BMI, waist circumference may need to be adapted for different ethnic groups.

WHY DO PEOPLE BECOME OBESE?

Obesity is a complex, multifaceted condition and is the result of an interplay between environmental and genetic factors. Many obese patients who have received dietetic advice still believe that there is nothing they can do to lose weight, and often feel that 'it is in all in their genes'. It is beyond this chapter to discuss the genetic influence in obesity risk in detail.

Apart from a few exceptional cases as seen in monogenic and/or syndromic obesity (e.g., disorder of the hypothalamic leptin-melanocortin system), findings from genome wide associations studies suggest that identified genetic factors make only a small contribution to obesity risks to the majority of people. This genotyping technology involves scanning of many thousands of single nucleotide polymorphisms in the human genome.

Genetic predisposition to obesity can be overcome by lifestyle changes. Genetic changes alone are unlikely to explain the growing obesity epidemic. So, if our genes have stayed largely the same, what has changed to explain the rapidly increasing incidence of obesity seen globally?

A suggestion is the obvious change to our environment, both with respect to food supply and demand and with respect to energy expenditure (EE) (physical exercise and work). There has been an increased intake of energy-dense foods that are high in fat and sugars and a reduction in physical activity due to an increasingly sedentary lifestyle, changing modes of transportation and increasing urbanisation. So fundamentally the cause of obesity is due to an energy imbalance between calories consumed and calories expended. Notwithstanding this, it would be prudent to suggest that the development of obesity and its related comorbidities is a result of the interplay of genetics, epigenetics (where genes are activated/switched off by an environmental stimulus at an earlier point in a person's life course) and our environment. Epigenetic mechanisms could potentially offer a logical explanation for the growing epidemic of obesity over the past few decades without a radical change in our gene pool. Environmental factors can affect the epigenetic programming of foetal and early postnatal development and through the various periods of life, affecting one's risk of developing obesity.

Relationship Between Energy Requirements and Energy Expenditure

There are a number of different components to EE. The bulk of EE is due to our resting metabolic rate or basal metabolic rate, defined as the amount of calories your body needs to accomplish its most basic (basal) life-sustaining functions, including respiration, circulation, digestion and cell production. The resting metabolic rate can account for 60%–80% of the total of daily EE. The other components of EE are the thermic effect of feeding which is the energy required to digest and dispose of nutrients and their metabolites from food. The thermic effect of feeding can be altered by dietary composition by up to 50% (e.g., increased by increasing protein intake) but as it only contributes typically 10%–15% of EE, the overall effect is quite modest. The remainder is mainly related to physical work or activity, including both voluntary and involuntary physical activity or NEAT (nonexercise activity thermogenesis). NEAT varies among individuals with the voluntary component influenced by recreational, occupational, transport actions and activities of daily living related to physical activity and exercise. NEAT can contribute between 10% and 75%+ of the total EE, but typically contributes up to 20%–40% of EE.

Generally, in obese individuals, body weight-adjusted NEAT is lower. It is therefore plausible that the increase in NEAT could be an important therapeutic target to increase caloric expenditure and facilitate weight loss. Reducing sedentary time is another potential target. Research has shown that obese individuals spend significantly more time sitting and less time standing as compared with leaner people, and data support the role of reducing sedentary time and the potential solution of adopting active workplaces and standing desks.

CONTROL OF FEEDING BEHAVIOURS: ROLE OF HORMONES

Ensuring adequate nutrition is key to our basic survival; it is therefore not surprising that there is tight neurological control of human feeding behaviour through a number of control centres in the brain. There are two main pathways involved. The first one is known as homeostatic regulation. It acts in response to the perceived energy needs required by our bodies. The second pathway is known as the hedonic pathway, which regulates our feeding based on reward circuits and other sensory cues that are not related to energy needs.

The brain receives a wide variety of signals from neurotransmitters (e.g., neuropeptide Y, opioids) gastrointestinal hormones (e.g., peptide YY, cholecystokinin) and other peptides. The receptors for these peptides and hormones are found in the central nervous system as well as in the gastrointestinal system. In total over 30 hormones, peptides and other substances have been identified as having a role in appetite in humans and other animals. Table 7.1 has a simplified summary of the action of hormones in influencing our feeding behaviour. Leptin is the most studied of these hormones, in part due to its potential as an antiobesity treatment.

Leptin was discovered in 1994. It is a hormone produced from adipose tissue and is important in the control of appetite. The largest expression of its receptors is found in the ventral basal hypothalamus. Leptin acts to reduce our appetite and reduce our food intake. It does not affect food intake from meal to meal but, instead, acts to alter food intake and control EE over the long term. As leptin is produced by fat cells, the amount of leptin released is directly related to the amount of body fat; so the more fat an individual has, the more leptin they will have circulating in their blood. Leptin levels increase if an individual increases their fat mass over a period of time and, similarly, leptin levels decrease if an individual decreases their fat mass over a period of time.

Obese people have unusually high levels of leptin. This may be because in some obese individuals, the brain does not appear to respond to leptin, so they keep eating, a concept known as leptin resistance, though its mechanism is still unclear. People lacking leptin or those with ineffective leptin receptors are severely obese.

NONHOMEOSTATIC REGULATION OF FEEDING BEHAVIOUR

Humans do not eat just to satisfy their energy needs; they also eat for pleasure. Eating is influenced by many different types of cues. For example, some people eat more when they feel stressed. Or they may feel hungry when they see pictures of certain foods or certain cues like the logos or symbols of fast-food companies such as the golden arches (McDonald's) or the colonel image (KFC), or even the smells and sounds associated with these foods and outlets (e.g., hearing someone eating a packet of potato crisps). These reinforced learned behaviours can easily 'override' our homeostatic-based signals, resulting in us eating much more than what our body needs.

TABLE 7.1 ■ **Summary of Peptides and Hormones and Receptors Involved in Satiation and Appetite**[5]

Peptide or Hormone	Main Site of Release	Main Function With Respect to Satiation and Appetite
Cholecystokinin	I cells in duodenum	Limits the amount of food consumed; acts on vagal afferents (CCK1R) and CNS, hypothalamic (e.g., arcuate) nuclei (CCK2R)
Ghrelin	Mostly stomach	Stimulates food intake; stimulates appetite via secretion of NPY and orexin
Leptin	Adipose tissue (also placenta and skeletal muscle)	Decreased levels induce hunger (starvation reduces leptin and drives appetite); regulates feeding behaviour and short- and long-term satiation.
GLP-1	Intestinal L cells (along with PYY)	Enhances satiety and fullness
NPY	hypothalamus and intestinal neurons	Stimulated by leptin and ghrelin to suppress appetite
PP	D cell in pancreas	Experimentally has anorectic effects with PP
PYY	Intestinal L cells	Activates ileal break and via hypothalamic ARC nucleus regulates food intake
OXM	Intestinal L cells	Acts via GLP-1 to decrease food intake
Apo A-IV	intestinal enterocytes	Linked to lipid absorption, decreases food intake in rodent models

Apo A-IV, Apolipoprotein A-IV; *ARC*, arcuate nucleus; *CCK*, cholecystokinin; *CNS*, central nervous system; *GLP-1*, glucagon-like peptide 1; *NPY*, neuropeptide Y; *OXM*, oxyntomodulin; *PP*, pancreatic peptide; *PYY*, peptide YY.

Modified from Camilleri M. Peripheral mechanisms in appetite regulation. *Gastroenterology* 2015;148(6): 1219–1233.

DISEASES ASSOCIATED WITH OBESITY

In addition to the well-recognised association of obesity with diseases mentioned previously including diabetes, hypertension and cardiovascular disorders, there are other less well-recognised associations, including sleep apnoea, osteoarthritis and psychological disorders due to psychosocial stigma.

Sleep Apnoea

Though the pathology is not 100% clear, the hypothesis is that increased fatty deposits around the neck or pharyngeal regions in obese individual can cause obstruction during sleep, resulting in increased snoring, a condition known as obstructive sleep apnoea, that is more common in men than women. Lung volume may also be reduced due to increased abdominal pressure on the diaphragm in patients with central obesity.

Osteoarthritis

Diseases of the bones, joints, connective tissue and skin have been commonly linked to obesity adding to the significant health costs attributed to being overweight. There is extensive literature on the role of obesity and T2DM as risk factors for developing an arthritic condition. The link between obesity and osteoarthritis is related to both the direct effect of excess mechanical load on the cartilages, especially of the weight-bearing joints such as hips and knees, and indirect, referring to the metabolic effects of the adipose tissue. Adipocytes produce and release adipokines, which are inflammatory mediators that act locally and systemically, creating a proinflammatory mechanism that can damage cartilages, bones and synovial tissue. This low-grade chronic inflammation resulting from chronic hyperglycaemia and insulin resistance reaches the joint through the subchondral vascular network and plays an important role in the initiation and perpetuation of the osteoarthritis process. Leptin, the major adipokine discussed previously, in addition to effects on decreasing appetite stimulates chondrocyte apoptosis. High glucose concentration has a pro-inflammatory and prodegradative effect on human chondrocytes, decreasing the joint's mechanical properties of stiffness and resistance. Moreover, diabetes is known to decrease bone remodelling and microvascular disease leads to decreased nutrient delivery to the bone and synovium.

Psychosocial Stigma

One of the adverse health outcomes which may not be visible but can be very debilitating for the individuals is the psychosocial aspects of obesity. For instance, obese individuals may experience more stigmatisation affecting education or employment and causing subsequent mental trauma. The stigmatisation may be worse for obese women compared with men and create increased psychological distress due to societal pressures to be thin. The result of emotional disability due to stigmatisation is a large increase in health care costs related to mental health issues in the obese.

The stigma directed toward obese people has been identified as a barrier to seeking health care. Health professionals have been shown to have the same level of stigma toward people living with obesity as the general public. Misconceptions can include attributing all health issues to obesity or disregarding the challenges of living at a higher body weight and the difficulties of losing weight; all of these aspects can prevent individuals from improving their health and well-being.

MANAGEMENT AND TREATMENT OF OBESITY

There are currently three main approaches to the management of obesity, all of which should ideally be supported with behavioural interventions. In addition to the period of active weight loss, the maintenance period is equally important, as is evidenced in that the majority of individuals attempting to lose weight regain the weight in the following 1–2 years.

The three primary approaches to weight loss are:

- Lifestyle changes – diet and exercise
- Pharmacotherapy
- Bariatric surgery

Founding principles of a successful weight loss programme include:

- Positive lifestyle changes including support of behaviour change.
- Weight loss goal of 0.5–1 kg a week, allowing steady weight loss with minimised loss of lean tissue. The goal should be linked to realistic weight loss targets, although in individuals with BMI 40+ kg/m^2 a more rapid weight loss might be indicated.
- Longer-term goal to lose 5%–10% of body weight which, if sustained, is associated with significant reduced risk of morbidity and mortality.

Physical Activity

Physical activity can help increase energy deficit, although evidence suggests it is not an optimal way to lose weight in the absence of dietary modification. In addition to the benefit of weight loss, load-bearing exercise and especially resistance exercise may have the benefit of helping to maintain lean tissue mass during caloric restriction. The primary goal regarding physical activity in the obese person is increasing physical activity and reducing sedentary time. Most governments generally recommend for adults a minimum of 30 minutes of moderate intensity exercise on 5 or more days a week. The activity can be in one session or several sessions lasting 10 minutes or more.

Dietary Approaches

Evidence suggests that there is not one best diet when it comes to weight loss, the key being long-term sustainability, similar to the concept for control of blood glucose in people with diabetes. However, all approaches rely on energy restriction to some extent. Some advocates of low-carbohydrate or even ketogenic diets suggest that the metabolic action of ketones facilitates fat metabolism; however, the effects of this dietary approach may simply be by reducing the food sources which typically contribute to 50% of dietary energy intake, and only partially replacing this dietary energy with highly satiating, high-fat substitutes, resulting in a significant energy deficit.

Common dietary approaches for weight loss include:

- The 500 kcal/day deficit diet: individuals vary in metabolic efficiency and a 500 kcal per day deficit may not lead to a weekly 0.5-kg weight loss in all individuals. This can be achieved by decreasing portion sizes, so individuals reduce intake of a number of foods to achieve the energy deficit without making any macronutrient category 'forbidden'.
- Low-calorie diets (1000–1600 kcal/day), with the consideration that they may not be nutritionally complete and may not lead to prolonged dietary habit change.
- Very-low-calorie diets (less than 1000 kcal/day) under clinical supervision. These can be in the form of food or meal replacement products such as milkshakes as total meal replacements. Same concerns as with low-calorie diets.

Regardless of the dietary approach recommended to support weight loss, it is essential to incorporate maintenance programs that mitigate against weight regain after the initial weight loss program ends.

Role of Medication and Surgery in Obesity Management

Managing obesity with medication should be considered only for patients who have not reached their target weight loss or have reached a plateau on lifestyle changes. Antiobesity medications approved by the Food and Drug Administration include:

- Orlistat (Alli, Xenical), which works via inhibiting fat absorption, requires adherence to a low-fat diet, otherwise the side effect is profound diarrhoea or oily stools.
- Phentermine and topiramate (Qsymia) suppress appetite and can lead to dry mouth and rarely cardiovascular side effects.
- Bupropion and naltrexone (Contrave) suppresses appetite and can alter mood in a negative way.
- Liraglutide (Saxenda, Victoza) mimics Glucagon-like Peptide-1 to delay gastric emptying and suppress appetite. Side effects include nausea, vomiting, dehydration and possible kidney failure.

Bariatric surgery may be considered when most or all of the following criteria are fulfilled:

- BMI is 40 kg/m^2 or more, or between 35 kg/m^2 and 40 kg/m^2 (may be lower in people of Asian ethnicity) and
- The person has other significant comorbidities including T2DM or hypertension.
- Appropriate nonsurgical measures have been tried but have failed to achieve or maintain adequate, clinically beneficial weight loss for at least 6 months.
- The person is fit for anaesthesia and surgery.
- The person is willing to adopt lifelong lifestyle changes.
- Of note, surgery can be recommended as a first-line option for adults with a BMI of more than 50 kg/m^2 in whom surgical intervention is considered appropriate.

Bariatric surgery includes a range of procedures that can require lifelong vitamin and mineral supplementation. Prior to surgery, dietetic and psychological support is required. Following surgery diet needs to be carefully managed including (depending on type of procedure) a liquid diet followed by introduction of meals of very small volume.

Gut Microbiota and Obesity

The connection between gut microbiome and obesity was recognised following microbiome transplantation experiments performed in mice. Transplantation from an overweight adult twin to its germ-free mice sibling led to rapid increases in body and fat mass, while mice receiving the lean twin microbiome maintained normal weight. The theory that bacterial composition affects weight is also supported by studies comparing the gut microbiota of obese and lean people. Observations from these studies revealed higher proportion of Firmicutes (F) and lower prevalence of Bacteroidetes (B) in obese individuals, suggesting that the F/B ratio could be used as a biomarker indicative of obesity susceptibility. However, with the rapid accumulation of data looking at the human gut microbiome and obesity, studies could not find a clear trend between the F/B ratio and obesity status, suggesting that the complexity of how gut microbiome modulates obesity is much more than a simple imbalance between two gut bacterial strains.

The hypothesis that antibiotics can alter gut microbiota has also been explored. Childhood obesity has been linked to antibiotics exposure in infancy, suggesting a potential role of a healthy gut microbiome in the control of body weight.

Diabetes Mellitus

OUTLINE AND EPIDEMIOLOGY

Diabetes mellitus can be defined as a range of metabolic disorders which are typified by hyperglycaemia, resulting from either an absolute or relative insulin insufficiency. T1DM is an autoimmune disorder that results in the destruction of the insulin-secreting beta cells of the pancreas, whereas T2DM results from insulin resistance associated with obesity and excessive adiposity. Prevalence of T2DM is higher in certain communities and is linked to ethnicities, being more common in individuals of African and Asian descent compared with those of European descent. These latter observations are confounded by the effects of adverse social determinants that can increase susceptibility including greater levels of nutritional deprivation. The incidence of T2DM has also been strongly associated with increasing age. Historically, T2DM was called maturity onset diabetes, before it was reclassified as non-insulin-dependent diabetes. However, increasing rates of obesity (especially at earlier points in the life course) and increasing use of adjunctive insulin therapy have made both terms obsolete and confusing. Despite this, both terms can still be seen in older publications and are occasionally used by people living with diabetes. The incidence of diabetes in populations is around 5%–10% of adults in most economically developed countries, with a number of countries, typically Pacific Island nations that have a very high incidence of obesity reporting an incidence of 20% or more. With age, incidence increases, with individuals over 75 years of age being 2–4 times more likely to be living with diabetes.[6]

Assessment of diabetes control can be made using the HbA1c, a reference to glycated haemoglobin that is used as an indicator of blood glucose control over the previous 8–12 weeks. Glucose in the blood binds to red blood cells in a directly proportionate way with increased glucose leading to more being bound to red blood cells. Bound glucose stays on the red blood cells throughout their life span of around 16 weeks. Diabetes is defined as an HbA1c >48 mmol/mol or two blood glucose measurements consisting of a fasting glucose >7.0 mmol/L or a random glucose >11.1 mmol/L or the same levels from an oral glucose tolerance test (75 g glucose) either fasting or after 2 hours. There are also interim levels of glucose which indicate impaired fasting glucose and impaired glucose tolerance (Table 7.2).

TABLE 7.2 ■ **National Institute for Health and Care Excellence Diagnostic Criteria for Diabetes Mellitus and Gestational Diabetes**

Parameter Measured	Impaired Fasting Glucose	Impaired Glucose Tolerance	Diabetes Mellitus	Gestational Diabetes
HbA1c	42%–47% suggestive refer for OGTT		>48 mmol/L	Not appropriate in pregnancy
Fasting glucose	>6.0 mmol/L (IDΓ) >5.6 mmol/L (ADA)	Requires OGTT to confirm	>7.0 mmol/L with symptoms or on 2 occasions	NICE UK >5.6 mmol/l (typical part of OGTT)
Random glucose	Not applicable	Not applicable	>11.1 mmol/L with symptoms or on 2 occasions	Not applicable
2 hours following 75-g glucose (OGTT)	Not applicable	>7.8 mmol/L	> 11.1 mmol/L	> 7.8 mmol/L

ADA, American Diabetes Association; *IDF*, International Diabetes Federation; *NICE*, National Institute for Health and Clinical Excellence; *OGTT*, oral glucose tolerance test.

CLASSIFICATION OF DIABETES

Most individuals living with diabetes have T2DM, accounting for 85% of cases, with T1DM and the similar but slower-onset latent autoimmune diabetes in adults making up the rest of the cases. Although with increasing duration and age T2DM can appear to clinically behave like T1DM, in the majority of cases, due to the differing pathology and clinical management, the focus for nutritional interventions should vary. Gestational diabetes mellitus (GDM), a type of hyperglycaemia which encompasses levels of glycaemia associated with diabetes along with impaired fasting glucose and impaired glucose tolerance, is seen in more than 15% of pregnancies and will be discussed late in this chapter.[7] As well as being a risk factor for future development of T2DM, it is also strongly associated with age, obesity, ethnicity and levels of deprivation with some communities reporting 40%–50% of pregnancies complicated by GDM.

Another form of diabetes is classified as maturity-onset diabetes in youth (MODY). The underlying pathophysiology represents different genetic conditions which typically influence how insulin is secreted (directly or indirectly) or alters glucose metabolic pathways. Most cases may respond to sulphonylurea therapy and do not require insulin, and in some cases, MODY may not be associated with risk of complications associated with T1DM and T2DM. Most cases of MODY are the result of one of four genetic defects, the most common ones include defects in in hepatocyte nuclear factor 1 homeobox A or glucokinase proteins; the former is very sensitive to sulphonylurea, and the later typically only results in modest hyperglycaemia which outside of pregnancy, rarely requires active treatment.

Additionally, there are a number of rarer causes of diabetes, which may have additional implications when it comes to nutrition, such as cystic fibrosis. Other causes include Leprechaunism (Donohue syndrome), acromegaly and hereditary haemochromatosis which may have genetic causes, but the diabetes is a result of the pathological processes, relating to the effect of growth hormone or iron on tissues increasing insulin resistance in the cases of acromegaly and haemochromatosis, respectively.

GENETICS AND THE ENVIRONMENT

Both T1DM and T2DM have inherited components, although in both the pattern of inheritance is complex. With T1DM the genetic risk has been associated with the Human Leukocyte Antigen genes, which are responsible for cell surface antigen recognition, and therefore defects could result in autoimmune responses. Genetic factors associated with T2DM are located across a number of chromosomes and may also interact with genes increasing the risk of obesity. To date genetic markers for T2DM have not been fully defined. MODY, which is also described as monogenic diabetes, is linked to specific genes as described previously.

Environmental factors can alter the effects of insulin, glucose and fat metabolism, altering insulin secretion or adipose, liver and/or response to insulin and therefore glucose metabolism.

Environmental factors have also been associated with risk of T2DM, with smoking now accepted as a risk factor associated with a 30%–40% increased risk for T2DM. Smoking is now included in a number of diabetes risk scores. Although the mechanism is less clear with respect to air pollution, there is increasing evidence of a causal association in both humans and animal models. Environment also interacts with lifestyle, especially diet and physical activity, to increase risk of developing T2DM, with poverty and aspects of housing also being linked with increased risk and poorer health outcomes.

Although the risk factors for T1DM are less well defined, there have been reported links to latitude, with northerly latitudes being associated with increased incidence of T1DM. The mechanism and causal nature of this association has not been confirmed. Other associated risk factors include infection with a number of viruses including Coxsackievirus B and in some populations, early exposure to cow's milk as observed only in Finnish cohorts.

EPIGENETICS, OBESITY AND MORBIDITY

Alongside genetic factors, a number of environmental triggers can alter gene expression, potentially increasing the risk of developing T2DM. Initial evidence for epigenetic influence on diabetes risk came from long-term follow-up of the children born to mothers who lived through the Dutch Hunger Winter in the 1940s and children born in the UK in the 1920s. These studies found that a challenging in utero environment linked to reduced food availability or a large placenta relative to the birth weight of the baby was associated not only with increased risk of developing obesity and T2DM later in life, but also with hypertension and cardiovascular disease in their offspring.

Additionally, it has been noted that an individual's risk for developing T2DM is increased by 40%–70% if one or both parents have the disease.[8] The risk of an individual having dysglycaemia or T2DM is increased if their mother has any form of diabetes during pregnancy (T1DM, T2DM or GDM). This is postulated to be a response to the increase in glucose supply during pregnancy altering gene expression, especially postpartum, where the infant needs to adjust from a nutrient-rich to a relatively nutrient-poor environment. These examples of the plasticity of the genome in response to environmental stress suggest that epigenetic factors can significantly increase future risk of T2DM, which would be of particular importance in the management of childhood undernutrition, as historically the focus has been on rapid recovery and regaining of body mass. It is not clear whether this approach will alter the individual's risk of developing diabetes later in life nor how reversible these alterations to gene expression are and if more conservative and measured nutrition interventions can moderate this risk. The epigenetic changes resulting from changes in nutrient environment are believed to underlie the 'thrifty' gene or Barker hypothesis and are used to explain not only the early origins of disease later in life such as T2DM, but also why some communities within different ethnic groups may be at greater risk of developing T2DM, especially when migrating from rural to urban environments, where there is an increased exposure to refined carbohydrates and less opportunity for physical activity.

MICROVASCULAR AND MACROVASCULAR CONSEQUENCES

Complications of diabetes can be classified as being either microvascular or macrovascular, with potential overlap between the two, despite subtle differences between pathological mechanisms. Macrovascular complications affect the large blood vessels, increasing risk of cardiovascular, cerebrovascular and peripheral vascular disease. Microvascular disease can lead to disease in the smaller vessels which can lead to disease in the eye, kidney and other tissues. Microvascular complications include retinopathy, nephropathy and neuropathy.

Risk factors for microvascular and macrovascular complications in diabetes vary slightly between individuals with T1DM and T2DM. The majority of the evidence in T1DM is that glycaemic control is the major determining factor that influences risk of complications. In T2DM due to the presence of metabolic syndrome, a combination of glycaemic control and lipid and blood pressure management is necessary to mitigate risk of both macrovascular and microvascular complications.

HYPOGLYCAEMIA AND NUTRITION

Risks of hypoglycaemia are strongly related to medication, in that diabetes managed with insulin is associated with the highest risk of hypoglycaemia. Risk of hypoglycaemia with oral agents used in the management of T2DM is predominantly linked to sulphonylureas and insulin secretagogues. The half-life of insulin and the oral agents can lead to prolonged episodes of hypoglycaemia which can be resistant to treatment or result in the hypoglycaemic episode recurring. The risk of hypoglycaemia can be exacerbated by the effects of alcohol which reduces the ability of the liver to synthesise glucose either from glycogenolysis or gluconeogenesis.

Clinical definition of hypoglycemia can be defined in three levels. Level one (mild) has a glucose concentration of less than 70 mg/dL (<3,9 mmol). Level two (moderate) has a glucose concentration of less than 54 mg/dL (<3 mmol) while the third and last level (severe), the individual is unable to function to do mental or physical changes as the blood glucose concentration may drop below 40 mg/dL (<2.2 mmol).[9] Depending on a number of factors, including habitual levels of glycaemia and hypoglycaemia awareness, people living with diabetes can feel hypoglycaemic at different levels. Typically, if habitual levels are elevated, then the threshold for feeling symptoms is altered, meaning some individuals may report feeling hypoglycaemic with glucose levels within or even above the normal range. Equally, with increased duration, especially with T1DM, hypoglycaemia awareness can be reduced, so that symptoms may not appear until glucose levels are low enough to induce neuroglycopenic symptoms. Hypoglycaemic unawareness can be very dangerous to the individual if they are driving or operating machinery and can lead to death if episodes occur while the patient is sleeping.

Despite only a limited number of agents being associated with hypoglycaemia, many people living with diabetes (both T1DM and T2DM) report experiencing episodes of hypoglycaemia that can lead to compensatory eating of foods containing carbohydrate in an attempt to try to avoid hypoglycaemia. The resulting dual side effect is weight gain and increased medication and insulin requirements, creating a vicious cycle. It is important that focused nutritional education about the risk of hypoglycaemia (including symptoms, testing and management), interaction between diet (physical activity) and insulin requirements and effect on weight be available. Although insulin and to some extent sulphonylureas are associated with weight gain, careful support and education can help weight management.

It can be challenging to provide information with respect to hypoglycaemia as the symptoms and perception can result in individuals tending to consume greater than the recommended loads of rapidly absorbed glucose, resulting in at least transient hyperglycaemia. Recommendations for hypoglycaemia avoidance can be based on a standard of 15–20 g of rapidly absorbed carbohydrate, which is then followed by a repeat fingerstick test 15 minutes later. If the measured glucose does not increase, carbohydrate dosing needs to be repeated. There is emerging evidence for the use of different strategies for carbohydrate management of hypoglycaemia based on the amount of carbohydrate per kilogram body weight. The higher the patient's weight, the more carbohydrate it takes to raise blood sugar. For someone with a weight between 48 and 76 kg, 1 g of carbohydrate raises blood glucose by 0.22 mmol/L. People weighing between 77 and 105 kg will raise their blood glucose by 0.17 mmol/L after consuming 1 g of carbohydrate.

It is important to note that oral carbohydrate should only be used to manage hypoglycaemia in conscious individuals. In unconscious individuals whose hypoglycaemia is not linked to alcohol intoxication, it is possible to use intramuscular glucagon to initially manage hypoglycaemia, although that can result in nausea, vomiting and headaches. In inpatient settings and in alcohol-intoxicated individuals, due to the inhibition of glycogenolysis by alcohol, intravenous glucose is used to manage hypoglycaemia.

DIETARY APPROACHES TO GLYCAEMIC CONTROL

Type 1 Diabetes

T1DM has been historically a disease where the dietary approach has been carbohydrate restriction. With modern insulin analogues and continuous subcutaneous insulin infusion systems or pumps, it is possible to flexibly and rapidly dose insulin, allowing diet to be quantified with respect to its carbohydrate content, so that insulin doses can be selected, and as such the dietary approach can flexible based on an individual's preferences and other health needs.[10]

That said, increasingly there are individuals who have chosen to reduce their carbohydrate intake as an approach to managing their T1DM. There are reports of individuals, both adults and children, successfully managing T1DM from a glycaemic perspective with low- or very-low-carbohydrate diets. This approach must be weighed against the risks associated with hypoglycaemia. Especially with children, low-carbohydrate diets need to be considered with caution due to limited data on how growth can be affected.

Type 2 Diabetes

Prevention of T2DM, including the reduction in risk of impaired glucose tolerance and impaired fasting glucose, is managed with a similar approach as that taken for T1DM, with the focus on weight reduction of at least 7 kg with 10 kg recommended for people who are overweight or obese. The DIRECT study suggests that, depending on the duration of the T2DM, the nature of the underlying pathology and degree of beta-cell dysfunction, a sustained weight loss of 15 kg or more over 2 years can result in remission, defined as medication-free normoglycaemia, in up to 36% of patients.[11] If remission is not achieved, weight loss, or more specifically loss of metabolically active fat mass, is associated with significant improvements in glycaemia.

When considering glycaemic control, although weight management is the cornerstone of control there is little evidence to suggest that any one dietary strategy is superior to another. When evaluating the effectiveness of a dietary intervention for T2DM, it is worth considering the potential to significantly improve glycaemia and the possibility to reverse the pathological processes driving insulin resistance and relative insulin deficiency; however, the primary predictor is the ability of the patient to sustain the dietary intervention. Despite the lack of evidence for any one dietary approach or even optimal proportions of macronutrients in the diet of a person living with T2DM, a number of dietary approaches have good evidence of efficacy and should be discussed as potential options for individuals based on their personal preferences and the nature of their diabetes.

Type 2 Diabetes Remission. Although not an entirely new concept, cases of spontaneous remission of T2DM have been reported since the 1960s. However, more recently a number of studies have been designed specifically in an attempt to achieve remission. Definition of remission and reversal have been developed, although not entirely agreed upon as an international consensus. It is generally accepted that remission is defined as a HbA1c of less than 48 mmol/mol, achieved for at least 6–12 months without medication. In addition, some studies have added a category of diabetes reversal, which is similar to remission, with the exception that metformin can be continued as the only therapy employed.[12]

The studies which have sought to achieve remission as the primary outcome have focused on weight loss either by bariatric surgery or total meal replacement. In addition, a number of secondary analyses have shown the potential of the Mediterranean diet, low-carbohydrate diets and plant-based diets to achieve remission. As previously mentioned, remission is most likely when weight loss of 15 kg or more occurs.[11] With very-low-carbohydrate diets, there are data that suggest that a reduction to HbA1c levels compatible with remission can be achieved without weight loss, although whether this remission can be sustained or whether the low-carbohydrate dietary pattern must be maintained is unclear.

SPECIFIC APPROACHES TO MANAGING TYPE 2 DIABETES

Total Meal Replacements

Meal replacements have been used for a number of years in the management of weight and more recently in studies of T2DM, including the DIRECT study, with a view to inducing remission. The principle of this approach is to replace all meals with complete nutrient shakes, with a severe caloric restriction of around 800 kcal per day. There is less evidence to support a solid food-based approach. Prior to the development of remission protocols, total meal replacements were used cautiously as there was a history of adverse events linked to inadequate protein quality. However, modern formulations appear to be safe, with suitability of use now focusing more on risk/benefit relating to medication and comorbidities. Often significant reductions in sulphonylureas and insulin are required to minimise risk of hypoglycaemia, and close monitoring by a specialist is suggested. With respect to comorbidities, one should be aware that this approach can have a mild diuretic effect and a review of diuretic medication is worthwhile, and the approach is not recommended for patients with chronic kidney disease except in concert with a specialist in that area due to the potential for electrolyte abnormalities. It is also important to recognise that rapid weight loss may increase the risk of gallstone formation and alteration in vegetable intake may alter International Normalized Ratio for patients treated with warfarin.

Although over a third of individuals at 2 years can maintain remission from T2DM, prolonged remission depends on the initial amount of weight lost and maintenance of the loss. Despite the data supporting the use of total meal replacements to achieve remission from T2DM, the approach is not a long-term solution. To maintain the benefits, a long-term dietary approach is needed to help maintain weight loss. Research suggests that male subjects, younger people and individuals with shorter duration of T2DM are predictors of greater likelihood of an individual having success in achieving sustained remission.

Bariatric Surgery

Data from systematic reviews of studies of people with T2DM who have undergone bariatric surgery suggest 58%–95% can achieve remission.[13] Although as is true of other approaches that induce remission, the finding is primarily driven via weight loss, with additional influence of endocrine changes associated with bariatric procedures, including those observed after gastric bypass surgery. Remission of diabetes may be secondary to altered delivery of nutrients to the small bowel, stimulating incretin secretion, including increased levels of GLP-1. GLP-1 is in incretin that supports insulin secretion and suppresses glucagon along with alteration of the vagal tone, slowing gastric emptying. It may also reduce insulin resistance.

Mediterranean Diet

The Mediterranean diet has been suggested to be one of the healthiest diets in the world, associated with a reduced incidence of cardiovascular disease and cancer in populations where the diet is prevalent. With respect to T2DM, a recent network meta-analysis suggested that a Mediterranean diet was the most efficacious way to improve glycaemic control when compared with nine other types of diet (including low-fat, vegetarian, high-protein, moderate-carbohydrate, low-carbohydrate, Palaeolithic diets).[14]

When considering the Mediterranean diet, it is important to understand what this dietary pattern is and what it is not. The Mediterranean diet is a cultural dietary pattern that includes eating food that is available and seasonal, originally based on the food that was available in rural Crete in the 1950s, which involved vegetables and fruit, with pulses, whole grains, fish and fermented dairy. The main fat source used was olive oil, and meat was not regularly available and alcohol, predominantly wine, was consumed in moderation. Therefore, the principles of this simple plant-based diet with moderate amounts of animal-based foods should perhaps be more of a focus than the regular consumption of extra virgin olive oil and nuts which is often cited due to the data from the PREDIMED study.[15]

Low-Carbohydrate Diets

Evidence suggests that low-carbohydrate diets, including very-low-carbohydrate diets, can be effective in the short- to medium-term glycaemic management of T2DM for up to 3–6 months.[16] These diets in some cases may be low enough to induce ketogenesis, containing below 5% (or 50 g per day) energy from carbohydrate. The so called ketogenic diets have been controversial, although they have a long history in the management of diabetes before the discovery of insulin, but they have increasingly been accepted as one of the options in T2DM dietary therapy. There is a lack of evidence to show superiority over other dietary approaches, but they may become an option for some individuals who are highly motivated to try them.

Energy-Restricted Diets

Energy restricted diets have been the basis of management of type 2 diabetes since the 1980s when there was a move away from counting carbohydrates and fats. Although theoretically effective, long-term sustainability of these approaches may impede their effectiveness. Some advocates of other approaches suggest that this method is less ideal as only focusing on energy restriction does not consider dietary quality.

Plant-Based Diets

A number of studies have shown that vegan diets can be effective in controlling T2DM with only very limited evidence with respect to achieving remission. This dietary approach needs to be carefully planned so that it is nutritionally adequate, especially as regards vitamin B12 intake. It is likely that less stringent forms of plant-based eating, such as lacto-ovo vegetarian, pescatarian and flexitarian diets, the latter of which are similar to the Mediterranean Diet mentioned previously, will also be helpful. With rising interest in plant-based eating, an increasing number of highly processed plant-based foods are now available, and patients should be educated regarding their consumption as they may make this type of diet less healthy. The challenge of reducing intake of highly processed foods is not unique to plant-based diets, but the issue of the health halo associated with these foods may lead to consumers being less aware of the overall health effects of highly processed plant-based foods, including a tendency to be very high in salt or added sugars.

DIABETES, AGEING AND FRAILTY

The prevalence of diabetes increases in the population with age, with over half the people living with diabetes being over 65 years in economically more developed countries, and over a quarter over 75 years. In the United States, around one in four adults aged over 65 years of age has diabetes, compared with around 5%–10% of adults overall.[17] Despite the large number of older people with diabetes, due to these individuals also living with comorbidities, they are often excluded from clinical trials, and therefore there are very limited data on the best way to support older people with diabetes.

With increasing age, as is the case with people who do not have diabetes, there is an increased risk of both dementia and frailty. Frailty is recognised as a significant risk factor for morbidity and mortality of people living with diabetes. It also appears that extremes of glycaemia (both hypoglycaemia and hyperglycaemia) are associated with increased risk of frailty for people with diabetes. Diabetes has also been acknowledged as being a risk factor for both developing dementia and the risk of mild cognitive impairment progressing to dementia.[18]

Because of the increased risk of developing frailty and dementia with diabetes, especially if control is poor, as part of clinical management dietary strategies that reduce risk of frailty and dementia should be attempted. These strategies on the whole are highly compatible with many dietary recommendations for people with diabetes, which include basing meals on minimally processed foods and adding servings of vegetables and fruit as part of a Mediterranean-style diet. What might be slightly more controversial is that evidence in older adults suggests that higher protein requirements are needed to maintain muscle function and overall health. Historically, albeit based on limited evidence, recommendations for people with diabetes were to consume a moderate amount of protein due to concerns that higher protein intakes might increase risk of progressive kidney dysfunction; however, recent data suggest that the type of protein may be more important than quantity in progressive kidney disease (see Chapter 9). An increased protein intake can increase insulin requirements and may have a modest effect on glycaemia, but it can also increase the satiating effect of the meal, so it is important in individuals at risk of undernutrition and frailty that nutrient density is optimised so that dietary plans are designed to minimise risk of unintended consequences including malnutrition.

DIABETES COPRESENTING WITH OTHER COMORBIDITIES

It is important to note that with increasing age and diabetes the likelihood that multiple comorbidities will coexist also increases. Given that comorbidities also tend to exclude people from research, this means there is very limited data on the optimal approach to manage people with diabetes who have cardiovascular disease, kidney disease or other complications. There are a number of guidelines regarding cardiovascular rehabilitation and enteral feeding. The primary principle is that dietary interventions should be considered to balance the clinical need and the personal preferences of the person with diabetes to optimise both their physical health and their quality of life.

THYROID DISORDERS

Thyroid disorders are amongst the most common endocrine diseases. Left untreated, underlying thyroid disease can increase the risks of developing heart disease, neuropathy and mental health issues. The thyroid gland, an important endocrine organ, plays a vital role in the regulation of metabolism and body weight as well as growth and development. Its effects are mediated by the thyroid hormones, triiodothyronine (T3) and thyroxine (T4). T4, which is the main form of thyroid hormone circulating in the blood, is produced by the thyroid gland. Levels of T4 are controlled by another hormone known as the thyroid-stimulating hormone (TSH) which is produced in the pituitary gland. The production of TSH and T4 is tightly controlled by negative feedback as part of homeostatic processes in our bodies. When there is very little circulating T4 in the body, the pituitary gland will produce more TSH to stimulate the thyroid gland to produce more T4. Once the T4 in the plasma exceeds a normal concentration, the pituitary's production of TSH is supressed under normal conditions.

Classification and Screening

Patients with thyroid disease are typically classified according to the results of thyroid function tests. In most healthy individuals, a normal level of TSH means that the functioning of the thyroid gland is also normal. Changes in TSH often occur before any changes in the levels of T4 and T3. Primary hypothyroidism refers to patients with elevated TSH, one possible sign that the thyroid gland is not producing enough thyroid hormone, and low thyroxine (T4) levels. On the other hand, hyperthyroidism is diagnosed when the thyroid is producing an excess of T4 and the TSH level is low. The measurement of thyroid antibodies may also help to diagnose the cause of some specific thyroid problems (Table 7.3).

Autoimmune Disorders of Thyroid and Thyroiditis

Autoimmune disease, such as Hashimoto thyroiditis, can cause hypothyroidism. Another autoimmune condition, known as Graves disease, is a type of hyperthyroidism. Short-lived symptoms of hyperthyroidism can occur with a condition called thyroiditis, which can be caused by a viral or a bacterial infection. It is usually quite rare and can be either associated with a weakened immune system or a problem with the development of the thyroid gland.

Thyroid Disorder and Weight Regulation

It has been observed that individuals with thyroid disorders can have problems regulating their body weight as low thyroid hormone levels are shown to be associated with low basal metabolic rates and, hence, reduced daily EE. The approach, in addition to replacement of thyroid hormone, should be similar to the approaches to obesity referred to earlier in this chapter if the patient is overweight.

TABLE 7.3 ■ **Diagnosis of Thyroid Disorders Using TSH and T4 Levels**[19]

Medical Condition	TSH	Free T4
Primary hypothyroidism (e.g., Hashimoto thyroiditis)	High	Low
Thyrotoxicosis (e.g., Graves disease)	Low	High

T4, Thyroxine; *TSH*, thyroid-stimulating hormone.

Iodine Deficiency

Iodine is essential for the production of thyroid hormones; as our bodies do not synthesise iodine, it is necessary to consume iodine as part of a nutritionally balanced diet. Sources of iodine include seafood (fish, crustaceans and shellfish along with seaweed), dairy products (especially when cattle feed is supplemented) and in some countries iodised salt.

Iodine deficiency measured as urinary iodine concentration less than 100 µg/L in average adults can lead to birth defects, goitre and hypothyroidism. Although the introduction of iodised salt has helped to eliminate iodine deficiency in most parts of the world, about 30% of the world's population remains at risk for iodine deficiency. Iodine deficiency continues to be a challenging public health nutrition problem especially for populations who are living in remote mountainous regions and who eat a predominantly vegetarian diet.

In some parts of rural India, iodine deficiency is still prevalent. Whilst oral iodine supplements are available, they are not taken due to suspicion of foreign medication. To overcome this problem, a company developed a skin patch using the same technology as nicotine patches for smokers. This skin patch is shaped as a little red dot containing iodine for women to wear on the centre of their forehead, allowing it to be worn as a common daily accessory for married women in India. It is reported that on average women wearing the skin patch absorb about 12% of their daily requirement of iodine. While these skin patches may be culturally acceptable, the efficacy in preventing hypothyroidism or endemic cretinism has not been established.

Nutritional Considerations for Managing Thyroid Disease

Due to the potential effect of thyroid function on weight, is it important for individuals with an underactive thyroid to be effectively counselled regarding expectations of weight stabilisation and weight loss along with how thyroxine dose will be initiated and titrated. Patients must be counselled about the risks of increasing thyroxine dose too rapidly and above what is required to normalise function with respect to the negative cardiovascular, bone and psychological harmful effects. Adherence to treatment can also be a challenge in those with hyperthyroidism as weight gain and fatigue may be associated with carbimazole and other medical therapies that can induce transient hypothyroidism. Along with support to maintain adherence to therapy as prescribed, it is sensible to provide the appropriate dietary advice to help individuals manage any weight change.

Thyroxine therapy availability can be inhibited by concomitant iron or calcium intake; this is most often seen in pregnancy as thyroxine dose often requires upward titration and there is coadministration with iron or calcium supplements. If an individual requires both thyroxine and iron or calcium, it is sensible to take them several hours apart. It should be noted that adequate iron levels are required for normal thyroid function as haem is a cofactor in the synthesis of thyroxine by the thyroid. Thyroxine synthesis also requires glutathione, so selenium is another nutrient which may influence thyroid function. Other potential nutritional factors that are worth considering include soy and isoflavone supplements which may alter thyroxine synthesis or affect its action, as may excessive brassica intake, including broccoli. Although commonly discussed in the lay literature, the effects are modest effects at best and may only need consideration if no other cause is apparent.

GLUCOCORTICOIDS

Cushing Syndrome and Nutrition

Cushing syndrome is also known as hypercortisolism and can be either primary or iatrogenic, secondary to continued and possibly excessive use of cortisol therapy as may occur in asthma or rheumatologic disease. Primary hypercortisolism can also occur due to endogenous cortisol production, the most common cause being an ACTH (adrenocorticotrophic hormone) producing pituitary adenoma which stimulates the production of cortisol from the adrenal glands, situated on top of the kidney. Hypercortisolism from pituitary adenoma is also known as Cushing disease in contrast to Cushing syndrome which, in addition to iatrogenic causes, can also result from ectopic ACTH syndrome, by benign adrenal adenomas or occasionally malignant tumours, and very rarely familial Cushing syndrome.

Independent of the cause of the Cushing syndrome, the symptoms are typically similar, in that there is a tendency for muscles to atrophy and fat to be deposited in a classic pattern. There is muscle wasting typically of the limbs, with fat deposition around the face, between the shoulder blades and above the clavicle (supraclavicular fat pad, also called Buffalo hump). Additionally, there can be hirsutism and male pattern baldness in women, with bruising and purple striae. Cushing syndrome can also increase the risk of depression, hypertension and dysglycaemia along with negatively impacting tissue viability and inhibiting wound healing. Treatment of Cushing syndrome is achieved by the removal of the underlying cause, which can involve surgery, radiation or other oncologic treatments if the cause is a tumour for example. If the cause is related to steroid therapy, then typically the condition will partially or totally resolve when treatment ceases.

Dysglycaemia and diabetes related to steroid treatment result from increased insulin resistance. Glucose patterns may follow the pattern of drug delivery. When prednisolone is given in the morning, the greatest insulin resistance and hence hyperglycaemia occurs around 6–8 hours later. Although there is little evidence for how best to manage glucose intolerance due to steroid administration, medications including use of insulin or a modified dietary pattern with reduced carbohydrate intake during the middle of the day have been tried. Counselling may also be required to discuss the effects of steroid therapy with respect to muscle loss and adipose tissue gain, especially the distress of bodily changes along with any potential increase in appetite associated with steroid therapy. Due to the effect of steroid treatment on insulin action, care needs to be taken when planning to cease steroid therapy, in that dose of exogenous insulin needs to be systematically stepped down to avoid reactive hypoglycaemia.

Addison Syndrome

Addison syndrome, also known as adrenal insufficiency or hypocortisolaemia, is a rare endocrine condition in which there is inadequate secretion of glucocorticoids. It can occur as an isolated pathology or in some instances as part of Schmidt syndrome or autoimmune polyendocrine syndrome occurring with other autoimmune endocrine conditions including T1DM and/or autoimmune hypothyroidism. Addison syndrome requires replacement of cortisol with hydrocortisone therapy, often in a timed fashion, as endogenous secretion typically follows a diurnal pattern, increasing in the early hours of the morning with a second smaller rise in the afternoon. Without this pattern of secretion of cortisol, the normal morning rise in glucose will not occur, and if the patient also has T1DM, there is an increased risk of early morning hypoglycaemia due to the requirement for exogenous insulin. Hypoglycaemia can be managed by either adjusting insulin or early morning dosing with hydrocortisone and/or increasing dietary carbohydrate intake.

OSTEOPOROSIS

Osteoporosis is a condition of low bone density typically associated with advanced age, especially in postmenopausal women, although increasingly it is being identified in men. It is a part of a continuum that begins with normal bone health and progresses through osteopenia to osteoporosis and is associated with increased risk of fractures. The most effective way to minimise risk of bone demineralisation is to achieve optimal bone mass which occurs around the age of 25–30 years. Demineralisation occurs more rapidly in women postmenopause as the protective effect of oestrogen is lost.

The endocrinology of bone metabolism is in part influenced by the availability of calcium, which is also required for a number of other cellular functions including muscle contractility. Dietary calcium is one factor that affects bone mineralisation, but as with any metabolic concept, excretion and reabsorption of calcium by the kidney, along with transportation in the blood, is important as most calcium in plasma is bound to protein, mostly albumin, with free calcium being very tightly controlled. The level of calcium in the circulating pool is controlled by parathyroid hormone produced by the four coffee bean-sized glands sitting within the thyroid, and vitamin D, a nutrient with hormonelike functions. The absorption of calcium is enhanced by calcitriol, the active form of vitamin D, which is activated by an enzyme in the kidney, 1-alpha hydroxylase. Dietary sources of vitamin D, in the form of cholecalciferol, are limited to oily fish, egg yolks, red meat, offal and fortified foods, whereas plant sources including certain algae contain ergocalciferol. In addition, vitamin D can be synthesised from cholesterol metabolites in the skin to form cholecalciferol, which must undergo hydroxylation by both the liver and kidney before it becomes active calcitriol. Levels of vitamin D vary throughout the year, being highest toward the end of summer and lowest during spring. For this reason, many countries recommend supplementary vitamin D for individuals with limited sunlight exposure, including older adults and individuals who expose a limited amount of skin to sunlight and/or have a darker skin tone and all adults through the winter months. Despite a lot of interest in wider effects of vitamin D with respect to metabolic health and immune function, there lacks robust evidence to support a higher dose for a vitamin D supplement than 10 mcg per day (15–20 mcg/d in the United States).[20] It is important that patients be counselled to take their vitamin D supplement with fatty foods and not on an empty stomach, unless it is dissolved in oil, because vitamin D is a fat-soluble vitamin.

The dietary approaches to reduce the risk of developing osteoporosis include calcium and vitamin D intake as part of a diet rich in plants (vegetables, fruit, pulses, nuts and seeds) and adequate protein intake. Although some studies have suggested that high-protein diets can increase urinary calcium losses, there is no evidence it negatively impacts upon bone mineral density, and the opposite may in fact be true. Alongside a suitable diet, physical activity is essential for optimising bone mass, specifically load-bearing exercise, which applies moderate stress to the bone to encourage remodelling and which helps to maximise its strength. Patients should be warned that excessive aerobic exercise, which can result in amenorrhea in younger persons, can result in decreased bone density due to hypooestrogenism (see later in this chapter).

Risk of osteoporosis is also increased by a number of health conditions, including hyperthyroidism, due to the effect of increased thyroid hormone on osteoclast activity remodelling and bone resorption at a rate which exceeds the rate of osteoblasts' capacity to deposit bone. This is not just a consideration with respect to clinical hyperthyroidism; it can be significant where inappropriate thyroxine is administered as part of a weight loss strategy. The effect of weight loss on bone mass also needs to be considered, further supporting the role of exercise, including resistance exercise. Another disease that can affect bone mass is coeliac disease. It is recommended that individuals with coeliac disease should have at least 1000 mg of calcium per day to counteract any effect villous atrophy may have on absorption of calcium to minimise the risk of osteoporosis seen in people with this disease.

Reproductive Endocrinology

EFFECT OF WEIGHT ON MALE AND FEMALE FERTILITY

The start of puberty from a biological perspective may be prompted when an adolescent reaches a certain body weight. This observation has been associated with the reduction in average age for onset of puberty and increasing levels of childhood obesity. It is especially the case in women that as well as a reasonably adequate dietary intake, a minimum body fat is required to support menstruation and therefore fertility. This observation may be linked to the fact that a minimum body weight and dietary intake of certain nutrients (particularly energy intake) is necessary for the synthesis of sex hormones, but this influence varies between individuals and different ethnic groups.

Due to the relationship between body weight and body fat on fertility, amenorrhea can be observed in females and infertility in both males and females at low body weight. This effect is perhaps most often observed clinically in patients with eating disorders and in particular anorexia nervosa. Additionally, the low body weight can also contribute to bone mineral demineralisation and osteoporosis because of the lower load on bones (see earlier discussion).

NUTRITION REQUIREMENTS OF PREGNANCY AND LACTATION

Although increased nutritional requirements are associated with both pregnancy and lactation, it is important that nutritional status preconception and periconception are also considered. Fertility can be reduced by both a high and low body weight, and with metabolic disease including diabetes and thyroid disease, both of which need to be optimally managed to help to achieve the best pregnancy outcome. With respect to preconception and periconceptional nutrition, the role of folic acid supplementation is perhaps the most well-known public health message, due to studies which demonstrated a reduction in neural tube defects with supplementation.[21] Most women are encouraged to consume 400 mcg per day and those at higher risk encouraged to consume 5 mg per day starting at the time they try to conceive up until the end of the first trimester. The window of supplementation is longer than the time between conception and the closure of the neural tube as this time point is difficult to predict. In addition, it is important to consider the nutritional stores of the woman prior to pregnancy, as the shifts in metabolism that occur in pregnancy result in a drive of nutrients from the mother to the foetus. For this reason, nutrients such as calcium can become of concern in women who conceive a number of times within a short time span. Increasingly, due to its role in brain development, supplementation of iodine intake is being increasingly recommended during pregnancy, as dietary sources can be limited in areas where there is less in local water supplies, it is not supplemented in feed for dairy cattle or salt is not routinely iodised. Although iron supplements are routinely prescribed during pregnancy, it is important to note that it is normal for haemoglobin levels to fall in pregnancy due to increased plasma volume. Therefore, many national guidelines suggest recommending iron supplementation (typically using iron sulphate) when haemoglobin is below 110 g/L in the first trimester and below 100 g/L in the final trimester. It is important also to screen for haemoglobinopathies and treat based on ferritin levels and not routinely offer iron supplements to all pregnant women, as they can worsen constipation and contribute to other digestive issues.

The nutritional requirements associated with pregnancy change through the course of pregnancy. In the first trimester metabolic requirements tend to increase, but slightly decrease in the third trimester. The effect of the placenta on metabolism and how nutrients are supplied to the foetus is also essential for its development. The placenta not only has effects on nutrient availability, but also has endocrine effects which can contribute to insulin resistance. If increased insulin demands cannot be met, the woman will develop GDM as previously discussed. Lactation is also associated with increased nutrient demands, and, in general, the nutrient composition of breast milk will tend to be maintained at the expense of the mother. Therefore, extra energy and nutrient requirements are required to maintain maternal stores.

GESTATIONAL DIABETES

GDM is a condition which affects 5%–50% of pregnancies depending on the age and ethnic background of the maternal population as previously mentioned. It is defined as diabetes first presenting in pregnancy. Globally, definitions vary but typically it is glycaemia above the normal range (e.g., a fasting glucose of >5.5 mmol/L) or following an oral glucose tolerance test (75 g glucose) > 7.8 mmol/L at 2 hours (see Table 7.2). A glucose tolerance test is required for diagnosis, as HbA1c is not reliable due to the change in plasma volume and rate of haemoglobin turnover.

Risk of developing GDM is increased in women who are over 28 years of age and obese, have previously had GDM or a large baby, have a family history of diabetes or are of south Asian or African origin. The aim of treatment is to optimise glucose levels, often using self-blood glucose monitoring both pre- and postprandial to aim to keep glucose within normal levels. Typically, to achieve tight glucose control, dietary changes are needed which are similar to those used to manage T2DM. A range of strategies are also used, that can include controlling carbohydrate serving sizes, looking to reduce glycaemic load, and some centres even advocating low carbohydrate at breakfast as the greatest glycaemic excursion is typically in the morning. When dietary management can no longer control glucose levels, metformin is used in some countries prior to the initiation of insulin, which can be a combination of basal insulin and prandial dosing. Typically, following the delivery of the baby, glycaemia returns to normal. Because GDM is associated with increased risk for the development of T2DM, the patient should be screened for diabetes after about 6 weeks postpartum and then yearly. Good intrapartum glycaemic control is aimed to reduce the risk of macrosomia which can lead to birth complications including shoulder dystocia and even stillbirth.

POLYCYSTIC OVARY SYNDROME

Polycystic ovary syndrome is a common endocrine disorder in women linked to inappropriate levels of free testosterone. It can be considered both a gynaecological and an endocrine condition, with the condition linked to weight gain and insulin resistance. The mechanism is complex and includes an effect of adiposity leading to a decrease in steroid-binding hormone globulin, which results in increased free testosterone. The increase in testosterone, coupled with insulin resistance leading to hyperinsulinemia, affects theca cell formation and can lead to multiple cysts. The presence of multiple ovarian cysts as well as increased testosterone levels can lead to amenorrhea, infertility and hirsutism.

The pharmaceutical management options for polycystic ovary syndrome are limited, although metformin is commonly used. Lifestyle management is a primary therapeutic approach. The primary focus is the support of weight loss followed by weight maintenance through a change in diet and increased physical activity. A range of dietary approaches can be used as with obesity and T2DM, with a low glycemic index or carbohydrate approach being useful given that the goal is to reduce energy intake and reduce drivers of insulin secretion.

EARLY MENOPAUSE

There is limited evidence to suggest dietary intake plays a role in risk of early menopause, defined as the occurrence of menopause before a woman is 45 years old. However, with early menopause, there is decreased oestrogen and secondary risk of reduction in bone density resulting in osteopenia and osteoporosis. The recommendation is that women in menopause have a calcium intake of 1000 mg per day and vitamin D supplementation of 10 mcg per day (Recommendations in the United States for calcium is 1200 mg with 20 mcg Vitamin D).

References

1. World Health Organization. Obesity and overweight. 2021. Available at: https://www.who.int/news-room/fact-sheets/detail/obesity-and-overweight.
2. Wells JC, Sawaya AL, Wibaek R, et al. The double burden of malnutrition: Aetiological pathways and consequences for health. *Lancet*. 2020;395(10217):75–88.

3. Basen-Engquist K, Chang M. Obesity and cancer risk: Recent review and evidence. *Curr Oncol Rep.* 2011;13(1):71–76.
4. Sattar N, McInnes IB, McMurray JJV. Obesity is a risk factor for severe COVID-19 infection. *Circulation.* 2020;142(1):4–6.
5. Camilleri M. Peripheral mechanisms in appetite regulation. *Gastroenterology.* 2015;148(6):1219–1233.
6. Saeedi P, Petersohn I, Salpea P, et al. Global and regional diabetes prevalence estimates for 2019 and projections for 2030 and 2045: Results from the International Diabetes Federation Diabetes Atlas, 9th ed. *Diabetes Res Clin Pract.* 2019;157:107843.
7. International Diabetes Federation. Care & Prevention: Gestational Diabetes. Available at: https://www.idf.org/our-activities/care-prevention/gdm.
8. Ali O. Genetics of type 2 diabetes. *World J Diabetes.* 2013;4(4):114–123.
9. Endocrine society. Severe hypoglycemia. 2022. Available at: https://www.endocrine.org/patient-engagement/endocrine-library/severe-hypoglycemia.
10. Dyson PA, Twenefour D, Breen C, et al. Diabetes UK evidence-based nutrition guidelines for the prevention and management of diabetes. *Diabet Med.* 2018;35(5):541–547.
11. Lean MEJ, Leslie WS, Barnes AC, et al. Durability of a primary care-led weight-management intervention for remission of type 2 diabetes: 2-year results of the DiRECT open-label, cluster-randomised trial. *Lancet Diabetes Endocrinol.* 2019;7(5):344–355.
12. Knowler WC, Barrett-Connor E, Fowler SE, et al. Reduction in the incidence of type 2 diabetes with lifestyle intervention or metformin. *N Engl J Med.* 2002;346(6):393–403.
13. Sheng B, Truong K, Spitler H, Zhang L, Tong X, Chen L. The long-term effects of bariatric surgery on type 2 diabetes remission, microvascular and macrovascular complications, and mortality: A systematic review and meta-analysis. *Obes Surg.* 2017;27(10):2724–2732.
14. Schwingshackl L, Chaimani A, Hoffmann G, Schwedhelm C, Boeing H. A network meta-analysis on the comparative efficacy of different dietary approaches on glycaemic control in patients with type 2 diabetes mellitus. *Eur J Epidemiol.* 2018;33(2):157–170.
15. Basterra-Gortari FJ, Ruiz-Canela M, Martínez-González MA, et al. Effects of a Mediterranean eating plan on the need for glucose-lowering medications in participants with type 2 diabetes: A subgroup analysis of the PREDIMED Trial. *Diabetes Care.* 2019;42(8):1390–1397.
16. Feinman RD, Pogozelski WK, Astrup A, et al. Dietary carbohydrate restriction as the first approach in diabetes management: critical review and evidence base. *Nutrition.* 2015;31(1):1–13.
17. Kirkman MS, Briscoe VJ, Clark N, et al. Diabetes in older adults. *Diabetes Care.* 2012;35(12):2650–2664.
18. Albai O, Frandes M, Timar R, Roman D, Timar B. Risk factors for developing dementia in type 2 diabetes mellitus patients with mild cognitive impairment. *Neuropsychiatr Dis Treat.* 2019;15:167–175.
19. Croker EE, McGrath SA, Rowe CW. Thyroid disease: Using diagnostic tools effectively. *Aust J Gen Pract.* 2021;50(1–2):16–21.
20. SACN. Update of rapid review: Vitamin D and acute respiratory tract infections PHE; 2020. Available at: https://www.gov.uk/government/publications/sacn-rapid-review-vitamin-d-and-acute-respiratory-tract-infections.
21. MRC Vitamin Study Group Prevention of neural tube defects: Results of the Medical Research Council Vitamin Study. *Lancet.* 1991;338(8760):131–137.

CHAPTER 8

Nutrition in Gastrointestinal and Hepatobiliary Medicine

Dominic Crocombe ■ Lisa Sharkey

LEARNING POINTS

By the end of this chapter, you should be able to:

- Describe the nutritional aspects of common inflammatory gastrointestinal (GI) conditions, including coeliac disease, inflammatory bowel disease (IBD) and eosinophilic oesophagitis
- Describe the role of nutrition in motility and functional GI disorders, including gastroparesis, chronic constipation, and irritable bowel syndrome (IBS)
- Define short bowel syndrome (SBS) and be aware of the principles of nutritional management in patients with SBS
- Describe the nutritional aspects of acute and chronic liver disease, including alcohol-related liver disease (ALD) and nonalcoholic fatty liver disease, liver failure and cirrhosis
- Describe the nutritional aspects of common pancreatobiliary conditions, including gallstone disease, bile acid malabsorption, acute pancreatitis and pancreatic exocrine insufficiency

CASE STUDIES

Gastrointestinal Case Example: Coeliac Disease

A 19-year-old man presents to his general practitioner (GP) with 6-month history of fatigue, 5 kg of weight loss, vague abdominal discomfort, and occasional loose bowel motions. He is not sure if there has been any blood in his stool. He describes a profoundly itchy, blistering rash on his arms. He has no significant past medical history and takes no regular medications. His mother has hypothyroidism. He works in a cafe and is physically active, has never smoked, and drinks 16 units of alcohol per week, typically lager with friends at the weekends. He describes his diet as 'balanced', consisting predominantly of ready-made meals and the occasional takeaway. He does not consciously exclude any foods.

On physical examination his height is 1.85 m, weight 62 kg and body mass index (BMI) 18.1 kg/m^2. He has subconjunctival pallor. There is an excoriated, vesicular rash on both elbows. There are no aphthous ulcers. His cardiovascular and respiratory systems are unremarkable. His abdomen is soft and nontender with no organomegaly. There is no peripheral oedema.

The GP arranges a panel of tests that reveal normal capillary blood glucose, a microcytic anaemia, normal renal and liver panels. His ferritin level is in the lower end of the normal range, and vitamin B12 and folate levels are replete. Thyroid function tests are normal. Antitissue transglutaminase (anti-TTG) is positive and total immunoglobulin A levels are normal. Faecal calprotectin is negative. Total vitamin D level is 32 nmol/L. The patient remains on his usual diet, and he undergoes an upper GI endoscopy.

Duodenal biopsies show partial villous atrophy, which confirm a diagnosis of coeliac disease. His GP explains the need for him to follow a lifelong gluten-free diet and prescribes vitamin D, calcium and iron supplementation. He is referred to a registered dietitian who gives advice about naturally gluten-free foods, substitute foods, the principles of healthy diet and the importance of nutrition and vitamin D for bone health, and together they devise a holistic meal plan and follow up. He is advised to join a patient

CASE STUDIES —(Continued)

association such as Coeliac UK for further information he can explore. After 1 year his symptoms have settled, his BMI is 24 kg/m^2, and he undergoes a repeat endoscopy and biopsy, which show recovery of villous architecture. Because coeliac disease puts him at risk of osteopenia, a routine bone density scan is arranged that shows normal bone density.

Gastrointestinal Case Example: Inflammatory Bowel Disease

A 17-year-old girl presents to the emergency department with an abdominal mass. She reveals a 6-week history of diarrhoea, weight loss and mouth ulcers. Physical examination reveals a temperature of 37.7°C and a tachycardia of 112 beats per minute. Her BMI is 17 kg/m^2. Pregnancy testing is negative, but C-reactive protein (CRP) is 35 mg/L, haemoglobin is 110 g/L and erythrocyte sedimentation rate is 55 mm/h.

She is reviewed by the surgical team, and an abdominal ultrasound is arranged to look for appendicitis. This shows a normal appendix, but a thickened terminal ileum and a possible collection, in keeping with a new diagnosis of Crohn disease. Care is transferred to the gastroenterology team, and she is started on antibiotics. Immunosuppression for IBD is not yet started, as there is an active infection and no tissue biopsy to confirm a diagnosis. A magnetic resonance imaging scan of the small bowel subsequently shows a 20-cm segment of terminal ileal thickening and confirms a collection with a few locules of gas within.

The registered dietitian is asked to review the patient because of weight loss and suggests exclusive enteral nutrition, for treatment and for nutrition support. The patient agrees to this as she is concerned about the side effects of medication. She is provided with elemental diet drinks and tolerates these orally. She is discharged after 4 days, continuing an elemental diet and antibiotics with plans for a subsequent outpatient ileo-colonoscopy and follow-up.

At clinic review 6 weeks later, she has gained 7 kg in weight and the abdominal mass has resolved. She has had an endoscopy and terminal ileal biopsies confirmed a histological diagnosis of Crohn disease. She is eating a healthy balanced diet. After further counselling she starts on immunomodulatory treatment with azathioprine and is followed up regularly in the IBD clinic.

Gastrointestinal Case Example: Irritable Bowel Syndrome

A 45-year-old schoolteacher seeks help from her GP for increasingly bothersome abdominal symptoms. She gets lower abdominal pains 3–4 times per week and struggles with a bowel habit that is 'all over the place'. On deeper questioning by the GP, she describes straining to pass hard stool for some of the week and then passing looser motions at other times. There is no rectal bleeding or weight loss. Her symptoms have been present for at least 6 years but have worsened over the past 6 months. Over this time, she has taken on extra responsibilities at work and has had to care for her elderly father.

The GP arranges some tests; her full blood count, electrolytes, liver function and CRP are normal. A faecal calprotectin is negative. Whilst waiting for her results to come back, she does her own research and starts a low FODMAP (fermentable oligosaccharides, disaccharides, monosaccharides and polyols) diet. On follow-up from the GP she reports this diet had no effect. The GP suggests seeking guidance from a registered dietitian and refers her to a local dietitian-led IBS clinic. The dietitian reviews her symptoms and investigations and makes a positive diagnosis of IBS. They agree a second trial of a low FODMAP diet with a structured reintroduction phase, which the patient had not done during her first trial. Reintroducing honey causes a recurrence of symptoms suggesting fructose is a trigger for this lady. Other reintroductions such as onions, garlic, green vegetables, beans and dairy are more successful. Long term, she is able to comfortably eat a healthy balanced diet whilst minimising intake of foods high in fructose to prevent recurrence of her symptoms.

Hepatobiliary Case Example: Nonalcoholic Fatty Liver Disease

A 56-year-old woman presents to her GP for a scheduled 6 monthly review of her type 2 diabetes (T2DM). She has no new symptoms. She works in an office and does not smoke or drink alcohol, and her only regular physical activity is light gardening and the occasional weekend walk. Her weight is stable, she has a BMI of 36 kg/m^2 and her latest HbA1c is 65 mmol/mol despite metformin and insulin therapy. She also has hypertension, for which she takes ramipril, and she takes a statin based on a cardiovascular risk calculation.

Continued

CASE STUDIES —(Continued)

Her GP is concerned as her blood tests today are as follows:

	Today	6 Months Ago	Normal Range
Bilirubin	12	8	0–17 µmol/L
alanine aminotransferase	70	24	10–40 IU/L
aspartate aminotransferase	64	30	10–40 IU/L
AST:ALT ratio	0.91	–	–
Alkaline phosphatase	46	52	30–130 IU/L
Albumin	36	37	32–50 g/L
Haemoglobin	140	138	115–150 g/L
Platelets	278	304	150–450 × 10^9/L
Urea and electrolytes	Normal	Normal	

ALT, Alanine transaminase; *AST*, aspartate transaminase

On examination there is central adiposity, no hepatomegaly and no clinical signs of chronic liver disease.

The GP refers her to the local hepatology service. A basic noninvasive liver aetiology screen (autoantibodies and immunoglobulins, hepatitis B and C serology, iron studies) are all normal. Ultrasound of the liver shows increased echogenicity consistent with hepatic steatosis; no biliary tree abnormalities; no focal lesions. The hepatologist confirms the diagnosis of nonalcoholic fatty liver disease (NAFLD). Her FibroScan result is 6 kPa, which suggests a low risk of advanced fibrosis. The diagnosis is explained and the hepatologist advises weight loss, signposts to the website of a local weight loss service and gives brief advice regarding a Mediterranean dietary pattern and increasing physical exercise to help improve overall metabolic health.

A referral to a registered dietitian is made to help with implementing dietary modifications. A brief dietary history reveals she does not restrict any food groups. She eats three regular meals per day with regular snacking of crisps, biscuits, and small cakes during the day. A typical breakfast would be a medium-sized bowl of sugar-sweetened breakfast cereal with semiskimmed milk or two slices of toast with butter and jam. A packed lunch usually consists of sandwiches, crisps, sweetened yoghurt and a piece of fruit or chocolate bar. A typical dinner would be cooked meal (e.g., sausages and mashed potatoes, pasta, meat, or fish pie, with sides of vegetables and occasionally a small dessert).

The dietitian devises a meal plan based on principles of reducing her overall calorie intake and following a Mediterranean diet modified to optimise protein and lower excess saturated fat and excess carbohydrate intake, prioritising whole foods, fibre and protein with the goal of being satiating and nutrient dense without providing excess energy. Some simple suggestions include swapping her current breakfast choices of cereal or toast for reduced fat Greek yoghurt and berries, or eggs. She is given guidance on portion control and advised to base her main meals on lean meat, fish or meat alternatives, a variety of whole vegetables and fewer 'white' carbohydrates. She is advised to use olive oil for cooking. She is encouraged to replace calorie-dense snacks with healthier options such as fruit, nuts, boiled egg, small pieces of chicken or other meats or unsweetened yoghurt. She enrols herself in a local weight loss service and finds benefit in the group sessions and peer support. She starts walking more regularly and encourages her family to join her.

At her next 6-month GP appointment she has managed to lose 6 kg (7% of body weight) and her BMI is 32 kg/m^2. She feels better in herself and feels she has more energy than before. Her HbA1c is 46 and she can reduce her insulin dose. Her liver blood tests have normalised. The GP acknowledges and congratulates her on these achievements and encourages her to continue, setting new goals ahead of her next appointment.

CASE STUDIES —(Continued)

Hepatobiliary Case Example: Decompensated Cirrhosis

A critically unwell 39-year-old man is brought to the resuscitation area of the emergency department with large-volume haematemesis and melaena. He drinks up to 1 L of vodka per day. On examination he has jaundice, spider naevi and ascites. At emergency upper GI endoscopy, the gastroenterologist identifies and successfully treats bleeding oesophageal varices. The unifying diagnosis is decompensated cirrhosis secondary to alcohol-related liver disease (ALD).

A weaning regimen of chlordiazepoxide is used to prevent alcohol withdrawal syndrome. Intravenous Pabrinex (containing B vitamins) is given to prevent Wernicke encephalopathy. Due to his unstable condition, it is not safe to weigh him accurately so the nurse measures ulna length and mid-upper arm circumference to estimate his Malnutrition Universal Screening Tool score, which recognises his high risk of malnutrition.

Once stabilised and recovering on the ward, he is reviewed by the registered dietitian. His body weight is 64 kg, height 180 cm, and BMI 19.7 kg/m^2. He gives a brief dietary history of minimal food intake, eating predominantly white bread, chips or crisps or the occasional ready-made sandwich, and drinking 750–1000 mL vodka per day. Triceps skin fold measurement and mid-upper arm circumference are done and, according to the Royal Free Hospital Global Assessment, he is severely malnourished. He has sarcopenia. His estimated nutritional requirements are 2,600 kcal and 100 g protein per day. He is able to swallow safely so is encouraged to eat three calorie- and nutrient-dense meals per day with regular snacks alongside branched-chain amino acid (BCAA)-enriched oral nutrition supplement drinks. The physiotherapist advises him regarding simple resistance exercises to encourage muscle development.

He undergoes abdominal paracentesis, which removes 6000 mL ascitic fluid. Following this, his actual weight is 58 kg. His electrolytes are closely monitored, and his weight is measured regularly to monitor changes. During the admission he develops a chest infection and subsequent grade 1 hepatic encephalopathy (HE). This reduces his oral intake for 3 days, so a nasogastric tube is placed and feeding regimen commenced to meet his nutritional requirements. Antibiotics successfully treat his infection, and he can return to an oral diet. He is also given regular lactulose to treat HE and prevent its recurrence.

Two weeks later, his weight is 62 kg and he is safely discharged home. He is given a nutrition support plan and oral nutrition supplements to continue his recovery at home. He is enrolled in the local alcohol cessation service. For his ascites, he is started on low-dose spironolactone and advised about a low-salt (sodium) diet. He is followed up in the medical hepatology clinic.

Hepatobiliary Case Example: Gallstone Pancreatitis

A 66-year-old woman presents to the surgical assessment unit complaining of acute severe epigastric pain radiating to her back, nausea and vomiting. Further history reveals intermittent epigastric/right upper quadrant pains for the last 3 months for which she is awaiting an outpatient ultrasound scan.

On examination she is febrile, hypotensive and tachycardic, and she has jaundice and epigastric tenderness on palpation. Her height is 160 cm, weight is 75 kg, and BMI is 29.2 kg/m^2 (overweight). Blood amylase is 6000 U/L and (computed tomography) CT imaging confirms acute pancreatitis, multiple gallstones in the gallbladder and an obstructing stone in the common bile duct with signs of cholangitis.

Other blood tests reveal:

Investigation	Result	Normal range
Magnesium	0.34	0.70–1.00 mmol/L
Adjusted calcium	1.45	2.20–2.60 mmol/L
Phosphate	1.00	0.70–1.45 mmol/L
Potassium	3.1	3.5–5.0 mmol/L
Sodium	137	135–145 mmol/L

She is resuscitated on the high-dependency unit with intravenous fluids and treated with intravenous antibiotics. Her 12-lead electrocardiogram shows sinus tachycardia. Serum magnesium, calcium and

Continued

CASE STUDIES —(Continued)

potassium are replaced intravenously under continuous cardiac monitoring. She is unable to keep fluids down so a nasogastric tube is placed for early enteral feeding.

She undergoes urgent endoscopic retrograde cholangiopancreatography to remove the gallstone obstructing the common bile duct. This relieves her jaundice, and her inflammatory markers drop dramatically over the next 48 hours. She is discharged 6 days later and is followed up in the general surgery clinic. Three months later she undergoes elective laparoscopic cholecystectomy.

The following year she is referred to her local gastroenterology service for investigation of chronic persistent diarrhoea and steatorrhoea. A selenium homocholic acid taurine test is negative, effectively ruling out bile acid malabsorption. A faecal elastase test is very low, and a diagnosis of pancreatic exocrine insufficiency is confirmed. Blood tests for vitamin A, D, E and K reveal multiple deficiencies, which require replacement with oral supplements. She is started on pancreatin supplementation in the form of Creon, which she is advised to take with meals and snacks. Her dietitian recommends a healthy balanced and nonrestrictive dietary pattern focused on prioritising protein and adequate calories, whilst being careful not to include too much fibre (as this can impair the action of pancreatin).

Introduction

Good nutrition is essential to human health, and the gastrointestinal (GI) and hepatobiliary systems are essential to good nutrition. The GI tract, consisting of a hollow tube connecting the mouth to the anus, is a complex organ responsible for the breakdown of food into nutrients that can be absorbed into the circulation. Food is eaten by mouth, passes the pharynx and enters the oesophagus under volitional control. From there, autonomic pathways take over and entero-endocrine hormones signal various processes, including GI motility and satiety. Most of the digestion of food particles occurs in the proximal gut (stomach and duodenum) while absorption mainly occurs in the jejunum and ileum. The colon processes the remainder into waste and absorbs a remarkable amount of fluid. The hepatobiliary system, consisting of the liver, pancreas and biliary system, provides digestive enzymes, hormones and other substances that are integral to the digestion and absorption of nutrients. Venous blood containing nutrients absorbed from the GI tract passes, via the portal vein, to the liver where the nutrients undergo further processing.

Dysfunction of any part of the GI tract can affect the ability of the body to absorb, digest and process nutrients. It has been estimated that GI complaints account for 10% of the work of GPs. The commonest benign conditions are gastro-oesophageal reflux disease (GORD), irritable bowel syndrome (IBS) diverticular disease, coeliac disease, and inflammatory bowel disease (IBD). Oesophageal, gastric, colorectal and pancreatic cancers are, respectively, the sixth, fourth, seventh and third most common cancers worldwide amounting to a huge disease burden. Many dietary and lifestyle factors are implicated in the pathogenesis of these cancers.

The majority of GI and hepatobiliary conditions are best managed in a multidisciplinary manner, with doctors, dietitians, specialist nurses and other health care professionals working as a team to ensure optimal outcomes for every individual patient.

Disorders of the Oesophagus

The oesophagus is the first part of the GI tract to encounter food. Its function is to transport food into the stomach. The upper third contains striated muscle, under voluntary control, while the lower two thirds consist of smooth muscle innervated by the sympathetic and parasympathetic nervous system, which coordinate contractions to propel food boluses forward. The upper and lower muscular sphincters are present to prevent aspiration into the lungs and GORD, respectively.

GASTRO-OESOPHAGEAL REFLUX

Reflux of gastric contents into the oesophagus is actually a very common event but is usually short-lived and postprandial. However, pathological reflux can lead to unpleasant symptoms, oesophageal damage and severe complications in some. It is estimated that 5%–10% of adults suffer with GORD, and it is one of the most common GI complaints seen in primary and secondary care. The classic symptoms overlap and are often difficult for patients to verbalise, but may include heartburn, regurgitation, retrosternal discomfort, water brash or coughing.

The diagnosis can be made clinically, but older patients, those not responding to proton pump inhibitor (PPI) therapy or those with alarm symptoms (dysphagia, weight loss, haematemesis) should undergo endoscopic investigation with oeosphago-gastric duodenoscopy (OGD). In some cases, oesophageal pH studies or impedance studies are required to make the diagnosis.

First-line medical treatment is acid suppression with PPI, but lifestyle and dietary modifications can also help. Known dietary triggers include caffeine, tea, spicy foods, alcohol, carbonated drinks, onions, tomatoes,[1] peppermint and citrus foods, and trials avoiding these may improve symptoms in some people. Keeping a food and symptom diary can help patients identify dietary triggers and track their response to dietary modification. A reduction in meal size and attention to the timing of meals, for example, avoiding eating late in the evening, can also help.[2]

Obesity is associated with erosive reflux, Barrett oesophagus, and oesophageal cancer with odds ratios of 1.59, 1.24 and 2.45, respectively.[3] Overweight patients should be supported to lose excess weight, as the increased intra-abdominal pressure associated with obesity promotes reflux.

The presence of a hiatus hernia is also common in patients with reflux. A hiatus hernia occurs when the stomach rises through the diaphragm into the thoracic cavity; the most common form is a sliding hiatus hernia in which the gastro-oesophageal junction moves up. These contribute to reflux by widening the gap in the diaphragmatic crura and causing proximal movement of the lower oesophageal sphincter. Ingested contents can also become stagnant in a moderate or large hiatus hernia, forming a sump for reflux into the upper oesophagus. For patients with a hernia and GORD not relieved by medication, surgery in form of fundoplication may be needed. This procedure, now commonly performed laparoscopically, forms a complete or partial wrap from the gastric fundus around the gastro-oesophageal junction. A randomised multicentre trial in the UK comparing fundoplication to medical management demonstrated a low complication rate and favourable 1-year follow-up data in the surgery in terms of medication use and overall health outcomes.[4]

EOSINOPHILIC OESOPHAGITIS

Eosinophilic oesophagitis is an allergic disorder characterised by cell-mediated hypersensitivity to foodborne allergens that has been increasing in incidence since the 1990s and is now estimated to affect 1 in 2000 people. The usual presentation is with dysphagia, and the occurrence of repeated food bolus obstruction should strongly raise suspicion of eosinophilic oesophagitis. Diagnosis is by OGD and biopsy.[5] Commonly (44%), characteristic stacked circumferential rings can be seen endoscopically—so-called trachealisation of the oesophagus. There may also be linear furrows (48% of cases), white papules (27%), or strictures (21%).[6] Histologically, the presence of more than 15 eosinophils per high-power field is diagnostic; however, this finding can be seen in the lower oesophagus in GORD, so biopsies should be taken from the upper, mid and lower oesophagus with consistent findings of eosinophils seen in each biopsy.

Treatment options include medical therapy with topical or systemic steroids, and PPIs. However, dietary therapy can also be effective. The six-food elimination diet, which is designed to exclude the most common allergens of milk, eggs, nuts, wheat, soy and seafood, achieves histological remission of oesophageal eosinophilia in up to 72% of cases.[7] Four- and two-food elimination diets also have good response rates and are likely to be associated with better compliance.[8] It is not yet clear whether the endpoint of treatment should be clinical or histological remission.

Disorders of the Stomach

The main functions of the stomach are to act as a reservoir for food, facilitating controlled entry of ingested material into the small intestine, and to begin the process of digestion. This digestion is partly mechanical, using gastric contractions to break food into smaller particles, and partly chemical, via gastric acid secreted by parietal cells and pepsinogen secreted by chief cells. Acid secretion is stimulated partly by vagal activation but mainly by gastrin secretion from G cells in the gastric antrum. The stomach also secretes intrinsic factor, which is necessary for vitamin B12. Gastric emptying requires peristaltic movement toward an open pylorus. The presence of dietary lipid in the duodenum slows gastric emptying, probably due to increased levels of cholecystokinin and peptide YY,[9] hence low-fat diets are often recommended in patients with delayed gastric emptying (gastroparesis).

GASTRITIS AND PEPTIC ULCER DISEASE

Peptic ulcer disease (PUD) refers to the presence of ulceration (breaks in the mucosa) affecting the stomach or duodenum, which is most commonly associated with nonsteroidal anti-inflammatory drugs (NSAIDs) or infection with *Helicobacter pylori*. With an increased awareness of these risk factors, PUD is less common now than 50 years ago, with annual incidence rates of 0.03%–0.19%.[10]

H. pylori is a Gram-positive spiral bacillus with which around 50% of the worldwide population become infected at some point in their lifetime. It is adapted to survive in the acidic environment of the stomach and is implicated in the pathogenesis of acute gastritis, chronic gastritis, PUD, gastric lymphoma and gastric adenocarcinoma.[11] It can be tested for with blood serology, breath testing, or rapid urease testing performed on gastric biopsy taken during endoscopy.

NSAIDs inhibit cyclo-oxygenase-1, which leads to a relative deficiency of prostaglandins within the stomach, resulting in an increase in gastric acid secretion and less mucus production. Hence the gastric lining is exposed directly to acid, causing injury and inflammation. The various types of NSAIDs have differing risks of gastric injury, and newer selective cyclo-oxygenase-2 inhibitors have the same systemic anti-inflammatory effects but are more gastroprotective.

Treatment for gastritis and PUD involves eradication of *H. pylori* if present. Eradication treatment follows well-established protocols, usually a 7-day course of two antibiotics and a PPI. PPIs are also used in the treatment of gastritis and PUD not associated with HP infection. Smoking is associated with an increased risk of ulcers and *H. pylori* infection, so smoking cessation should be advised as part of both treatment and prevention. There is weak evidence that a high-fibre diet may protect against the formation of duodenal ulcers.[12] Before the widespread use of acid-suppression medication, a bland diet incorporating milk was often recommended for patients with gastritis or PUD; however, there is no good evidence to support this and it is no longer advised.

GASTRIC MOTILITY DISORDERS

In the fasted state the gastric migratory motor complex describes a series of gastric contractions of various amplitudes and frequencies, which are designed to clear any residual food or chyme ready for the next meal. It is mediated by the gut hormone motilin and 5HT3 receptors. Following ingestion of a meal, the gastric fundus relaxes, partly mediated by vagal activity and partly by distension detected by mechanoreceptors. Hormonal signals also contribute, particularly cholecystokinin. In the gastric antrum, synchronised contractions occur at a rate of three per minute (slow waves), to break down food into smaller particles. These are controlled by the interstitial cells of Cajal, which form the 'pacemaker' of the stomach, and numbers of these cells are reduced in some types of gastroparesis.[13]

TABLE 8.1 ■ **Conditions Associated With Gastroparesis**

Condition	Comments
Diabetes mellitus	Type 1 or type 2, related to length of diagnosis and level of glycaemic control
Idiopathic gastroparesis	No other causes identified
Postviral	Usually resolves within 2 years
Postsurgery	Postvagotomy (ulcer surgery, some lung surgeries, e.g., lung transplant), gastric surgery for obesity
Medications	Alcohol, anticholinergics, calcium channel antagonists, opiates, THC, TCAs
Systemic diseases	Parkinson, scleroderma, muscular dystrophy, amyloidosis, hypothyroidism

TCA, Tricyclic antidepressant; *THC*, tetrahydrocannabinol.

Gastroparesis or Delayed Gastric Emptying

Gastroparesis, or delayed gastric emptying, causes intermittent and variable symptoms of nausea, vomiting, early satiety, upper abdominal pain and bloating. The associated conditions are shown in Table 8.1, with diabetes and idiopathic gastroparesis accounting for the majority of cases. There is some overlap between gastroparesis and cyclical vomiting syndrome, a condition which manifests with similar symptoms, but they are episodic, with patients able to eat and drink normally for weeks or months between episodes. Clinicians should also be vigilant for patients with an undiagnosed eating disorder presenting as gastroparesis. Indeed, such patients can have abnormalities of gastric emptying on testing but will not get better without appropriate psychiatric care.

The gold standard test for diagnosing gastroparesis is gastric scintigraphy—the patient ingests a 99m-Tc-containing standard meal, usually scrambled eggs, and the rate of loss of food from the stomach is measured. In normal controls, 40%–80% of a solid meal will have emptied in 2 hours and almost all the meal by 4 hours. OGD is often required prior to scintigraphy to exclude any structural disease, particularly if there are any features suggesting PUD or upper GI cancer. Clues to gastroparesis at endoscopy include retained food and fluid residue despite a prolonged period of fasting prior to the test. New-generation wireless capsule endoscopy systems can measure pH, pressure and temperature changes as well as recording images, so can measure gastric emptying time.

The management of gastroparesis is largely dietary.[14] The types of food consumed and the timing of meals are important. Fat and fibre empty more slowly from the stomach so generally patients are advised a low-fat and low-fibre diet. A 'grazing' diet, where small meals are consumed more often, can also help manage symptoms. Some patients with difficult symptoms may need to take in more of their calories in liquid form and should be supported by a registered dietitian.

For people with diabetes mellitus, improved glycaemic control helps normalise gastric motility, and patients should have their medications reviewed by a specialist to facilitate this. For all patients, any medication which is known to inhibit gastric emptying should be discontinued. Prokinetic medications are often only useful in the short term. Metoclopramide and domperidone are dopamine antagonists: the former acts on central and peripheral receptors and the latter on peripheral receptors only. Dopamine inhibits gastric emptying but stimulates colonic motility. The major adverse effect of metoclopramide is tardive dyskinesia, a movement disorder which can be irreversible and is related to the duration of treatment; therefore, it is not recommended beyond

12 weeks of use unless the risk of tardive dyskinesia is significantly outweighed by therapeutic benefit. Domperidone does not cause tardive dyskinesia but can cause prolongation of the QT interval and cardiac arrhythmias. Precautions were introduced in 2014 relating to this, and domperidone should be used at the lowest effective dose for the shortest time possible and should not be used in patients with hepatic impairment, those taking other drugs which prolong the QT interval, or people with cardiac disease. Erythromycin, a macrolide antibiotic, acts via motilin receptors in the stomach to stimulate gastric emptying; however, tachyphylaxis is common so is only effective for short periods (around 2–3 weeks).

In refractory cases of gastroparesis, patients may need artificial nutritional support via nasojejunal feeding tube, which passes through the stomach to deliver feed into the jejunum. This may need to be converted to a permanent jejunostomy if there is no resolution of symptoms.[14] Injection of botulinum toxin (Botox) into the pylorus can be helpful in selected cases, and studies have demonstrated an improvement in symptoms in around 50% of patients with diabetic and idiopathic gastroparesis.[15] Gastric electrical stimulation (GES) therapy, also called the gastric pacemaker, has shown improvements in symptoms in some trials, but these came alongside large placebo response rates, and gastric electrical stimulation therapy was not associated with a demonstrable change in measured gastric emptying.

Rapid Gastric Emptying

Following partial gastrectomy for PUD or cancer, gastric bypass for obesity, or Whipple operation (pancreaticoduodenectomy), rapid gastric emptying and dumping syndrome can occur[16] secondary to loss of normal control by the pylorus. The early phase is caused by unregulated 'dumping' of food and fluid into the small intestine, which overwhelms its absorptive capacity and causes release of various enterohormones and insulin. These cause physical symptoms of pain, bloating, wind and diarrhoea and vasomotor symptoms of flushing, palpitations/tachycardia and sweating, within an hour of eating. The late phase is characterised by rebound hypoglycaemia in response to the surge of insulin released. Typically around 4 hours after eating patients might experience light headedness, hunger, weakness, and confusion.

Managing symptoms of dumping syndrome can be tricky. Patients are advised to avoid drinking too much fluid with meals and to consume mainly high-protein, high-fibre and high-fat meals whilst limiting carbohydrate intake to reduce the insulin spike and rebound. In particular, simple sugars and foods containing refined carbohydrates should be avoided. Some experts advise lying down after eating, as this also slows gastric motility.

Disorders of the Small Intestine

The small intestine is a truly remarkable organ; of course, its main function is digestion and absorption of food but it must also protect the body from the outside world by forming a barrier to microbes, and it secretes a variety of hormones that regulate ingestion, digestion and GI motility. The surface area of the small intestinal mucosa is enormous, expanded by villi and microvilli to around 250 m^2, commonly quoted as around the size of a tennis court!

COELIAC DISEASE

Coeliac disease is an autoimmune gluten-sensitive enteropathy. Autoimmune diseases are thought to develop following an environmental trigger in genetically sensitive individuals. However, unlike most other autoimmune diseases, the environmental trigger in coeliac disease is known: gluten. Ingested gluten contains gliadin peptides, which are deamidated and cross-linked by tissue transglutaminase and presented by the appropriate major histocompatibility complex—usually major histocompatibility complex DQ2—to reactive T cells. Hence, for coeliac disease to occur, the person usually has the appropriate DQ haplotype, circulating antitissue transglutaminase (anti-TTG) antibodies and ingestion of gluten. A minority of individuals have seronegative coeliac disease; that is, they do not have anti-TTG antibodies and the gliadin peptides are possibly less immunogenic in such cases.

Coeliac disease affects up to 1 in 100 people, depending on the population, though in many cases it remains undiagnosed. The highest rates are seen in Europe, America and Australia, and it remains quite rare in Asia and sub-Saharan Africa.[17] Certain individuals are at higher risk and should be screened —first-degree relatives of someone with coeliac, patients with type 1 diabetes, autoimmune thyroid conditions, people with Turner syndrome or Down syndrome.

The 'classic' presentation of coeliac disease with steatorrhoea, malabsorption, and failure to thrive is now rarely seen. Patients may have nonspecific symptoms, such as bloating, diarrhoea, fatigue, or may be completely asymptomatic.

The only available management strategy for coeliac disease is complete dietary exclusion of gluten. There are studies investigating the use of enzymes to digest gliadin into nontoxic peptides, TTG blockers and tight junction regulators, but until these are proven to be useful, dietary management is the sole therapy, and patients must be seen by an experienced dietitian. They can also find useful and practical information from patient groups, such as Coeliac UK.

Patients need to be educated on key principles of dietary management of coeliac disease, including:

1. Naturally gluten-free foods
2. Substitute foods
3. 'Hidden' gluten and oats
4. Cross-contamination
5. Eating out
6. Ensuring adequate dietary intake of key nutrients (folate, iron and vitamin D may require supplementation)

Complications of coeliac disease include iron deficiency, osteopaenia and osteoporosis and, very rarely, small bowel adenocarcinoma and lymphoma. The lymphoma is a specific subtype, termed enteropathy-associated T-cell lymphoma, which can arise in patients known to have coeliac disease or can be the presenting feature in some. Response rates to conventional lymphoma chemotherapy are poor, with average overall survival of only 7 months reported.[18]

Many women are diagnosed with coeliac disease whilst of childbearing age. There are conflicting data on female fertility and fecundity, but women who have had recurrent miscarriages or have unexplained infertility should probably be screened for coeliac disease.[19]

SMALL INTESTINAL BACTERIAL OVERGROWTH

The small intestine is generally microbe-free, with only 10^3 organisms/mL. However, several disparate conditions can promote expansion of these numbers, leading to small intestinal bacterial overgrowth (SIBO). These are summarised in Table 8.2. This is probably more common than appreciated due to poor diagnostic tests, lack of clinician awareness and symptom overlap with common conditions like IBS. Bacterial overgrowth leads to malabsorption of fats and fat-soluble vitamins. However, vitamin K deficiency is rare, due to intraluminal synthesis by bacteria, which can also synthesise folate. Hence, SIBO can be characterised by vitamin A, D, E and B12 deficiency (as bacteria compete for B12), but a normal prothrombin time and normal or high folate level.

The gold standard for diagnosis is a jejunal aspirate and culture, with a positive finding being the presence of $>10^5$ colony forming units per millilitre. Noninvasive breath tests measuring hydrogen or carbon dioxide production by bacteria after ingestion of a radiolabelled carbohydrate (lactose or glucose) are more freely available but suffer with high false-positive and false-negative rates.

TABLE 8.2 ■ **Conditions Associated With Bacterial Overgrowth**

Medical	GI Dysmotility	Anatomical	Postsurgical
PPI therapy	Scleroderma	SB diverticula	Gastrojejunostomy
Immunodeficiency syndromes	Chronic pseudo-obstruction	Enteric fistula	Pancreas transplant with roux loop
Cirrhosis	Diabetic autonomic neuropathy		Absence of ICV

GI, Gastrointestinal; *ICV*, ileocaecal valve; *PPI*, proton pump inhibitor; *SB*, small bowel.

Management is with antibiotics, either a nonabsorbable antibiotic like rifaximin, which can be given long term, or a rotating course of two or three antibiotics (to avoid the development of resistance). Various regimens are available.[20] Vitamin deficiencies should be checked for and replaced. Pre- and probiotics have not demonstrated consistent results in this area, and further work is needed to establish the optimal treatment for SIBO.

LACTOSE INTOLERANCE

Lactase enzymes are present on the tips of microvilli in the small intestine and break down ingested lactose into glucose and galactose. Primary lactose intolerance is extremely common, affecting up to 80% of Asian and northern European populations, though it is less frequent in other parts of the world.[21] Secondary lactase deficiency can arise from any condition causing damage to intestinal villi—IBD, coeliac disease, and certain enteric infections such as *Giardia*.

Lactase deficiency does not always cause symptoms but in some individuals the undigested lactose causes bloating, wind and diarrhoea. Diagnosis can be made by dietary exclusion and the consequent improvement in symptoms or a lactose hydrogen breath test. Management is usually by changing to lactose-free foods, which are now widely available, but care should be taken to ensure sufficient calcium intake, and a review by a dietitian may be needed. Substitute lactase enzymes can also be taken with meals.

IRON-DEFICIENCY ANAEMIA

Iron-deficiency anaemia is the commonest cause of anaemia worldwide, partly related to the body's inability to store much iron (total body stores are only 3–5 g) and the prevalence of GI diseases, which cause poor absorption or GI loss of iron.[22]

Absorption, metabolism and transport of iron is a complex process, so there are multiple pathologies which can interfere with this. Sufficient iron must be ingested. People following vegetarian and vegan diets are therefore at risk of deficiency as nonhaem sources of iron (vegetables, beans, pulses) are less well absorbed than haem sources, for example, from red meat. Gastric acid helps in keeping iron in the more easily absorbed ferrous (Fe^{2+}) rather than ferric (Fe^{3+}) state. Nonhaem iron is absorbed into enterocytes in the duodenum and proximal jejunum via the divalent metal transporter 1, where it is then reduced to ferric iron by ferroportin. Haem iron probably enters enterocytes as a metalloporphyrin, then is degraded within enterocytes. Both sources of iron then cross the basolateral membrane and bind to transferrin in plasma. Transferrin is synthesised in the liver and transports both absorbed dietary iron and recycled iron from breakdown of old erythrocytes to the bone marrow for erythrocyte synthesis. Small amounts of iron are stored as ferritin or haemosiderin in reticuloendothelial calls, hepatocytes and skeletal muscle.

Iron deficiency causes a microcytic, hypochromic anaemia with low serum iron, low transferrin saturation, low ferritin, and high total iron binding capacity. Care must be taken in interpreting iron studies in the context of acute illness as ferritin is an acute phase reactant and levels may be nonspecifically raised in systemic disease. Similarly, inflammation causes an artificially low serum iron level.

Common causes of iron-deficiency anaemia are outlined in Table 8.3. A thorough history will usually point toward the cause, but if not, minimum investigations in newly diagnosed iron-deficiency anaemia include a urine dipstick to check for blood loss, OGD with duodenal biopsies to check for coeliac disease and a colonoscopy to check for colorectal cancer for anyone aged >45 years with GI symptoms or weight loss.

Even when the cause has been established, many patients will need to take supplemental iron, at least in the short term. There are various forms of oral iron available; most have GI side effects which limit tolerability. For the minority unable to tolerate any preparation, intravenous iron formulations are available.

SHORT BOWEL SYNDROME

The average length of the human small bowel is around 600 cm, though it ranges from 280 cm to 800 cm and depends upon the method of measurement (on cadavers, intraoperatively or using radiological imaging). There is a lot of redundancy, and people can undergo massive resections without any loss of function. However, there is a critical point at which the length of bowel is inadequate for maintaining nutritional requirements and individuals need to adapt their food and fluid intake or rely on parenteral nutritional support. Such cases are characteristic of SBS.

In SBS, caloric balance is determined by the residual small bowel length, whereas fluid balance is determined by the presence or absence of the colon in continuity with the small bowel. Fluid management in SBS is often mismanaged by both clinicians and patients. The proximal small bowel is mainly secretory, relying on the distal small bowel and colon to absorb most of the luminal fluid. In addition to ingested fluid and the 0.5 L of saliva produced per day, gastric acid volumes are usually around 1.5–2 L per day and biliopancreatic secretions another 1–1.5 L, meaning that over 6 L of fluid pass into the distal small bowel every day. In SBS, the sodium

TABLE 8.3 ■ **Common Causes of Iron Deficiency**

Inadequate Intake	Inadequate Absorption	Increased Losses
Vegetarian or vegan diet	Coeliac disease	Menstruation
Anorexia nervosa and other eating disorders	Hypochlorhydria	Regular blood donation
Poor-quality diet	Postsurgical (gastrectomy, gastric bypass)	Gastric ulcer
	Hookworm infection	GI malignancy
	Inflammatory bowel disease	Inflammatory bowel disease
		Angiodysplasia (anywhere in GI tract)
		Renal tract cancers
		Malaria

GI, Gastrointestinal.

content of ingested fluids becomes critical to fluid balance. Ingested fluids need to contain at least 90 mmol/L of sodium to match the intracellular sodium content of jejunal enterocytes. If the fluid in the jejunal lumen is hypotonic to this, sodium moves down an osmotic gradient into the lumen, drawing water with it, resulting in net sodium and water losses in stomal effluent. This is a common cause for high-output ileostomy. Patients with SBS affected in this way need careful education about the importance of fluid balance, avoidance of hypotonic fluids and the role of glucose-electrolyte mixes in managing this problem.[23]

Hypomagnesaemia is a common problem as unabsorbed fatty acids in the gut lumen chelate magnesium and the secondary hyperaldosteronism commonly seen in SBS patients (due to volume depletion) causes renal excretion of magnesium. Replacement of oral magnesium salts usually exacerbates stomal losses. Low doses of magnesium oxide given at night, when motility is slower, can be used. Some patients require occasional or regular intravenous magnesium replacement.

Patients with a jejuno-colic anastomosis (formed following surgical resection of the ileum ± part of the colon) are prone to two specific conditions—oxalate renal stones and D-lactic acidosis. Undigested fatty acids bind to luminal calcium, which is then not freely available to bind to dietary oxalate. Luminal oxalate can then be easily absorbed in the colon and accumulates in the kidneys, causing oxalate stones or a diffuse nephrocalcinosis leading to chronic renal failure over time. Dehydration and high dietary fat intake can exacerbate this process. Restriction of oral oxalate-rich foods is required to prevent this occurrence; these include spinach, rhubarb, beetroot, chocolate and strawberries.

D-lactic acidosis occurs when colonic bacteria ferment undigested carbohydrates, forming D-lactate, which is absorbed into the circulation and is difficult to metabolise. It can cross the blood–brain barrier and cause dysphasia, ataxia, altered mental status and, in severe cases, reduced level of consciousness. Patients will have a high anion gap metabolic acidosis with normal measured lactate (as this can only detect the usual L-isomer). Dietary restriction of simple carbohydrates is the main form of management.

Following massive intestinal resection, physical and hormonal adaptations occur to maximise residual function; however, this can take 1–2 years to fully develop. Therefore, patients with SBS requiring parenteral nutrition support may be able to be weaned off it over time. The combination of medical treatments and dietary modifications designed to maximise the residual function of the short bowel and encourage adaptation are designated 'intestinal rehabilitation', which is now the preferred term to 'intestinal failure'. Some patients will benefit from additional treatment in the form of growth factors such as GLP-2 analogues, intestinal lengthening surgery or intestinal transplantation.[24]

Disorders of the Colon and Rectum

CONSTIPATION

The term 'constipation' is used widely and often incorrectly. The definition is infrequent passage of stools (generally less than three bowel movements per week) or difficult passage of stools (need to strain or passage of hard stools). There are numerous secondary causes of constipation which may need to be excluded in certain patients (Table 8.4). Patients with 'red flag' symptoms (rectal bleeding, weight loss, abdominal mass, aged over 50) need urgent investigation for any new change in bowel habit.

Functional constipation is defined under the reviewed Rome (IV) criteria[25] and is estimated to affect 17% of adults in the community.[26] The diagnosis requires that a person has at least two of these symptoms for at least 3 months (plus additional stipulations that the criteria for IBS are not met and loose stools are rarely present without the use of laxatives):

- Straining required for at least 25% of defaecations
- Lumpy or hard stools (Bristol stool chart type 1 or 2) during at least 25% of defaecations

TABLE 8.4 ■ **Secondary Causes of Constipation**

Condition	Clues	Investigations Needed
Colorectal cancer	Age > 50, weight loss, blood in stools	Colonoscopy, CT scan
Colonic stricture	History of cancer, IBD, diverticulosis plus abdominal distension, vomiting	CT scan
Medication	Common culprits include iron, opiates, antacids, antiparkinsonian agents, calcium antagonists, tricyclic antidepressants	Medication review
Hypothyroidism		Thyroid function tests
Autonomic neuropathy	PMH of diabetes	Consider transit studies
Parkinson disease	Slow motility, slow speech, cogwheel rigidity	
Multiple sclerosis	Relapsing-remitting or progressive motor or sensory symptoms	
Constipation predominant IBS	Concurrent abdominal pain related to defaecation	History
Hypercalcaemia	History of renal failure, hyperparathyroidism	Serum calcium
Anorectal disorders (anal fissure, haemorrhoids)	Bright red rectal bleeding, anal pain on defaecation, history of haemorrhoids	Rectal examination

CT, Computed tomography; *IBD*, inflammatory bowel disease; *PMH*, past medical history.

- Sensation of incomplete evacuation after at least 25% of defaecations
- Sensation of anorectal obstruction/blockage for at least 25% of defaecations
- Manual manoeuvres required (manual support of pelvic floor, manual digital evacuation) during at least 25% of defaecations
- Less than three spontaneous bowel movements per week

General lifestyle and dietary advice for patients with chronic constipation often includes increased exercise, fluid intake and fibre intake. Although there is little conclusive evidence that physical activity improves bowel function, it does improve quality of life and overall symptom scores in IBS patients including constipation-predominant IBS (IBS-C). Studies on probiotics for functional constipation have generally been small and compared one strain of probiotic to placebo, rather than another. This also hampers systematic reviews of the evidence, and such reviews in paediatric populations have been negative overall. In adults, a systematic review and meta-analysis of 1182 patients demonstrated particular benefits for *Bifidobacterium lactis*.[27] Currently the evidence is generally too weak to recommend probiotics for functional constipation, but they are unlikely to cause any harm.

An increase in dietary fibre intake is part of first-line recommendations in most guidelines on constipation in adults and children. Daily intake amounts recommended vary from 25 to 30 g for women and 30 to 38 g for men. Many modern diets fall far short of these recommendations, which is why fibre supplements are so commonly used.

Laxatives are divided into groups based on their mechanism of action – osmotic, stool softeners, bulk-forming and stimulant laxatives. Bulk-forming laxatives are generally first line as many modern diets are low in fibre. Ispaghula (also called psyllium) husk is a soluble plant fibre, whilst methylcellulose is a type of insoluble fibre. Both hold water and provide bulk and soften stools but insoluble fibre supplementation may cause bloating and increased gas, which some patients will find intolerable. A 2011 systematic review of fibre supplementation compared with placebo showed that soluble fibre led to an improvement in number of stools per week, stool consistency and global symptoms (85.5% in treated group versus 47.4% in placebo group).[28]

Nonabsorbable osmotic laxatives draw water in from the GI lumen and make stools easier to pass. They include magnesium salts, lactulose and polyethylene glycol. Sodium docusate and arachis oil can soften stools but are often ineffective as single agents. Over-the-counter stimulant laxatives include senna and bisacodyl, whilst sodium picosulphate is generally reserved for bowel preparation prior to radiological or endoscopic procedures. Stimulant laxatives can be most effective for slow transit constipation, though they can cause cramping due to their mechanism of action. High doses of stimulant laxatives have been subject to misuse as a weight loss mechanism, which can cause severe electrolyte abnormalities.

New directly acting drugs for constipation are available for selected patients. Prucalopride is a selective 5HT4 agonist licensed for use in chronic constipation when the patient has already failed to respond to at least two other laxatives. Lubiprostone was a chloride channel activator licensed for chronic idiopathic constipation but was withdrawn from the UK market in 2018. Linaclotide is available for constipation-predominant IBS (see later).

DIVERTICULAR DISEASE OF THE COLON

Diverticulosis (the presence of diverticula) of the colon has an increasing incidence with age: <2% of people under age 30 are affected, compared with 50%–66% of those aged over 80.[29,30] Diverticula occur at areas of relative weakness where the vasa recta blood vessels pass through the muscular colonic wall. They are most common in the left colon (sigmoid and descending colon). Data from multiple epidemiological and animal studies has provided evidence that a low intake of dietary fibre is implicated in the development of diverticular disease.[31–33] Prospective dietary cohort studies have confirmed this finding.[34] Smoking has not been found to be implicated in the development of diverticulosis but does seem to increase the risk of developing complications.[33,35] Most patients do not develop complications, but those who do can suffer with recurrent episodes of diverticulitis (infection and inflammation), diverticular abscess or colonic perforation which can require surgery.

Diagnosis can be via endoscopic procedure (colonoscopy or sigmoidoscopy) or cross-sectional imaging such as CT. It is often noted incidentally on CT scans done for other reasons. Simple diverticulosis should be managed by a combination of a balanced diet including whole grains, fruit and vegetables, increased fluid intake, physical activity, stopping smoking and avoiding constipation with dietary measures or bulk-forming laxatives.

Diverticular disease occurs when the patient with diverticulosis develops symptoms—often left lower quadrant abdominal pain, tenderness, and a change in bowel habit. It is important to exclude other causes, particularly colonic cancer, if a patient has new change in bowel habit, has new rectal bleeding or weight loss and is over 50 years old. Management is as described previously plus simple analgesia or antispasmodic medications for pain. NSAIDs should be avoided as they have been associated with a higher risk of complications, including perforation, in patients with diverticular disease.[36]

Acute diverticulitis may be managed in primary care, if not severe, or in hospital if severe or the patient has not responded to antibiotics at home or developed complications. Patients admitted to hospital with fever, raised inflammatory markers or systemic sepsis should have a contrast enhanced CT scan within 24 hours of admission to confirm the diagnosis.[37] During an episode of acute diverticulitis patients may be placed on a liquid only diet or a low-fibre diet, though there are almost no studies to evidence this recommendation.

Inflammatory Bowel Disease

MALNUTRITION IN INFLAMMATORY BOWEL DISEASE: PREVALENCE, CAUSES, CONSEQUENCES

Malnutrition of any kind (protein-energy, micronutrient) is a common problem in IBD. The historical rates of malnutrition in IBD are quoted as high as 80% but more recent estimates are much more conservative, which may be related to increased patient and clinician awareness, more effective treatments, more multiprofessional teamwork or other factors. Nutrition screening studies have identified between 16% and 29.1% of all IBD patients attending outpatient clinics to be at mild or moderate nutrition risk using the various screening tools.[38–41] The prevalence rates published do vary somewhat depending on which tools are used and the patient groups selected. In a 2002 study of IBD patient awaiting surgery, the rates of malnutrition varied from 25% to 42% using different screening tools.[42] Other studies have looked at sarcopenia in IBD patients with rates as high as 42% for patients in hospital, and even patients in clinical remission can display reduced muscle strength.[43]

There are numerous potential causes of malnutrition in patients with IBD and for many it will depend on the site, activity, and extent of disease. Some will have significantly increased energy and nutritional requirements, increased GI losses of micronutrients, reduced intake of food due to disease-related anorexia or fear of exacerbating symptoms, and a minority will have malabsorption.

Patients with IBD who are malnourished have higher risks of complications including admissions to hospital, surgery, venous thromboembolism, length of hospital stay and mortality.[44–47]

THE ROLE OF DIET IN THE PATHOGENESIS OF INFLAMMATORY BOWEL DISEASE

The pathogenesis of IBD is incompletely understood, but it is likely to involve altered immune responses to one or more environmental factors in genetically susceptible individuals. The environmental factors may relate to the gut microbiota, foodborne antigens, smoking, medications or a combination of some or all of these. Dietary intake and the gut microbiome are intrinsically linked, and there is evidence of dysbiosis in many individuals with IBD. Fewer Firmicutes and more Proteobacteria and Bacteroides are seen in IBD compared with healthy controls.[48,49]

A systematic review of the role of diet in IBD was published in 2011.[50] It demonstrated an increased risk of Crohn disease and ulcerative colitis (UC) with high dietary intake of polyunsaturated fatty acids (PUFAs), omega-6 fatty acids and meat. There was a reduced risk of developing Crohn disease with higher dietary fruit intake (73%–80% reduced risk), though there may be confounding factors as diets high in fruit tend to have less fat and more fibre. The role of fibre was examined in prospective cohort studies of nurses' health,[51] which showed a hazard ratio of 0.59 of developing Crohn disease in the group consuming a median of 24 g fibre per day. Higher consumption of fruit was associated with less risk of developing UC (odds ratio 0.69) and Crohn (odds ratio 0.57).[52]

In the Nurses Health studies, dietary intake of zinc was negatively associated with the risk of developing Crohn disease but not UC.[53] Vitamin D deficiency is more common in IBD patients than the general population[54] and there are presumed causes for this—restricted dietary intake, lack of sun exposure for patients taking immunosuppressants, malabsorption and chronic inflammation. 1,25-(OH)-D2 has a number of immunomodulatory effects, including stimulation of nucleotide-binding oligomerisation domain 2 in animal models.[55] Nucleotide-binding oligomerisation domain 2 was the first genetic marker of Crohn disease, and it is involved in microbial sensing within the gut lumen.

MICRONUTRIENT DEFICIENCIES IN INFLAMMATORY BOWEL DISEASE

Patients with IBD should be screened for anaemia, vitamin D and zinc deficiency on an annual basis, and some may require more detailed micronutrient testing depending on their individual circumstances (Table 8.5).

NUTRITION AS TREATMENT FOR INFLAMMATORY BOWEL DISEASE

Nutrition support with oral supplements or enteral or parenteral nutrition should be offered to IBD patients for the usual indications. However, there is also evidence for the use of diet as *therapy* for active Crohn disease following a small case series in the 1970s, mainly conducted in children, that demonstrated an improvement in inflammation and nutritional parameters with an enteral nutrition diet.[56,57]

As with many nutrition studies, interpreting the evidence is challenging—the studies were observational, there were often no placebo arms and various enteral feeding regimens were used (exclusive or

TABLE 8.5 ■ **Micronutrients in IBD**

Micronutrient	Risk Factors for Deficiency	Clinical Features of Deficiency	Diagnosis
Iron	Chronic GI blood loss Inadequate intake Malabsorption	Fatigue, pallor, exertional breathlessness, glossitis, nail changes	Serum ferritin <30 ng/mL or transferrin saturation <15%
Vitamin B12	Ileal resection, active ileal disease	Macrocytic anaemia Peripheral neuropathy	Serum B12 <200 pg/mL
Folate	MTX Inadequate intake Malabsorption	Macrocytic anaemia	Plasma folate < 4.5 nmol/L or red cell folate <140 ng/mL
Vitamin D	Inadequate intake Malabsorption	Abnormalities in bone metabolism	Total serum 25OH-D <30 nmol/L
Vitamin A	Inadequate intake Malabsorption	Night blindness, xerophthalmia	Serum vitamin A level <1.3 µmol/L
Magnesium	Diarrhoea	Muscle cramps, arrhythmias	Serum magnesium <0.7 mmol/L
Vitamin K	Absence of colon	Easy bruising, mucosal bleeding	Raised prothrombin time or INR
Selenium	Inadequate intake Malabsorption	Cardiomyopathy	Plasma red cell selenium <0.75 µmol/L Or low glutathione peroxidase activity
Zinc	High GI losses Inadequate intake Malabsorption	Reduced wound healing	Serum zinc <11 µmol/L

Reference ranges refer to adults only. Ferritin, selenium and zinc are affected by the acute phase response.
GI, Gastrointestinal; *INR*, International Normalized Ratio; *MTX*, methotrexate.

nonexclusive enteral nutrition, elemental or semielemental formulas, via different methods of delivery, e.g., oral or via nasogastric tube, for varying lengths of time). A Cochrane review in 2018 demonstrated steroids were superior to enteral nutrition for induction of remission in Crohn disease in adults (73% compared with 45%) but enteral nutrition was superior to steroids in children (83% versus 61%), although the evidence was of low quality.[58] There was no difference between elemental, semielemental and polymeric formulas. In current clinical practice, enteral nutrition is used more widely in paediatric IBD, in whom there are increased concerns about the effect of corticosteroids on growth and development. Use of enteral nutrition as therapy for maintenance of remission is hindered by the unpalatability of the formulae and/or patient aversion to long-term nasogastric tube placement.

OBESITY IN INFLAMMATORY BOWEL DISEASE

As rates of obesity rise generally, the prevalence of obesity in IBD patients is also currently high. Two US-based retrospective cohort studies showed rates of obesity in patients with Crohn disease and UC were between 30.3% and 35.2%.[59,60] A UK population-based study carried out in Scotland showed 38% of IBD patients were overweight and 18% obese.[61] There is no evidence that obesity is associated with increased hospitalisations, complications, or rates of surgery. However, if patients with obesity require surgery they may be at an increased risk of longer operating times, higher conversion rates from laparoscopic to open approach and postoperative complications including wound infections and pulmonary complications.[62–64]

Irritable Bowel Syndrome

PREVALENCE, AETIOPATHOLOGY AND DIAGNOSIS OF INFLAMMATORY BOWEL DISEASE

IBS is one of the most common GI disorders seen in general practice and in gastroenterology clinics. The prevalence is around 10% in the general population.[65] It is associated with significant health costs due to its prevalence and can have profound effects upon an individual's quality of life. The pathophysiological mechanisms that potentially underlie IBS have been extensively investigated, and current consensus is that IBS represents a collection of disorders of gut–brain interaction that lead to disturbances of GI motility, hypersensitivity of the GI tract, and abnormal central nervous system processing.[66] Diagnosis and subclassification into diarrhoea-predominant IBS, IBS-C, or mixed IBS is made according to the Rome IV criteria (Box 8.1).[25] If a patient's symptoms meet the Rome IV criteria and there are no additional red flag symptoms (Box 8.2), then clinicians should make a positive diagnosis of IBS. In the absence of red flag symptoms, minimal testing with full blood count, C-reactive protein, anti-TTG antibody and faecal calprotectin is all that is required, and further investigations are unnecessary.

BOX 8.1 ■ Rome IV Diagnostic Criteria for Irritable Bowel Syndrome[67]

Recurrent abdominal pain on average at least 1 day/week in the last 3 months, associated with two or more of the following criteria:

1. Related to defaecation
2. Associated with a change in frequency of stool
3. Associated with a change in form (appearance) of stool

Criteria fulfilled for the last 3 months with symptom onset at least 6 months prior to diagnosis

Further criteria for subclassification into diarrhoea-predominant irritable bowel syndrome, constipation-predominant irritable bowel syndrome, and mixed irritable bowel syndrome not included

BOX 8.2 ■ Red Flag Lower Gastrointestinal Symptoms[68]

Age > 45 years
Rectal bleeding (not previously investigated)
New change in bowel habit for more than 6 weeks
Weight loss
Abdominal mass or distension
History of previous cancer
Family history of colorectal cancer

DIETARY THERAPY FOR INFLAMMATORY BOWEL DISEASE: FIRST-LINE DIETARY ADVICE, FIBRE, AND PROBIOTICS

Following a positive diagnosis of IBS, first-line dietary advice should be based around general principles of a healthy, balanced diet, for example, the British Dietetic Association fact sheet of dietary advice in IBS.[69] Reducing the intake of ultra-processed foods, alcohol, caffeine and foods containing sugar alternatives (such as sorbitol and mannitol) may help symptoms, although the formal evidence base for this is limited.[68] Some patients may identify trigger foods for their symptoms, and it is important that they are counselled to ensure their eating habits do not become overly restrictive of essential food groups. There is currently no evidence-based role for blood tests to identify food intolerances or food allergies in IBS, yet there are many commercially available.

The relationship of fibre intake and IBS is complex, not least because soluble and insoluble fibre play different roles. In general, dietary fibre has beneficial effects on the gut; however, in many patients with IBS, it triggers symptoms, particularly pain, bloating and wind. A systematic review of randomised control trials demonstrated global symptom benefit from supplementing soluble fibre (ispaghula) but not insoluble fibre (bran) in patients with IBS.[70] Patients with diarrhoea-predominant IBS may find symptomatic benefit from reducing dietary fibre, whereas patients with IBS-C may benefit from the opposite. Some patients with IBS may find benefit from adopting a low-fibre diet concomitant with taking a soluble fibre supplement, such as ispaghula. Supplementation with insoluble fibre, such as bran, is unlikely to be beneficial and is more likely to exacerbate pain and bloating so is not usually recommended.[68]

There is weak evidence that probiotics may help reduce symptoms in IBS; however, it is not clear which strains or combinations of species are likely to be of benefit. Therefore, probiotics are not generally recommended, but patients with IBS may wish to trial a combination probiotic for a defined period of time and assess symptom response.[68]

DIETARY THERAPY FOR INFLAMMATORY BOWEL DISEASE: LOW FODMAP

The low FODMAP diet was developed specifically for the management of IBS symptoms and involves restriction of foods containing certain carbohydrates, namely fermentable oligosaccharides, disaccharides, monosaccharides and polyols (FODMAPs). These are found in varying quantities in certain fruits and vegetables, wheat and dairy products. Whilst not inherently unhealthy, FODMAPs are poorly absorbed compounds that ferment when they enter the colon, causing gas production and drawing water into the colonic lumen. In most adults they do not cause symptoms, so again visceral hypersensitivity is probably involved in the generation of symptoms in people with IBS. A 2018 systematic review and meta-analysis of low FODMAP trials concluded the diet resulted in a global reduction in IBS symptoms, with a relative risk of 0.69.[71]

Any patient starting a low FODMAP diet for IBS should be supported by a trained health care professional, usually a dietitian or doctor, to optimise the chance of success through the three key stages: restriction, reintroduction and personalisation. The restriction phase consists of 6–8 weeks of excluding certain FODMAP containing foods and assessing symptom response. In the reintroduction phase, certain foods will be reintroduced in a stepwise way (usually one new food weekly) and symptom response monitored. Finally, the information gleaned from the prior phases will guide a personalised dietary plan to ensure nutritional adequacy whilst minimising IBS symptoms.

DIETARY THERAPY FOR INFLAMMATORY BOWEL DISEASE: EXCLUSION DIETS

Many patients will themselves identify trigger foods, but if not, they can be asked to keep a food and symptom diary for 1–2 weeks, which they can then interrogate together with a specialist GI dietitian. Wheat is a commonly identified culprit here, but trials have not concluded any difference in global symptoms between a gluten-containing and a gluten-free diet in IBS. Wheat contains fructans (a type of FODMAP) which confounds interpretation. It is important to consider coeliac disease in any patient who reports a link of symptoms to wheat gluten ingestion.

Disorders of the Liver

The liver is the major organ of nutrient metabolism in the body. Its essential functions include protein metabolism and synthesis, lipid metabolism including cholesterol synthesis, glucose homeostasis including gluconeogenesis and glycogenolysis and bilirubin and bile acid metabolism. Therefore a malfunctioning liver has major negative consequences for maintaining a healthy nutritional state via various mechanisms. Clinicians caring for patients with liver disease should proactively anticipate and address protein-energy malnutrition (i.e., undernutrition), sarcopenia and micronutrient deficiencies.[72,73]

Liver damage can be acute, for example, from viral hepatitis or hepatotoxic drug injury, or chronic, most commonly secondary to chronic alcohol excess, NAFLD, also called metabolic-associated fatty liver syndrome, and chronic viral hepatitis B and C. Less common aetiologies of chronic liver disease include autoimmune (autoimmune hepatitis, primary biliary cirrhosis and primary sclerosing cholangitis) and hereditary metabolic conditions such as Wilson disease and haemochromatosis. In some cases, more than one aetiology will be present simultaneously.

The liver is a resilient organ and can regenerate following cellular injury but severe damage that is either acute and fulminant or chronic and progressive can lead to liver failure, which is associated with high rates of morbidity and mortality. Managing the nutritional requirements of patients with liver failure can be particularly challenging. Metabolic features of liver failure include hypoglycaemia resulting from deranged glucose metabolism and rapid depletion of hepatic glycogen stores, and hyperammonaemia as the normal hepatic conversion of ammonia to urea is impaired.

ALCOHOL-RELATED LIVER DISEASE

ALD is perhaps the aetiology most strongly associated with undernutrition, particularly sarcopenia. Individuals who chronically consume excessive alcohol often derive most of their calorie requirements from refined carbohydrates and alcohol itself, with poor dietary intake of protein and micronutrients. Alcohol can dysregulate the metabolic functions of skeletal muscle, including to the action of insulin, and can lead directly to muscle loss. Chronic excess alcohol increases resting energy expenditure by 25% but abstinence can reduce this back to normal within days.[74]

Abstinence from alcohol is the single most important factor for reducing liver-related morbidity and mortality and is essential to a holistic nutritional approach in patients with ALD. However, sudden alcohol cessation in people who are physically dependent can precipitate alcohol withdrawal syndrome. Clinically this presents on a spectrum from tremor, sweating and mild agitation, to the medical emergencies of delirium tremens and/or seizures. Alcohol withdrawal syndrome is prevented using tapered protocols of benzodiazepines under medical supervision.

Clinicians should have a high clinical suspicion of micronutrient deficiency in patients with ALD, particularly of vitamins B1 (thiamine) and B12 (cobalamin), vitamin D, and the electrolytes potassium, magnesium, and phosphate. These should be tested where appropriate and replaced accordingly.[72] Thiamine deficiency may manifest clinically as Wernicke encephalopathy characterised by a triad of ophthalmoplegia with nystagmus, ataxia and confusion. This is reversible with thiamine replacement. Korsakoff syndrome is the irreversible equivalent to Wernicke encephalopathy. On clinical assessment, distinguishing between alcohol intoxication, alcohol withdrawal, hepatic encephalopathy (HE), and Wernicke-Korsakoff syndrome can be challenging.

For patients who are at high risk of Wernicke-Korsakoff syndrome, prophylactic thiamine should be given promptly, for example, intravenously for 3 days followed by oral supplementation in the longer term. Thiamine is often given in combination with other vitamins, for example as intravenous Pabrinex, which contains thiamine, riboflavin (B2), pyridoxine (B6), nicotinamide (B3), ascorbic acid (vitamin C) and glucose.

Alcoholic steatohepatitis (ASH) is the inflammatory stage of ALD that drives progression to fibrosis and cirrhosis. Patients with ASH who are unable to meet caloric requirements through oral diet should be offered individualised nutritional supplementation. This has been shown to improve rates of mortality and complications, including infection, HE and synthetic liver dysfunction.[72,75] In severe ASH there is a risk of hypoglycaemia following periods of fasting, for example, overnight or prior to hospital procedures, as hepatic glycogen stores are quickly depleted. Intravenous glucose therapy may be required to maintain normoglycaemia in such situations.[72]

Nutritional considerations for patients with cirrhosis are discussed in the later section of this chapter.

NONALCOHOLIC FATTY LIVER DISEASE

Nonalcoholic fatty liver disease (NAFLD), also called metabolic-associated liver disease, refers to a spectrum of liver disorders in people without a history of hazardous or harmful alcohol consumption. An estimated 24% of adults in developed countries have NAFLD.[76] Most cases of NAFLD are at the least severe end of the spectrum with simple hepatic steatosis (nonalcoholic fatty liver), which is benign and asymptomatic. Of these, approximately 15% will develop into the inflammatory form, nonalcoholic steatohepatitis (NASH), that drives progression to liver fibrosis and cirrhosis. At liver biopsy, hepatic steatosis is present when >5% of hepatocytes contain macrovesicular lipid deposits (made up predominantly of triglyceride) and NASH is characterised by hepatocellular ballooning, lobular inflammation and fibrosis.[77] In practice, diagnosis of NAFLD is usually made without biopsy but with noninvasive methods such as liver function blood tests and ultrasound imaging. Diagnosing and staging NASH and fibrosis are challenging without biopsy; existing noninvasive scoring systems can diagnose advanced NAFLD fibrosis but are of limited value in picking up mild to moderate disease.[78]

NAFLD is strongly associated with the metabolic syndrome, obesity and insulin resistance, thus diet is a key factor in its prevention and management. Globally, over half of patients with type 2 diabetes (T2DM) have NAFLD.[79] Environments that foster sedentary lifestyles and easy access to calorie-dense, nutrient-poor and ultra-processed foods and sugar-sweetened beverages underscore the epidemic of metabolic syndrome and NAFLD.

Dietary Fat in NAFLD

At the individual level, free fatty acids in the liver that are not oxidised for energy are esterified and stored in hepatocytes. These fatty acids can originate from the body's endogenous stores of visceral and subcutaneous adipose tissues that are broken down by lipolysis in the fasting state or from dietary macronutrients: fat and carbohydrate. In patients with NAFLD, the ratio of hepatic fat from each source is approximately 60% from body adipose tissue, 25% from dietary carbohydrate and 15% from dietary fat.[80] Excessive habitual energy intake, especially of refined sugars and saturated fat in combination, promotes excessive liver fat accumulation.[81]

Digested fat is absorbed from the gut and packaged into chylomicrons, which circulate and deposit fatty acids around the body. Dietary saturated fatty acids (for example, from meat, dairy, coconut oil, palm oil) lead to liver fat deposition when consumed in excess, even in controlled, isocaloric conditions.[82] This does not appear to be the case with unsaturated fatty acids: monounsaturated fatty acids (MUFAs) and polyunsaturated fatty acids (PUFAs). Dietary MUFAs (for example, from olive oil and tree nuts, also seafood, poultry and some other animal products) appear to be protective against NAFLD, perhaps even in the absence of weight loss.[83] PUFAs (for example from cold water fish, seed oils, dairy) may also be protective but the evidence is limited and ideal omega-3-to-omega-6 ratios are not well described in this context.[84] It is worth noting that most whole-food sources of dietary fat contain varying combinations of saturated fatty acids, PUFAs and MUFAs. Also, the fatty acid composition of the diet consumed by livestock will impact the fatty acid profile of the meat, dairy and eggs produced.

Dietary Carbohydrate and Sugars in NAFLD

Dietary carbohydrate can be synthesised into fatty acids via the process of de novo lipogenesis (DNL) in the liver. This demonstrably leads to hepatic steatosis predominantly when overall dietary energy intake exceeds physiologic requirements (i.e., in a state of caloric excess).[85,86] A higher rate of DNL is observed in the presence of NAFLD and insulin resistance.[87,88] Refined sugars, for example, sucrose and fructose found in sodas and processed foods, are potent substrates for DNL and subsequent liver fat deposition.[89,90] High consumption of fructose is also associated with proinflammatory pathways, altered gut permeability and lipotoxicity that may contribute to hepatic inflammation in NASH.[91] In contrast, whole-food sources of complex carbohydrates, namely whole vegetables and fruits, are less culpable, which suggests a possible protective mechanism for dietary fibre against NAFLD; however, outcomes from interventional trials of fibre in NAFLD are limited.

Dietary Protein in NAFLD

Optimising dietary protein can protect against the fattening effects of both saturated fat and sugars on the liver in NAFLD,[92] even in patients with T2DM,[93] at least in the short term. Obese sarcopenia is common in NAFLD patients, suggesting suboptimal protein intake and suboptimal skeletal muscle conditioning. A habitual diet higher in protein and low to moderate in fat and carbohydrate has been shown to improve NAFLD and insulin resistance.[94] This may in part be due to the higher satiating effect that protein has over carbohydrate and fat in addition to its effects on the health of skeletal muscle, which is a key tissue in insulin sensitivity. Physical exercise is likely to potentiate the benefit from dietary protein on skeletal muscle and insulin sensitivity.

Nutritional Approaches to NAFLD Management

For patients with NAFLD, including NASH, who are overweight or obese, the most effective intervention to prevent and reverse disease progression is one that reduces excess body weight.

Weight loss of between 5% and 10% body weight is associated with improvements in hepatic steatosis, inflammation, and liver enzymes. Patients who lose more than 10% are more likely to see additional improvements in stage of fibrosis.[95] For severely obese patients with NAFLD, bariatric surgery has the strongest evidence base for weight loss and leads to resolution of hepatic steatosis in approximately 92% and resolution of NASH in approximately 70% of patients.[96] Novel endoscopic bariatric and metabolic therapies are also available and in development for NAFLD.[97]

Dietary approaches to weight loss for NAFLD should follow the general principles of dietary approaches to overweight and obesity (Chapter 7). Current formal guidelines for NAFLD management advocate hypocaloric dietary patterns and do not favour restriction of either dietary carbohydrate over fat or vice versa.[72,95] A combined lifestyle approach of dietary modification plus physical exercise is likely to be most effective for NAFLD.[98] Nonetheless, physical exercise alone can improve hepatic steatosis, insulin resistance and overall health and should be encouraged in patients with NAFLD whether overweight or normal weight.[99] The mode of exercise should be tailored to patient preference to maximise chances of long-term maintenance.

Overall dietary pattern and food quality are of upmost importance in the management of NAFLD. Broadly speaking, high-calorie, low-micronutrient foods, especially those containing excess fructose, sucrose and saturated fat, should be minimised to facilitate a caloric deficit. Ideally, whole complex carbohydrate foods (such as fruits, vegetables and unrefined whole grains) should be the primary source of dietary carbohydrate, and the intake of processed foods, refined grains, refined sugars and sugar-sweetened beverages should be minimal. Replacing some dietary carbohydrate with protein is likely to be of overall benefit to hepatic fat content.[100–103] In place of saturated fats and *trans*-fats, unsaturated fats, particularly MUFAs, should be prioritised alongside sufficient protein and micronutrients. Alcohol should be avoided in NAFLD, and indeed in chronic liver disease of any aetiology, to reduce the risk of progression to cirrhosis.[104]

Compared with the standard Western diet, a Mediterranean diet is generally considered to be the best and most sustainable dietary pattern for improving body weight, insulin sensitivity, hepatic steatosis and fibrosis for patients with NAFLD.[72,95] It also has benefits for cardiovascular risk and other metabolic conditions (Chapters 6 and 7). The Mediterranean diet is usually described as consisting of whole vegetables, fruit and whole grains supplemented with seafood, poultry, dairy and olive oil. However, defining and replicating the diet accurately is not straightforward. There is much heterogeneity across studies, and the ideal components and macronutrient composition of the Mediterranean diet are not standardised.

Low-carbohydrate diets have been shown to rapidly improve hepatic steatosis, potentially independent of weight loss.[105–107] Clinical studies confirm benefit from a low-carbohydrate diet in patients with NAFLD, at least in the short term.[103,108,109] Mediterranean diets modified by lowering carbohydrate content are also effective in NAFLD.[110,111] Another dietary approach that has shown short-term benefit in NAFLD is intermittent fasting, specifically the 5:2 diet.[108] It is important to note that low-carbohydrate and intermittent fasting diets have not been tested and may not be safe for patients with cirrhosis, in whom glucose metabolism and hepatic glycogen storage is typically impaired. Patients following any new dietary pattern should be counselled and supervised by a trained professional to ensure adequate intake of essential nutrients.

Nutritional Supplements in NAFLD

Vitamin E supplementation in patients with NASH has been shown to improve histological inflammation and liver enzyme derangement but has no impact on fibrosis.[112] Several other dietary supplements have been trialled in NAFLD, including vitamin C, resveratrol, anthocyanin, bayberries and omega-3-fatty acids but there is currently not enough evidence of clinical benefit for any of these to be widely recommended.[72,113]

Other Considerations in NAFLD

NAFLD should not be considered alone, and management should be tailored to individual preferences and culture, taking into account comorbidities such as T2DM, obesity and cardiovascular disease. This is particularly important as cardiovascular disease is the major cause of death amongst patients with NAFLD. In NAFLD, as in all liver disease, unexplained weight loss warrants further investigation to rule out underlying malignancy. Patients with NAFLD-related cirrhosis, especially decompensated cirrhosis, will have further nutritional requirements and considerations. These are covered in the later section on cirrhosis.

Whilst most cases of NAFLD are associated with overnutrition, fatty liver disease can also be caused by severe protein-calorie undernutrition. Most reports are in malnourished children from low-income countries[114]; however, clinicians caring for patients with anorexia nervosa and other eating disorders should be aware of this possibility.[115] The degree of hepatic steatosis can be severe but tends to resolve with refeeding.[116]

WILSON DISEASE

Wilson disease is a rare genetic disorder of toxic accumulation of copper in the liver resulting from impaired copper excretion from hepatocytes (autosomal recessive transmission; *ATP7B* gene). It typically presents before the age of 40 years and is characterised by neurological and psychiatric, renal and hepatic complications. It can present as acute liver failure (ALF) requiring liver transplantation.

The rate of gastric and intestinal copper absorption, which is fairly stable regardless of intake, remains normal in Wilson disease. In fact, normal homeostatic mechanisms increase the amount of copper absorbed when dietary copper levels are low, and less copper is absorbed when higher amounts of copper are consumed.[117] Furthermore, many healthful foods such as meat, seafood, vegetables, mushrooms and fruits contain small amounts of copper. Avoiding copper-containing foods can be burdensome and lead to highly restrictive dietary patterns with no proven benefit to disease progression.[118] Therefore, copper-restricted diets are not generally recommended in Wilson disease with the exception of avoiding foods that contain markedly high amounts of copper, for example, shellfish and liver, which should be avoided in the first year of treatment.[118–120] Treatment is with copper chelating agents such penicillamine, which promotes urinary copper excretion. Penicillamine also interferes with the action of vitamin B6 (pyridoxine), which should be supplemented (25–50 mg/d) in patients taking this medication. Zinc supplementation can also be used in Wilson disease as it reduces copper absorption in the GI tract.

HEREDITARY HAEMOCHROMATOSIS

Hereditary haemochromatosis is an autosomal recessive disease characterised by an abnormally high rate of intestinal iron absorption (most commonly a result of C282Y mutation on *HFE* gene). This leads to toxic deposition of iron, and subsequent dysfunction, in the liver and other organs. The cornerstone of treatment is regular phlebotomy, which reduces the risk of developing cirrhosis. Dietary factors that affect iron absorption include vitamin C intake, which increases iron absorption by converting ferric iron to ferrous in the digestive tract, and polyphenols in tea and coffee, which can reduce iron absorption.[121] Restricting sources of dietary iron, for example, red meat, may be helpful[122]; however, there are no specific dietary interventions with strong clinical evidence of effectiveness on outcomes in hereditary haemochromatosis.

ACUTE LIVER FAILURE

ALF usually occurs in patients without preexisting liver disease and can present on a spectrum of severity. Viral, drug-induced (e.g., paracetamol overdose) and autoimmune hepatitis are the commonest aetiologies. Most patients will have normal nutritional status at presentation but fulminant hepatocellular damage causes synthetic and metabolic dysfunction and may be further complicated by multiorgan failure. Impaired carbohydrate, lipid and protein metabolism may manifest as hypoglycaemia, hyperlactataemia and hyperammonaemia, all of which are poor prognostic signs. Several mechanisms underlie hypoglycaemia in ALF: glycogen stores are depleted, hepatocyte damage leads to impaired gluconeogenesis and circulating glucose can also be reduced by hyperinsulinaemia secondary to pancreatic hypersecretion and impaired hepatic metabolism of insulin.[123]

Patients who are (or who are at risk of) underweight, sarcopenia and/or micronutrient deficiency should be fed promptly. ALF leads to an increase in resting energy expenditure by up to 30%.[124] In acute hospital and intensive care settings, the nutritional approach to patients with ALF should follow similar principles to those used in other critically unwell patients. Therefore, unless contraindicated, oral, enteral or parenteral nutrition should be used to meet nutritional requirements as per their usual indications and contraindications.[72] Whilst protein restriction is not generally recommended in ALF, in a small proportion of patients with hyperacute, fulminant liver failure and severe hyperammonaemia driving HE, it may be appropriate to restrict protein in the initial phase (for example up to 48 hours) until arterial ammonia levels are controlled. The principal objectives of nutritional therapy in ALF as outlined by European Society for Clinical Nutrition and Metabolism are in Box 8.3.

A small proportion of individuals with ALF may be appropriate candidates for liver transplant.[125] Severe obesity and undernutrition are both risk factors for requiring liver transplantation in ALF.[126] Nutritional considerations in liver transplantation are considered later in this chapter.

CIRRHOSIS

The natural history of most chronic liver diseases includes the progression to cirrhosis, which is characterised by irreversible, nodular fibrosis and synthetic dysfunction. Due to the typically slow progression of chronic liver disease to cirrhosis, the onset of symptoms and signs of cirrhosis may be slow. Once established, patients with cirrhosis may develop decompensated disease, which has several hallmark manifestations including jaundice, ascites, spontaneous bacterial peritonitis, HE, variceal haemorrhage, and hepatorenal syndrome. Decompensated liver disease dramatically increases rates of morbidity and mortality.

Nutritional Principles in Cirrhosis

Both undernutrition and severe obesity are associated with poorer outcomes in cirrhosis.[127,128] Therefore, at the very least, all patients with liver disease should be accurately weighed and

BOX 8.3 ■ Principal Objectives of Nutritional Therapy in Acute Liver Failure[72]

- Ensure adequate provision of energy by providing glucose, lipid, vitamins and trace elements.
- Ensure optimal rates of protein synthesis by providing adequate protein or amino acids.
- Avoid metabolic complications of nutritional therapy through ensuring euglycaemia and preventing hyperammonaemia (which can manifest as cerebral oedema and hepatic encephalopathy) and hypertriglyceridaemia.

screened for malnutrition using a validated tool such as Malnutrition Universal Screening Tool, or the liver disease-specific Royal Free Hospital Nutrition Prioritising Tool.[129,130] In patients with cirrhosis with high BMI, clinicians should beware of inaccuracies due to ascites and fluid retention (this is accounted for by the Royal Free Hospital Nutrition Prioritising Tool) and remain vigilant for sarcopenia. If available, bioelectrical impedance analysis or simple bedside testing such as handgrip strength can be used to assess nutritional status and confer prognostic value. The Royal Free Hospital Global Assessment is a validated predictive method of assessing nutritional status in cirrhosis that uses the measures of BMI, mid-arm muscle circumference and brief dietary intake assessment.[131] The European Association for the Study of the Liver provides useful stepwise guidance on nutritional screening and assessment for inpatients with cirrhosis (Fig. 8.1).[73] Radiological methods exist to formally assess for sarcopenia. In all cases of liver disease, involvement of a registered dietitian is of utmost value to assess nutritional status and requirements and tailor a nutrition plan for the patient.

The prevalence of protein-calorie malnutrition, sarcopenia and micronutrient deficiencies are high in patients with cirrhosis, regardless of aetiology.[132] This is likely multifactorial. Patients who are dependent on alcohol are more likely to have inadequate nutritional intake from poor-quality

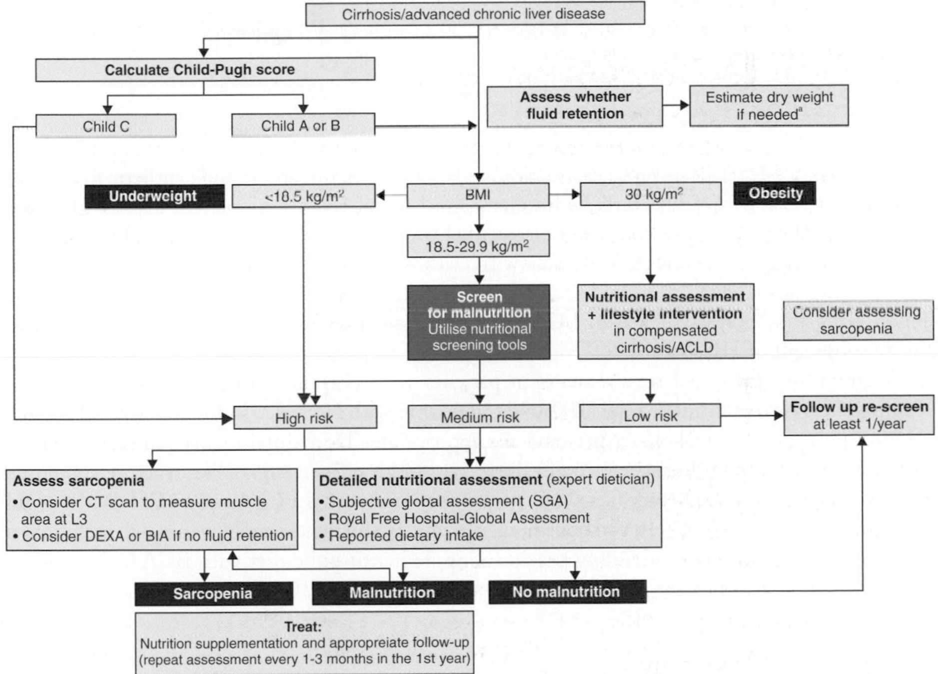

Fig. 8.1 European Association for the Study of the Liver guideline for nutritional screening and assessment in patients with cirrhosis.[73] All patients should undergo a rapid screening of malnutrition using validated, accepted tools. A liver-specific screening tool which takes into consideration fluid retention may be advisable (Royal Free Hospital Nutritional Prioritizing Tool). Patients found to be at high risk of malnutrition should undergo a detailed nutritional assessment, and based on the findings they should receive either supplementation or regular follow-up. [a]In a case of fluid retention, body weight should be corrected by evaluating the patient's dry weight by postparacentesis body weight or weight recorded before fluid retention if available, or by subtracting a percentage of weight based upon severity of ascites (mild, 5%; moderate, 10%; severe, 15%), with an additional 5% subtracted if bilateral pedal oedema is present. *ACLD*, advanced chronic liver disease; *BIA*, bioelectrical impedance analysis; *BMI*, body mass index; *CT*, computed tomography; *DEXA*, dual-energy X-ray absorptiometry.

TABLE 8.6 ■ **Guide to Nutritional Requirements in Cirrhosis**[72,73,135]

Nutritional Recommendations for Malnutrition in Cirrhosis	
Daily calories	30–40 kcal/kg per day and avoid periods of prolonged fasting
Protein	1.2–1.5 g/kg per day with increased BCAAs (0.2–0.25 g/kg per day or 30 g per day)
Carbohydrates	50%–70% of daily calories but avoid simple sugars (especially fructose); consider late evening carbohydrate snack
Lipids	10%–20% of daily calories with increased MUFAs and PUFAs
Special Considerations	
Hepatic encephalopathy	Maintain protein intake, increase BCAAs
Ascites	Reduced sodium diet (≤ 2 g per day) and water restriction when necessary/possible
Oesophageal varices	These are not a contraindication for placing a nasogastric tube; however, PEG tube placement is associated with higher risk of complications

BCAA, Branched-chain amino acid; *MUFA*, monounsaturated fatty acid; *PEG*, percutaneous endoscopic gastrostomy; *PUFA*, polyunsaturated fatty acid.

diets. As progressive fibrosis replaces functioning hepatocytes, metabolic and synthetic liver function deteriorates. This means carbohydrate and lipid metabolism is impaired, hepatic glycogen stores are depleted and the production of essential proteins, including albumin and micronutrient carriers, declines. Therefore, for people with cirrhosis periods of fasting, including overnight, can lead to muscle catabolism and worsen sarcopenia. Also, increased production of aromatic amino acids and decreased levels of BCAAs—valine, leucine and isoleucine—can contribute to the development of HE.

A guide for nutritional requirements in patients with cirrhosis can be found in Table 8.6. Resting energy expenditure is typically higher in people with cirrhosis, so higher targets for daily calorie intake (i.e., 30-40 kcal/kg per day) are appropriate. To maintain glycogen stores, carbohydrate should be the primary source of calories, although refined sugars like fructose should be avoided where possible. Dietary fats should prioritise unsaturated PUFAs and MUFAs. To avoid glycogen depletion and protein catabolism, regular meals and snacks are encouraged, including a late evening carbohydrate-containing snack.[133] Supplementing the diet with BCAAs has shown to improve HE and protein metabolism but not mortality.[134] BCAA-enriched drinks are not considered particularly palatable.

Hepatic Encephalopathy

Ammonia is a nitrogenous neurotoxin produced in the GI tract from the bacterial metabolism of protein. In the healthy liver it is converted to urea, which is water soluble and renally excreted. In liver failure this process is impaired and results in hyperammonaemia, which can cause HE. HE can complicate nutritional intake, particularly when high grade, as conscious level and cough and swallow functions can become compromised. Low-grade HE can cause disordered sleep and confusion that affects normal eating patterns. Treatment is with laxatives (lactulose) to minimise stasis within the GI tract and antibiotics (rifaximin). Protein-restricted diets are no longer considered helpful in most cases of HE.[72] BCAA-enriched nutritional supplementation has been shown to improve HE in some patients with cirrhosis.[134]

Ascites, Fluid Balance and Albumin

Whole-body water retention can be difficult to manage in patients with cirrhosis. The presence of ascites can cause early satiety due to pressure on the GI tract. A low-salt diet (≤2 g sodium/day) is often recommended in patients with cirrhotic ascites but may be unpalatable and difficult to adhere to. The use of herbs and spices can help maintain flavour when preparing food without salt. Total daily water restriction may also be appropriate, but clinical status and serum electrolytes should be closely monitored when advised alongside diuretic medications.

Serum albumin level correlates with liver synthetic function and is used in severity scores of cirrhosis, such as Child-Pugh.[136] Hypoalbuminaemia is often incorrectly used as a marker of malnutrition but serum albumin level does not correlate well with clinical nutritional status.[137] Intravenous replacement of human albumin solution is a common inpatient intervention that may benefit patients with spontaneous bacterial peritonitis, hepatorenal syndrome or cirrhotic ascites requiring large volume paracentesis. Otherwise, the administration of intravenous albumin to raise serum albumin to 'normal' levels in patients with cirrhosis is of no clinical benefit.[138]

LIVER TRANSPLANTATION

Patients with cirrhosis who undergo liver transplantation should be nutritionally optimised prior to surgery to improve chance of a successful outcome.[125] Malnutrition, sarcopenia, and obesity are all associated with a higher risk of poor outcomes after liver transplantation.[139,140] A high-protein, nutrient-dense diet, alongside physical exercise, may be beneficial in preventing sarcopenia and maintaining muscle mass prior to surgery.[141]

After liver transplantation, the metabolic dysfunction associated with cirrhosis does not automatically resolve, highlighting the importance of other organs (namely the pancreas, adrenal glands and GI tract) and tissues (skeletal muscle and visceral fat) in metabolic health.[142] Nutritional requirements are likely to be increased in the immediate weeks to months posttransplantation owing to an increased basal energy expenditure plus increased protein and micronutrient requirements for wound healing.[143] In the longer term, posttransplantation weight gain is common, as are sarcopenic obesity, persistence of pretransplant glucose dysregulation and the development of the metabolic syndrome.[144,145] One contributing factor is commonly used immunosuppressive medication, particularly corticosteroids and calcineurin inhibitors, that are independently associated with weight gain and insulin resistance. Therefore, liver transplantation should not be viewed as a cure-all for patients with cirrhosis, especially from a nutritional perspective. An individualised and flexible nutrition plan guided by specialist nutrition professionals is likely to be beneficial for patients who have received a liver transplant as their nutritional requirements and risks change over time.

Parenteral Nutrition-Related Liver Disease

Recognised complications in patients on long-term parenteral nutrition include steatohepatitis and cholestatic liver disease, which can progress to cirrhosis. For more information see the chapter 4 on nutrition support.

Disorders of the Biliary System and Pancreas

GALLSTONES

Obesity is a risk factor in gallstone formation, as is rapid weight loss (greater than 1.5 kg loss per week). Other risk factors for gallstones related to weight loss include following a very-low-calorie diet with no dietary fat, long periods of fasting, and high serum triglycerides.[146] Gallstone disease is more common in Western countries, suggesting a role for the standard Western diet in gallstone formation. Dietary cholesterol, saturated and *trans*-fatty acids, refined carbohydrates and sugars and possibly legumes may increase the risk.[147,148] There may be a protective effect against gallstone formation from fibre, vegetables, coffee, unsaturated fatty acids and vitamin C supplementation; however, the evidence for these is not strong.[149] Patients with gallstone disease should avoid foods and drinks that trigger their symptoms, although these vary widely between individuals and identifying trigger foods is not always straightforward.

Most patients with symptomatic and complicated gallstone disease will be offered cholecystectomy. Patients are often advised to follow a low-fat diet following cholecystectomy; however, there is little evidence that this is beneficial in terms of improving persistent symptoms such as diarrhoea or bloating.[150]

BILE ACID MALABSORPTION

Bile contains bile salts, acids, pigments, cholesterol and lecithin. It is produced by the liver and is secreted via the bile ducts into the duodenum. Its primary function is food digestion, particularly the emulsification of fats and thus the absorption of the fat-soluble vitamins A, D, E and K. Bile acids are reabsorbed into the circulation at the terminal ileum. If the terminal ileum is damaged, for example by coeliac disease, IBD, radiotherapy, or surgical resection, bile acid malabsorption may result. Instead, bile acids will enter the colon where they are broken down and stimulate intraluminal water and electrolyte secretion that manifests clinically as chronic watery diarrhoea. Approximately one-third of patients have idiopathic bile acid malabsorption, which may be due to hormone-dependent overproduction of bile.[151] There is a large overlap with diarrhoea-predominant IBS and bile acid malabsorption. Diagnosis is confirmed with the nuclear medicine test, selenium homocholic acid taurine.

The mainstay of treatment of bile salt malabsorption is with bile salt sequestrant medications (colesevelam or colestyramine). A low-fat diet, defined as taking no more than 20% of daily energy from fat, is the most commonly recommended dietary intervention and has been shown to improve symptoms.[152]

PANCREATITIS

Acute Pancreatitis

Acute pancreatitis typically causes severe, acute epigastric pain, nausea and vomiting. It can be secondary to complicated gallstones, alcohol excess, certain viruses, toxins or hypertriglyceridaemia. The underlying pathology is complex but involves autodigestion of pancreatic parenchyma due to premature activation of the digestive enzymes produced by the exocrine cells of the pancreas. Most cases will resolve with supportive treatment but around 20% progress to severe, necrotising pancreatitis associated with local complications, multiorgan failure and high mortality. A highly catabolic condition, fluid and nutrition demands increase with disease severity. Therefore, fluid, electrolyte and nutritional status should be monitored and corrected accordingly. Severe hypocalcaemia can occur in severe disease; however, calcium is implicated in the pathogenesis of acute pancreatitis so replacement should be undertaken with caution. Impaired endocrine function can lead to deranged glucose homeostasis, typically hyperglycaemia. Approximately 25% of patients with acute pancreatitis will develop pancreatic exocrine insufficiency in the future.[153]

Despite historical concerns about oral nutrition in acute pancreatitis, it has been shown that early eating and drinking is safe and can shorten length of hospital stay, especially in mild disease.[154] A softened, low-fat diet may be easier tolerated in the early stages. If oral feeding is contraindicated or not tolerated, enteral nutrition is associated with significantly better outcomes than parenteral nutrition, especially in severe disease.[155] Pancreatic enzyme supplementation is not usually required in acute pancreatitis.

Acute pancreatitis can be caused by hypertriglyceridaemia (serum triglycerides >1000 mg/dL), for which intravenous insulin is often used in the acute setting. On recovery, these patients should receive long-term dietary and lifestyle advice, for example, to follow a low-fat diet, with the aim of reducing circulating triglyceride levels and thus risk of recurrence.[156]

Chronic Pancreatitis and Pancreatic Exocrine Insufficiency

Chronic pancreatitis is characterised by prolonged and/or recurrent bouts of pancreatic inflammation with resulting fibrosis and loss of endocrine and exocrine functions. Malnutrition in chronic pancreatitis is common and multifactorial. Abdominal pain is a dominant symptom and, along with nausea and vomiting, often causes anorexia. The clinical manifestations of impaired exocrine function relate to maldigestion of dietary fat and malabsorption: diarrhoea, steatorrhoea, bloating, weight loss and nutritional deficiencies, especially of fat-soluble vitamins. Endocrine dysfunction can result in secondary diabetes mellitus. Alcohol excess is the most common aetiology of chronic pancreatitis and confers a higher risk of malnutrition earlier in the disease course than other aetiologies. There is also clinical overlap between patients with chronic pancreatitis and SIBO.

Pancreatic exocrine insufficiency is tested with faecal elastase levels (which are low) and treated with pancreatic enzyme supplementation (pancreatin, for example Creon) taken with food. Pancreatin capsules contain pancreatic enzymes (lipase, amylase and protease) encased in a pH-sensitive casing able to withstand exposure to gastric acid before breaking down in the alkaline duodenum. Most contain porcine-derived pancreatic enzymes and patients should be informed of this for religious or cultural reasons.

Consensus guidelines recommend patients with chronic pancreatitis consume high-protein, high-energy foods in the form of five to six small regular meals per day. A low-fat diet is not usually required in patients taking pancreatic enzyme supplements unless persistent steatorrhoea is a troublesome symptom.[154] Dietary fibre can impair the effects of pancreatin; therefore, patients should be advised to avoid too much fibre in the diet.[157]

Serum levels of potassium, magnesium, iron, zinc, selenium and fat-soluble vitamins (A, D, E and K) may be low in chronic pancreatitis and should be tested and replaced as needed. Of particular importance is vitamin D as most patients will have insufficient levels. This, alongside other lifestyle factors (alcohol, smoking, physical inactivity) and chronic inflammation, make patients with chronic pancreatitis highly susceptible to osteopenia and osteoporosis. Vitamin D and calcium supplementation plus regular weight-bearing or resistance exercise are important components of holistic management in improving bone health.

Summary

- The GI and hepatobiliary systems are essential for the digestion and absorption of nutrients into the body.
- Common disorders of the oesophagus include GORD, which is more common in obesity, and eosinophilic oesophagitis, which can be effectively controlled with elimination of common dietary allergens.
- The stomach acts as a temporary reservoir for food. There is little consensus on specific dietary approaches in the management of PUD. Both delayed gastric emptying (gastroparesis) and rapid gastric emptying can often be managed with dietary modification of macronutrient content and meal timing.
- The small bowel is the primary site of nutrient absorption. Coeliac disease is an autoimmune enteropathy triggered by gluten that necessitates a lifelong gluten-free diet. Iron deficiency

is the commonest cause of anaemia globally and should prompt careful investigation to exclude causes of malabsorption or blood loss and supplementation.

- Surgical resection of the small bowel to an extent that surpasses the body's compensatory capacities leads to SBS, which requires specialist nutrition support. High-output ileostomy is often best managed with hypertonic glucose-electrolyte solutions, and hypomagnesaemia can be particularly difficult to treat in SBS. Jejuno-colic anastomosis can lead to two specific nutritional complications: oxalate renal stones and D-lactic acidosis.
- IBD can affect any part of the GI tract and dietary factors may play a role in pathogenesis but are poorly understood. Malnutrition is common in patients with IBD. Enteral nutrition is a useful treatment for induction of remission in Crohn disease and is commonly used in paediatrics.
- IBS is a disorder of gut–brain interaction that causes lower GI symptoms. Dietary fibre may benefit or worsen symptoms dependent on subclassification of IBS and fibre type. The low-FODMAP diet has proven benefit in IBS and patients should be supported by a trained professional to optimise results.
- The liver is the major organ of nutrient metabolism, and liver failure leads to major derangement in metabolic function. Malnutrition and sarcopenia are common in patients with liver disease and are major risk factors for morbidity and mortality. Features of decompensated cirrhosis, such as HE and ascites, pose additional challenges to managing fluid and nutrition in these patients.
- ALD, NAFLD and chronic viral hepatitis are the commonest causes of liver disease. Most NAFLD is caused by excessive caloric intake, associated with T2DM and the metabolic syndrome. Management relies on lifestyle modification with the view to weight loss of at least 5%–10% body weight. A Mediterranean diet, low-carbohydrate diet, and intermittent fasting all have an evidence base for benefit in improving hepatic steatosis in NAFLD, at least in the short term.
- Acute pancreatitis can cause major metabolic and electrolyte disturbance; early feeding with oral or enteral nutrition is now considered best practice. Chronic exocrine insufficiency necessitates pancreatic enzyme supplementation with meals.

Selected Key References

- Arias et al. 2014.[7] Efficacy of dietary interventions in patients with eosinophilic esophagitis
- Nightingale et al. 2006.[23] British Society of Gastroenterology guidelines for management SBS
- Narula et al. 2018.[58] Cochrane review of enteral nutrition for inducing remission in Crohn
- Holtmann et al. 2016.[66] Overview of pathophysiology in IBS
- Black and Ford. 2021.[68] Best management for IBS
- Dionne et al. 2018.[71] Systematic review and meta-analysis of gluten-free and low FODMAP diets for IBS
- Plauth et al. 2019.[72] ESPEN Guideline on clinical nutrition in liver disease
- Merli et al. 2019.[73] European Association for the Study of the Liver. European Association for the Study of the Liver Clinical practice guideline on nutrition in chronic liver disease
- Chakravarthy et al. 2020.[102] Review article of macronutrients and micronutrients in NAFLD
- Sanyal et al. 2010.[112] Pioglitazone vs Vitamin E for the treatment of non-diabetic patients with non-alcoholic steatopancreatitis trial of vitamin E in NASH
- Perumpail et al. 2017.[135] Optimising nutrition in cirrhosis
- Arvanitakis et al. 2020.[154] ESPEN Guideline on nutrition in acute and chronic pancreatitis

References

1. Du J, Liu J, Zhang H, Yu C-H, Li Y-M. Risk factors for gastroesophageal reflux disease, reflux esophagitis and non-erosive reflux disease among Chinese patients undergoing upper gastrointestinal endoscopic examination. *World J Gastroenterol.* 2007;13(45):6009–6015. https://doi.org/10.3748/wjg.v13.45.6009.
2. Kang JH-E, Kang JY. Lifestyle measures in the management of gastro-oesophageal reflux disease: Clinical and pathophysiological considerations. *Ther Adv Chronic Dis.* 2015;6(2):51–64. https://doi.org/10.1177/2040622315569501.
3. Singh S, Sharma AN, Murad MH, et al. Central adiposity is associated with increased risk of esophageal inflammation, metaplasia, and adenocarcinoma: A systematic review and meta-analysis. *Clin Gastroenterol Hepatol.* 2013;11(11):1399–1412.e7. https://doi.org/10.1016/j.cgh.2013.05.009.
4. Grant AM, Wileman SM, Ramsay CR, et al. Minimal access surgery compared with medical management for chronic gastro-oesophageal reflux disease: UK collaborative randomised trial. *BMJ.* 2008;337(2): a2664–a2664. https://doi.org/10.1136/bmj.a2664.
5. Rank MA, Sharaf RN, Furuta GT, et al. Technical review on the management of eosinophilic esophagitis: A report from the AGA Institute and the Joint Task Force on Allergy-Immunology Practice Parameters. *Gastroenterology.* 2020;158(6):1789–1810.e15. https://doi.org/10.1053/j.gastro.2020.02.039.
6. Kim HP, Vance RB, Shaheen NJ, Dellon ES. The prevalence and diagnostic utility of endoscopic features of eosinophilic esophagitis: A meta-analysis. *Clin Gastroenterol Hepatol.* 2012;10(9):988–996.e5. https://doi.org/10.1016/j.cgh.2012.04.019.
7. Arias A, González-Cervera J, Tenias JM, Lucendo AJ. Efficacy of dietary interventions for inducing histologic remission in patients with eosinophilic esophagitis: A systematic review and meta-analysis. *Gastroenterology.* 2014;146(7):1639–1648. https://doi.org/10.1053/j.gastro.2014.02.006.
8. Molina-Infante J, Arias Á, Alcedo J, et al. Step-up empiric elimination diet for pediatric and adult eosinophilic esophagitis: The 2-4-6 study. *J Allergy Clin Immunol.* 2018;141(4):1365–1372. https://doi.org/10.1016/j.jaci.2017.08.038.
9. Little TJ, Russo A, Meyer JH, et al. Free fatty acids have more potent effects on gastric emptying, gut hormones, and appetite than triacylglycerides. *Gastroenterology.* 2007;133(4):1124–1131. https://doi.org/10.1053/j.gastro.2007.06.060.
10. Sung JJY, Kuipers EJ, El-Serag HB. Systematic review: The global incidence and prevalence of peptic ulcer disease. *Aliment Pharmacol Ther.* 2009;29(9):938–946. https://doi.org/10.1111/j.1365-2036.2009.03960.x.
11. Uemura N, Okamoto S, Yamamoto S, et al. *Helicobacter pylori* infection and the development of gastric cancer. *N Engl J Med.* 2001;345(11):784–789. https://doi.org/10.1056/NEJMoa001999.
12. Ryan-Harshman M, Aldoori W. How diet and lifestyle affect duodenal ulcers. Review of the evidence. *Can Fam Physician Med Fam Can.* 2004;50:727–732.
13. Zárate N, Mearin F, Wang X-Y, Hewlett B, Huizinga JD, Malagelada J-R. Severe idiopathic gastroparesis due to neuronal and interstitial cells of Cajal degeneration: Pathological findings and management. *Gut.* 2003;52(7):966–970. https://doi.org/10.1136/gut.52.7.966.
14. Camilleri M, Parkman HP, Shafi MA, Abell TL, Gerson L, American College of Gastroenterology. Clinical guideline: Management of gastroparesis. *Am J Gastroenterol.* 2013;108(1):18–37; quiz 38. https://doi.org/10.1038/ajg.2012.373.
15. Coleski R, Anderson MA, Hasler WL. Factors associated with symptom response to pyloric injection of botulinum toxin in a large series of gastroparesis patients. *Dig Dis Sci.* 2009;54(12):2634–2642. https://doi.org/10.1007/s10620-008-0660-9.
16. Berg P, McCallum R. Dumping syndrome: A review of the current concepts of pathophysiology, diagnosis, and treatment. *Dig Dis Sci.* 2016;61(1):11–18. https://doi.org/10.1007/s10620-015-3839-x.
17. Kang JY, Kang AHY, Green A, Gwee KA, Ho KY. Systematic review: Worldwide variation in the frequency of coeliac disease and changes over time. *Aliment Pharmacol Ther.* 2013;38(3):226–245. https://doi.org/10.1111/apt.12373.
18. Sieniawski M, Angamuthu N, Boyd K, et al. Evaluation of enteropathy-associated T-cell lymphoma comparing standard therapies with a novel regimen including autologous stem cell transplantation. *Blood.* 2010;115(18):3664–3670. https://doi.org/10.1182/blood-2009-07-231324.
19. Downey L, Houten R, Murch S, Longson D, Guideline Development Group. Recognition, assessment, and management of coeliac disease: Summary of updated NICE guidance. *BMJ.* 2015;351:h4513. https://doi.org/10.1136/bmj.h4513.

20. Dukowicz AC, Lacy BE, Levine GM. Small intestinal bacterial overgrowth: A comprehensive review. *Gastroenterol Hepatol*. 2007;3(2):112–122.
21. Storhaug CL, Fosse SK, Fadnes LT. Country, regional, and global estimates for lactose malabsorption in adults: A systematic review and meta-analysis. *Lancet Gastroenterol Hepatol*. 2017;2(10):738–746. https://doi.org/10.1016/S2468-1253(17)30154-1.
22. Pasricha S-R, Tye-Din J, Muckenthaler MU, Swinkels DW. Iron deficiency. *Lancet*. 2021;397(10270):233–248. https://doi.org/10.1016/S0140-6736(20)32594-0.
23. Nightingale J, Woodward JM, Small Bowel and Nutrition Committee of the British Society of Gastroenterology. Guidelines for management of patients with a short bowel. *Gut*. 2006;55(Suppl 4): iv1–12. https://doi.org/10.1136/gut.2006.091108.
24. Allan P, Lal S. Intestinal failure: A review. *F1000Res*. 2018;7:85. https://doi.org/10.12688/f1000research.12493.1.
25. Lacy BE, Mearin F, Chang L, et al. Bowel disorders. *Gastroenterology*. 2016;150(6):1393–1407.e5. https://doi.org/10.1053/j.gastro.2016.02.031.
26. Choung RS, Locke Iii GR, Schleck CD, Zinsmeister AR, Talley NJ. Cumulative incidence of chronic constipation: A population-based study 1988-2003: Cumulative incidence of chronic constipation. *Aliment Pharmacol Ther*. 2007;26(11–12):1521–1528. https://doi.org/10.1111/j.1365-2036.2007.03540.x.
27. Dimidi E, Christodoulides S, Fragkos KC, Scott SM, Whelan K. The effect of probiotics on functional constipation in adults: A systematic review and meta-analysis of randomized controlled trials. *Am J Clin Nutr*. 2014;100(4):1075–1084. https://doi.org/10.3945/ajcn.114.089151.
28. Suares NC, and Ford AC, (2011), Systematic review: the effects of fibre in the management of chronic idiopathic constipation. *Alimentary Pharmacology & Therapeutics*, 33:895–901. https://doi.org/10.1111/j.1365-2036.2011.04602.x.
29. Parks TG. Reappraisal of clinical features of diverticular disease of the colon. *Br Med J*. 1969;4(5684):642–645. https://doi.org/10.1136/bmj.4.5684.642.
30. Hughes LE. Postmortem survey of diverticular disease of the colon. I. Diverticulosis and diverticulitis. *Gut*. 1969;10(5):336–344. https://doi.org/10.1136/gut.10.5.336.
31. Manousos O, Day NE, Tzonou A, et al. Diet and other factors in the aetiology of diverticulosis: An epidemiological study in Greece. *Gut*. 1985;26(6):544–549. https://doi.org/10.1136/gut.26.6.544.
32. Painter NS, Burkitt DP. Diverticular disease of the colon: A deficiency disease of Western civilization. *Br Med J*. 1971;2(5759):450–454. https://doi.org/10.1136/bmj.2.5759.450.
33. Aldoori WH, Giovannucci EL, Rimm EB, Wing AL, Trichopoulos DV, Willett WC. A prospective study of alcohol, smoking, caffeine, and the risk of symptomatic diverticular disease in men. *Ann Epidemiol*. 1995;5(3):221–228. https://doi.org/10.1016/1047-2797(94)00109-7.
34. Crowe FL, Appleby PN, Allen NE, Key TJ. Diet and risk of diverticular disease in Oxford cohort of European Prospective Investigation into Cancer and Nutrition (EPIC): Prospective study of British vegetarians and non-vegetarians. *BMJ*. 2011;343:d4131. https://doi.org/10.1136/bmj.d4131.
35. Papagrigoriadis S, Macey L, Bourantas N, Rennie JA. Smoking may be associated with complications in diverticular disease. *Br J Surg*. 1999;86(7):923–926. https://doi.org/10.1046/j.1365-2168.1999.01177.x.
36. Wilson RG, Smith AN, Macintyre IM. Complications of diverticular disease and non-steroidal anti-inflammatory drugs: A prospective study. *Br J Surg*. 1990;77(10):1103–1104. https://doi.org/10.1002/bjs.1800771008.
37. National Institute for Health and Clinical Excellence. Diverticular disease: Diagnosis and management (Clinical Guideline 147). 2019. Available at: https://www.nice.org.uk/guidance/ng147. Accessed March 4, 2021.
38. Hartman C, Eliakim R, Shamir R. Nutritional status and nutritional therapy in inflammatory bowel diseases. *World J Gastroenterol*. 2009;15(21):2570–2578. https://doi.org/10.3748/wjg.15.2570.
39. Sumi R, Nakajima K, Iijima H, et al. Influence of nutritional status on the therapeutic effect of infliximab in patients with Crohn's disease. *Surg Today*. 2016;46(8):922–929. https://doi.org/10.1007/s00595-015-1257-5.
40. Csontos ÁA, Molnár A, Piri Z, Pálfi E, Miheller P. Malnutrition risk questionnaire combined with body composition measurement in malnutrition screening in inflammatory bowel disease. *Rev Esp Enferm Dig*. 2017;109(1):26–32. https://doi.org/10.17235/reed.2016.4557/2016.

41. Haskey N, Peña-Sánchez JN, Jones JL, Fowler SA. Development of a screening tool to detect nutrition risk in patients with inflammatory bowel disease. *Asia Pac J Clin Nutr*. 2018;27(4):756–762. https://doi.org/10.6133/apjcn.112017.01.
42. Fiorindi C, Luceri C, Dragoni G, et al. GLIM criteria for malnutrition in surgical IBD patients: A pilot study. *Nutrients*. 2020;12(8). https://doi.org/10.3390/nu12082222.
43. Bamba S, Sasaki M, Takaoka A, et al. Sarcopenia is a predictive factor for intestinal resection in admitted patients with Crohn's disease. *PLoS One*. 2017;12(6):e0180036. https://doi.org/10.1371/journal.pone.0180036.
44. Ananthakrishnan AN, McGinley EL. Infection-related hospitalizations are associated with increased mortality in patients with inflammatory bowel diseases. *J Crohns Colitis*. 2013;7(2):107–112. https://doi.org/10.1016/j.crohns.2012.02.015.
45. Ananthakrishnan AN, McGinley EL, Binion DG, Saeian K. A novel risk score to stratify severity of Crohn's disease hospitalizations. *Am J Gastroenterol*. 2010;105(8):1799–1807. https://doi.org/10.1038/ajg.2010.105.
46. Wallaert JB, De Martino RR, Marsicovetere PS, et al. Venous thromboembolism after surgery for inflammatory bowel disease: Are there modifiable risk factors? Data from ACS NSQIP. *Dis Colon Rectum*. 2012;55(11):1138–1144. https://doi.org/10.1097/DCR.0b013e3182698f60.
47. Takaoka A, Sasaki M, Nakanishi N, et al. Nutritional screening and clinical outcome in hospitalized patients with Crohn's disease. *Ann Nutr Metab*. 2017;71(3–4):266–272. https://doi.org/10.1159/000485637.
48. Swidsinski A, Weber J, Loening-Baucke V, Hale LP, Lochs H. Spatial organization and composition of the mucosal flora in patients with inflammatory bowel disease. *J Clin Microbiol*. 2005;43(7):3380–3389. https://doi.org/10.1128/JCM.43.7.3380-3389.2005.
49. Seksik P, Rigottier-Gois L, Gramet G, et al. Alterations of the dominant faecal bacterial groups in patients with Crohn's disease of the colon. *Gut*. 2003;52(2):237–242. https://doi.org/10.1136/gut.52.2.237.
50. Hou JK, Abraham B, El-Serag H. Dietary intake and risk of developing inflammatory bowel disease: A systematic review of the literature. *Am J Gastroenterol*. 2011;106(4):563–573. https://doi.org/10.1038/ajg.2011.44.
51. Ananthakrishnan AN, Khalili H, Konijeti GG, et al. A prospective study of long term intake of dietary fiber and risk of Crohn's disease and ulcerative colitis. *Gastroenterology*. 2013;145(5):970–977. https://doi.org/10.1053/j.gastro.2013.07.050.
52. Li F, Liu X, Wang W, Zhang D. Consumption of vegetables and fruit and the risk of inflammatory bowel disease: A meta-analysis. *Eur J Gastroenterol Hepatol*. 2015;27(6):623–630. https://doi.org/10.1097/MEG.0000000000000330.
53. Ananthakrishnan AN, Khalili H, Song M, Higuchi LM, Richter JM, Chan AT. Zinc intake and risk of Crohn's disease and ulcerative colitis: A prospective cohort study. *Int J Epidemiol*. 2015;44(6):1995–2005. https://doi.org/10.1093/ije/dyv301.
54. Fletcher J. Vitamin D deficiency in patients with inflammatory bowel disease. *Br J Nurs Mark Allen Publ*. 2016;25(15):846–851. https://doi.org/10.12968/bjon.2016.25.15.846.
55. Wang T-T, Dabbas B, Laperriere D, et al. Direct and indirect induction by 1,25-dihydroxyvitamin D3 of the NOD2/CARD15-defensin beta2 innate immune pathway defective in Crohn disease. *J Biol Chem*. 2010;285(4):2227–2231. https://doi.org/10.1074/jbc.C109.071225.
56. Voitk AJ, Echave V, Feller JH, Brown RA, Gurd FN. Experience with elemental diet in the treatment of inflammatory bowel disease. Is this primary therapy? *Arch Surg 1960*. 1973;107(2):329–333. https://doi.org/10.1001/archsurg.1973.01350200189039.
57. Logan RF, Gillon J, Ferrington C, Ferguson A. Reduction of gastrointestinal protein loss by elemental diet in Crohn's disease of the small bowel. *Gut*. 1981;22(5):383–387. https://doi.org/10.1136/gut.22.5.383.
58. Narula N, Dhillon A, Zhang D, Sherlock ME, Tondeur M, Zachos M. Enteral nutritional therapy for induction of remission in Crohn's disease. *Cochrane Database Syst Rev*. 2018;4:CD000542. https://doi.org/10.1002/14651858.CD000542.pub3.
59. Flores A, Burstein E, Cipher DJ, Feagins LA. Obesity in inflammatory bowel disease: A marker of less severe disease. *Dig Dis Sci*. 2015;60(8):2436–2445. https://doi.org/10.1007/s10620-015-3629-5.
60. Seminerio JL, Koutroubakis IE, Ramos-Rivers C, et al. Impact of obesity on the management and clinical course of patients with inflammatory bowel disease. *Inflamm Bowel Dis*. 2015;21(12):2857–2863. https://doi.org/10.1097/MIB.0000000000000560.

61. Steed H, Walsh S, Reynolds N. A brief report of the epidemiology of obesity in the inflammatory bowel disease population of Tayside, Scotland. *Obes Facts.* 2009;2(6):370–372. https://doi.org/10.1159/000262276.
62. Krane MK, Allaix ME, Zoccali M, et al. Does morbid obesity change outcomes after laparoscopic surgery for inflammatory bowel disease? Review of 626 consecutive cases. *J Am Coll Surg.* 2013;216(5):986–996. https://doi.org/10.1016/j.jamcollsurg.2013.01.053.
63. Causey MW, Johnson EK, Miller S, Martin M, Maykel J, Steele SR. The impact of obesity on outcomes following major surgery for Crohn's disease: An American College of Surgeons National Surgical Quality Improvement Program assessment. *Dis Colon Rectum.* 2011;54(12):1488–1495. https://doi.org/10.1097/DCR.0b013e3182342ccb.
64. Klos CL, Safar B, Jamal N, et al. Obesity increases risk for pouch-related complications following restorative proctocolectomy with ileal pouch-anal anastomosis (IPAA). *J Gastrointest Surg.* 2014;18(3):573–579. https://doi.org/10.1007/s11605-013-2353-8.
65. Spiller R, Aziz Q, Creed F, et al. Guidelines on the irritable bowel syndrome: Mechanisms and practical management. *Gut.* 2007;56(12):1770–1798. https://doi.org/10.1136/gut.2007.119446.
66. Holtmann GJ, Ford AC, Talley NJ. Pathophysiology of irritable bowel syndrome. *Lancet Gastroenterol Hepatol.* 2016;1(2):133–146. https://doi.org/10.1016/S2468-1253(16)30023-1.
67. Schmulson MJ, Drossman DA. What Is new in Rome IV. *J Neurogastroenterol Motil.* 2017;23(2):151–163. https://doi.org/10.5056/jnm16214.
68. Black CJ, Ford AC. Best management of irritable bowel syndrome. *Frontline Gastroenterol.* 2021;12(4):303–315. https://doi.org/10.1136/flgastro-2019-101298.
69. BDA. Irritable bowel syndrome food fact sheet. Accessed October 29, 2021. Available at: https://www.bda.uk.com/resource/irritable-bowel-syndrome-diet.html.
70. Moayyedi P, Quigley EMM, Lacy BE, et al. The effect of fiber supplementation on irritable bowel syndrome: A systematic review and meta-analysis. *Am J Gastroenterol.* 2014;109(9):1367–1374. https://doi.org/10.1038/ajg.2014.195.
71. Dionne J, Ford AC, Yuan Y, et al. A systematic review and meta-analysis evaluating the efficacy of a gluten-free diet and a low FODMAPs diet in treating symptoms of irritable bowel syndrome. *Am J Gastroenterol.* 2018;113(9):1290–1300. https://doi.org/10.1038/s41395-018-0195-4.
72. Plauth M, Bernal W, Dasarathy S, et al. ESPEN guideline on clinical nutrition in liver disease. *Clin Nutr.* 2019;38(2):485–521. https://doi.org/10.1016/j.clnu.2018.12.022.
73. Merli M, Berzigotti A, Zelber-Sagi S, et al. EASL clinical practice guidelines on nutrition in chronic liver disease. *J Hepatol.* 2019;70(1):172–193. https://doi.org/10.1016/j.jhep.2018.06.024.
74. Levine JA, Harris MM, Morgan MY. Energy expenditure in chronic alcohol abuse. *Eur J Clin Invest.* 2000;30(9):779–786. https://doi.org/10.1046/j.1365-2362.2000.00708.x.
75. Cabré E, Rodríguez-Iglesias P, Caballería J, et al. Short- and long-term outcome of severe alcohol-induced hepatitis treated with steroids or enteral nutrition: A multicenter randomized trial. *Hepatology.* 2000;32(1):36–42. https://doi.org/10.1053/jhep.2000.8627.
76. Younossi Z, Anstee QM, Marietti M, et al. Global burden of NAFLD and NASH: Trends, predictions, risk factors and prevention. *Nat Rev Gastroenterol Hepatol.* 2018;15(1):11–20. https://doi.org/10.1038/nrgastro.2017.109.
77. Kleiner DE, Brunt EM, Natta MV, et al. Design and validation of a histological scoring system for non-alcoholic fatty liver disease. *Hepatology.* 2005;41(6):1313–1321. https://doi.org/10.1002/hep.20701.
78. Buzzetti E, Lombardi R, De Luca L, Tsochatzis EA. Noninvasive assessment of fibrosis in patients with nonalcoholic fatty liver disease. *Int J Endocrinol.* 2015;2015:1–9. https://doi.org/10.1155/2015/343828.
79. Younossi ZM, Golabi P, de Avila L, et al. The global epidemiology of NAFLD and NASH in patients with type 2 diabetes: A systematic review and meta-analysis. *J Hepatol.* 2019;71(4):793–801. https://doi.org/10.1016/j.jhep.2019.06.021.
80. Donnelly KL, Smith CI, Schwarzenberg SJ, Jessurun J, Boldt MD, Parks EJ. Sources of fatty acids stored in liver and secreted via lipoproteins in patients with nonalcoholic fatty liver disease. *J Clin Invest.* 2005;115(5):1343–1351. https://doi.org/10.1172/JCI23621.
81. Sobrecases H, Lê K-A, Bortolotti M, et al. Effects of short-term overfeeding with fructose, fat and fructose plus fat on plasma and hepatic lipids in healthy men. *Diabetes Metab.* 2010;36(3):244–246. https://doi.org/10.1016/j.diabet.2010.03.003.

82. Rosqvist F, Kullberg J, Ståhlman M, et al. Overeating saturated fat promotes fatty liver and ceramides compared with polyunsaturated fat: A randomized trial. *J Clin Endocrinol Metab*. 2019;104(12):6207–6219. https://doi.org/10.1210/jc.2019-00160.
83. Errazuriz I, Dube S, Slama M, et al. Randomized controlled trial of a MUFA or fiber-rich diet on hepatic fat in prediabetes. *J Clin Endocrinol Metab*. 2017;102(5):1765–1774. https://doi.org/10.1210/jc.2016-3722.
84. Bjermo H, Iggman D, Kullberg J, et al. Effects of n-6 PUFAs compared with SFAs on liver fat, lipoproteins, and inflammation in abdominal obesity: A randomized controlled trial. *Am J Clin Nutr*. 2012;95(5):1003–1012. https://doi.org/10.3945/ajcn.111.030114.
85. Chiu S, Mulligan K, Schwarz J-M. Dietary carbohydrates and fatty liver disease: De novo lipogenesis. *Curr Opin Clin Nutr Metab Care*. 2018;21(4):277–282. https://doi.org/10.1097/MCO.0000000000000469.
86. Neuschwander-Tetri BA. Carbohydrate intake and nonalcoholic fatty liver disease. *Curr Opin Clin Nutr Metab Car*. 2013;16(4):446–452. https://doi.org/10.1097/MCO.0b013e328361c4d1.
87. Parks EJ. Dietary carbohydrate's effects on lipogenesis and the relationship of lipogenesis to blood insulin and glucose concentrations. *Br J Nutr*. 2002;87(S2):S247–S253. https://doi.org/10.1079/BJN/2002544.
88. Ameer F, Scandiuzzi L, Hasnain S, Kalbacher H, Zaidi N. De novo lipogenesis in health and disease. *Metabolism*. 2014;63(7):895–902. https://doi.org/10.1016/j.metabol.2014.04.003.
89. Maersk M, Belza A, Stødkilde-Jørgensen H, et al. Sucrose-sweetened beverages increase fat storage in the liver, muscle, and visceral fat depot: A 6-mo randomized intervention study. *Am J Clin Nutr*. 2012;95(2):283–289. https://doi.org/10.3945/ajcn.111.022533.
90. Geidl-Flueck B, Hochuli M, Németh Á, et al. Fructose- and sucrose- but not glucose-sweetened beverages promote hepatic de novo lipogenesis: A randomized controlled trial. *J Hepatol*. Published online March 6, 2021. https://doi.org/10.1016/j.jhep.2021.02.027.
91. Jegatheesan P, De Bandt J-P. Fructose and NAFLD: The multifaceted aspects of fructose metabolism. *Nutrients*. 2017;9(3). https://doi.org/10.3390/nu9030230.
92. Bortolotti M, Kreis R, Debard C, et al. High protein intake reduces intrahepatocellular lipid deposition in humans. *Am J Clin Nutr*. 2009;90(4):1002–1010. https://doi.org/10.3945/ajcn.2008.27296.
93. Markova M, Pivovarova O, Hornemann S, et al. Isocaloric diets high in animal or plant protein reduce liver fat and inflammation in individuals with type 2 diabetes. *Gastroenterology*. 2017;152(3):571–585.e8. https://doi.org/10.1053/j.gastro.2016.10.007.
94. Drummen M, Dorenbos E, Vreugdenhil ACE, et al. Long-term effects of increased protein intake after weight loss on intrahepatic lipid content and implications for insulin sensitivity: A PREVIEW study. *Am J Physiol Endocrinol Metab*. 2018;315(5):E885–E891. https://doi.org/10.1152/ajpendo.00162.2018.
95. European Association for the Study of the Liver (EASL), European Association for the Study of Diabetes (EASD), European Association for the Study of Obesity (EASO). EASL-EASD-EASO Clinical practice guidelines for the management of non-alcoholic fatty liver disease. *J Hepatol*. 2016;64(6):1388–1402. https://doi.org/10.1016/j.jhep.2015.11.004.
96. Mummadi RR, Kasturi KS, Chennareddygari S, Sood GK. Effect of bariatric surgery on nonalcoholic fatty liver disease: Systematic review and meta-analysis. *Clin Gastroenterol Hepatol*. 2008;6(12):1396–1402. https://doi.org/10.1016/j.cgh.2008.08.012.
97. Abu Dayyeh BK, Bazerbachi F, Graupera I, Andres C. Endoscopic bariatric and metabolic therapies for non-alcoholic fatty liver disease. *J Hepatol*. 2019;71:1246–1248. https://doi.org/10.1016/j.jhep.2019.07.026.
98. Kenneally S, Sier JH, Moore JB. Efficacy of dietary and physical activity intervention in non-alcoholic fatty liver disease: A systematic review. *BMJ Open Gastroenterol*. 2017;4(1):e000139. https://doi.org/10.1136/bmjgast-2017-000139.
99. Storck LJ, Imoberdorf R, Ballmer PE. Nutrition in gastrointestinal disease: Liver, pancreatic, and inflammatory bowel disease. *J Clin Med*. 2019;8(8):1098. https://doi.org/10.3390/jcm8081098.
100. Winters-van Eekelen E, Verkouter I, Peters HPF, et al. Effects of dietary macronutrients on liver fat content in adults: a systematic review and meta-analysis of randomized controlled trials. *Eur J Clin Nutr*. 75, 588–601 (2021). https://doi.org/10.1038/s41430-020-00778-1.
101. De Chiara F, Ureta Checcllo C, Ramón Azcón J. High protein diet and metabolic plasticity in non-alcoholic fatty liver disease: Myths and truths. *Nutrients*. 2019;11(12):2985. https://doi.org/10.3390/nu11122985.

102. Chakravarthy MV, Waddell T, Banerjee R, Guess N. Nutrition and nonalcoholic fatty liver disease. *Gastroenterol Clin North Am*. 2020;49(1):63–94. https://doi.org/10.1016/j.gtc.2019.09.003.
103. Skytte M, Samkani A, Petersen A, et al. A carbohydrate-reduced high-protein diet improves HbA1c and liver fat content in weight stable participants with type 2 diabetes: A randomised controlled trial. *Diabetologia*. 2019:62. https://doi.org/10.1007/s00125-019-4956-4.
104. Rehm J, Taylor B, Mohapatra S, et al. Alcohol as a risk factor for liver cirrhosis: A systematic review and meta-analysis. *Drug Alcohol Rev*. 2010;29(4):437–445. https://doi.org/10.1111/j.1465-3362.2009.00153.x.
105. Mardinoglu A, Wu H, Bjornson E, et al. An integrated understanding of the rapid metabolic benefits of a carbohydrate-restricted diet on hepatic steatosis in humans. *Cell Metab*. 2018;27(3):559–571.e5. https://doi.org/10.1016/j.cmet.2018.01.005.
106. Browning JD, Baker JA, Rogers T, Davis J, Satapati S, Burgess SC. Short-term weight loss and hepatic triglyceride reduction: Evidence of a metabolic advantage with dietary carbohydrate restriction. *Am J Clin Nutr*. 2011;93(5):1048–1052. https://doi.org/10.3945/ajcn.110.007674.
107. Ryan MC, Abbasi F, Lamendola C, Carter S, McLaughlin TL. Serum alanine aminotransferase levels decrease further with carbohydrate than fat restriction in insulin-resistant adults. *Diabetes Care*. 2007;30(5):1075–1080. https://doi.org/10.2337/dc06-2169.
108. Holmer M, Lindqvist C, Petersson S, et al. Treatment of NAFLD with intermittent calorie restriction or low-carb high-fat diet—a randomized controlled trial. *JHEP reports : innovation in hepatology*, 3(3), 100256. 2021;0(0). https://doi.org/10.1016/j.jhepr.2021.100256.
109. Schwimmer JB, Ugalde-Nicalo P, Welsh JA, et al. Effect of a low free sugar diet vs usual diet on nonalcoholic fatty liver disease in adolescent boys: A randomized clinical trial. *JAMA*. 2019;321(3):256. https://doi.org/10.1001/jama.2018.20579.
110. Salvia R, D'Amore S, Graziano G, et al. Short-term benefits of an unrestricted-calorie traditional Mediterranean diet, modified with a reduced consumption of carbohydrates at evening, in overweight-obese patients. *Int J Food Sci Nutr*. 2017;68(2):234–248. https://doi.org/10.1080/09637486.2016.1228100.
111. Gepner Y, Shelef I, Schwarzfuchs D, et al. Effect of distinct lifestyle interventions on mobilization of fat storage pools: CENTRAL Magnetic Resonance Imaging Randomized Controlled Trial. *Circulation*. 2018;137(11):1143–1157. https://doi.org/10.1161/CIRCULATIONAHA.117.030501.
112. Sanyal AJ, Chalasani N, Kowdley KV, et al. Pioglitazone, vitamin E, or placebo for nonalcoholic steatohepatitis. *N Engl J Med*. 2010;362(18):1675–1685. https://doi.org/10.1056/NEJMoa0907929.
113. Bjelakovic G, Gluud LL, Nikolova D, Bjelakovic M, Nagorni A, Gluud C. Meta-analysis: Antioxidant supplements for liver diseases—the Cochrane Hepato-Biliary Group. *Aliment Pharmacol Ther*. 2010;32(3):356–367. https://doi.org/10.1111/j.1365-2036.2010.04371.x.
114. Mclean AE. Hepatic failure in malnutrition. *Lancet*. 1962;2(7269):1292–1294. https://doi.org/10.1016/s0140-6736(62)90847-4.
115. Rosen E, Bakshi N, Watters A, Rosen HR, Mehler PS. Hepatic complications of anorexia nervosa. *Dig Dis Sci*. 2017;62(11):2977–2981. https://doi.org/10.1007/s10620-017-4766-9.
116. Waterlow JC. Amount and rate of disappearance of liver fat in malnourished infants in Jamaica. *Am J Clin Nutr*. 1975;28(11):1330–1336. https://doi.org/10.1093/ajcn/28.11.1330.
117. Turnlund JR, Keyes WR, Kim SK, Domek JM. Long-term high copper intake: Effects on copper absorption, retention, and homeostasis in men. *Am J Clin Nutr*. 2005;81(4):822–828. https://doi.org/10.1093/ajcn/81.4.822.
118. Russell K, Gillanders LK, Orr DW, Plank LD. Dietary copper restriction in Wilson's disease. *Eur J Clin Nutr*. 2018;72(3):326–331. https://doi.org/10.1038/s41430-017-0002-0.
119. European Association for the Study of the Liver. EASL clinical practice guidelines: Wilson's disease. *J Hepatol*. 2012;56(3):671–685. https://doi.org/10.1016/j.jhep.2011.11.007.
120. Roberts EA, Schilsky ML. Diagnosis and treatment of Wilson disease: An update. *Hepatology*. 2008;47(6):2089–2111. https://doi.org/10.1002/hep.22261.
121. Radford-Smith DE, Powell EE, Powell LW. Haemochromatosis: A clinical update for the practising physician. *Intern Med J*. 2018;48(5):509–516. https://doi.org/10.1111/imj.13784.
122. Moretti D, van Doorn GM, Swinkels DW, Melse-Boonstra A. Relevance of dietary iron intake and bioavailability in the management of HFE hemochromatosis: A systematic review. *Am J Clin Nutr*. 2013;98(2):468–479. https://doi.org/10.3945/ajcn.112.048264.

123. Vilstrup H, Iversen J, Tygstrup N. Glucoregulation in acute liver failure. *Eur J Clin Invest.* 1986;16(3):193–197. https://doi.org/10.1111/j.1365-2362.1986.tb01328.x.
124. Schneeweiss B, Pammer J, Ratheiser K, et al. Energy metabolism in acute hepatic failure. *Gastroenterology.* 1993;105(5):1515–1521. https://doi.org/10.1016/0016-5085(93)90159-a.
125. Millson C, Considine A, Cramp ME, et al. Adult liver transplantation: A UK clinical guideline—part 1: Pre-operation. *Frontline Gastroenterol.* 2020;11(5):375–384. https://doi.org/10.1136/flgastro-2019-101215.
126. Dick AAS, Spitzer AL, Seifert CF, et al. Liver transplantation at the extremes of the body mass index. *Liver Transpl.* 2009;15(8):968–977. https://doi.org/10.1002/lt.21785.
127. Sam J, Nguyen GC. Protein-calorie malnutrition as a prognostic indicator of mortality among patients hospitalized with cirrhosis and portal hypertension. *Liver Int.* 2009;29(9):1396–1402. https://doi.org/10.1111/j.1478-3231.2009.02077.x.
128. Álvares-da-Silva MR, Reverbel da Silveira T. Comparison between handgrip strength, subjective global assessment, and prognostic nutritional index in assessing malnutrition and predicting clinical outcome in cirrhotic outpatients. *Nutrition.* 2005;21(2):113–117. https://doi.org/10.1016/j.nut.2004.02.002.
129. Tandon P, Raman M, Mourtzakis M, Merli M. A practical approach to nutritional screening and assessment in cirrhosis. *Hepatology.* 2017;65(3):1044–1057. https://doi.org/10.1002/hep.29003.
130. Wu Y, Zhu Y, Feng Y, et al. Royal Free Hospital-Nutritional Prioritizing Tool improves the prediction of malnutrition risk outcomes in liver cirrhosis patients compared with Nutritional Risk Screening 2002. *Br J Nutr.* 2020;124(12):1293–1302. https://doi.org/10.1017/S0007114520002366.
131. Morgan MY, Madden AM, Soulsby CT, Morris RW. Derivation and validation of a new global method for assessing nutritional status in patients with cirrhosis. *Hepatology.* 2006;44(4):823–835. https://doi.org/10.1002/hep.21358.
132. Peng S, Plank LD, McCall JL, Gillanders LK, McIlroy K, Gane EJ. Body composition, muscle function, and energy expenditure in patients with liver cirrhosis: A comprehensive study. *Am J Clin Nutr.* 2007;85(5):1257–1266. https://doi.org/10.1093/ajcn/85.5.1257.
133. Plank LD, Gane EJ, Peng S, et al. Nocturnal nutritional supplementation improves total body protein status of patients with liver cirrhosis: A randomized 12-month trial. *Hepatology.* 2008;48(2):557–566. https://doi.org/10.1002/hep.22367.
134. Gluud LL, Dam G, Les I, et al. Branched-chain amino acids for people with hepatic encephalopathy. *Cochrane Database Syst Rev.* 2017;5:CD001939. https://doi.org/10.1002/14651858.CD001939.pub4.
135. Perumpail BJ, Li AA, Cholankeril G, Kumari R, Ahmed A. Optimizing the nutritional support of adult patients in the setting of cirrhosis. *Nutrient.* 2017;9(10):1114. https://doi.org/10.3390/nu9101114.
136. Ballmer PE, Walshe D, McNurlan MA, Watson H, Brunt PW, Garlick PJ. Albumin synthesis rates in cirrhosis: Correlation with Child-Turcotte classification. *Hepatology.* 1993;18(2):292–297.
137. Bharadwaj S, Ginoya S, Tandon P, et al. Malnutrition: Laboratory markers vs nutritional assessment. *Gastroenterol Rep.* 2016;4(4):272–280. https://doi.org/10.1093/gastro/gow013.
138. China L, Freemantle N, Forrest E, et al. A randomized trial of albumin infusions in hospitalized patients with cirrhosis. *N Engl J Med.* 2021;384(9):808–817. https://doi.org/10.1056/NEJMoa2022166.
139. Kalafateli M, Mantzoukis K, Choi Yau Y, et al. Malnutrition and sarcopenia predict post-liver transplantation outcomes independently of the Model for End-stage Liver Disease score. *J Cachexia Sarcopenia Muscle.* 2017;8(1):113–121. https://doi.org/10.1002/jcsm.12095.
140. Rutherford A, Davern T, Hay JE, et al. Influence of high body mass index on outcome in acute liver failure. *Clin Gastroenterol Hepatol.* 2006;4(12):1544–1549. https://doi.org/10.1016/j.cgh.2006.07.014.
141. Spengler EK, O'Leary JG, Te HS, et al. Liver transplantation in the obese cirrhotic patient. *Transplantation.* 2017;101(10):2288–2296. https://doi.org/10.1097/TP.0000000000001794.
142. Plank LD, Metzger DJ, McCall JL, et al. Sequential changes in the metabolic response to orthotopic liver transplantation during the first year after surgery. *Ann Surg.* 2001;234(2):245–255. https://doi.org/10.1097/00000658-200108000-00015.
143. Hammad A, Kaido T, Aliyev V, Mandato C, Uemoto S. Nutritional therapy in liver transplantation. *Nutrients.* 2017;9(10):E1126. https://doi.org/10.3390/nu9101126.
144. Laryea M, Watt KD, Molinari M, et al. Metabolic syndrome in liver transplant recipients: Prevalence and association with major vascular events. *Liver Transpl.* 2007;13(8):1109–1114. https://doi.org/10.1002/lt.21126.

145. Tietge UJF, Selberg O, Kreter A, et al. Alterations in glucose metabolism associated with liver cirrhosis persist in the clinically stable long-term course after liver transplantation. *Liver Transpl.* 2004;10(8):1030–1040. https://doi.org/10.1002/lt.20147.
146. Erlinger S. Gallstones in obesity and weight loss. *Eur J Gastroenterol Hepatol.* 2000;12(12):1347–1352. https://doi.org/10.1097/00042737-200012120-00015.
147. Gaby AR. Nutritional approaches to prevention and treatment of gallstones. *Altern Med Rev.* 2009;14(3):258–267.
148. Stokes CS, Krawczyk M, Lammert F. Gallstones: Environment, lifestyle and genes. *Dig Dis.* 2011;29(2):191–201. https://doi.org/10.1159/000323885.
149. Di Ciaula A, Garruti G, Frühbeck G, et al. The role of diet in the pathogenesis of cholesterol gallstones. *Curr Med Chem.* 2019;26(19):3620–3638. https://doi.org/10.2174/0929867324666170530080636.
150. Ribas Blasco Y, Pérez Muñante M, Gómez-Fernández L, Jovell-Fernández E, Oms Bernad LM. Low-fat diet after cholecystectomy: Should it be systematically recommended? *Cir Esp (Engl Ed).* 2020;98(1):36–42. https://doi.org/10.1016/j.ciresp.2019.05.009.
151. Walters JRF. Bile acid diarrhoea and FGF19: New views on diagnosis, pathogenesis and therapy. *Nat Rev Gastroenterol Hepatol.* 2014;11(7):426–434. https://doi.org/10.1038/nrgastro.2014.32.
152. Jackson A, Lalji A, Kabir M, et al. The efficacy of a low-fat diet to manage the symptoms of bile acid malabsorption—outcomes in patients previously treated for cancer. *Clin Med.* 2017;17(5):412–418. https://doi.org/10.7861/clinmedicine.17-5-412.
153. Hollemans RA, Hallensleben NDL, Mager DJ, et al. Pancreatic exocrine insufficiency following acute pancreatitis: Systematic review and study level meta-analysis. *Pancreatology.* 2018;18(3):253–262. https://doi.org/10.1016/j.pan.2018.02.009.
154. Arvanitakis M, Ockenga J, Bezmarevic M, et al. ESPEN guideline on clinical nutrition in acute and chronic pancreatitis. *Clin Nutr.* 2020;39(3):612–631. https://doi.org/10.1016/j.clnu.2020.01.004.
155. Al-Omran M, Albalawi ZH, Tashkandi MF, Al-Ansary LA. Enteral versus parenteral nutrition for acute pancreatitis. *Cochrane Database Syst Rev.* 2010(1):CD002837. https://doi.org/10.1002/14651858.CD002837.pub2.
156. Adiamah A, Psaltis E, Crook M, Lobo DN. A systematic review of the epidemiology, pathophysiology and current management of hyperlipidaemic pancreatitis. *Clin Nutr.* 2018;37(6):1810–1822. https://doi.org/10.1016/j.clnu.2017.09.028.
157. Dutta SK, Hlasko J. Dietary fiber in pancreatic disease: Effect of high fiber diet on fat malabsorption in pancreatic insufficiency and in vitro study of the interaction of dietary fiber with pancreatic enzymes. *Am J Clin Nutr.* 1985;41(3):517–525. https://doi.org/10.1093/ajcn/41.3.517.

CHAPTER 9

Nutrition in Hypertension and Kidney Medicine

Mariana Markell ■ Joanna Bond ■ James Bradfield ■ Elaine MacAninch

LEARNING POINTS

By the end of this chapter, you should be able to:

- Describe the nutritional factors that may help to prevent or delay the progression of chronic kidney disease (CKD) (stage 1–5) to end-stage kidney disease (ESKD)
- Describe the main nutritional factors that are involved in the management of late-stage CKD (stage 4–5)
- Explain the role of diet in the prevention and management of kidney stones
- Compare and contrast the differences in nutritional management among CKD, acute kidney injury (AKI) and nephrotic syndrome
- Apply patient data to formulate a basic nutrition management plan
- Determine when to refer on to a dietitian and the relevant patient data to communicate
- Understand the importance of a doctor's role in nutrition care within the multiprofessional kidney disease team
- Identify common challenges (client and professional aspects) that may arise when agreeing on a nutrition management plan and in making dietary changes

CASE STUDY 9.1 Chronic Kidney Disease (CKD) Stage 1–3

Harry is a 38-year-old man who rarely visits his general practitioner. While visiting his doctor with a sprained ankle he was found to have elevated blood pressure and has gained 3 kg since his son was born 3 months. He reports a family history of hypertension and cardiovascular disease, so you decide to do some further investigation and order blood tests. Harry is a nonsmoker and drinks one or two bottles of beer most evenings. He is a bus driver and finds it hard to find the time for exercise.

Vital Signs and Anthropometrics

Blood pressure (BP) 155/90; height 1.78 m; weight 90 kg; waist circumference 107 cm (42 inches); body mass index (BMI) 28

LABORATORY RESULTS (FASTING)

Test	Results	Reference Range
HbA1c	6.2	4.7–5.4
Triglycerides	200 mg/dL	<150 mg/dL

CASE STUDY 9.1 Chronic Kidney Disease (CKD) Stage 1–3—(Continued)

LABORATORY RESULTS (FASTING)

Test	Results	Reference Range
Total cholesterol	225 mg/dL	<200 normal 200–239 borderline >239 High
Uric acid	8.2 mg/dL	male: 3.5–7.2 mg/dL
Blood urea nitrogen	17 mg/dL	5–20 mg/dL
Creatinine	1.2 mg/dL	male: 0.7–1.3 mg/dL
K	4.1 mEq/L	3.3–5.3 mEq/L
Mg	2.5 mg/dL	1.8–3.0 mg/dL

Plan

You prescribe hydrochlorothiazide 25 mg daily to treat his hypertension.

DIET (24-HOUR RECALL)

Meal	Food
Breakfast	Cereal with milk
Snack	Coffee and 3 sugars and a bag of crisps (potato chips)
Late morning snack	Large coffee and 3 sugars
Lunch	Ham and cheese with lettuce and mustard on rye bread, can of Coca-Cola and an apple
Snack	Snicker's bar and coffee with milk and 3 sugars
Dinner	Pasta with meat sauce, side salad with mayonnaise, 2 bottles of beer
Snack	4 chocolate chip cookies and coffee and 3 sugars

Think about how you may approach a conversation on diet with Harry.

1. What do you think the opportunities may be to incorporate nutrition into the consultation when treating his hypertension? How might the medication choice affect your recommendations?
2. You notice that his HbA1c is also elevated and he is at risk of type 2 diabetes mellitus (T2DM). Thinking back to Chapter 7, 'Nutrition in Endocrine (Obesity/Diabetes) and Reproductive Medicine,' what do you think the main dietary messages are to reduce BP and reduce the risk of T2DM, and how do you think this may compare to the advice appropriate for CKD prevention?
3. How may you approach a discussion on risk with your patient?

CASE STUDY 9.2 Low Clearance (CKD 4–5)

Harry is now 47 years old. He and his wife have three children, ages 9, 5, and 1. They have been extremely busy raising their children and working to make ends meet. About 3 years before, Harry noticed that his legs were getting swollen, so you prescribed diuretics (Frusemide). Harry began to go to the bathroom more frequently, especially at night. He was also waking up at night with leg cramps, which he associated with taking frusemide and therefore reduced his dose. Gradually he started taking Frusemide less and less regularly. The oedema (swelling) would come and go. As Harry was really busy he did not attend his BP checks with you.

CASE STUDY 9.2 Low Clearance (CKD 4–5)—(Continued)

Harry subsequently noted that he was gaining weight, but he really did not feel like he was eating any more than usual. He tried to maintain a low sodium intake. During a medical assessment at work he was stunned to find that his BP was 180/105 and his weight was 95kg. He made an appointment to see you and you increase the dosages of his BP medication and Frusemide and refer him to a nephrologist.

LABORATORY RESULTS (FASTING)

Test	Results Reference	Range
Triglycerides	220mg/dL	<150mg/dL
Total cholesterol	325mg/dL	<200 desirable; 200–239 borderline high; >239 high
Uric acid	8.9mg/dL	male: 3.5–7.2mg/dL
Blood urea nitrogen	65mg/dL	5–20mg/dL
Creatinine	3.4mg/dL	Male: 0.7–1.3mg/dL
Estimated glomerular filtration rate	25.3mL/min per 1.73 m^2	>60mL/min
K	3.2 mEq/L	3.3–5.3 mEq/L
Mg	1.6mg/dL	1.8–3.0mg/dL
Ca	7.7mg/dL	8.4–9.8mg/dL
P	5.7mg/dL	2.5–4.8mg/dL
Intact parathyroid hormone	250pg/mL	10–65pg/mL
Hemoglobin	11.8g/dL	12.6–16.1g/dL
Albumin	3.5g/dL	2.7- 4.7g/dL 2.8
Urinalysis		
pH	6.1	5–7
Specific gravity	1.010	1.002–1.030
Protein	Negative	Negative
Glucose	Negative	negative

The nephrologist explains to Harry that his kidneys are beginning to fail and made the following recommendations:

Medications

- Enalapril 20mg daily
- Frusemide 80mg daily
- Phosphate binder with meals
- calcitriol 0.25mcg daily

Medication Nutrition Therapy

- 0.8g of protein per kg ideal body weight (IBW)
- Kilocalories per registered dietitian (RD) recommendation
- 2g sodium/day
- Phosphate-restricted diet
- No potassium restriction
- No fluid restriction
- A referral to the renal dietitian

CASE STUDY 9.2 Low Clearance (CKD 4–5)—(Continued)

1. Which results are significant regarding Harry's current health status?
2. Make sure you understand the rationale and nutritional implications for the recommendations that the doctor made for Harry.
3. What kinds of foods will Harry have to increase or decrease?

CASE STUDY 9.3 Renal Replacement Therapy

Here is information from a food record that Harry kept for several days prior to the next meeting with the dietitian.

Meal	Food
Breakfast	Porridge with cinnamon and sugar, large banana, coffee with milk
Snack	Glass of milk and apple
Lunch	Cup lentil soup, cheddar cheese sandwich with mayonnaise, low-fat yoghurt, Diet Coke, coffee with milk
Snack	Latte
Dinner	Beef steak, baked potato with butter, broccoli, salad with balsamic dressing, slice of cake
Snack	Glass of milk and 2 biscuits, 3 beers

Harry and his wife meet with a renal dietitian. Following that visit Harry was very conscientious about his dietary choices, and he started losing weight and felt well for the next year. However, over time he started to feel more tired and would get weak after doing easy tasks. He began to experience anorexia, headaches and nausea. He went back to his nephrologist, and updated lab results revealed that he had reached ESKD and he would have to start dialysis.

Medication Plan

- Continue phosphate binders
- Adjust antihypertensive medications as indicated as dialysis proceeds
- Start erythropoietin intravenously with dialysis
- Continue Frusemide as long as he has urine output
- Begin water-soluble vitamins and change to active vitamin D with dialysis

New Nutrition Goals

- 1.2–1.3 g of protein per kg IBW
- 2 g sodium
- Fluid intake = urine output + 500 mL (1000 mL)

Harry was admitted to have an arteriovenous fistula created in his arm to provide access for dialysis. After 3 weeks of dialysis his weight dropped from 95 kg to 91 kg.

When Harry first began dialysis, he became depressed and anxious. He was convinced that his condition would only worsen and he was having a difficult time functioning at work and at home. He is struggling to follow dietary restrictions although he has no appetite due to his depression. He is finding the fluid restriction especially hard and is gaining 3.5 kg between his dialysis sessions.

QUESTIONS

1. Harry was encouraged to increase his energy and protein once he started haemodialysis (HD). Why is this? Looking at his food log, which foods will have to increase and which should he decrease to achieve these goals? Are there specific types of protein that might be better?
2. What do you think Harry's risk of malnutrition is? What may the challenges be in assessing this?
3. How might you approach a conversation on the importance of following his prescribed potassium, phosphate and fluid restriction?
4. What may make it challenging or may make it easier for Harry to follow nutrition advice?

CASE STUDY 9.4 Kidney Transplant

Harry's sister was able to donate a kidney to him. He was given prednisone and tacrolimus with mycophenolate mofetil for immunosuppression. His hypertension returned and he again required treatment. He gained 10 kg within 6 months following the transplant. His fasting labs at 6 months posttransplant were as follows:

LABORATORY RESULTS

Test	Results Reference	Range
Glucose	119 mg/dL	65–100 mg/dL
Triglycerides	289 mg/dL	<150 mg/dL
Total cholesterol	280 mg/dL	<200 desirable; 200–239 borderline high; >239 high
Blood urea nitrogen	20 mg/dL	5–20 mg/dL
Creatinine	1.1 mg/dL	Male: 0.7–1.3 mg/dL
K	5.4 mEq/l	3.3–5.3 mEq/l
Mg	1.3 mg/dL	1.8–3.0 mg/dL
Haematocrit	44%	38%–47.7%

QUESTIONS

1. What are Harry's medical issues now? How do you explain his laboratory findings? His weight gain?
2. What dietary recommendations would you make for him?
3. After his transplant, Harry is feeling much better but slips back into poor eating habits. How do you react to a regression by the patient? What feelings does it evoke in you? What do you think is going on for him?

Introduction

Chronic kidney disease (CKD) ranks in the top 10 noncommunicable diseases contributing to disease and disability and occurs in an estimated 10% of the global population. Stages of CKD are classified as CKD 1 to 5 according to National Institute for Health and Clinical Excellence (NICE) in the UK. Although there are different systems of classification across the world, it is important to recognise that treatment, including nutritional interventions, will vary depending on the stage of CKD (Table 9.1).

Summary of Nutritional Issues

Nutrition and dietary interventions may be used to lower the risk of CKD, slow progression of existing disease, and manage complications at every stage of CKD. There is no one-size-fits-all generic renal diet; dietary treatment must be individualised and appropriate to the stage of kidney disease, biochemistry, other health conditions and pharmacologic and kidney replacement therapies. Social determinant and cultural factors must also be considered. In these case progressions, we illustrate how nutritional management may change for one individual to highlight the importance of regular screening and adapting advice for clinical needs. In this chapter, we will also cover several specific kidney diseases that require different nutritional approaches, including acute kidney injury (AKI), nephrotic syndrome and kidney stone disease.

TABLE 9.1 ■ **Classification of Chronic Kidney Disease Using GFR and ACR Categories**

	ACR Categories (mg/mmol) Description and Range			Increasing Risk
GFR categories (mL/min per 1.73 m^2), description and range	**<3 Normal to Moderately Increased A1**	**3–30 Moderately Increased A2**	**>30 Severely Increased A3**	
≥90 Normal and high	G1	No CKD in the absence of markers of kidney damage*		
60–89 Mild reduction related to normal range for a young adult	G2			
45–59 Mild-moderate reduction	G3a			
30–44 Moderate–severe reduction	G3b			
15–29 Severe reduction	G4			
≤15 Kidney failure	G5			
Increasing risk				

**ACR*, Albumin-to-creatinine ratio; *CKD*, chronic kidney disease; *GFR*, glomerular filtration rate.
Modified fom 'Kidney Disease: Improving Global Outcomes (KDIGO) CKD Work Group' (2013).

WHAT IS THE ROLE OF A RENAL DIETITIAN AND THE ROLE OF A DOCTOR WITHIN THE MULTIPROFESSIONAL TEAM?

As diet is an essential part of the treatment, renal dietitians are an important part of the multiprofessional team. People living with CKD have a need for specific nutrition assessment and often have multimorbidities leading to complex dietary requirements. Dietary restrictions may also influence nutritional status and need to be individualised to avoid adverse consequences. Specialist renal dietitians take a holistic approach, tailoring dietary advice and prioritising nutritional goals to the person's clinical, physical, social and psychological status.

In the UK a dietitian review is recommended every 6 months for all patients with CKD4 and over and every 2–3 months if on renal replacement therapy (RRT). These recommendations may vary by country with monthly dietitian reviews recommended in the United States. Individualised dietary advice from specialist renal dietitians improves patient outcomes. Specialist renal dietitians hold central responsibility for nutritional assessment and dietary therapy in the prevention and management of CKD and in more advanced stages of AKI. However, as nutrition is such a vital part of the treatment, it is important that all members of the multidisciplinary team have an understanding of the importance of nutrition. This includes nutrition assessment and an understanding of first line advice and, most importantly, when to refer to a dietitian.

Nutritional Issues as Kidney Disease Progresses

CKD 1–3

A 2020 systematic review of modifiable lifestyle factors in the primary prevention of CKD, higher intake of potassium and vegetables, lower intake of sodium, increased physical activity, moderate alcohol consumption, and avoidance of tobacco smoking were found to be consistently associated with lower risk of CKD. However, it was noted that the current quality of evidence was low to very low. These identified dietary factors are in line with previous reviews suggesting higher diet quality and overall healthier diet pattern like Dietary Approaches to Stop Hypertension (DASH) and Mediterranean dietary guidelines are protective against CKD. Adherence to a dietary pattern rich in whole grains, vegetables, fruit, legumes, nuts and fish and lower intake of red and processed meats, sodium, and sugar-sweetened beverages has been associated with lower odds of CKD incidence. The nutrition recommendations for CKD therefore are in line with the evidence for T2DM and cardiovascular prevention as discussed in Chapter 6. Although to date most of the research into nutrition and CKD prevention is focused on DASH and Mediterranean dietary patterns, it is possible that other patterns, for example vegetarian diets, may be protective but to date there are few clinical studies available.

The most common cause of CKD is T2DM, with one in three people living with diabetes likely to develop CKD due to diabetic nephropathy after 15–20 years. The second most common cause is hypertension, although it is recognised that elevated BP can be either a cause or a consequence of CKD. Other important risk factors include older age and family history of CKD.

However, in other causes of CKD the impact of diet on disease progression is less clear, including polycystic kidney disease, obstructive uropathy, glomerular nephrotic and nephritic syndromes such as focal segmental glomerulosclerosis, membranous nephropathy, lupus nephritis, amyloidosis and rapidly progressive glomerulonephritis.

In the case of hypertension with type 1 diabetes mellitus or T2DM, dietary intervention to improve glycaemic control and reduce BP will also reduce CKD risk. Therefore the best practice recommendation to reduce glycaemic and cardiac risk and hypertension will include guidance on decreasing alcohol and salt intake and decreasing weight if overweight, aiming for at least a 5%–10% weight loss. The effect other dietary approaches to T2DM such as low-carbohydrate diets or very-low-caloric diets have not been studied regarding effects on CKD risk. For those with prediabetes, effective dietary interventions can significantly reduce the risk of developing T2DM and are likely to therefore reduce CKD risk too.

During early stages CKD 1–3 is generally managed in primary care and, depending on the underlying cause, with careful monitoring and management CKD may not progress any further. For those with an estimated glomerular filtration rate (eGFR) of 44–59 mL/min, the lifetime risk of end-stage renal disease was 7.51% for men and 3.21% for women but for those with diabetes or glomerulonephritis, the risk of progressing to end-stage renal disease is higher. The management of all newly diagnosed CKD 1–3 should include regular monitoring of all modifiable risk factors for CKD and associated conditions such as hypertension, vascular disease and diabetes (Table 9.2).

The management of all newly diagnosed patients with CKD 1–3 should include regular monitoring of serum creatinine, eGFR and albumin-to-creatinine ratio and treatment of any underlying disease process. The treatment of individual glomerular diseases is complex and beyond the scope of this chapter.

In the 2020 Kidney Disease Outcomes Quality Initiative (KDOQI) clinical nutrition guidelines, few intervention studies of dietary patterns in CKD are identified. However, observational studies on dietary patterns containing fruits, vegetables, whole grains, lean meats, low-fat dairy and low added salt led to improved clinical outcome and, in particular, CKD mortality.

TABLE 9.2 ■ **Summary of Modifiable Risk Factors and Nutrition Management CKD 1–3**

• Optimise blood glucose levels in patients with diabetes
• Meticulous control of hypertension (<140/90 or lower)
• Careful monitoring of antihypertensive agents alongside dietary interventions (ACE inhibitors may need to be changed as GFR declines as they can increase potassium or worsen kidney function)
• DASH/Mediterranean style or possibly plant-based diet
• Reduce dietary sodium (Na) to 2.3g SODIUM
• Smoking cessation if appropriate
• Regular exercise (30min/day moderate activity)
• Reduction in alcohol consumption
• Antiplatelet and anticoagulant drugs if appropriate for reduction of cardiovascular risk CVD
• Weight loss (if overweight)
• Lipid lowering if appropriate for cardiovascular risk

ACE, Angiotensin-converting enzyme; *CKD*, chronic kidney disease; *CVD*, cardiovascular disease; DASH, Dietary Approaches to Stop Hypertension; *GFR*, glomerular filtration rate.

Energy Requirements in CKD 1–3

Target: Current guidelines recommend 25–35 kcal/kg, which is the same as the general population.

Protein Requirements in CKD 1–3

Benefits of lower protein intakes are of interest in patients in CKD stages 3–5, but there are no specific guidelines to restrict lower than 0.8–1 g per kilogram ideal body weight (IBW) in stages 1–3. Recommendations therefore match those made for the general public.

Potassium/Phosphate

Most people will not require a restriction in CKD 1–3. Indeed, adequate potassium intake has been linked to improved BP, with the ratio between sodium and potassium identified as a potentially important factor in reducing hypertension, such as is found in a DASH-style dietary pattern. It is therefore important not to restrict potassium prematurely. However, general guidance can be offered on avoiding potassium containing salt substitutes and limiting manufactured/processed foods (which are higher in both phosphate and sodium).

Fruits and Vegetables

As kidney function declines, net acid retention in the residual nephrons leads to metabolic acidosis which may accelerate decline in kidney function and lead to muscle wasting as is seen in later stage CKD.

To reduce net endogenous acid production (NEAP), patients may be prescribed bicarbonate. Several studies have also shown that increasing fruit and vegetables can also reduce NEAP. To reduce the rate of decline of residual kidney function, increasing fruit and vegetables in early kidney disease may be beneficial with one study suggesting that the beneficial as early as CKD 2.

Sodium

Target: Reduce dietary sodium (Na) to < 100 mmol/day (<2.3 g or 6 g salt) (KDOQI 2020).

Reducing sodium has been demonstrated to improve hypertension, although this effect is potentiated with higher fruit and vegetables and dairy as in DASH, as well as reducing alcohol, cessation of smoking, decreasing weight if overweight and increasing physical activity. General advice can be given on reducing high-salt processed foods and replacing salt with herbs and spices to enhance flavours.

CKD 3–5 NOT ON DIALYSIS

When kidney function continues to decline to moderate to severe CKD (generally defined as below 30 mL per minute eGFR), patients will be referred to a specialist renal unit, where they should have access to a renal dietitian. Discussions on potential RRT will include patient assessment and education to plan future treatment. Nutrition interventions may now need to be balanced with potassium and phosphate restrictions if these values start to move out of range.

Energy Requirements

Target: 25–35 kcal/kg per IBW

Of patients with stage 3–5 CKD, 20%–40% have protein energy wasting, associated with increased risks of infection/poor healing and reducing life expectancy and quality of life.

However, weight gain may increase BP, glucose and cardiovascular risk and therefore may also accelerate the decline in kidney function; thus control of energy intake while maintaining excellent nutrition is important.

Energy metabolism may also be impaired in patients with late-stage CKD and may fluctuate depending on health status, for example, when acutely ill or influenced by hyperparathyroidism, hyperglycaemia or chronic inflammation. Although several trials in CKD 3–5 suggest that predialysis 30–35 kcal per kilogram of IBW helps to maintain neutral nitrogen balance and nutritional status, it is important that energy recommendations be personalised. Regular assessment of weight, appetite and general nutrition status should be performed so recommendations can be adjusted.

Protein

Target: 0.8–1.0 g/kg

Protein is required for adequate growth in children and maintenance and repair in adults. Eight of the amino acid building blocks are considered essential for human health. By-products of protein catabolism include urea and creatinine, which is a by-product of muscle catabolism specifically. Both are normally cleared by the kidneys and excreted in urine and increase as kidney function declines. A low-protein diet may lower workload of the kidneys and reduce hyperfiltration, although long-term effects must be weighed against the risk of muscle loss and sarcopenia.

As kidney disease progresses, catabolism and loss of lean body mass occurs. As urea starts to rise with progression of disease, patients can begin to experience uraemic symptoms, which combined with acute or chronic inflammatory responses can increase nausea, lethargy and taste changes and may contribute to the high levels of protein energy malnutrition found in this patient group.

Currently protein recommendations for CKD 3–5 predialysis vary depending on country, and this topic is currently being debated, although the general consensus is a target of 08–1.0 g/kg in both the United States and UK.

The 2019 UK guidelines suggesting a target of 0.8–1.0 g/kg IBW per day for patients with stage 4–5 CKD not on dialysis in an attempt to reduce the prevalence of undernutrition and because of insufficient evidence to routinely recommend low-protein diets. In contrast, 2020 US guidelines suggest a low-protein diet of 0.55–0.60 g dietary protein/kg body weight per day, or a very-low-protein diet providing 0.28–0.43 g dietary protein/kg body weight per day with additional keto acid/amino acid analogs. However, the proviso is that this recommendation is only for those who are metabolically stable and under close clinical supervision. The rationale is to reduce risk for ESKD/death and improve quality of life, but as the evidence is not strong, few US nephrologists would prescribe such a severe restriction clinically.

Low-protein diets (0.6 g/kg or less) are rarely prescribed for patients with CKD in current dietetic practice in the UK with NICE advising not to use diets below 0.6 to 0.8 g protein/kg. A 2018 Cochrane review concluded that very-low-protein diets (0.3–0.4 g/kg per day) may delay the need for dialysis, but concordance with these diets was difficult. A more modest protein restriction (0.5–0.6 g/kg per day) did not have an effect; furthermore, maintaining the prescribed level may be difficult in practice. In each case, however, these broad recommendations should be considered in conjunction with the patient's biochemical results, nutritional status, comorbidities and protein intake individually recommended in accordance with these.

Potassium

Varies depending on patient's clinical status; <2 g/day if hyperkalaemic. Remember severe hyperkalaemia is a medical emergency.

Target: UK Renal Association (local guidelines may vary):

Potassium restriction is required when > 5.5 mmol/L or 6 mmol/L.

Potassium supplementation may be required if potassium is <3.5 mmol/L.

Potassium has an essential role in controlling BP and mediating cellular, vascular and neuromuscular function. Elevated potassium does not always result in symptoms but anecdotally some people describe tingling, heavy limbs or gastrointestinal hypermotility. However, if untreated, hyperkalaemia can lead to muscle weakness, arrhythmias, cardiac arrest, and death which means close and careful monitoring and advice is vital.

In the UK, renal association guidelines classify hyperkalaemia as mild (5.5–5.9 mmol/L), moderate (6.0–6.4 mmol/L) or severe (≥6.5 mmol/L), although local guidelines may differ.

The requirement for or the extent of potassium restriction needs to be individualised depending on biochemistry, medication and dietary assessment. In the United States, the use of exchange resins such as sodium-zirconium cyclosilicate and patiromer has increased, allowing patients a less strict potassium restriction.

If distal tubular function and urine output are maintained, most patients do not become hyperkalaemic until end stage, unless they are given an angiotensin-converting enzyme (ACE) inhibitor (ACEi), angiotensin receptor blocker (ARB) or mineralocorticoid antagonist. If distal tubular function is impaired, however, as is seen with diabetic kidney disease (type IV renal tubular acidosis (RTA)) or sickle cell nephropathy, serum potassium levels may rise secondary to reduced potassium excretion by the kidneys despite continued urine output.

Many foods including fruit, vegetables, legumes, nuts, potatoes, meat, fish and milk contain significant amounts of potassium (see Table 9.6). These foods are also important sources of fibre, vitamins and minerals important for overall health. It is therefore essential that overall diet and health goals are individualised. A renal dietitian can help to maintain nutritional balance in line with other medical priorities such as avoiding adverse effects on NEAP (as discussed previously), protein energy malnutrition, cardiovascular risk or maintaining blood glucose levels. Advice can be targeted to restrict foods highest in potassium to avoid overly restrictive diets.

When treating hyperkalaemia, clinicians are advised to first try to identify contributing nondietary factors that can be corrected which include:

- Antihypertensive medicines such as mineralocorticoid antagonists (spironolactone) or ACEi and angiotensin receptors blockers (ARB), and occasionally beta blockers
- Metabolic acidosis (may be corrected with sodium bicarbonate prescription)
- Decline in residual tubular function
- Requirement for dialysis
- Catabolism
- Infection
- Haemolysed blood sample
- Constipation
- Adrenal insufficiency

PHARMACOLOGICAL TREATMENT OF HYPERKALAEMIA

Emergent treatment of hyperkalaemia is beyond the scope of this chapter. Insulin and dextrose can be administered in the short term to treat severe hyperkalaemia by redistributing potassium into the intracellular space, but caution should be observed as insulin kinetics are prolonged with kidney failure, and severe hypoglycaemia may result, with deaths reported in patients who were not closely observed after administration.

In the long term, potassium binders (sodium-zirconium cyclosilicate, calcium polystyrene sulphonate or patiromer) can be taken with meals to aid the patient to maintain safe serum potassium levels.

Phosphate

Varies depending on patient's clinical status, 0.8–1 g/day.

Target: UK Renal Association (local guidelines may vary).

Stage 3–5: Maintain levels in the normal range: 0.9–1.5 mmol/L.

Phosphorus is an essential mineral necessary for bone growth and mineralisation, as well as for regulation of acid-base homeostasis. However, as kidney function declines (typically as eGFR decreases to <45 mL/min), the kidneys are unable to clear phosphate sufficiently and blood levels can start to rise. It is recommended that assessment of dietary phosphorus intake should be initiated when a patient reaches CKD stage 3.

Previous guidelines advised restricting phosphate to 800 to 1000 mg (25–32 mmol) phosphorus per day in Europe. In 2020, KDOQI suggested that rather than specific dietary phosphate ranges, individualised treatments based on patient needs and clinical judgment should be created. In particular, an emphasis should be placed on replacing animal with vegetable protein-based dietary phosphorus and on reducing phosphorus additives found within processed foods.

It should be noted that phosphorous and phosphate are different measurements. In food, phosphorus is measured in milligrams but in blood, phosphate is measured in millimoles. To convert phosphorus in milligrams to phosphate in millimoles, divide by 31 (which is the atomic weight of phosphorus), for example: 800 mg / 31 = 26 mmol.

Limiting protein intake automatically results in a reduction in phosphorus intake, as will limiting processed foods. In addition, the absorption of phosphorus from plant-based proteins is lower than animal proteins, with one study showing improved phosphate results on a vegetarian diet. Swapping from processed foods high in phosphate additives to fresh ingredients or more vegetarian proteins where phosphate is less bioavailable can actually improve nutrient density. Phosphate-restricted diets can therefore be achieved without too much effect on dietary quality.

NICE recommends monitoring to ensure avoidance of malnutrition by maintaining a protein intake at or above the minimum recommended level.

Some patients with CKD 4–5 requiring a low-phosphate diet may need phosphate binders, which are calcium based or made of a phosphate-binding polymer. It is important to refer to current or national latest guidance for recommended types and doses. In the UK, for example, NICE CG157 and in the US Kidney Disease Improving Global Outcomes. Phosphate binders should be taken at mealtimes to reduce the amount of phosphate absorbed from the gastrointestinal tract into the blood. It is important that patients receive appropriate education regarding timing and dose of binders and ensure this is regularly reviewed. An increased dose may be required with higher phosphate meals.

Sodium

Target: <100 mmol/day (<2.3 g sodium or 5.8 g salt) (KDOQI 2020).

In all stages of CKD, a high sodium intake is associated with worsening hypertension. Sodium recommendations are the same as CKD 1–3 (unless salt losing nephropathy is present, which is very rare).

Renal Replacement Therapy

Nutrition requirements and goals will vary depending on the type of RRT. Multiple factors can impact an individual patient's ability to follow dietary recommendations (Table 9.3). Detailed analysis of each dialysis modality is beyond the scope of this chapter but broadly there are two main types, haemodialysis (HD) and peritoneal dialysis (PD).

HAEMODIALYSIS

HD can be performed at a renal unit or at home. Blood is passed over a semipermeable membrane and waste products diffuse from the high concentration in the blood to the low concentration in a dialysate solution. For those attending a dialysis unit, a typical prescription would be three times a week for 4 hours, although this can vary and will be individualised. For those dialysing at home

TABLE 9.3 ■ **Summary of Potential Barriers and Enablers to Nutrition Plans for Patients With Kidney Disease**

Summary of Barriers	Enablers
Poor appetite secondary to uraemia, nausea or taste changes Mood changes, depression or anxiety related to the demands of treatment and symptoms Conflicting information on diet and health Contradicting or confusing dietary messages related to multiple health conditions such as diabetes and renal restrictions Treatment fatigue Demanding treatment schedules reducing time for meal preparation Lethargy Social problems such as reduced income/reduced social connections Multiple dietary and fluid restrictions	Accurate, timely and consistent nutrition care from all health professionals (referring to the dietitians' care plan) Access to counselling services Food provision during dialysis Involvement of supporting services such as meal delivery companies, social care, third-sector organisations Involvement of family and carers to assist with shopping, preparation and meal provision

many people choose to have more frequent but shorter dialysis, for example, 5–6 times a week. With more frequent dialysis, patients often experience fewer uraemic symptoms and it is easier to keep potassium, phosphate and fluid in balance, allowing them more freedom in their dietary choices.

PERITONEAL DIALYSIS

PD needs to be done daily and also occurs at home. Continuous ambulatory PD involves passing a dialysate into the peritoneal cavity and the peritoneum acts as a filter through which metabolic waste products including electrolytes, urea, creatinine and fluid are drawn from the bloodstream. The dialysate is then drained from the peritoneum via a catheter. The exchanges are normally done four times a day and take approximately 30 minutes. Aseptic technique via a closed system minimises the risk of infection. Automated PD is similar to continuous ambulatory PD but the exchanges are automated, being managed by a machine called a cycler, and normally take place whilst the patient is asleep, making it an ideal therapy for children, who often grow better on the modality compared with HD. It is important to note that the dialysate contains glucose and absorption leads to increased caloric load as well as alteration of blood sugar in patients with diabetes.

Energy

HD target: 30–35 kcal/kg per IBW
PD target: 30–35 kcal/kg per IBW (This includes calories from dialysate.)

Protein energy undernutrition is common, affecting 28%–54% of dialysis patients, and is associated with reduced quality of life and a decline in life expectancy. This finding is likely due to a number of reasons including associated symptoms of uraemia, the burden of long dialysis sessions and frequent hospital visits that can make it challenging to find time for shopping and preparing food and the potential loss of income and financial impact on disposable income, which may affect diet quality. As mentioned previously, patients receiving PD are likely to absorb glucose from their dialysis fluid, which, when taken into account, can result in lower dietary energy requirements. As will be discussed under general nutrition assessment of the patient with CKD, care must be taken when assessing the risk of malnutrition which can be masked by oedema.

Protein

Target: HD and PD: 1.0–1.4 g/kg per IBW

Protein requirements in HD and PD are based on data which suggests intakes less than 0.8 g/kg and more than 1.4 g/kg have been associated with increased risk of mortality. Protein requirements can increase during periods of illness and decreased intake is associated with factors mentioned earlier.

For patients having PD, peritonitis can be a complication. During a period of peritonitis infection and treatment, protein losses into peritoneal fluid can result and requirements increase. Dietary protein intake of 1.5 g/kg per IBW per day or higher is recommended.

Potassium

Target: Pre-HD 4–6 mmol/L

As before it is important to base dietary advice according to serum potassium levels and dietary assessment. Other causes of hyperkalaemia as outlined previously should be corrected. In some instances, such as when patients are underdialysed and are waiting to have access issues resolved, dietary potassium restrictions may need to be tightened temporarily. Regular monitoring is essential, with guidelines recommending that predialysis bloods are taken at least once a month. It is also important to avoid low potassium levels which can exacerbate weakness. Patients with hypokalaemia should have their diet and other potential causes reviewed. Low potassium levels can be the result of undernutrition.

Phosphate and Calcium

HD target, phosphate: Aim to keep pre dialysis levels between 1.1 and 1.7 mmol/L.

It is important that reducing dietary phosphate does not compromise protein intake. Some patients, especially those with poor appetite, may have low phosphate levels and may need dietary advice to reduce their risk of malnutrition as well as a reduction or even discontinuation of phosphate-binding medication.

Fluid

HD target: Most people on thrice weekly HD will need to restrict the amount of fluid they drink as urine output declines. The calculation of fluid allowance should consider individual patient features such as weight and comorbidity as well as symptoms and tolerance to HD. To help establish daily fluid allowance, patients may be requested to do a 24-hour urine collection to measure the volume. A common recommendation is 500–750 mL + equivalent of previous days urine output.

PD target: Fluid management on PD is less of an issue because of the more regular ultrafiltration of fluid during the exchanges. Fluid targets are advised on an individual basis, and fluid can be managed by altering the concentration of osmotically active substance in the dialysate.

Excessive fluid weight gains can cause shortness of breath, hypertension and increased cardiovascular risk. The UK Renal Nutrition Group 2019 guidelines advise clinical assessment of fluid status quarterly to determine a patient's 'dry weight' or their actual weight without excess fluid. Predialysis any weight above the target is seen as 'fluid gain' and during dialysis fluid is removed to try and achieve the target weight. However, if the patient is significantly higher in weight, fluid may need to be removed more gradually over a few dialysis sessions. Clinical assessment of fluid status involves looking for any signs of overhydration such as oedema or breathlessness and any signs of weight loss, especially after intercurrent illness. Clinicians are also advised to use a validated objective measurement, such as bioimpedance, at regular intervals and when clinical assessment is unclear. The weight gained between dialysis sessions is referred to as interdialytic weight gain; this will be individually set for each patient but typically is set as no more than 1–2 kg between sessions, and patients are advised on limiting fluid to achieve this. It is difficult to remove more than 3–4 kg at one dialysis session. Rapid fluid removal may result in cramping, nausea, vomiting or even hypotension or syncope. To help reduce thirst, it is important to also reduce hyperglycaemia if present and to advise on reducing salt.

It is important to note that fluid restrictions can be extremely challenging and as urine output declines, with those anuric often restricted to less than 500 mL per day. Support and guidance are especially important during hot weather or during times of celebration in which sharing a hot drink or an alcoholic or a nonalcoholic drink is a part of many cultures. For example, using cups with a small fluid volume, avoiding high-liquid foods such as soups and jellies and using ice cubes or lemon sweets/candies rather than a long drink may help quench thirst.

Sodium

Target: As previously for sodium (Na), to <100 mmol/day (2.3 g sodium or 5.8 g salt).

As salt intake can increase thirst, it is important that patients with normal or high BP requiring advice on reducing fluids are also given advice on the importance of reducing salt. However, this advice may vary as some dialysis patients with autonomic neuropathy become hypotensive and require salt tablets plus mineralocorticoid therapy to maintain adequate BP.

Micronutrients

Water-soluble vitamin and essential trace element supplements are advised for all patients on HD. This is due to the removal of micronutrients during dialysis, as well as dietary restriction. Low levels of various micronutrients have been found in patients on HD and patients on PD.

Post–Kidney Transplant

Following transplantation many dietary restrictions including fluid, potassium and phosphorous restriction may be relaxed, although they may be necessary on an individual basis. For instance, in some cases calcineurin inhibitor therapy can lead to hyperkalaemia. Patients are advised to follow a healthy diet to reduce the cardiovascular risk factors such as hyperlipidaemia and forestall the development of T2DM which can occur de novo following transplantation.

BONE HEALTH

Preexisting bone disease can be exacerbated by steroid treatment posttransplant and refractory hyperparathyroidism. The risk of bone fractures may be four times higher for kidney transplant patients compared with the general population, although the fractures tend to be acral (hands and feet) rather than spine or hip. Nutrition interventions to minimise bone mineral density loss include advice on achieving 1000 mg/day dietary calcium (1300 mg/day postmenopause) or a calcium supplement, daily vitamin D (the dose to determined individually), regular weight bearing exercise, maintaining a normal weight and avoiding smoking or excessive alcohol intake.

PHOSPHATE

Hypophosphatemia is common, particularly in the first 3–6 months posttransplant due to increased urine, increased levels of the phosphatonin FGF23, hyperparathyroidism and immunosuppressive treatment. Patients may be advised to increase dietary phosphate temporarily. Phosphate supplementation may be used for short periods but is not recommended in the long term. Blood phosphate, calcium and parathyroid hormone levels need to be monitored regularly. Patients need to be counselled regarding normalisation of phosphate intake, as some will rigidly stick to their dialysis dietary recommendations despite normal kidney function, exacerbating hypophosphatemia.

WEIGHT GAIN

Weight gain is extremely common in the first year following successful transplantation and can be as great as 6–10 kg with a change in BMI between 2 and 3.8 kg/m^2. Contributing factors include use of steroids, easing of dietary restrictions and an increased appetite associated with an improved sense of well-being. As well as increasing cardiovascular and diabetes risk, excessive weight gain has also been shown to be associated with reduced life span of the renal allograft.

NEW-ONSET DIABETES MELLITUS AFTER KIDNEY TRANSPLANTATION

New-onset diabetes mellitus after kidney transplantation occurs in around 15%–30% of people at 1 year post-kidney transplant. Risk factors include use of steroids and calcineurin inhibitors, family history of diabetes, age and weight gain/presence of obesity. There is a lack of published data on dietary interventions to help reduce new-onset diabetes mellitus after kidney transplantation. At this time standard diabetes prevention guidelines as discussed in Chapter 7 should be applied.

FOOD SAFETY

Basic food safety principles are more important posttransplant due to risks related to immunosuppressive therapy, including the risk of foodborne infections such as *Escherichia coli*, Listeria or Salmonella. For most transplant patients this means following general public health guidance to reduce the risk of food poisoning. In the UK this guidance is governed by the food standards agency.

Specific Nutrition Assessment in Patients With CKD

NUTRITION ASSESSMENT ADAPTED FROM THE BRITISH DIETETIC ASSOCIATION 2020

A well-structured and thorough nutrition assessment is crucial to all populations and disease states, and this is true for those suffering with all aspects of kidney disease. While there is an entire chapter in this book that deals with nutritional screening and assessment as topics, there are some aspects which are specific to kidney disease and therefore need to be discussed to ensure that patients receive the best care available to them. It is also important to note and recognise the situations where conventional screening and assessment methods may lead to some patients' needs being overlooked and therefore missing out on nutritional therapy that they require.

A reminder: As outlined in Chapter 2, nutritional screening is the application of simple, rapid and validated nutritional screening tools, which are reproducible with minimal training, while nutritional assessment is a clinical skill used to identify specific issues related to potential poor nutrition. Nutritional screening may be carried out by a range of stakeholders in health care, including the patients themselves, whereas nutritional assessment must be carried out by a trained professional like an RD. There are multiple models used to carry out nutritional assessment, and the one which will be discussed here is the ABCDEF model, as recommended by the British Dietetic Association (BDA). This acronym stands for Anthropometry, Biochemistry, Clinical, Dietary, Environmental and Functional factors. Ultimately the method used will vary from practitioner to practitioner but the most important thing is that the information is collected in a systematic and comprehensive form. Doctors play an important role in the assessment and identification of nutritional issues. While a dietitian can perform a more detailed nutrition assessment, doctors can help with early identification and appropriate onward referral.

Anthropometry

Anthropometry includes but is not limited to a patient's height, weight, BMI and weight gain/loss percent (if applicable). If these measurements are not possible, for example, in the case of a patient who may be bedbound or unable to stand on weighing scales, other anthropometric measurements may be recorded such as ulna length and mid-upper arm circumference. These latter measurements may then be compared with reference standards which can provide an estimate of height and weight for use in BMI calculations. Importantly in kidney disease, there are several factors to consider when trying to accurately measure anthropometry.

Malnutrition Universal Screening Tool

As previously discussed in Chapter 2, the Malnutrition Universal Screening Tool (MUST) is used to quickly screen patients at risk of malnutrition. However, caution must be applied in interpretation for patients with kidney disease. In those patients with kidney disease who suffer from fluid

TABLE 9.4 ■ **Contribution of Ascites and Oedema to Body Weight**

	Ascites	Oedema
Minimal	2.2 kg	1.0 kg
Moderate	6.0 kg	5.0 kg
Severe	14.0 kg	10.0 kg

Adapted from Parenteral and Enteral Group of the British Dietetic Association. *A Pocket Guide to Clinical Nutrition*, 5th edition. Updated 2018. British Dietetic Association; 2018.

retention in the form of oedema or fluid shifts during dialysis, fat and muscle loss or muscle wasting may not be evident. In addition, it is important to note if patients have undergone amputations due to diabetes and/or peripheral vascular disease. Although these adjustments are beyond the scope of this chapter, they can be found in the MUST instruction booklet. The Parenteral and Enteral Nutrition Group of the BDA provide a guide for estimating the contribution of oedema and/or ascites to body weight in the absence of amputations (Table 9.4).

It may well be important to explore measures of muscle mass and strength rather than relying on weight alone. One simple, cost-effective, and quick way of doing so is by measuring a patient's handgrip strength using a dynamometer. This measurement reflects the strength of muscles in the upper extremities and gives a functional measure of a patients' nutritional status. This technique has been used in the diagnosis of sarcopenia, or loss of muscle mass, a condition that affects up to 63% of patients with CKD, depending on their age, stage of CKD, method of measurement and what cutoffs are used. In a study of patients referred onto a specialist kidney ward, half of those at risk of malnutrition were not identified by MUST when compared with Subjective Global Assessment, which is a more detailed nutrition assessment tool requiring specialist dietitian input.

KIDNEY (RENAL)-SPECIFIC NUTRITIONAL PLAN

The Renal Inpatient Nutritional Screening Tool is a specific screening tool developed to include questions on appetite, intake and supplement use in addition to weight changes and BMI. It helps correct for the challenges in obtaining an oedema free weight. In a multicentre clinical trial, the Renal Inpatient Nutritional Screening Tool identified 50% of patients admitted into the kidney ward as malnourished compared with 45% with the gold standard Subjective Global Assessment full nutrition assessment.

The nutrition impact score does not require a weight and instead uses a patient questionnaire to gather information on appetite or barriers to intake, such as taste changes, bowel change and nausea.

As previously noted, CKD-related malnutrition is common, affecting 20%–40% of patients in stage 4 and 5 CKD, 28%–54% of patients in dialysis and an estimated 50% of kidney ward admissions (compared with overall 29% of all hospital admissions). The reasons include:

- Potential dietary and fluid restrictions limiting patient choice
- Poor appetite secondary to uraemia, anaemia and taste changes
- The treatment burden with multiple medications, many hospital appointments and if on dialysis, long treatment sessions which may limit time for food preparation and shopping

- Managing multimorbid conditions including a high incidence of depression or mood disorders and/or frailty
- Protein energy wasting secondary to accelerated protein catabolism associated with acidosis, insulin resistance and chronic inflammation
- Coexisting atherosclerosis, hypertension or diabetes
- Micronutrient deficiencies in relation to nutrient losses during dialysis or secondary to medications

CKD and Obesity

For patients with obesity, it is important to support them in losing weight while not leaving them malnourished. Achieving a target weight may slow progression of kidney disease by improving risk factors such as uncontrolled hypertension or diabetes or it may ensure that patients are eligible to be put on a transplant list. Although current guidelines do not specify a BMI cutoff, a national survey revealed significant variability of BMI threshold for transplant centres. Moreover, in a recent review of kidney transplant outcomes, it was shown that despite those with higher BMIs having an increased risk of delayed graft function, longer-term (5–10 year) graft survival rates were no different for those with a higher BMI. The authors concluded that weight alone should not be a reason for precluding someone from transplantation and other factors, such as age, difficulties on dialysis and cardiovascular risk should also be taken into consideration.

Using Laboratory Results in the Formulation of Your Care Plan

As in many clinical conditions, analyses of blood samples are extremely useful in formulating, monitoring and reviewing nutritional interventions in kidney disease. Parameters most often affected by kidney disease are shown in Table 9.5.

Because of the role that the kidneys play in overall homeostasis and fluid balance, any damage or loss of function may have systemic effects which are frequently reflected in blood biochemistry. For those suffering from either an AKI or CKD, there will be a rise in creatinine (by definition) most often with a rise in blood urea nitrogen as well. As by-products of creatine and protein (amino acid) metabolism, respectively, both of these compounds are found at high concentrations due to reduced clearance by the kidneys.

As eGFR decreases and the kidneys become progressively less efficient at filtering the blood, they are also less efficient at excreting acid. If there is insufficient bicarbonate to buffer retained acid, this results in increased NEAP, with higher NEAP being associated with accelerated CKD progression to ESKD. Bicarbonate should therefore be closely monitored and corrected to maintain serum levels within the targets included in Table 9.5. Low level of bicarbonate could also result in higher potassium levels, as acidosis drives potassium from the intracellular to the extracellular compartment, and correction of acidosis can help modulate potassium levels.

Measurement and monitoring of electrolytes is crucial in kidney disease as has been previously discussed. Ineffective clearance of sodium leads to increased fluid retention and worsening hypertension. In more advanced stages of CKD, potassium, phosphate and magnesium levels may rise. Parathyroid levels increase in response to retention of phosphate and decrease in ability of the kidney to activate vitamin D. Increases in intact parathyroid hormone often occur as early as CKD stage 3.

Albumin levels may fall in diseases where the glomerular barrier is disrupted and nephrotic syndrome ensues, such as the nephroses, including diabetic nephropathy, and diseases associated with systemic lupus erythematosus, sickle cell disease and intrinsic kidney diseases beyond the scope of this chapter. Low albumin leads to fluid retention and oedema. High cholesterol is also a hallmark of nephrotic syndromes, possibly resulting from loss of regulatory proteins in the urine. Nephrotic syndrome will be discussed in detail later.

TABLE 9.5 ■ **Standard Reference Ranges for Biochemical Parameters Often Affected by Chronic Kidney Disease**

	UK	USA
Na	133–146 mmol/L	135–145 mEq/L
K	3.5–5.3 mmol/L	3.5–5 mEq/L
Urea	2.5–7.8 mmol/L	8–20 mg/dL (blood urea nitrogen)
Creatinine	6–120 µmol/L	0.7–1.3 mg/dL
Corrected Ca	2.2–2.6 mmol/L	8.5–10.2 mg/dL
Bicarbonate	22–29 mmol/L	23–28 mEq/L
PO_4	0.8–1.15 mmol/L	3.0–4.5 mg/dL
Mg	0.7–1.15 mmol/L	1.5–2.4 mg/dL
Albumin	35–50 g/L	3.5–5.4 g/dL
HbA1C	18–46 mmol/mol	4.7%–6.5%
Hemoglobin	130–180 g/L (males) 115–165 g/L (females)	14–17 g/dL (males) 12–16 g/dL (females)
Estimated glomerular filtration rate	90–120 mL/min per 1.73 m^2	90–120 mL/min per 1.73 m^2
Parathyroid hormone (when normocalcaemic)	1.6–6.9 pmol/L	14–65 pg/mL

Anaemia is also common in the patient with CKD, due to decreased production of erythropoietin by the kidneys, as well as iron deficiency anaemia that can occur with blood loss during HD or due to dietary restriction. Attention to the presence of vitamin deficiencies especially of the B vitamins should be addressed in CKD patients with anaemia.

Clinical

The assessment of a patients' clinical status is essential in kidney disease, as it is in all other conditions. However, similarly to evaluation of biochemistry values, a number of considerations are especially important to bear in mind. Though all aspects of the clinical status are important, focus should also be on those factors which may have an effect on dietary intakes, including upcoming tests and scans, some of which may occur at meal times, leading to a reduced oral intake.

The first aspect to consider is the extent of the patient's kidney disease. Assessment of the presenting complaint may well inform the dietary requirements that are likely to be present and give an indication of a patient's risk of malnutrition. Patients with high levels of urea in their system (uraemia) as a result of reduced clearance often suffer from uraemic anorexia and may be suffering from nausea and/vomiting, thus reducing their interest in food or desire to eat. This is especially important when considering that given the metabolic stresses associated with ill health, the need to eat and supply the body with energy and other nutrients is at its highest.

A clinical assessment should also include speaking with the patient and examining some physical features. Presence of oedema, weight loss and/or cachexia; information about bowel habits and urine output; catheterisation; presence of nausea or vomiting; taste changes; fluid restrictions;

frequency of dialysis (if applicable) and medications should all be noted to give a complete picture of a patients' clinical status. Many of these factors will contribute to the nutritional care plan. For example, presence of oedema may necessitate fluid restriction, which in turn may require lower volume, concentrated nutritional supplements (if indicated).

Dietary

A good dietary assessment should provide as much detail as possible on both quantitative and qualitative elements of nutritional intakes, including foods, fluids and supplements as covered in Chapter 2. Special attention should be given to sources of protein in the diet, regardless of what type/stage of renal disease the patient has, as well as the patient's fluid intakes. For those with a fluid restriction, sources of sodium in the diet should be noted, bearing in mind that 75% of the sodium in the diet is already in the foods we eat while just 25% is added in cooking and before eating. Salty foods increase thirst and lead to greater fluid intakes. Additionally, foods high in potassium and phosphate should be noted if the patient is hyperkalaemic or hyperphosphatemic. Table 9.6 includes a list of foods high in potassium, sodium and phosphate.

It is worth investigating how dietary intakes vary according to whether a patient receives dialysis and how efficient the treatment is as underdialysis can also reduce appetite. Some patients may avoid eating during dialysis due to nausea or lethargy or to reduce the risk of low BP. BP is more likely to drop in patients who require a lot of fluid to be removed during their dialysis session as previously mentioned. If the patient requires dialysis 3 days during the week, this factor has a significant impact on energy and protein requirements.

A final consideration in the diets of those with advanced CKD may be vitamin D and calcium intakes. Kidneys are responsible for the hydroxylation of 25-hydroxyvitamin D to 1, 25-dihydroxyvitamin D (the active form in humans), which is essential for the uptake of dietary calcium. Therefore, damage to the kidneys and reduced function may lead to secondary and subsequently tertiary hyperparathyroidism, with resultant renal osteodystrophy, a condition characterised by altered bone morphology. Patients should receive supplementation with active vitamin D preparations unless they are hypercalcaemic.

Recommendations for Specific Kidney Diseases

ACUTE KIDNEY INJURY

AKI is characterised by sudden reductions in the eGFR and an associated reduction in the kidneys' ability to filter waste products from the blood. There are a number of common causes of AKI which can be divided into three subsections:

- Prerenal, due to reduced perfusion to the kidneys resulting in decreased eGFR such as hypovolaemia, reduced cardiac output and use of certain medications such as diuretics and nonsteroidal antiinflammatory drugs
- Intrinsic renal, due to physical damage to the kidney structure such as by drugs (e.g., chemotherapy), inflammation or cancers (e.g., myeloma), or intrinsic kidney diseases such as rapidly progressive glomerulonephritides
- Postrenal, due to an increased pressure within the tubules of the kidney because of a physical obstruction to urine flow such as by an enlarged prostate, cancer, a blocked catheter or kidney stones

A nutritional assessment should take into account the source of the AKI as it may well change the management. It is important to note that patients suffering from CKD may also experience a rapid increase in their serum creatinine. While this may be a progression of their CKD, it may also suggest the presence of an AKI (51), which is frequently diagnosed as AKI on CKD. AKI is managed medically until resolved, but there are a number of nutritional considerations such as supporting oral intakes during the acute illness.

TABLE 9.6 ■ **Foods That May Need to Be Restricted in Chronic Kidney Disease**

High-Salt Foods[a]
Salted meats and processed meat products such as ham, bacon, sausages, pate or salami
Ready-made and powdered soups
Ketchup, soy sauce, mayonnaise, pickles
Stock cubes, gravy powder and salted flavourings
Tinned food containing salt
Smoked meat and fish, prawns and anchovies
Meat and yeast extracts
Cheese
Salted snacks like crisps, nuts, biscuits, popcorn
Ready meals, sauces and takeaway meals
Pasta sauce
Bread and breakfast cereals
High-Phosphate Foods[b]
Many processed foods have phosphate additives in them, so try to reduce the amount of these foods that you eat:
Dairy products
Bony fish
Shellfish
Nuts
Chocolate
Drinks such as cola, malted drinks and milky drinks such as Ovaltine and hot chocolate
High-Potassium Foods[c]
Bananas, avocado, oranges, currants, dried fruit (raisins, sultanas, dates, dried apricots)
Beetroot, tomato puree, sundried tomatoes, dried and fresh mushrooms, spinach
Beans and pulses (e.g., kidney beans, chickpeas, lentils, soya beans) are high in potassium but can be used instead of meat or if you are vegetarian
Jacket or baked potatoes, oven, microwave or shop-bought chips, manufactured potato products such as hash browns, potato waffles, frozen roast potatoes or potato wedges
Fried cassava, yam or sweet potato
Taro, plantain and parsnip
Breakfast cereals containing lots of dried fruit, nuts or chocolate (e.g., muesli, granola, fruit and fibre bran-based breakfast cereals, such as All Bran, Bran Flakes)
Potato crisps, chocolate, fudge, nuts; biscuits and cakes containing lots of dried fruit, nuts or chocolate
High-potassium foods to limit: Coffee (limit to 1 cup a day), malted milk drinks for example Ovaltine or Horlicks, hot chocolate, fruit and vegetable juices, smoothies, wine (limit to 1 small glass white wine), beer, cider
Limit milk to ½ pint per day (300 mL)
Limit yoghurt to 3 small pots per week
Condensed milk, evaporated milk and milk powders

[a]Modified from British Dietetic Association. Salt: food fact sheet. Available at: https://www.bda.uk.com/resource/salt.html.
[b]Modified from Kidney Care UK. Chronic kidney disease mineral bone disease (CKD-MBD). Available at: https://www.kidneycareuk.org/about-kidney-health/conditions/chronic-kidney-disease-mineral-bone-disease-ckd-mbd/.
[c]Modified from Kidney Care UK. Lowering your potassium levels. Available at: https://www.kidneycareuk.org/about-kidney-health/living-kidney-disease/kidney-kitchen/lowering-your-potassium-levels/.

Up to 42% of patients who present to hospital with AKI are also suffering from malnutrition, highlighting the need for nutrition support throughout the illness. In identification of malnutrition among this population group, please refer to the previous section on anthropometry for the specific considerations in kidney disease. The main aim of nutrition support during the period of acute illness is to maintain nutritional status, preventing any decline in nutritional stores while minimising side effects of the condition.

From a nutrition and diet perspective, AKI can either be experienced in a catabolic or noncatabolic state. Typically, those who present with pre- or postrenal AKI experience a noncatabolic state of AKI. They will likely meet their nutritional requirements with diet alone or with a combination of diet and oral nutritional supplements. Their requirements are displayed in Table 9.7. These patients should be advised on a low-salt diet to reduce thirst and support less fluid intake. In practice, however, fluid and electrolyte balance is usually medically managed and will be guided by the patients' recent blood biochemistry. Calcium may be low in these patients as a result of either high phosphate or reduced levels of albumin, thus making the adjusted, or corrected, calcium figure more relevant or requiring the measurement of ionised calcium, which is the free form.

Meanwhile, AKIs experienced in a catabolic state are more likely to present accompanied by trauma and sepsis. RRT is common in this cohort, which is often managed in an intensive care unit. RRT may be intermittent or continuous which will affect nutritional requirements. Because many patients are sedated and intubated, artificial nutrition is common (enteral in the first instance, parenteral if indicated). Nutritionally dense, low-volume supplements and feeds are important for these patients due to the need to closely monitor fluid retention. These patients generally have higher nutritional requirements given that they are in a catabolic state and these are displayed in Table 9.7. It is also worth pointing out that when patients are sedated, any calorie-containing medicines, such as propofol (a short-acting anaesthetic), must be factored into calculations.

For patients who go on to require some form of RRT, there are a number of nutritional considerations. Depending on the type of dialysis they receive, protein requirements are altered as is shown in the table. This is largely due to the extracorporeal losses of amino acids during filtration. These patients may also experience electrolyte imbalances, such as elevated potassium and the aforementioned elevated phosphate. There are no generic requirements for electrolytes in this population group, but rather, interventions should be driven by recent blood biochemistry.

Dietitians can provide advice around low-potassium and low-phosphate diets; however, they are less commonly prescribed than in the later stages of CKD because a diet low in phosphate may hamper attempts at effective nutrition support and effective nutritional maintenance. It is also important to remember that hypophosphatemia may hinder attempts at extubation due to weakness of respiratory muscles. There is poor evidence that the provision of micronutrients in patients with AKIs are beneficial and current guidelines do not typically advise additional supplementation.

Much like in noncatabolic AKI, patients with catabolic AKI requiring RRT will need strict control of fluid balance to prevent overload, which will likely be medically managed using monitoring techniques such as daily weights rather than traditional fluid requirement equations. Finally, it is very important to observe for recovery of kidney function, as the recovering kidney has impairment of nutrient reabsorption as well as maintenance of fluid balance, and patients often develop polyuria with hypocalcaemia, hypokalaemia and hypophosphatemia which should be addressed individually.

NEPHROTIC SYNDROME

Nephrotic syndrome is a collection of signs and symptoms resulting from abnormality of the glomerular podocyte. This leads to albumin and other proteins leaking into the urine which in turn leads to oedema. Hypercholesterolemia is often observed as well as hypoalbuminemia. Hypercoagulability can occur due to loss of clotting inhibitors in the urine. Nephrotic-range proteinuria is defined as >3 g/m^2 per 24 hours. The syndrome requires the presence of nephrotic

TABLE 9.7 ■ **Nutritional Requirements in AKI**

	Noncatabolic (No RRT)	Noncatabolic (on IHD)	Noncatabolic (on CRRT)	Catabolic (No RRT)	Catabolic (on IHD)	Catabolic (on CRRT)
Protein (g/kg BW[a]/day)	0.8–1.0	Minimum 1.1	1.2–1.5[b]	1.0–1.3[b] Gradually increase to 1.3	1.0–1.5 1.5–2.0	Up to 1.7 in hypercatabolism 1.5–2.5/kg per day in critically ill patients with AKI
Energy	Tailored to individual requirements and clinical state. (Some authors suggest 20–30 kcal/kg per day even in the critical settings.)					
Fluid	Fluid requirements require individual medical assessment. Standard fluid equations are unlikely to be helpful. Fluid balance and daily weights should be monitored closely.					
Electrolytes	Monitor and adjust intake as required. These will vary depending on disease state and type of treatment.					
Micronutrients	Requirements are not well documented. Lipid-soluble vitamin levels and antioxidant status are low. CRRT has negative effect on balance of some water-soluble vitamins (such as thiamine, folate and vitamin C) and trace elements (copper, zinc, selenium. Whether micronutrient supplementation improves outcomes remain unknown.					

[a]All recommendations for kg/body weight (BW) refer to actual body weight; however, special considerations to avoid overfeeding and underfeeding should be taken into account in individual who are underweight or obese.

[b]There is currently no evidence to support these protein requirements and values are provided based on the expert opinion of the authors. If protein provision is increased further, close monitoring of kidney function, patient condition and nitrogen balance will be required. A target of 1.3 g/kg per day should be reached progressively in patients on intensive care unit with AKI and should be adapted to the clinical conditions.

AKI, Acute kidney injury; *BW*, body weight; *CRRT*, Continuous Renal Replacement Therapy; *IHD*, intermittent haemodialysis; *RRT*, renal replacement therapy.

Singer P. (2020) Protein metabolism and requirements in the ICU. Clin Nutr ESPEN. 38:3-8 range proteinuria as well as three of the following: hypertension, hypoalbuminemia, oedema, or hypercholesterolemia.

It can be caused by a range of primary diseases which target the kidneys directly such as focal segmental glomerulosclerosis or membranous nephropathy. It can also be due to secondary systemic diseases that affect the whole body such as diabetes, sickle cell disease and systemic lupus erythematosus. Diabetes is the most common cause of nephrotic syndrome. The medical management of nephrotic syndrome can include the following:

- Use of ACEi or ARBs to manage BP while reducing proteinuria
- Diuretics to reduce oedema and help with BP control
- Cholesterol medication if cholesterol is elevated
- Management of the underlying disease process (e.g., control of blood glucose)
- Other approaches, including mineralocorticoid antagonists which have been reported to decrease proteinuria, if not hyperkalaemic
- Use of SGLT2 inhibitors, which have been reported to decrease proteinuria and possibly decrease progression to end ESKD
- Use of steroids to treat certain primary glomerulopathies (membranous, IgA, focal segmental glomerulosclerosis (FSGS)), and calcineurin inhibitors (FSGS) and mycophenolate mofetil (systemic lupus erythematosus)

Nutrition Goals

- Moderate protein intake
  - 0.8–1 g/kg IBW
  - Despite low albumin levels, avoid a high-protein intake which has been associated with worsening proteinuria
- No added salt
  - At most 6 gm salt (2400 mg sodium) a day
- A fluid restriction may be needed due to oedema based on the individual or if the patient develops hyponatremia due to excess free water intake in the setting of increased antidiuretic hormone (ADH) because of intravascular volume depletion
- Healthy eating principles (e.g., The EatWell Guide)
- Aim for normal BMI range
- Tight diabetes control if appropriate
- Advice on potassium based on the individual
- Levels may drop due to aggressive diuretic therapy or hypomagnesemia
  - Levels may increase secondary to ACEi/ARBs and/or tubular dysfunction which is commonly seen in patients with diabetes or sickle cell disease (type 4 renal tubular acidosis (RTA))

KIDNEY STONES

It is estimated that 9%–10% of people will have symptoms of kidney stones at some point of their life with men being slightly more affected than women. There are several types of kidney stones including:

- Calcium stones (account for 60%–80% of stones)
  - Calcium oxalate
  - Calcium phosphate
- Struvite stones
  - 10%–15% of stones
- Uric acid stones
  - 5%–10% of stones

- Cystine stones
    - 1% of stones
- Others
    - 1% of all

Calcium oxalate stones may occur due to primary hypercalciuria, hyperoxaluria or hypocitraturia. They are also seen following bariatric surgery or in any disease where fat malabsorption occurs, due to binding of calcium to fat which prevents its binding to oxalate and allows more oxalate to be absorbed, subsequently making its way to the kidneys. Struvite stones are most commonly the result of recurrent urinary infections with *Proteus mirabilis*.

It is important to differentiate the composition of stones so as to target diet therapy appropriately. Dietary treatment, including avoidance of high oxalate foods, is more useful in preventing the recurrence of calcium oxalate stones (Table 9.8), although all types of stones benefit from high fluid intake, reduced salt and moderate animal protein intake.

For calcium oxalate stones, the following nutrition goals apply:

- Drink 2.5–3 L fluid intake aiming to keep urine dilute
    - Limit carbonated drinks
    - Limit pure fruit juices
    - Limit tea and coffee
    - Include a bedtime drink to stop urine concentrating overnight (The patient can also be told to drink some fluid every time they wake up to urinate during the night.)
    - Add lemon juice to water, which helps to increase the citrate level of the urine which prevents calcium oxalate crystallising
- Moderate protein intake
    - 0.8–1 g/kg IBW
    - Recent evidence shows a vegetarian diet is beneficial due to making the urine pH more alkaline so meat-free days should be encouraged
- No added salt (6 g salt (2400 mg sodium) a day)
- Normal calcium intake
    - Do not restrict
    - Calcium supplements are not recommended

TABLE 9.8 ■ **NICE Renal and Ureteric Stones: Assessment and Management 2019**

High-Oxalate Foods
Tea Chocolate including cakes, cocoa, biscuits and spread Malted drinks Nuts and nut butters Strawberries Rhubarb Beetroot Spinach Parsley
250 mg calcium
200 mL milk 200 mL of calcium enriched soya milk 125 g pot of yogurt 30 g cheese 60 g oily fish with bones (e.g., sardines/pilchards)

- Limit oxalate rich foods; remind patients that 'green smoothies' are often extremely high in oxalate because of concentrated intake of spinach, kale and other high oxalate foods
- Avoid large doses of vitamin C (>2000 mg) from over-the-counter supplements as at high dose vitamin C is metabolised to oxalate
- Encourage a BMI in the normal range

Conclusion

In this chapter we have discussed the importance of individual assessment to determine the most appropriate nutrition advice for those living with kidney disease. Appropriate advice depends on the type of kidney disease, comorbid conditions, the stage of disease and other medications, renal replacement or other therapies. As demonstrated within the progressive Case Study, nutrition is an essential part of medical care relevant to all stages of kidney disease. In some cases nutrition intervention may help to slow kidney decline, reduce the risk of complications, and improve symptoms. It may be essential to patient safety and can enhance both longevity and enhance quality of life. It is therefore essential that all members of the health care team can recognise and treat nutrition problems as they arise with the help of renal dietitians. Changing dietary requirements and demanding treatment schedules and symptoms can be challenging for those living with kidney disease, and empathic, accurate and practical nutrition support from health professionals is a key to quality, evidence-based care.

References

1. Bikbov B, Purcell C, Levey A, et al. Global, regional, and national burden of chronic kidney disease, 1990–2017: a systematic analysis for the Global Burden of Disease Study 2017. *Lancet*. 2020;395(10225):709–733.
2. National Institute for Health and Care Excellence. Chronic kidney disease: assessment and management. NICE guideline NG203. 2021. Available at: https://www.nice.org.uk/guidance/ng203/resources/chronic-kidney-disease-assessment-and-management-pdf-66143713055173. Accessed September 7, 2021.
3. British Renal Society. A multi-professional renal workforce plan for adults and children with kidney disease. Available at: https://ukkidney.org/sites/renal.org/files/FINAL-WFP-OCT-2020_compressed.pdf. Accessed September 7, 2021.
4. Kelly J, Su G, Zhang L, et al. Modifiable lifestyle factors for primary prevention of CKD: a systematic review and meta-analysis. *J Am Soc Nephrol*. 2020;32(1):239–253.
5. Bach K, Kelly J, Palmer S, Khalesi S, Strippoli G, Campbell K. Healthy dietary patterns and incidence of CKD. *Clin J Am Soc Nephrol*. 2019;14(10):1441–1449.
6. James S, Abate D, Abate K, et al. Global, regional, and national incidence, prevalence, and years lived with disability for 354 diseases and injuries for 195 countries and territories, 1990–2017: a systematic analysis for the Global Burden of Disease Study 2017. *Lancet*. 2018;392(10159):1789–1858.
7. Pugh D, Gallacher P, Dhaun N. Management of hypertension in chronic kidney disease. *Drugs*. 2019;79(4):365–379.
8. Gheith O, Othman N, Nampoory N, Halimb M, Al-Otaibi T. Diabetic kidney disease: difference in the prevalence and risk factors worldwide. *Journal of the Egyptian Society of Nephrology and Transplantation*. 2016;16(3):65.
9. Diabetes U.K. Evidence-based nutrition guidelines for the prevention and management of diabetes. Available at: https://www.diabetes.org.uk/professionals/position-statements-reports/food-nutrition-lifestyle/evidence-based-nutrition-guidelines-for-the-prevention-and-management-of-diabetes. Accessed September 9, 2021.
10. National Institute for Health and Care Excellence. Hypertension in adults: diagnosis and management. NICE guideline NG136. Available at: https://www.nice.org.uk/guidance/ng136/resources/hypertension-in-adults-diagnosis-and-management-pdf-66141722710213. Accessed September 7, 2021.
11. Diabetes Prevention Program Research Group The 10-year cost-effectiveness of lifestyle intervention or metformin for diabetes prevention: an intent-to-treat analysis of the DPP/DPPOS. *Diabetes Care*. 2012;35(4):723–730.

12. Lindstrom J, Louheranta A, Mannelin M, et al. The Finnish Diabetes Prevention Study (DPS): lifestyle intervention and 3-year results on diet and physical activity. *Diabetes Care*. 2003;26(12):3230–3236.
13. Turin T, Tonelli M, Manns B, et al. Lifetime risk of ESRD. *J Am Soc Nephrol*. 2012;23(9):1569–1578.
14. National Institute for Health and Care Excellence. Type 2 diabetes in adults: management. NICE guideline NG28. Available at: https://www.nice.org.uk/guidance/ng28/resources/type-2-diabetes-in-adults-management-pdf-1837338615493. Accessed September 9, 2021.
15. National Institute for Health and Care Excellence. Type 1 diabetes in adults: diagnosis and management. NICE guideline NG17. Available at: https://www.nice.org.uk/guidance/ng17/resources/type-1-diabetes-in-adults-diagnosis-and-management-pdf-1837276469701. Accessed September 9, 2021.
16. National Institute for Health and Care Excellence. Cardiovascular disease: risk assessment and reduction, including lipid modification. Clinical guideline CG181. Available at: https://www.nice.org.uk/guidance/cg181/resources/cardiovascular-disease-risk-assessment-and-reduction-including-lipid-modification-pdf-35109807660997. Accessed September 7, 2021.
17. Kelly J, Palmer S, Wai S, et al. Healthy dietary patterns and risk of mortality and ESRD in CKD: a meta-analysis of cohort studies. *Clin J Am Soc Nephrol*. 2016;12(2):272–279.
18. Ikizler T, Burrowes J, Byham-Gray L, et al. KDOQI clinical practice guideline for nutrition in CKD: 2020 update. *Am J Kidney Dis*. 2020;76(3):S1–S107.
19. Public Health England. Government recommendations for energy and nutrients for males and females aged 01–18 years and 19+ years. Available at: https://assets.publishing.service.gov.uk/government/uploads/system/uploads/attachment_data/file/618167/government_dietary_recommendations.pdf. Accessed September 9, 2021.
20. Scialla J, Appel L, Astor B, et al. Net endogenous acid production is associated with a faster decline in GFR in African Americans. *Kidney Int*. 2012;82(1):106–112.
21. Kanda E, Ai M, Kuriyama R, Yoshida M, Shiigai T. Dietary acid intake and kidney disease progression in the elderly. *Am J Nephrol*. 2014;39(2):145–152.
22. He F, Li J, MacGregor G. Effect of longer term modest salt reduction on blood pressure: Cochrane systematic review and meta-analysis of randomised trials. *BMJ*. 2013;346(apr03 3). f1325–f1325.
23. Sacks F, Svetkey L, Vollmer W, et al. Effects on blood pressure of reduced dietary sodium and the Dietary Approaches to Stop Hypertension (DASH) diet. *N Engl J Med*. 2001;344(1):3–10.
24. Lodebo B, Shah A, Kopple J. Is it important to prevent and treat protein-energy wasting in chronic kidney disease and chronic dialysis patients? *J Ren Nutr*. 2018;28(6):369–379.
25. Wright M, Southcott E, MacLaughlin H, Wineberg S. Clinical practice guideline on undernutrition in chronic kidney disease. *BMC Nephrol*. 2019;20(1):370.
26. Hahn, D., Hodson, E. M., & Fouque, D. (2018). Low protein diets for non-diabetic adults with chronic kidney disease. The Cochrane database of systematic reviews, 10(10), CD001892. https://doi.org/10.1002/14651858.CD001892.pub4.
27. Wright M, Jones C. Renal association clinical practice guideline on nutrition in CKD. *Nephron Clin Pract*. 2011;118(s1):c153–c164.
28. Moranne O, Froissart M, Rossert J, et al. Timing of onset of CKD-related metabolic complications. *J Am Soc Nephrol*. 2008;20(1):164–171.
29. Goldsmith D, Covic A, Fouque D, et al. Endorsement of the Kidney Disease Improving Global Outcomes (KDIGO) Chronic Kidney Disease-Mineral and Bone Disorder (CKD-MBD) guidelines: a European Renal Best Practice (ERBP) commentary statement. *Nephrol Dial Transplant*. 2010;25(12):3823–3831.
30. Moe S, Zidehsarai M, Chambers M, et al. Vegetarian compared with meat dietary protein source and phosphorus homeostasis in chronic kidney disease. *Clin J Am Soc Nephrol*. 2010;6(2):257–264.
31. Ashby D, Borman N, Burton J, et al. Renal association clinical practice guideline on haemodialysis. *BMC Nephrology*. 2019;20(1):379.
32. Veenstra D, Best J, Hornberger J, Sullivan S, Hricik D. Incidence and long-term cost of steroid-related side effects after renal transplantation. *Am J Kidney Dis*. 1999;33(5):829–839.
33. British Dietetic Association. Dietary advice post renal transplantation. Available from: https://www.bda.uk.com/uploads/assets/26cfde56-7970-477a-a37ee481a1638b7d/dietaryadvicepostrenaltransplant-toolkit.pdf. Accessed September 14, 2021.
34. British Dietetic Association. Model and process for nutrition and dietetic practice. Available at: https://www.bda.uk.com/uploads/assets/1aa9b067-a1c1-4eec-a1318fdc258e0ebb/2020-Model-and-Process-for-Nutrition-and-Dietetic-Practice.pdf. Accessed September 9, 2021.

35. British Association for Parenteral and Enteral Nutrition. Malnutrition Universal Screening Tool. Available at: https://www.bapen.org.uk/pdfs/must/must_full.pdf. Accessed September 14, 2021.
36. Johansen K, Lee C. Body composition in chronic kidney disease. *Current opinion in nephrology and hypertension*. 2015;24(3):268–275. https://doi.org/10.1097/MNH.0000000000000120.
37. Parenteral and Enteral Group of the British Dietetic Association. *A Pocket Guide to Clinical Nutrition*. 5th ed. Updated 2018. British Dietetic Association; 2018.
38. Bohannon R, Peolsson A, Massy-Westropp N, Desrosiers J, Bear-Lehman J. Reference values for adult grip strength measured with a Jamar dynamometer: a descriptive meta-analysis. *Physiotherapy*. 2006;92(1):11–15.
39. Cruz-Jentoft A, Bahat G, Bauer J, et al. Sarcopenia: revised European consensus on definition and diagnosis. *Age Ageing*. 2018;48(1):16–31.
40. Sabatino A, Cuppari L, Stenvinkel P, Lindholm B, Avesani C. Sarcopenia in chronic kidney disease: what have we learned so far? *J Nephrol*. 2020;34(4):1347–1372.
41. Jackson H, MacLaughlin H, Vidal-Diez A, Banerjee D. A new renal inpatient nutrition screening tool (Renal iNUT): a multicenter validation study. *Clin Nutr*. 2019;38(5):2297–2303.
42. MacLaughlin H, Twomey J, Saunt R, Blain S, Campbell K, Emery P. The nutrition impact symptoms (NIS) score detects malnutrition risk in patients admitted to nephrology wards. *J Hum Nutr Diet*. 2018;31(5):683–688.
43. Carrero J, Thomas F, Nagy K, et al. Global prevalence of protein-energy wasting in kidney disease: a meta-analysis of contemporary observational studies from the international society of renal nutrition and metabolism. *J Ren Nutr*. 2018;28(6):380–392.
44. Jackson H. Nutrition screening in hospitalised patients—a renal perspective. *Journal of Kidney Care*. 2019;4(3):126–130.
45. British Association for Parenteral and Enteral Nutrition. Managing malnutrition to improve lives and save money. Available at: https://www.bapen.org.uk/pdfs/reports/mag/managing-malnutrition.pdf. Accessed September 14, 2021.
46. Kostakis I, Kassimatis T, Bianchi V, et al. UK renal transplant outcomes in low and high BMI recipients: the need for a national policy. *J Nephrol*. 2019;33(2):371–381.
47. British Dietetic Association. Salt: food fact sheet. Available at: https://www.bda.uk.com/resource/salt.html. Accessed September 14, 2021.
48. Kidney Care U.K. Chronic kidney disease mineral bone disease (CKD-MBD). Available at: https://www.kidneycareuk.org/about-kidney-health/conditions/chronic-kidney-disease-mineral-bone-disease-ckd-mbd/. Accessed September 14, 2021.
49. Kidney Care U.K. Lowering your potassium levels. Available at: https://www.kidneycareuk.org/about-kidney-health/living-kidney-disease/kidney-kitchen/lowering-your-potassium-levels/. Accessed September 14, 2021.
50. National Institute for Health and Care Excellence. Acute kidney injury: what causes it? Available at: https://111.wales.nhs.uk/Kidneyinjury,acute/#:~:text=Causes%20of%20acute%20kidney%20injury,or%20diarrhoea%2C%20or%20severe%20dehydration. Accessed September 14, 2021.
51. National Institute for Health and Care Excellence. Acute kidney injury: prevention, detection and management. Available at: https://www.nice.org.uk/guidance/ng148/resources/acute-kidney-injury-prevention-detection-and-management-pdf-66141786535621. Accessed September 14, 2021.
52. Think Kidneys. Nutritional considerations in adult patients with acute kidney injury. Available at: https://www.thinkkidneys.nhs.uk/aki/wp-content/uploads/sites/2/2021/03/Nutrition-Guide-2021.pdf. Accessed September 14, 2021.
53. Cano N, Fiaccadori E, Tesinsky P, et al. ESPEN guidelines on enteral nutrition: adult renal failure. *Clin Nutr*. 2006;25(2):295–310.
54. Gervasion JM, Garmon WP, Holowatyj MR. Nutrition support in acute kidney injury. *Nutr Clin Pract*. 2011;26(4):374–381.
55. Patel JJ, McClain CJ, Sarav M, Hamilton-Reeves J, Hurt RT. Protein requirements for critically ill patients with renal and liver failure. *Nutr Clin Pract*. 2017;32(1 suppl):101s–111s.
56. Naylor HL, Jackson H, Walker GH, et al. British Dietetic Association evidence-based guidelines for the protein requirements of adults undergoing maintenance haemodialysis or peritoneal dialysis. *J Hum Nutr Diet*. 2013;26:315–328.

57. Singer P, Blaser AR, Berger MM, et al. ESPEN guideline on clinical nutrition in the intensive care unit. *Clin Nutr*. 2019;38(1):48–79.
58. Fiaccadori E, Sabatino A, Barazzoni R, et al. ESPEN guideline on clinical nutrition in hospitalized patients with acute or chronic kidney disease (E-pub ahead of print). *Clin Nutr*. 2021 Feb 9;S0261-5614(21):00052-2 https://doi.org/10.1016/j.clnu.2021.01.028. PMID: 33640205.
59. KDIGO. Clinical practice guidelines for acute kidney injury Kidney International Supplements 2, 1. 2012. Available at https://kdigo.org/wp-content/uploads/2016/10/KDIGO-2012-AKI-Guideline-English.pdf. Accessed September 22, 2021.
60. Oh WC, Mafrici B, Rigby M, et al. Micronutrient and amino acid losses during renal replacement therapy for acute kidney injury. *Kidney Int Rep*. 2019;4(8):1094–1108.

CHAPTER 10

Nutrition in Musculoskeletal and Disability Medicine

Minha Rajput-Ray ■ David Armstrong

LEARNING POINTS

By the end of this chapter, you should be able to:

- Describe musculoskeletal metabolism and the burden of disease
- Understand dietary choices for osteoporosis in a postmenopausal woman
- Describe the relationship between vitamin D and bone health
- Understand how the multifactorial aspects of coeliac disease affect musculoskeletal health
- Describe how lifestyle factors (smoking, alcohol) may affect musculoskeletal health
- Explain the effects that eating disorders can have on musculoskeletal health

CASE STUDY 10.1 Dietary Choices for Osteoporosis in a Postmenopausal Woman

A 55-year-old postmenopausal woman with osteoporosis and history of fracture is concerned about repeated fracture risk. She is intolerant of oral calcium supplements, stating that 'it gives her a chalky taste and a sore stomach' and states that she did not want to take dairy produce. Her vitamin D level is noted to be 20 nmol/L. She is given information about dietary calcium sources, including nondairy products, and encouraged to take vitamin D supplements. After dual energy X-ray absorptiometry (DEXA) scanning and calculation of FRAX (Fracture Risk Assessment Tool) score, it is also recommended that she takes a weekly bisphosphonate tablet.

Discussion Points

- Adequate calcium and vitamin D intake are essential for good bone health. The UK RNI (Reference Nutrient Intake) for calcium is 700 mg per day. Many specialists and guidelines recommend 700–1200 mg for patients with osteoporosis.
- While it is possible to obtain sufficient calcium from the diet alone, many patients are prescribed a calcium and vitamin D supplement to ensure compliance. Some people find these supplements are unpalatable or that they cause gastrointestinal upset.
- Refer to the BDA food fact sheet on calcium for more information on achieving dietary requirements: https://www.bda.uk.com/uploads/assets/b1f5f83d-fdd0-41be-b7ef16c174fdcbc8/Calcium2017-food-fact-sheet.pdf.

Dairy produce is an excellent source of calcium (e.g., 200 mg in a glass of milk, 50 mg in a tablespoon of yoghurt; cheese, rice pudding and custard are also popular dairy sources). There are, however, many excellent nondairy sources of calcium including baked beans, sardines, tofu, figs, nuts, tahini (sesame) paste and leafy vegetables (kale, okra, and spinach).

There is a lot of useful information for patients about calcium intake from the Royal Osteoporosis Society website, https://theros.org.uk/, and an excellent online calculator at https://www.cgem.ed.ac.uk/research/

Drug doses as per British National Formulary

CASE STUDY 10.1 Dietary Choices for Osteoporosis in a Postmenopausal Woman—(Continued)

rheumatological/calcium-calculator/, from the University of Edinburgh. Additional advice is available from the British Dietetic Association https://www.bda.uk.com/ and the Vegan Society https://www.vegansociety.com/.

Several large meta-analyses have shown that increasing calcium alone does not increase bone density or reduce fracture risk. There is, however, good evidence for combination of calcium and vitamin D to increase bone mineral density (BMD) and reduce risk of fractures. This is especially true in certain high-risk groups such as older people living in residential care. Calcium supplements should therefore always be combined with vitamin D. Some studies have suggested correlations between increased all-cause mortality, heart disease and high calcium intakes, especially in men, but this remains controversial, especially in terms of establishing causation. It is fair to say though there is no need for extra supplemental calcium in subjects with a good dietary intake. Dairy produce remains an excellent source of calcium, protein, fat and calories, as well as other micronutrients, in vulnerable groups, especially the elderly.

CASE STUDY 10.2 Vitamin D and Bone Health

An 82-year-old woman who lives in a care home is assessed for general frailty. Her serum vitamin D level is found to be 10 ng/mL, severely deficient. Her Clinical Frailty Score is assessed as 4, vulnerable. She is referred to a local community team who arranges a full review including falls assessment, nutrition review and physiotherapy. She is prescribed 4000 IU of cholecalciferol (vitamin D3) daily for 10 weeks, after which she continues with 800 IU daily. Her dietary calcium intake is improved with the addition of extra dairy produce. Her general physical health slowly improves over the next 6 months.

Discussion Points

- Vitamin D is essential for good health, including bone and muscle strength, immune function and the neurological system.
- Low vitamin D is associated specifically with rickets in children and osteomalacia in adults; deficiency is common in patients with osteoporosis as well. Deficiency is also associated with muscle weakness, increased risk of falls and general frailty.

Several different regimes are used to correct deficiency. Most involve loading the patient with up to 300,000 IU vitamin D3 over 6–12 weeks, depending on other clinical conditions, choice and availability of different preparations. There is no evidence that single megadoses of vitamin D, for example, 100,000 IU or more, offer any benefit. UK National Health Service recommendations are that everyone considers taking 400 IU vitamin D from October to the end of March, as it is difficult to make adequate vitamin D in the skin during these months even with good sunlight exposure. Some people, such as those in residential care or who seldom go outdoors, or who cover their skin when outdoors or who have darker skin, are advised to take 400 IU throughout the year. However, many specialists recommend 800 IU in patients with frailty or bone or muscle disease, and in the United States the recommendation is 1000 IU (National Institutes of Health). Some patients require higher doses of vitamin D to achieve normal levels. These include those with obesity or malabsorption and people taking drugs such as antiepileptic medication, corticosteroids and some cancer treatments. Increasing dietary intake of foods rich in vitamin D can be helpful, such as cod liver oil, mushrooms, oily fish and fortified cereals, but cannot reverse severe deficiency.

A small number of patients will experience hypercalcaemia when vitamin D levels are corrected, because they were suffering from 'hidden' primary hyperparathyroidism, but for most patients with high parathyroid hormone (PTH) levels and low vitamin D, the hyperparathyroidism will remit once the vitamin D is corrected. Persistent hyperparathyroidism or hypercalcaemia should be investigated in the usual way by a physician.

- Patients who observe a strict vegan diet should be offered plant-based vitamin D2 (ergocalciferol) rather than animal-derived vitamin D3 (cholecalciferol).
- There is emerging evidence that correcting vitamin D deficiency improves muscle strength and reduces the risk of falls, although some controversies remain. It may be especially useful in elderly patients in this respect.
- As vitamin D is a fat-soluble vitamin, absorption is enhanced if it is taken with meals which will usually contain sources of dietary fat.

CASE STUDY 10.3 Multifactorial Aspects of Coeliac Disease Affecting Musculoskeletal Health

A 44-year-old man presents with insidious back pain. He reports no significant history of trauma other than 'knocks and bumps' in his occupation as a manual worker. He is diagnosed with an insufficiency fracture in L5. Further exploration of the history reveals a 3-year duration of gastrointestinal symptoms (diarrhoea, weight loss). Investigations also reveal anaemia related to folate deficiency and osteopenia on DEXA scan. Blood testing shows antitransglutaminase and antigliadin antibodies, and intestinal biopsy at endoscopy shows partial villous atrophy and inflammation. He is diagnosed with coeliac disease and referred to a registered dietitian, who advises him on a gluten-free diet. He is also noted to be deficient in vitamin D. An osteoporosis specialist recommends calcium and vitamin D supplementation and repeat of the DEXA after 2 years on a coeliac compliance diet.

Discussion Points

- Coeliac disease is a systemic autoimmune condition, not a 'food intolerance.'
- The body produces antibodies to gluten and other proteins in a range of foods including barley, wheat, oats and rye, which leads to inflammation in the small intestine, damage to the villi involved in absorption and chronic malabsorption.
- Many patients have had symptoms for years before diagnosis, and vitamin D deficiency, low BMD or even fracture may be the presenting sign. Coeliac disease should always be considered in younger patients with osteoporosis.
- While correction of calcium and vitamin D deficiency is important, the main treatment for the condition is strict observation of a gluten-free diet. Correction of nutritional deficiency, together with weight gain, can often cause increases in BMD without the need for bisphosphonates or other pharmaceutical intervention in the short term. Most patients are followed up at specialist Coeliac Disease clinics with DEXA scanning (https://www.coeliac.org.uk/).
- Body mass index (BMI): Many patients have low BMI, which is an independent risk for low bone density.
- Vitamin deficiency: Fat malabsorption may cause vitamin deficiencies including D and K. Calcium absorption may also be poor.
- Secondary hyperparathyroidism mobilises calcium from bone tissue to maintain serum levels, further reducing BMD.
- Chronic systemic inflammation: Circulating cytokines are associated with systemic inflammation, such as tumour necrosis factor alpha, and drive osteoclast-mediated bone loss. This is seen in other inflammatory conditions as well, including inflammatory bowel disease, rheumatoid arthritis and lupus.

CASE STUDY 10.4 Lifestyle Factors (Smoking, Alcohol) and Musculoskeletal Health

A 43-year-old man, who previously worked as a labourer on building sites but who has been unemployed for about 5 years, fractures his ankle in a fall after drinking 10 pints of beer over a 4-hour period. A review of his lifestyle reveals heavy daily alcohol consumption and smoking and poor diet including very little protein.

He is referred to the Fracture Liaison Service at his local hospital, where DEXA scan shows BMD in the osteopenia range, and he has a BMI of 22. After basic workup, he is referred for further investigation of raised liver enzymes, thought to be related to his alcohol intake. His calculated FRAX score is high enough for drug therapy to be recommended. He is offered referral to alcohol addiction and smoking cessation services but refuses both. He agrees to attend annually for an infusion of bisphosphonate but is told he must attend the dentist first for assessment, which he is reluctant to do.

He is referred to the hospital dietitian, whom he attends, and is given advice on increasing his intake of fruit and vegetables, protein, calcium and vitamin D. He is prescribed a calcium and vitamin D supplement, a multivitamin supplement and thiamine. He does not attend for review.

Discussion Points

- Tobacco smoking increases the risk of osteoporosis, fracture and poor healing after fracture. Smoking cessation is associated with a rise in BMD, partially related to increase in weight.
- Studies have shown that compared with complete abstinence, moderate alcohol consumption may be associated with a decreased risk of fracture, although similar findings are not seen in animal studies and there are possible confounders.

CASE STUDY 10.4 Lifestyle Factors (Smoking, Alcohol) and Musculoskeletal Health—(Continued)

- High alcohol intake is linked with increased risk of both osteoporosis and fracture, especially in younger subjects who may fail to reach peak bone mass and produce poorer quality bone.
- Heavy chronic alcohol consumption is associated with liver disease, which results in failure to properly convert hydroxylate cholecalciferol to 25-hydroxy vitamin D (calcidiol), and pancreatic disease leads to malabsorption of fat and thus a range of major and micronutrients including vitamin D and vitamin K. This contributes to poor bone health.
- More severe liver disease is also associated with hypogonadism in men and women, with falling levels of testosterone and oestrogen both contributing to increase bone loss and osteoporosis.
- Chronic heavy alcohol consumption can also contribute to nerve damage via deficiency of vitamin B1 (thiamine) and vitamin B12, increasing the risk of falls.
- Micronutrient deficiency is common in patients with poor diet and malabsorption leading to chronic malnutrition. Trace elements known to be important for bone health include boron (increases osteogenesis, regulates sex hormone production and prolongs vitamin D half-life), magnesium (regulates calcium hydroxyapatite crystal structure, regulates PTH and vitamin D function and reduces systemic inflammation), zinc (promotes osteoblast activity, reduces osteoclast function, and inhibits RANKL), copper, selenium and silicon.
- Some patients will not engage with services to help with addiction issues. Some will be willing to take a treatment or medication, but not be willing to modify their behaviour or lifestyle. Patient education, understanding and support are vital in addressing these issues.

CASE STUDY 10.5 Eating Disorder and Musculoskeletal Health

A 21-year-old woman presented weighing 45 kg and had a BMI of 16.5. Records suggested weight loss of around 15 kg over the previous year, and she had attended her general practitioner to discuss stress caused by exams and the death of a relative. She ran twice a day and admitted to skipping meals. She did not perceive herself to be underweight. DEXA scan showed low bone density for her age. Vitamin D levels was 35 nmol/L, in the insufficiency range. The diagnosis of an eating disorder was made, and she was referred to a specialist clinic, where she received psychological as well as nutritional support, including calcium and vitamin D supplementation. She gained 12 kg in weight over the next 2 years and developed a regular meal pattern. However, while out running she suffered a fracture of her metatarsal. Repeat DEXA showed no improvement in her BMD, although her vitamin D level was now normal. At the osteoporosis clinic, it was determined that she had not had a menstrual period for 3 years, and levels of oestrogen and testosterone were found to be low, in a prepubertal range. The risks and benefits of oestrogen replacement were discussed, and eventually a transdermal patch was prescribed. At follow-up in a further 2 years, BMD had increased by 15% but was still low for her age. She had no further fractures.

Discussion Points

- Low bone density is common in anorexia nervosa. Fractures related to excessive exercise, such as in the metatarsal bones, are sometimes seen.
- The causes of low bone density are complex and include the reduced weight bearing on bones due to low lean body mass, hypothalamic hypogonadotrophism, with loss of the normal suppressive effects of oestrogen on osteoclast mediated bone loss, and resistance to growth hormone. Vitamin D deficiency is common, and calcium intake may be low.
- Anorexia often presents in adolescent or young adult women, at a time when the rate of bone accrual is maximum, and therefore can dramatically affect peak bone mass.
- Improvement in total body weight alone is usually not enough to produce significant improvement in BMD, unless the menstrual cycle returns, as normal menstrual cycle (with oestrogen suppression of osteoclast activity) is crucial to reducing bone loss.
- Bisphosphonate use is generally not appropriate in young women, especially in those who have not yet reached peak bone mass, except for extreme or unusual cases. Supplementation with calcium and vitamin D, however, is widely recommended.
- Oestrogen replacement in the form of transdermal patch has been shown to improve BMD in anorexia but remains an individual choice in eating disorders; results from the oral contraceptive pill are mixed. However, most cases do not see a complete catch-up to normal bone density, and the patient will be at risk of osteoporosis and fragility fractures in later life.
- Exercise generally has a positive effect on bone health, but overexercise may be used to control weight and lead to amenorrhoea again. A balance must therefore be achieved.

Overview of Musculoskeletal Metabolism

BONE TISSUE, OSTEOPOROSIS AND FRACTURE RISK

Bone is living tissue and undergoes constant turnover. It comprises mainly protein (in the form of collagen) and calcium (in the form of calcium phosphate crystals, or calcium hydroxyapatite), although many other trace elements and minerals are important for healthy calcified tissue. Calcium crystals adhere to the collagen matrix and make up 60%–70% of bone by mass.

Bone matrix is produced by osteoblast cells and then calcified. Calcified bone tissue is resorbed by osteoclasts which adhere to the surface, establishing a turnover cycle. Osteoblasts and osteoclasts communicate via complex mechanisms including RANK ligand and osteoprotegerin.

Regulation of bone turnover is influenced by many factors including sex hormones, PTH, serum calcium levels, vitamin D, vitamin K, iron and a range of nutritional and lifestyle factors. The final clinical picture arising from the relationships between these factors can be quite complex. For example, high levels of iron, in overload conditions such as haemochromatosis, can result in oxidative stress leading to excess bone loss and osteoporosis; on the other hand, iron deficiency anaemia is also associated with low bone density, through effects on collagen, vitamin D metabolism and tissue hypoxia.

Vitamin D has two main forms, D_2 (ergocalciferol) and D_3 (cholecalciferol), that differ chemically in their side-chain structures. Both forms are well absorbed in the small intestine, through simple passive diffusion and intestinal membrane carrier proteins. The concurrent presence of fat in the gut enhances vitamin D absorption. Vitamin D promotes absorption of calcium from the gut and reduces urinary calcium loss. By maintaining serum calcium in the normal range, production of PTH is suppressed, and thus PTH-mediated bone resorption of calcium is attenuated. Low vitamin D levels can be associated with secondary hyperparathyroidism and mobilisation of calcium stores from the bone to maintain levels in the blood, and thus reduced bone mineral density (Table 10.1).

Vitamin K is vital in the carboxylation of osteocalcin, a protein produced by osteoblasts and important in the control of production and mineralisation of bone tissue, as well as other metabolic functions. Uncarboxylated osteocalcin is associated with low vitamin K, higher bone turnover and lower BMD.

The role of other major nutritional factors is discussed in the clinical cases.

Density of bone steadily increases through childhood, accelerating under the influence of sex hormones at puberty, and reaches a peak around the age of 25 (this tends to be higher in male than female subjects). Oestrogen has an important role in maintaining bone health in both men and women, acting as a potent inhibitor of bone turnover and thus bone loss. When oestrogen levels fall at menopause, women can lose bone density quite rapidly, and the risk of fracture increases. Men with normal testosterone levels but deficient oestrogen production related to rare conditions

TABLE 10.1 ■ **Definitions of Vitamin D Status**

Status	Serum 25(OH)D Concentration	
Severe vitamin D deficiency	<30 nmol/L	<12 ng/mL
Vitamin D deficiency	<50 nmol/L	<20 ng/mL
Vitamin D Sufficiency	>50 nmol/L	>20 ng/mL

Source: From Amrein K, Scherkl M, Hoffmann M, et al. Vitamin D deficiency 2.0: an update on the current status worldwide. *Eur J Clin Nutr* 2020;741498–1513. Available at: https://www.nature.com/articles/s41430-020-0558-y.

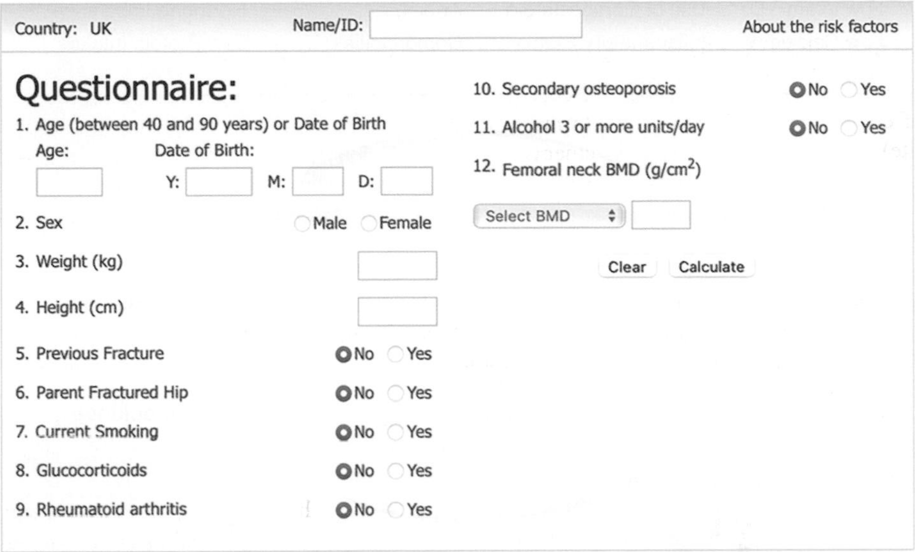

Country: UK Name/ID: About the risk factors

Questionnaire:

1. Age (between 40 and 90 years) or Date of Birth
   Age: Date of Birth: Y: M: D:
2. Sex Male Female
3. Weight (kg)
4. Height (cm)
5. Previous Fracture No Yes
6. Parent Fractured Hip No Yes
7. Current Smoking No Yes
8. Glucocorticoids No Yes
9. Rheumatoid arthritis No Yes
10. Secondary osteoporosis No Yes
11. Alcohol 3 or more units/day No Yes
12. Femoral neck BMD (g/cm^2)

Select BMD

Clear Calculate

Fig. 10.1 Online FRAX calculation tool. Source: National Osteoporosis Society. Fracture risk assessment tool. Available at: https://www.sheffield.ac.uk/FRAX/tool.aspx?country=1.

tend to have lower bone density, and in later life, male bone density correlates better with their levels of oestrogen than testosterone. Treatments which switch off the action of oestrogen and testosterone, such as long term medication for breast or prostate cancer, tend to have a strongly negative effect on bone density.

Low bone density is associated with higher risk of fracture. BMD is commonly measured by the process of DEXA, essentially a measure of how much radiation is absorbed by bone tissue exposed to a known small amount of radiation. Osteoporosis is defined as having BMD at either the hip or the lumbar spine more than 2.5 standard deviations below the average peak bone mass for a 25-year old, or a T score of <-2.5 on DEXA scanning. Although BMD on DEXA provides a good estimate of fracture risk, other factors are involved. Many patients will suffer fractures even with T scores greater then −2.5, while others with much lower BMD will not necessarily suffer from fractures, an observation that reflects the other factors related to bone quality as well as quantity. Such factors include the elasticity of the tissue and external risk factors such as frequency of falls. In recent years, an algorithm known as the FRAX score has been developed at the University of Sheffield (UK) to incorporate independent risk factors for fracture, including family history, previous fracture, tobacco and alcohol use, BMI, corticosteroid use and other comorbidities (Fig. 10.1). This produces a 10-year risk prediction for major osteoporotic fracture and specifically for hip fracture. The FRAX score is now widely used to guide management and can incorporate data from specific cohorts from most countries in the world.

MUSCLE TISSUE AND SARCOPENIA

Muscles and bones are intrinsically linked in terms of anatomy, development, function and nutritional health (Fig. 10.2). Both develop from the mesenchymal stem cell, and the attachment of muscles to bone on either side of a joint is essential to produce movement. Muscle cells (myocytes) contain numerous myofibrils made up of proteins including actin and myosin. Actin and myosin

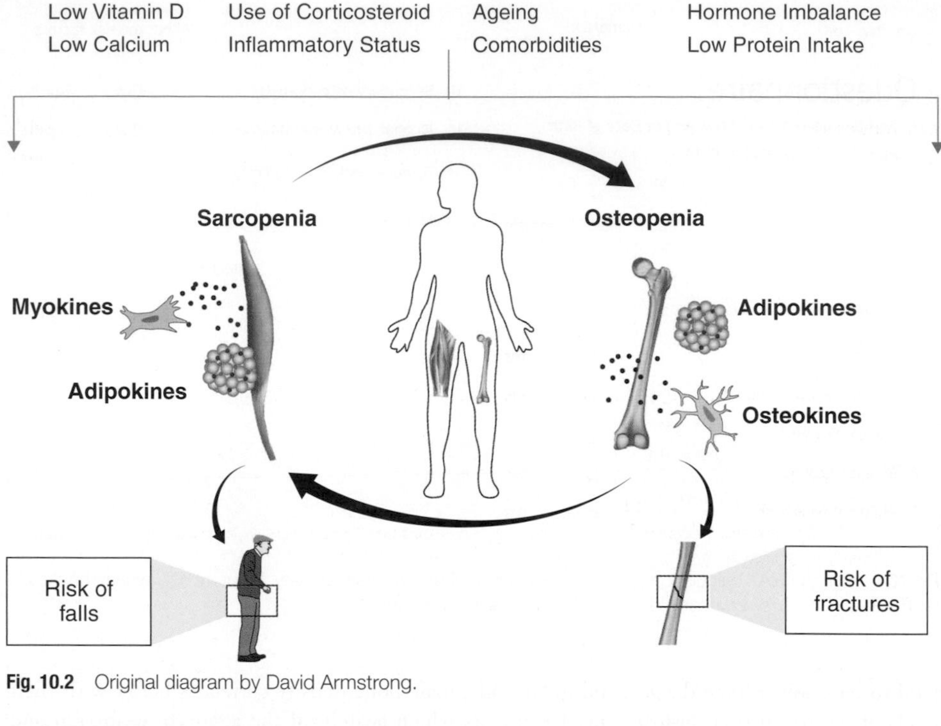

Fig. 10.2 Original diagram by David Armstrong.

TABLE 10.2 ■ **List of Food Rich in Vitamin D**

• Oily fish, like herring, salmon and mackerel
• Eggs
• Some pork products
• Lamb's liver
• Fortified bread
• Fortified yoghurts
• Specially processed mushrooms

Source: From Royal Osteoporosis Society. Vitamin D-rich food chooser. Available at: https://theros.org.uk/information-and-support/bone-health/vitamin-d-for-bones/vitamin-d-rich-food-chooser/.

slide past each other in an energy-dependent process involving the movement of calcium ions, causing the myocyte (and hence muscle) to contract and relax.

Many lifestyle and nutritional factors have similar effects on both muscle and bone tissue. Loss of muscle mass, known as sarcopenia, is associated with reduced power and often found in conjunction with osteopenia. While some regulators of bone and muscle health are specific to one tissue or the other, others, including adipokines derived from adipose tissue, can affect both. Protein intake is important for healthy muscle development, as it is for bone health, and negative nitrogen balance (when nitrogen loss exceeds intake) is associated with muscle loss. Protein supplements are often taken by those wishing to increase muscle mass and power, usually in association with physical exercise.

Vitamin D deficiency is associated with proximal muscle weakness and an increased risk of falls, and there is increasing evidence that supplementing vulnerable patients with vitamin D can reduce this risk. Glucocorticoid use can result in loss of both bone and muscle mass, with increased risk of both falls and fracture. Obesity, and the body habitus associated with secondary Cushing syndrome, can mask sarcopenia in some medical patients who have been taking steroids for years, and therefore both low muscle and bone mass should be considered in patients taking prescribed steroids in the long term, even with high BMI.

BOX 10.1 Summary of Key Points

- Bone is a living tissue and regulation of its turnover is influenced by many factors, such as sex hormones, parathyroid hormone, calcium, vitamin D, vitamin K, and iron levels, and a range of nutritional and lifestyle factors.
- Bone density highly falls in later life and more rapidly in females after menopause (due to the decreasing in oestrogen levels).
- Osteoporosis is defined as having bone mineral density at the hip or the lumbar spine more than 2.5 standard deviations below the average peak bone mass (e.g., for a 25-year-old woman on dual energy X-ray absorptiometry scanning, a T score of <−2.5.
- Protein intake is crucial for healthy muscle and bone development, and sarcopenia is low muscle mass, associated with reduced power.
- The burden of disability on musculoskeletal disorders as measured in terms of daily adjusted life-years is immense, from loss of independence and ability to manage daily tasks, to effects on employment and contribution to society.

Further Reading

Amrein K, Scherkl M, Hoffmann M, et al. Vitamin D deficiency 2.0: an update on the current status worldwide. *Eur J Clin Nutr* 2020;741498–1513. Available at: https://www.nature.com/articles/s41430-020-0558-y.

Compston J, Cooper A, Cooper C, et al. UK clinical guideline for the prevention and treatment of osteoporosis. *Arch Osteoporos*. 2017;12:43. https://doi.org/10.1007/s11657-017-0324-5.

Hsu E. Plant-based diets and bone health: sorting through the evidence. *Curr Opin Endocrinol Diabetes Obes*. 2020;27:248–252. https://doi.org/10.1097/MED.0000000000000552.

Maurel DB, Boisseau N, Benhamou CL, Jaffre C. Alcohol and bone: review of dose effects and mechanisms. *Osteoporos Int*. 2012;23:1–16. https://doi.org/10.1007/s00198-011-1787-7.

Micic D, Rao VL, Semrad CE. Celiac disease and its role in the development of metabolic bone disease. *J Clin Densitom*. 2020;23:190–199. https://doi.org/10.1016/j.jocd.2019.06.005.

Rizzoli R, Bischoff-Ferrari H, Dawson-Hughes B, Weaver C. Nutrition and bone health in women after the menopause. *Womens Health (Lond)*. 2014;10:599–608. https://doi.org/10.2217/whe.14.40.

Royal Osteoporosis Society. Vitamin D-rich food chooser. Available at: https://theros.org.uk/information-and-support/bone-health/vitamin-d-for-bones/vitamin-d-rich-food-chooser/.

Shams-White MM, Chung M, Du M, et al. Dietary protein and bone health: a systematic review and meta-analysis from the National Osteoporosis Foundation. *Am J Clin Nutr*. 2017;105:1528–1543. https://doi.org/10.3945/ajcn.116.145110.

Steinman J, Shibli-Rahhal A. Anorexia nervosa and osteoporosis: pathophysiology and treatment. *J Bone Metab*. 2019;26:133–143. https://doi.org/10.11005/jbm.2019.26.3.133.

van den Heuvel EGHM, Steijns JMJM. Dairy products and bone health: how strong is the scientific evidence? *Nutr Res Rev*. 2018;31:164–178. https://doi.org/10.1017/S095442241800001X.

CHAPTER 11

Nutrition in Haematology and Oncology

Pauline Douglas ■ Breanna Lepre ■ Laura Keaver

LEARNING POINTS

By the end of this chapter, you should be able to:

- Describe the role of nutrition in the prevention and management of cancer
- Describe evidence-based strategies for the management of nutritional anaemias
- Identify effects of cancer cachexia and describe pharmacological treatment
- List common nutrition-impact symptoms in the management of cancer
- Describe practical tips to mitigate common nutrition-impact symptoms in the management of cancer
- Demonstrate awareness of cancer survivorship as a distinct and important phase of the cancer journey

CASE STUDY 11.1 Nutritional Considerations in Radiotherapy

A 45-year-old man who has started receiving radiotherapy for head and neck cancer presents with the following:

Anthropometry	**Weight: 58.3 kg** **Weight (6 months ago): 67.2 kg** **Height: 1.74 m**	
Biochemistry	Na: K: Urea: Creatinine: Albumin:	**156 mmol/L** **4.4 mmol/L** **31.3 mmol/L** **263 μmol/L** **29 g/L**
Clinical		**Mucositis**

CASE STUDY 11.1 Nutritional Considerations in Radiotherapy—(Continued)

Dietary	Breakfast 2–3 spoons porridge made with skimmed milk Half cup of tea with skimmed milk Midmorning snack Half cup of tea with skimmed milk Lunch Few spoons of soup ½ slice of white bread Midafternoon snack Small milk pudding Dinner Minced steak with gravy Few spoons of mashed potatoes Little mashed carrot Evening Half cup of tea with skimmed milk Rich tea biscuit
	Other dietary information: No reported dislikes
Environmental	Lives alone
Functional	Increasing fatigue

Nutritional considerations. Weight loss: 13% of body weight in 6 months.
His current body mass index (BMI) is now 19 kg/m^2.
He has just started radiotherapy. How may this be affecting his intake? What would be the reason? How might this change as time goes on? What treatment might you consider offsetting his risks?
The nutritional impact symptoms are only starting to be evident with mucositis. Some weeks after the end of radiation his ability to eat may be significantly adversely affected. Note his altered biochemistry. His dietary intake is poor and will deteriorate. Need to ascertain dietary patterns before treatment and work with the client to help increase intake. Refer to Table 11.4. Consider social care referral and support. Also consider enteral feeding knowing that the effects of radiation will further impact his nutritional intake.

CASE STUDY 11.2 Nutritional Considerations in Mixed Anaemia (B12 and Intrinsic Factor Deficiency)

Sarah is a 38-year-old woman, who reported feeling nauseated and tired, and presented with the following:

Anthropometry	Weight: 51.1 kgs Weight (6 months ago): Unsure Height: 1.61 m BMI is 19.7 kg/m^2

Continued

CASE STUDY 11.2 Nutritional Considerations in Mixed Anaemia (B12 and Intrinsic Factor Deficiency)—(Continued)

Biochemistry	Red blood cells: 3.01 trillion cells/L White blood cells: 3.9 billion cells/L Platelet count: 131 × 10^9/L Haemoglobin: 5.2 g/dL Mean Corpuscular Volume: 112 fL Na: 140 mmol/L K: 4.4 mmol/L Urea: 4.5 mmol/L Creatinine: 0.70 mg/dL Albumin: 3.8 g/dL Homocysteine: 10 µmol/L Vitamin B12: 130 pg/mL Serum ferritin: 80 µg/L Serum folate: 3.1 ng/mL Bilirubin: 59 µmol/L
Clinical	Iron deficiency (5 years ago)
Dietary	**Breakfast** Cup of full-fat dairy free milk 1 slice of white bread Tablespoon of margarine (Nuttelex) **Midmorning snack** Cup of coffee with full-cream dairy free milk 2–3 salt and vinegar–flavoured rice cakes **Lunch** 2 slices of white bread ½ cup lettuce Vegan lentil patty (premade) 1 tablespoon eggless mayonnaise **Midafternoon snack** Apple, fresh, medium-sized **Dinner** 1 cup white pasta ½ cup tinned tomatoes ½ cup (raw) mushrooms ½ cup (raw) eggplant Tablespoon extra-virgin olive oil ½ clove of garlic **Evening** Cup of tea with full-cream dairy free milk Orange, fresh, sliced, medium
	Other dietary information: Vegan for 6 months
Environmental	Lives alone, single with no children Works as an architect in a busy office setting, mostly sitting down Lifetime nonsmoker, alcohol in small quantities
Functional	Nausea, fatigue, shortness of breath on exercise, yellow tinge to skin, possible weight loss (clothes feel loose)

What laboratory values are of concern? How might her habits be affecting these findings? What other investigations would you request? What are the hallmarks of the mixed diagnosis?

Consider food-based recommendations to increase the dietary diversity and nutrient quality of Sarah's diet. Further relevant information can be found throughout this chapter.

Introduction

ONCOLOGY

Cancer is defined as a group of diseases characterised by uncontrolled cellular growth. Cell and tissue division, differentiation and cell death are normally carefully regulated processes in the human body. Cancer can occur when a single cell has lost control of the balance between cell proliferation, death and differentiation. These abnormal cells can damage or invade surrounding tissue or spread to other parts of the body.

Cancers may be categorised into five basic types based on the cell of origin (Table 11.1). Cancer causes one in eight deaths worldwide and has now overtaken cardiovascular disease (CVD) as the leading cause of death in some parts of the world.[1] There were 17 million new cases of cancer and 9.6 million deaths from cancer worldwide in 2018, affecting populations in all countries and all regions. Approximately 70% of deaths from cancer occur in low- and middle-income countries.[2]

The most common cancers as of 2018 are lung (2.09 million cases), breast (2.09 million cases) and colorectal (1.80 million cases). The most common causes of cancer death are cancers of the lung (1.76 million deaths), colorectal system (862,000 deaths) and stomach (783,000 deaths).[2] By 2040, the global burden of cancer is expected to rise to 27.5 million new cases of cancer each year and 16.3 million cancer deaths.[3] The region of sub-Saharan Africa is projected to have a more than 85% increase in cancer incidence by 2030.[4]

The economic burden of cancer is significant on both individual and societal levels and is projected to increase in the future. The total cost of cancer in 2030, including direct medical costs, nonmedical costs and income losses, is projected to be $458 billion.[5] The economic burden of cancer poses a challenge to patients, their families, communities and governments internationally.

An individual's risk of developing cancer depends on many factors. Major risk factors for cancer worldwide include tobacco and alcohol use, poor diets (diets low in fruits, vegetables and whole grains, as well as those which contain high amounts of fast food, red and processed meat and sugar-sweetened beverages), elevated BMI and physical inactivity. These risk factors are also shared for other noncommunicable diseases such as CVD. Around one-third of deaths from cancer are linked to behavioural and diet-related risk factors.

HAEMATOLOGY

Haematology is the specialty responsible for the diagnosis and management of diseases related to the blood, including a wide range of benign and malignant disorders of the red and white blood cells, platelets, and the coagulation system. There are multiple red blood cell disorders, including anaemia, haemoglobinopathies, haemochromatosis, red cell enzyme deficiencies and red cell membrane disorders. White blood cells make up approximately 1% of total blood volume in a

TABLE 11.1 ■ **Types of Cancer**

Carcinomas	Arise from cells which cover external and internal body surfaces (epithelial tissue), for example, lung, breast and colon
Sarcomas	Arise from cells found in the supporting tissues of the body (connective tissues) such as muscle, bone, cartilage or fat
Lymphomas	Arise in the lymph nodes and tissues of the immune system
Leukaemias	Cancers of bone marrow, which creates blood cells
Myelomas	Arise in specific blood cells, for example B lymphocytes (B cells)

healthy adult. An unusually high or low number of white blood cells in the bloodstream can indicate a disorder. White blood cell disorders that involve neutrophils and lymphocytes are the most common (e.g., leukopenia and neutropenia). The most common types of blood disorders worldwide are haemophilia A and B and von Willebrand disease. In 2018, over 210,000 people worldwide were living with haemophilia and another 78,000 were living with von Willebrand disease. In sub-Saharan Africa, inherited haematological disorders are prevalent, due to malaria-causing *Plasmodium* parasites. Nutritional deficiencies and infections such as malaria, HIV and parasitic infections are considered common global causes of anaemia.[6]

NUTRITION AND CANCER

Nutritional factors can impact all cancer diagnoses at every stage of the disease (Fig. 11.1). The process by which normal cells mutate into invasive cancer cells and progress to clinically significant disease typically spans a period of many years. The cancer process is the result of complex interactions between diet, nutrition and physical activity, other lifestyle and environmental factors and host factors related to inheritance and prior exposure.[7] While this long latency period means that there are unlikely to be any foods or diets which cause acute or immediate effects on cancer diagnosis, there are several dietary considerations that may have a significant effect across the life course.

NUTRITION AND HAEMATOLOGY

Nutrition plays a role in the outcomes of blood-related processes.[8] Adequate nutrition enables blood coagulation, haematopoiesis and immunological functioning. Haematopoietic processes require high levels of energy; therefore, meeting nutritional needs for energy is a requirement for the fulfilment of haematopoietic processes. There are several vitamins and minerals required for normal blood formation and function, such as iron, copper, calcium, cobalt, zinc and vitamins A, C, E, K and several B vitamins. For example, calcium and Vitamin K play a key role in the activation of clotting factors II, VII, IX, X, protein C and protein S which are important for blood coagulation, while copper, iron, vitamin A, folate and B12 are required in erythropoiesis, the production of red blood cells. The roles of nutrients in key haematological processes can only be fulfilled when they are available in sufficient amounts. As inorganic elements, trace minerals are derived from diet. The majority of vitamins are derived through dietary intake although some, like vitamin K, can also synthesised within the body. Nutrient deficiencies can result in acute and

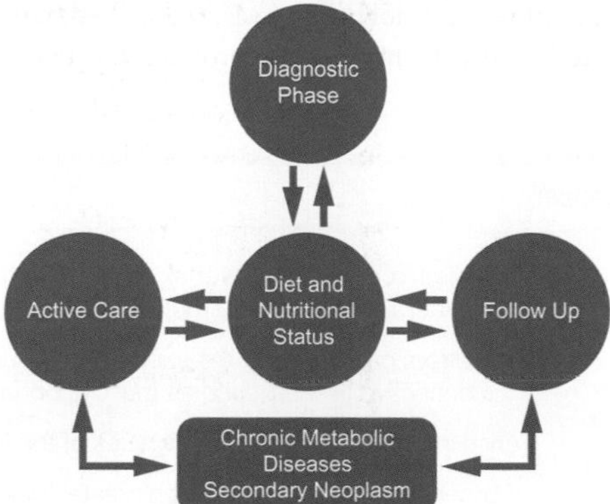

Fig. 11.1 From Nutrition and cancer. Adapted from Rosti G, Romano F, Secondino S, et al. The role of nutritional support in cured/chronic patients. *Nutrients*. 2020;12:3167.[11]

chronic conditions which require clinical management through pharmacological therapy, nutrition and patient education.[8]

Anaemia

PATHOLOGY AND DIAGNOSIS

Anaemia can be described as a reduction in the oxygen carrying capacity of the blood, caused by either a reduction in the haemoglobin concentration in the blood or a reduction in the number of circulating erythrocytes. It is estimated that 1.26 billion people globally have anaemia.[9] Anaemia develops through three main mechanisms—ineffective erythropoiesis, haemolysis and blood loss—and can be classified by the cause of the anaemia (e.g., nutritional: deficiency in iron and/or B12/folate), the morphology of red blood cells as well as the amount of haemoglobin. Nutritional deficiencies, diseases and genetic haemoglobin disorders are the most common contributors to anaemia.[8] A reduction in the oxygen-carrying capacity of red blood cells can have a significant impact on health. Signs and symptoms of anaemia are listed in Box 11.1.

INVESTIGATIONS

Pertinent points in the patient history include diet (e.g., vegetarian/vegan), nonsteroidal anti-inflammatory drug use, family history of haematologic disorders and recent potential causes of blood loss, as well as a history of gastrointestinal disease. Along with an assessment of diet and micronutrient status and the identification of aetiological factors, further evaluation can also include noninvasive screening for coeliac disease, *Helicobacter pylori* infection and autoimmune atrophic gastritis.[8,9]

Haemoglobin is known to vary by age, sex and physiological status (e.g., pregnancy). This makes defining the level at which anaemia is present difficult; however, a haemoglobin concentration below the cutoff values in Table 11.2 can be indicative of anaemia.[9]

NUTRITIONAL ANAEMIA

Nutritional anaemias can result when intake of certain nutrients is insufficient to meet demands for the synthesis of haemoglobin and erythrocytes. Iron-deficiency anaemia is the most common cause

BOX 11.1 ■ Signs and Symptoms of Anaemia

Fatigue
Pallor
Angina pectoris
Dyspnoea
Palpitations
Tachycardia
Dizziness
Insomnia
Ankle oedema
Decreased attention span
Irregular menstruation
Anorexia
Flatulence
Increased sensitivity to cold
Increased susceptibility to infection

TABLE 11.2 ■ **Haemoglobin Concentrations (Grams per Litre) for the Diagnosis of Anaemia and Assessment of Severity at Sea Level**

Population, Age	No Anaemia	Mild	Moderate	Severe
Children, 6–59 months	≥110	100–109	70–99	<70
Children, 5–11 years	≥115	110–114	80–109	<80
Children, 12–14 years	≥120	110–119	80–109	<80
Nonpregnant women, 15 years and above	≥120	110–119	80–109	<80
Pregnant women	≥110	100–109	70–99	<70
Men, 15 years and above	≥130	110–129	80–109	<80

Modified from World Health Organization. *Nutritional Anaemias: Tools for Effective Prevention and Control.* Geneva: World Health Organization; 2017.

(nutritional or otherwise) of anaemia.[8] Deficiencies of vitamins A, B2 (riboflavin), B6 (pyridoxine), B12 (cobalamin), C and E folate and copper can also result in anaemia, due to their specific roles in the production of haemoglobin or erythrocytes; whilst vitamin D deficiency does not cause anaemia per se, its presence is associated with iron-deficiency anaemia.[9] Other types of nutritional anaemia include megaloblastic anaemia, which stems from an inadequate vitamin B12 and folate supply in the body, and pernicious anaemia, whose aetiology involves antibodies to cells that synthesize intrinsic factor which is required for the absorption of vitamin B12. While inadequate dietary intake is a primary contributor to nutritional anaemia, it can also result from increased nutrient losses (e.g., haemorrhage associated with childbirth or heavy menstrual losses, which can lead to iron deficiency), impaired absorption (e.g., lack of intrinsic factor as previously mentioned diseases that affect intestinal absorption of vitamins or high intake of phytate), as well as altered nutrient metabolism (e.g., vitamin A deficiency or inflammation affecting mobilisation of iron stores).[9] There can also be pharmacological causes of nutritional anaemias (e.g., metformin and B12, oral contraceptives and B6, methotrexate and folate). These are not covered in detail within this text.

MANAGEMENT OF NUTRITIONAL ANAEMIAS

Treatment for anaemia has been shown to improve quality of life and physical condition, as well as alleviate fatigue and cognitive symptoms.[8,10] Interventions aim to address the most proximal causes of anaemia, such as poor dietary intake of haematopoietic nutrients (e.g., iron, B12 or vitamin A).[9] Interventions may include food-based strategies (e.g., to improve dietary diversity, bioavailability and intake of micronutrients), food fortification or micronutrient supplementation.[9] Social and behaviour-change communication strategies that aim to improve nutrition-related behaviour may also be considered part of the management approach (Table 11.3).

Cancer Prevention

The 10 Cancer Prevention Recommendations from the Diet, Nutrition, Physical Activity and Cancer—Third Expert Report are intended to reduce the incidence of cancer by providing evidence-based recommendations to help people to adopt and maintain a healthy lifestyle. While each individual recommendation is important in cancer prevention, the recommendations are most effective as a package of behaviours that, when applied together, promote a healthy lifestyle (Table 11.4).[7]

TABLE 11.3 ■ **Nutritional Management of Anaemia**

Food-Based Strategies	Recommendations
Dietary diversification and enhancing the bioavailability of micronutrients	• Increase the production and consumption of iron-rich foods, including meat (red meat where culturally acceptable and within safe levels), poultry and fish, but also iron-rich plant sources, such as legumes. • Increase the production and consumption of foods that are rich in vitamin A/carotenoid, such as green leafy vegetables, orange-fleshed fruits and vegetables (e.g., sweet potatoes), eggs, liver and fish oils. • Add fruits and vegetables that are rich in citric or ascorbic acids (e.g., citrus fruits) to the diet to increase the absorption of nonhaem iron. • Avoid combining known inhibitors of iron absorption with meals that are high in iron (e.g., separate tea and coffee drinking from mealtimes).
Infant and young child feeding practices (breastfeeding and complementary feeding)	• Infants should be exclusively breastfed for the first 6 months of life where possible, to achieve optimal growth and development. • After 6 months of age, infants should receive nutritionally adequate and safe complementary foods, while continuing to breastfeed for up to 2 years or beyond. • Low-birth-weight infants will need an external source of iron before 6 months of age.
Micronutrient Supplementation	**Recommendations**
Oral iron supplementation	Oral iron supplementation is readily available, inexpensive and convenient and is effective when intestinal uptake is intact. However, repletion occurs slowly with the use of oral iron supplementation, and the efficacy of oral iron is limited in some gastrointestinal conditions, such as inflammatory bowel disease, coeliac disease and autoimmune gastritis. In cases where faster repletion is desired, or where the haemoglobin level does not respond appropriately to treatment with oral iron supplementation, intravenous administration is the preferred route in the absence of infection.
Oral folic acid supplementation	Oral folic acid supplements may be used in the treatment of folate deficiency (megaloblastic) anaemia or macrocytic anaemia secondary to folic acid deficiency.
Oral iron and folic acid supplementation	Universal prenatal supplementation with iron or a combination of iron and folic acid is effective to prevent anaemia and iron deficiency at term.
Oral vitamin B12 supplementation	Oral vitamin B12 supplements may be used in the treatment of vitamin B12 deficiency and pernicious anaemia.
Intravenous iron	Intravenous iron is very effective in the treatment of iron-deficiency anaemia and should be considered when oral iron is ineffective, such as when uptake of iron through the gut is impaired or due to diminished patient compliance. Ferritin expression should increase shortly after administration and reaches higher levels than with oral iron supplementation. Intravenous iron should not be given in the setting of infection.

Continued

TABLE 11.3 ■ **Nutritional Management of Anaemia**

Food-Based Strategies	Recommendations
Intramuscular vitamin B12	Intramuscular vitamin B12 can be administered in two different forms: cyanocobalamin and hydroxocobalamin. Hydroxocobalamin is retained in the body longer and can be administered at intervals of up to 3 months. There is little difference in the cost of oral versus intramuscular vitamin B12 therapy; however, it is less convenient as it needs to be administered by a health professional.
Blood transfusion	Blood transfusion is generally restricted in chronic iron-deficiency anaemia and may be considered for patients with active bleeding who are hemodynamically unstable or for patients with critical anaemia (haemoglobin < 7 g/dL) or if all other treatments fail to correct the anaemia.

Modified from Abughaith J. The physiology of nutrition in haematology. *Int J Adv Res*. 2017;5:1424–1434 and World Health Organization. *Nutritional Anaemias: Tools for Effective Prevention and Control*. Geneva: World Health Organization; 2017.

TABLE 11.4 ■ **Recommendations from the Diet, Nutrition, Physical Activity and Cancer—Third Expert Report**

Recommendation	Goals	Additional Information
1. Be a healthy weight. Keep your weight within the healthy range and avoid weight gain in adult life.	• Ensure that body weight during childhood and adolescence projects toward the lower end of the healthy adult body mass index range. • Keep your weight as low as you can within the healthy range throughout life. • Avoid weight gain (body weight or waist circumference) throughout adulthood.	The healthy body mass index range for adults is defined by World Health Organization as 18.5–24.9 kg/m^2.
2. Be physically active. Be physically active as part of everyday life; walk more and sit less.	• Be at least moderately physically active, and follow or exceed national guidelines. • Limit sedentary habits.	Moderate physical activity is defined as any activity which increases the heart rate to about 60%–75% of its maximum.
3. Eat a diet rich in wholegrains, vegetables, fruits and beans. Make whole grains, vegetables, fruit and pulses (legumes), such as beans and lentils, a major part of your usual daily diet.	• Consume a diet that provides at least 30 g per day of fibre from food sources. • Include in most meals foods containing wholegrains, nonstarchy vegetables, fruit and pulses (legumes) such as beans and lentils. • Eat a diet high in all types of plant foods including at least five portions or servings (at least 400 g in total) of a variety of nonstarchy vegetables and fruit every day. • If you eat starchy roots and tubers as staple foods, eat nonstarchy vegetables, fruits and pulses (legumes) regularly too if possible.	

Continued

TABLE 11.4 ■ **Recommendations from the Diet, Nutrition, Physical Activity and Cancer—Third Expert Report—cont'd**

Recommendation	Goals	Additional Information
4. Limit consumption of fast foods and other processed foods high in fat, starches or sugars. Limiting these foods helps control calorie intake and maintain a healthy weight.	• Limit consumption of processed foods high in fat, starches or sugars, including fast foods, many preprepared dishes, snacks, bakery foods and desserts and confectionary (candy).	Fast foods are readily available convenience foods that are generally energy dense and have large portion sizes.
5. Limit consumption of red and processed meat. Eat no more than moderate amounts of red meat, such as beef, pork and lamb. Eat little, if any, processed meat.	• If you eat red meat, limit consumption to no more than about three portions per week (equivalent to about 350–500 g) cooked weight of red meat.	Red meat includes all types of mammalian muscle meat, such as beef, port, veal, lamb, mutton, horse and goat. The term 'processed meat refers' to meat that has been processed through salting, curing, fermentation, smoking or other processes to enhance flavour or improve shelf life.
6. Limit consumption of sugar-sweetened drinks. Drink mostly water and unsweetened drinks.	• Do not consume sugar-sweetened drinks.	Sugar-sweetened drinks are liquids sweetened by adding free sugars (e.g., sucrose, high-fructose corn syrup). This may include sugar-sweetened beverages, sports drinks, energy drinks and cordials among others.
7. Limit alcohol consumption. For cancer prevention, it's best not to drink alcohol.	• For cancer prevention, it's best not to drink alcohol. • If you do consume alcoholic drinks, do not exceed your national guidelines.	Children should not consume alcoholic drinks. Do not consume alcoholic drinks if you are pregnant.
8. Do not use supplements for cancer prevention. Aim to meet nutritional needs through diet alone.	• High-dose dietary supplements are not recommended for cancer prevention; aim to meet nutritional needs through diet alone.	A dietary supplement is defined as a product intended for ingestion that contains a dietary ingredient intended to increase consumption of micronutrients or other food components beyond what is usually achievable through diet alone. In some situations, for example, in women of childbearing age or in dietary inadequacy, supplements may be advisable. A qualified health professional can assess individual requirements as well as potential risks and benefits.

Continued

TABLE 11.4 ■ **Recommendations from the Diet, Nutrition, Physical Activity and Cancer—Third Expert Report—cont'd**

Recommendation	Goals	Additional Information
9. Breastfeed your baby, if you can. Breastfeeding is good for both mother and baby.	• The World Health Organization recommends infants be exclusively breastfed for 6 months then up to 2 years of age or beyond alongside appropriate and nutritious complementary foods.	Exclusive breastfeeding is defined as giving a baby only breastmilk and nothing else.
10. After a cancer diagnosis, cancer survivors should follow these recommendations if they can.	• All cancer survivors should receive nutritional care and support from trained professionals.	

Modified from World Cancer Research Fund/American Institute for Cancer Research. Diet, Nutrition, Physical Activity and Cancer: A Global Perspective. Continuous Update Project Expert Report 2018.

Cancer Diagnosis and Treatment

BODY WEIGHT

Overweight and obesity are defined by the World Health Organization as abnormal or excessive fat accumulation that presents a risk to health. A BMI of 25 kg/m^2 or more places a person within the overweight category while a BMI of 30 kg/m^2 or more places one within the obese category. There is consistent evidence that higher amounts of body fat are associated with increased risks of several cancers, including endometrial, liver and pancreatic cancers.[12]

It is also recognised that those with a higher BMI that are weight stable or with minimal weight loss have an increased rate of cancer survival.[13] Patients who cannot maintain their weight and have a weight loss of >2.4% have significantly reduced survival rate.[14]

BODY COMPOSITION

Cancer Cachexia

Cachexia or wasting syndrome can be diagnosed when there is an involuntary weight loss >6% over the last 6 months (in absence of starvation) *or* weight loss >2% with BMI <20 kg/m^2 or sarcopenia with a loss of skeletal muscle mass.[13] Unlike starvation in which fat stores from adipose tissue are depleted but are spared from skeletal muscle, neither fat nor protein is spared in cachexia. The loss of adipose tissue accounts for most of the weight loss but loss of muscle mass accounts for most of the morbidity and mortality. There is also higher resting energy requirement.

The cause of cachexia is multifactorial including systemic inflammation leading to changes in protein, fat, and carbohydrate metabolism.

Grip strength has been proposed as a measurement of nutritional status as the effectiveness of muscle function may be a more important determinant of survival than muscle size.

Effects of Cancer Cachexia

In cachexia, systemic proinflammatory processes are activated. See Table 11.5 which includes the impact of cytokines for which there is a related nutritional impact.

TABLE 11.5 ■ **Cytokines With Related Nutritional Impacts**

Cytokine	Affect	
Interleukin-1	Anorexia and weight loss	
Interleukin-6	Anorexia and weight loss	
Tumour necrosis factor-alpha	Anorexia and weight loss Possible increasing levels of corticotrophin-releasing hormone suppressing food intake	
Tumour lipid-mobilizing factor	Fat breakdown	Stimulation of cytokine production causing loss of appetite and decreased body weight
Proteolysis-inducing factor	Protein breakdown	
Tryptophan	Increased levels may cause nausea and reduced food intake	

An elevated C-reactive protein CRP (>10 g/L) and a decreased albumin (<35 mg/L) are considered to be an independent poor prognostic score—see The Glasgow Prognostic Score—although it is to be noted that albumin alone as a reverse acute phase reactant is not a reliable nutritional marker and prealbumin is more likely to demonstrate real-time changes reflecting undernutrition.[15]

Pharmacological Treatment of Cachexia

Eicosapentaenoic acid (EPA) is a polyunsaturated fatty acid. It has been associated with weight stabilisation in weight-losing patients with advanced cancer. EPA reduces production of cytokines interleukin (IL)-6, IL-1, and tumour necrosis factor. EPA blocks the substances produced by tumour cells such as tumour lipid-mobilising factor and proteolysis-inducing factor. These substances may stimulate cytokine production and therefore cause loss of appetite and body weight. Randomised controlled trial evidence is not definitive, and therefore it is not possible to reach any firm conclusion about optimal approaches to improve nutritional status/physical function in patients with cancer. While is it unclear if EPA prolongs survival in advanced cancer, some oral nutritional supplements now contain EPA. However, high-dose EPA requires caution due to potential side effects such as prolongation of bleeding time due to alteration of platelet function.

A recognised complication of cancer cachexia is decreased gastric and intestinal motility, which can lead to anorexia, chronic nausea, and early satiety. Metoclopramide can be used to help alleviate these symptoms, although data are sparse regarding effectiveness.

Megestrol acetate is a hormone treatment for breast and endometrial cancer, but it can also be used to stimulate appetite and promote weight gain. The increase in weight secondary to megestrol intake is associated with an increase in fat and body cell mass. The nutritional effects are dose related with a plateau in effect after 8 weeks of therapy. However, this agent (like other progestin analogues in this category) does have several side effects including alteration in menses in females.

The non-steroidal antiinflammatory drug ibuprofen has been shown to reduce the levels of IL-6 and cortisol. Research suggests ibuprofen can be used with megestrol acetate to enhance appetite.

Corticosteroid dexamethasone or prednisolone can be used for the short-term symptom management of anorexia and chronic nausea.

Sarcopenia

The prevalence of cancer increases with age, as does the prevalence of background sarcopenia which can further compound muscle loss independent of the impacts of cancer and/or the side effects of treatment.

Sarcopenic obesity can be prevalent and must be recognised. This is defined as muscle wasting that occurs alongside excess adiposity. The diagnosis of malnutrition can be difficult in sarcopenic obesity, because obesity makes it more difficult to detect the underlying muscle loss.

COMPLICATIONS OF SURGERY, RADIOTHERAPY AND CHEMOTHERAPY

Cytokines may decrease gastric motility and induce poor wound healing.

Multiple factors can affect nutritional intake after treatment for cancer, and some of them are outlined in Figure 11.2.

An individual receiving radiotherapy to the head and neck is more likely to experience mucositis, dysphagia and dysgeusia while someone with cancer of the lower gut may experience nausea and vomiting, diarrhoea and/or constipation.

NUTRITION IMPACT SYMPTOMS

For nutrition support, refer to Chapter 4.

Neutropenic Diets

There remains controversy due to limited evidence over the use of dietary restriction during immunosuppressive therapy.[16,17] Evidence of good food safety hygiene practices is emerging. An oncology dietitian will be able to provide the current evidence-based practices.

Cancer Survivorship

'Cancer survivor' can mean different things to different people. In this section we will use it to refer to those who have completed treatment and who are not under palliative care. Survival trends for cancer are generally increasing; in some countries, survival has increased by up to 5% for cancers of the liver, pancreas and lung.[18] The 5-year survival for breast cancer is over 80% in most countries.[18]

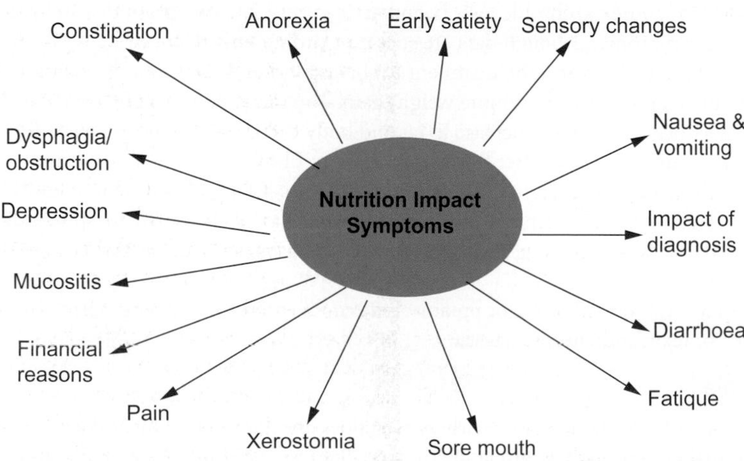

Fig. 11.2 Symptoms affecting nutrition.

These increases in survival are due to improvements in screening, as well as more effective and new cancer treatments. Five-year net survival is currently highest in the United States, Canada, Australia, New Zealand, Finland, Iceland, Norway and Sweden.[18]

Cancer survivorship is now regarded as a distinct and important phase of the cancer journey. In moving from being a 'cancer patient' to being a 'cancer survivor' there is a need to empower the individual and to improve overall awareness in relation to the importance of recovery and life with and beyond cancer. Survivors face numerous short- and long-term physical and mental health comorbidities[19] in addition to health issues brought about by the cancer, treatment received, impaired nutrition and physical status.[20]

CARDIOVASCULAR DISEASE AND PULMONARY EFFECTS

Cancer survivors are recognised as having an increased incidence of CVD risk factors, such as hypertension, diabetes, obesity and dyslipidaemia,[21,22] as well as an increased incidence of cardiovascular and pulmonary disease[23,24] compared with the general population. Cardiomyopathy, endothelial dysfunction and arrhythmias can occur due to chemotherapy induced toxicity.[24] Coronary artery disease, cardiomyopathy, arrhythmias and conduction disturbances, valvular disease and chronic pericardial disease can all occur secondary to radiotherapy induced toxicity while trastuzumab therapy (as one example of several chemotherapeutic agents, e.g., Adriamycin Doxorubicin is a classic example of an agent that can cause cardiac toxicity) is also associated with cardiac dysfunction.[24] Hypertension is a long-term consequence of many cancer therapies, including both chemotherapy and targeted agents.[25]

Prevention of future CVD includes adequate screening, continued use of antihypertensive agents, statin therapy and aspirin in persons when warranted for secondary cardiovascular prevention (often due to preexisting diagnoses), as well as lifestyle modifications such as increasing physical activity, consuming a healthy diet and weight loss as appropriate.[26] The World Cancer Research Fund (WCRF) recommendations[7] as outlined in Table 11.2 should be promoted.

Pulmonary toxicities that can occur, secondary to either chemotherapy or radiotherapy, are pulmonary fibrosis, radiation pneumonitis and an overall decrease in pulmonary function.[24] Pulmonary function tests are important for survivors; in a study of 20,483 5-year survivors of childhood cancer, survivors were 8.8 times more likely to die from a pulmonary cause.[27]

NUTRITION IMPACT SYMPTOMS

Nutrition impact symptoms can persist into survivorship and continue to have an impact on an individual's ability to eat as well as their quality of life. Fatigue, pain, and difficulty sleeping have been well documented.[28–32] Table 11.6 outlines some tips that can be provided to help alleviate some of these symptoms.

WEIGHT AND RECURRENCE

There is increasing evidence that being overweight or suffering from obesity, risk factors for numerous types of cancer, increases the risk of recurrence and decreases overall survival in those with cancer.[33–39] There is particularly strong evidence for breast cancer recurrence.[41,42] Those who are overweight should be encouraged and supported to achieve and maintain a healthy weight.

Some individuals, particularly those with breast, prostate or ovarian cancer, may experience weight gain because of their treatment. For those with breast cancer, chemotherapy has been associated with a 65% increased risk (95% confidence interval: 1.12–2.43) of significant weight gain ($\geq$5%) compared with women who did not receive chemotherapy.[40] Fewer than 10% of women who gain weight after diagnosis return to their prediagnosis weight within 6 years.[40]

TABLE 11.6 ■ **Practical Tips for Dealing With Common Side Effects Which Will Have a Nutritional Impact**

Tips for improving appetite	• Little and often: 2 small meals and 3 snacks daily • Full-fat milk[a] • Food fortification • Oral nutritional supplements • Fluids after meals • Plan meals to include favourite foods • Keep food visible and within easy reach • Energy-dense snacks, cheese and crackers, yoghurts, ready pot puddings
Advice for fatigue and early satiety	• Rest before meals • Timing of meals • Choose foods that are easy to prepare • Ready meals/freeze extra portions • Softer choices of protein, meats in casseroles, scrambled eggs, fish in sauces, dairy foods
Advice for dyspnoea	• Airway clearance • Rest before meals • Eat more slowly • Eat whilst sitting up • 5–6 small meals • Liquids after meals • Ready meals • Evaluate for O_2 supplementation • Pursed lip breathing
Advice for xerostomia (dry mouth)	• Identify and treat cause of dry mouth • Chew food well • Plenty of sauces/gravy with hot meals • Soft bread, moist/spreadable fillings • Sucking ice cubes • Rinse out mouth before and after meals
Advice for mucositis/sore mouth	• Keep mouth clean • Drink plenty of fluid • Chew food well • Plenty of sauces/gravy with hot meals • Soft bread, moist/spreadable fillings • Sucking ice cubes • Softer choices of protein, meats in casseroles, scrambled eggs, fish in sauces • Rinse out mouth before and after meals
Advice for dysgeusia (altered taste)	• Keep mouth clean • Choose foods you enjoy • Try all protein sources to see which ones work best for you • Use tart/sharp foods and drinks • Add herbs and flavourings (e.g., applesauce, mint jelly) • Cold or frozen foods may taste better than hot foods • Use plastic utensils and glass cookware
Nausea and vomiting	• Dry foods • Little and often (see above) • Use convenience foods if the smell of cooking affects you • Milk, milky drinks or oral nutritional supplements
Diarrhoea and constipation	• Drink plenty of fluids • Avoid foods/drinks that may cause diarrhoea • May need to change the amount of fibre consumed

[a]There is a wide range of milk alternatives available on the market, not all of which will have the same calorie or nutrient levels

Chemotherapy is also associated with a loss in muscle mass and increase in fat stores, independent of weight changes.[41] Androgen deprivation therapy, used in prostate cancer, has also been shown to have a similar effect.[42]

It should be noted that on the other end of the spectrum, some individuals will emerge post-treatment underweight or with a compromised nutritional status. Supportive care including access to a dietitian and potentially pharmacotherapy to relieve symptoms and improve appetite may be required.[44] For these individuals, continued weight loss will impair quality of life and increase the risk of complications. In this case, the focus should be on increasing food intake to achieve a positive energy balance and thus increase weight.[43,45–47]

DIET AND RECURRENCE

While there are health benefits to eating a varied and balanced diet, it is still not clear if diet alone can prevent recurrence of cancer. There is, however, strong evidence that a diet high in plant-based foods can reduce risk of cancer overall. Many epidemiological studies have shown that individuals who consume diets high in fruit, vegetables, and whole grains and low in meat and animal fats have lower rates of some cancers, including lung, breast, colon, and stomach.[48,49] A 43% reduction in overall mortality was observed in a study of breast cancer survivors in association with a dietary pattern characterized by the high intake of vegetables and whole grains,[48] while an observational study of 1000 colorectal cancer survivors reported that a diet higher in refined grains, red and processed meat and sugar-sweetened beverages was associated with poorer overall survival and a statistically significant increase in cancer recurrence.[49] While there is a suggestion that plant-based eating may have a beneficial effect, the evidence presented is preliminary and requires further study. There are different definitions of what constitutes a plant-based diet ranging from the reduction of total meat intake to total avoidance of all animal products. In addition, there are plant-based foods that would not be healthy if they were to form a significant proportion of the diet (e.g., fruit juices, refined grains, sweets and desserts). A dietitian can help support individuals who wish to consider this type of dietary pattern.

Another element in the diet that is often mentioned as relating to cancer is sugar. A high-sugar intake has not been shown to increase the risk or progression of cancer; however, foods with a high-sugar content add substantial calories to the diet and therefore could promote weight gain.[50] They also do not contribute many nutrients to the diet and can replace more nutritious foods, therefore their intake is recommended to be limited.

NUTRITION RECOMMENDATIONS FOR CANCER SURVIVORS

The WCRF recommends that cancer survivors follow the recommendations for cancer prevention (Table 11.4).[7] The main components of the WCRF recommendations are a focus on weight management and the consumption of a healthy diet (high in fruit, vegetable, and whole grains and low in saturated fat).[7]

Misinformation and Alternative Therapies

There is a large degree of misinformation targeted at those with cancer, leading to situations where as many as 4 in 10 individuals with cancer report believing that their cancer can be cured by alternative therapies alone.[51] Unfortunately, research has shown that those who pursue alternative cancer therapies have higher mortality rates than those who undergo traditional treatment.[52] In some cases, individuals raise large amounts of money to undertake treatments and regimens that have no proven evidence base, and in many cases are dangerous,[53,54] especially in individuals that are already cachectic and losing weight. This misinformation comes from a variety of sources, including social media influencers, individuals such as celebrity doctors or health 'gurus' who have perceived medical expertise, politicians, activists, mass media and alternative medicine practitioners.[55] Their reach is further amplified by the Internet which allows for the rapid spread of misinformation, at a rate much faster than accurate information.[57] In addition, those searching for credible advice on the Internet or through apps often find recommendations that are unfounded or negligent.[56,57] Thankfully, the public trust in medical scientists does appear to be high.[58] Therefore, it is vital that doctors and allied health professionals use their trustworthiness to steer those with cancer toward therapies and lifestyle measures that are evidence based. Referring to a dietitian will help to provide credible sources of information and support health care professionals and those with cancer.

Conclusion

The role of nutrition spans across all cancer diagnoses and at every stage of the disease.

- The 10 Cancer Prevention Recommendations (Table 11.4) are a package of behaviours that, when applied together, promote a healthy lifestyle. These recommendations are also suitable for cancer survivors.
- Treatment for cancer (surgery, radiotherapy and chemotherapy) can result in symptoms which affect nutrition (Fig. 11.2).
- Adequate nutrition is indispensable in the outcomes of haematopoietic processes.
- Nutritional anaemias can result when intake of certain nutrients is insufficient to meet demands for the synthesis of haemoglobin and erythrocytes. Common types of nutritional anaemia include:
  - Iron-deficiency anaemia
  - Megaloblastic anaemia
  - Pernicious anaemia
- Nutritional management of anaemia might include food-based strategies or nutrient supplementation (e.g., oral iron supplementation).
- There is a large amount of misinformation targeted at individuals with cancer. Referring to a dietitian will help to provide credible sources of nutrition information.

References

1. Cancer today. International Agency for Research on Cancer. 2016. Available at: https://gco.iarc.fr/today/home. Accessed November 19, 2020.
2. World Health Organization *Cancer*. Geneva; 2018. https://who.int/.
3. American Cancer Society. *Global Cancer Facts & Figures* https://www.cancer.org/research/cancer-facts-statistics/global.html. 4th ed. Atlanta; 2018.
4. Morhason-Bello IO, Odedina F, Rebbeck TR, et al. Challenges and opportunities in cancer control in Africa: A perspective from the African Organisation for Research and Training in Cancer. *Lancet Oncol.* 2013;14:e142–e151.
5. World Economic Forum *The Global Economic Burden of Non-communicable Diseases*. Geneva, Switzerland; 2011. https://www3.weforum.org/docs/WEF_Harvard_HE_GlobalEconomicBurden NonCommunicableDiseases_2011.pdf.
6. McGann PT, Williams AM, Ellis G, et al. Prevalence of inherited blood disorders and associations with malaria and anemia in Malawian children. *Blood Adv.* 2018;2(21):3035–3044.
7. World Cancer Research Fund/American Institute for Cancer Research https://www.wcrf.org/wp-content/uploads/2021/02/Summary-of-Third-Expert-Report-2018.pdf. Diet, nutrition, physical activity and cancer: A global perspective. Continuous Update Project Expert Report 2018. 2018.
8. Abughaith J. The physiology of nutrition in haematology. *Int J Adv Res.* 2017;5:1424–1434.
9. World Health Organization. *Nutritional Anaemias: Tools for Effective Prevention and Control.* Geneva, Switzerland: World Health Organization; 2017.
10. Jimenez K, Kulnigg-Dabsch S, Gasche C. Management of iron deficiency anemia. *Gastroenterol Hepatol (N Y).* 2015;11(4):241–250.

11. Rosti G, Romano Secondino S, et al. The role of nutritional support in cured/chronic patients. *Nutrients.* 2020;12:3167.
12. Lauby-Secretan B, Scoccianti C, Loomis D, et al. Body fatness and cancer—viewpoint of the IARC Working Group. *N Engl J Med.* 2016;375(8):794–798. https://doi.org/10.1056/NEJMsr1606602.
13. Fearon K, Strasser F, Anker SD, et al. Definition and classification of cancer cachexia; and international consensus. *Lancet Oncol.* 2011;12(5):489–495.
14. Martin L, Senesse P, Gioulbasanis I, et al. Diagnostic criteria for the classification of cancer associated weight loss. *J Clin Oncol.* 2015;33(1):90–99.
15. Proctor MJ, Morrison DS, Talwar D, et al. An inflammation-based prognostic score (mGPS) predicts cancer survival independent of tumour site: A Glasgow Inflammation Outcome Study. *Br J Cancer.* 2011;104(4):726–734.
16. Sonbol M, Jain T, Firwana B, et al. Neutropenic diets to prevent cancer infection: updated systematic review and meta- analysis. *BMJ Support Palliat Care 2019.* 2019;9:1–9.
17. Heng MS, Gauro JB, Yaxley A, Thomas J. Does a neutropenic diet reduce adverse outcomes in patients undergoing chemotherapy? *Eur J Cancer Care 2020.* 2020;29:e13155.
18. Group CW. Global surveillance of trends in cancer survival 2000–14 (CONCORD-3): Analysis of individual records for 37 513 025 patients diagnosed with one of 18 cancers from 322 population-based registries in 71 countries. *Lancet.* 2018;391(10125):P1023–P1075. https://doi.org/10.1016/S0140-6736(17)33326-3.
19. Miller KD, Siegel RL, Lin CC, et al. Cancer treatment and survivorship statistics, 2016. *CA Cancer J Clin.* 2016;66:271–289. https://doi.org/10.3322/caac.21349.
20. Carver JR, Shapiro CL, Ng A, et al. American Society of Clinical Oncology clinical evidence review on the ongoing care of adult cancer survivors: Cardiac and pulmonary late effects. *J Clin Oncol.* 2007;25:3991–4008.
21. Armenian SH, Xu L, Ky B, et al. Cardiovascular disease among survivors of adult-onset cancer: A community-based retrospective cohort study. *J Clin Oncol.* 2016;34(10):1122.
22. Strongman H, Gadd S, Matthews A, et al. Medium and long-term risks of specific cardiovascular diseases in survivors of 20 adult cancers: A population-based cohort study using multiple linked UK electronic health records databases. *Lancet.* 2019;394(10203):1041.
23. van Laar M, Feltbower RG, Gale CP, Bowen DT, Oliver SE, Glaser A. Cardiovascular sequelae in long-term survivors of young peoples' cancer: A linked cohort study. *Br J Cancer.* 2014;110(5):1338–1441.
24. Scholz-Kreisel P, Spix C, Blettner M, et al. Prevalence of cardiovascular late sequelae in long-term survivors of childhood cancer: A systematic review and meta-analysis. *Pediatr Blood Cancer.* 2017;64(7). Epub 2017 Feb 16.
25. Ky B, Kondapalli L, Lenihan DJ. Cancer survivorship: Cardiovascular and respiratory issues, UpToDate 2020. Available at: https://bit.ly/3pbgOnd.
26. Okwuosa TM, Anzevino S, Rao R. Cardiovascular disease in cancer survivors. *Postgraduate Med J.* 2017;93:82–90.
27. Armstrong GT, Liu Q, Yasui Y, et al. Late mortality among 5-year survivors of childhood cancer: a summary from the Childhood Cancer Survivor Study. *J Clin Oncol.* 2009;27(14):2328–2338.
28. Pertl MM, Quigley J, Hevey D. "I'm not complaining because I'm alive": Barriers to the emergence of a discourse of cancer-related fatigue. *Psychol Health.* 2014;29(2):141–161.
29. Corbett T, Groarke A, Walsh JC, McGuire BE. Cancer-related fatigue in post-treatment cancer survivors: Application of the common sense model of illness representations. *BMC Cancer.* 2016;16(1):919. https://doi.org/10.1186/s12885-016-2907-8.
30. Bower JE. Behavioral symptoms in patients with breast cancer and survivors. *J Clin Oncol.* 2008;26(5):768–777. https://doi.org/10.1200/JCO.2007.14.3248.
31. Boland EG, Ahmedzai SH. Persistent pain in cancer survivors. *Curr Opin Support Palliat Care.* 2017;11(3):181–190. https://doi.org/10.1097/SPC.0000000000000292.
32. Strollo SE, Fallon EA, Gapstur SM, Smith TG. Cancer-related problems, sleep quality, and sleep disturbance among long-term cancer survivors at 9-years post diagnosis. *Sleep Med.* 2020;65:177–185.
33. McTiernan A, Irwin M. Vongruenigen V. Weight, physical activity, diet, and prognosis in breast and gynecologic cancers. *J Clin Oncol.* 2010;28:4074–4080.
34. Wright ME, Chang SC, Schatzkin A, et al. Prospective study of adiposity and weight change in relation to prostate cancer incidence and mortality. *Cancer.* 2007;109:675–684.

35. Vrieling A, Kampman E. The role of body mass index, physical activity, and diet in colorectal cancer recurrence and survival: a review of the literature. *Am J Clin Nutr*. 2010;92:471–490.
36. Siegel EM, Ulrich CM, Poole EM, Holmes RS, Jacobsen PB, Shibata D. The effects of obesity and obesity-related conditions on colorectal cancer prognosis. *Cancer Control*. 2010;17:52–57.
37. Meyerhardt JA, Niedzwiecki D, Hollis D, et al. Cancer and Leukemia Group B 89803. Impact of body mass index and weight change after treatment on cancer recurrence and survival in patients with stage III colon cancer: Findings from Cancer and Leukemia Group B 89803. *J Clin Oncol*. 2008;26:4109–4115.
38. Protani M, Coory M, Martin JH. Effect of obesity on survival of women with breast cancer: Systematic review and meta-analysis. *Breast Cancer Res Treat*. 2010;123:627–635.
39. Patterson RE, Cadmus LA, Emond JA, Pierce JP. Physical activity, diet, adiposity and female breast cancer prognosis: a review of the epidemiologic literature. *Maturitas*. 2010;66:5–15.
40. Saquib N, Flatt SW, Natarajan L, et al. Weight gain and recovery of pre-cancer weight after breast cancer treatments: evidence from the Women's Healthy Eating and Living (WHEL) study. *Breast Cancer Res Treat*. 2007;105:177–186.
41. Kutynec CL, McCargar L, Barr SI, Hislop TG. Energy balance in women with breast cancer during adjuvant treatment. *J Am Diet Assoc*. 1999;99:1222–1227.
42. Smith MR, Finkelstein JS, McGovern FJ, et al. Changes in body composition during androgen deprivation therapy for prostate cancer. *J Clin Endocrinol Metab*. 2002;87(2):599–603.
43. Ravasco P, Monteiro-Grillo I, Vidal PM, Camilo ME. Dietary counseling improves patient outcomes: a prospective, randomized, controlled trial in colorectal cancer patients undergoing radiotherapy. *J Clin Oncol*. 2005;23:1431–1438.
44. Von Roenn J. Pharmacologic interventions for cancer-related weight loss. *Oncology Issues*. 2002;17:18–21.
45. Capuano G, Gentile PC, Bianciardi F, Tosti M, Palladino A, Di Palma M. Prevalence and influence of malnutrition on quality of life and performance status in patients with locally advanced head and neck cancer before treatment. *Support Care Cancer*. 2010;18:433–437.
46. Gupta D, Lis CG, Granick J, Grutsch JF, Vashi PG, Lammersfeld CA. Malnutrition was associated with poor quality of life in colorectal cancer: a retrospective analysis. *J Clin Epidemiol*. 2006;59:704–709.
47. Hopkinson JB, Wright DN, Foster C. Management of weight loss and anorexia. *Ann Oncol*. 2008;19(suppl 7):vii289–vii293.
48. Kwan ML, Weltzien E, Kushi LH, Castillo A, Slattery ML, Caan BJ. Dietary patterns and breast cancer recurrence and survival among women with early-stage breast cancer. *J Clin Oncol*. 2009;27:919–992.
49. Meyerhardt JA, Niedzwiecki D, Hollis D, et al. Association of dietary patterns with cancer recurrence and survival in patients with stage III colon cancer. *JAMA*. 2007;298:754–764.
50. Rock CL, Doyle C, Demark-Wahnefried W, et al. Nutrition and physical activity guidelines for cancer survivors. *CA Cancer J Clin*. 2012;62(4):243–274. https://doi.org/10.3322/caac.21142.
51. Kirkwood MK, Hanley A, Bruinooge SS, et al. The state of oncology practice in America, 2018: Results of the ASCO practice census survey. *J Oncol Pract*. 2018;14(7):e412–e420.
52. Johnson SB, Park HS, Gross CP, Yu JB. Use of alternative medicine for cancer and its impact on survival. *J Natl Cancer Inst*. 2018;110(1):121–124.
53. Caulfield T., Snyder J. When crowdfunding pays for bunk medical treatments. 2019. Available at: https://policyoptions.irpp.org/magazines/january-2019/when-crowdfunding-pays-for-bunk-medical-treatments/.
54. Snyder J, Adams K, Chen YY, et al. Navigating physicians' ethical and legal duties to patients seeking unproven interventions abroad. *Can Fam Physician*. 2015;61(7):584.
55. Larson HJ. The biggest pandemic risk? Viral misinformation. *Nature*. 2018;562(7726):309–310.
56. Keaver L, Loftus A, Quinn L. A review of iPhone and Android apps for cancer patients and survivors: Assessing their quality, nutrition information and behaviour change techniques. *J Hum Nutr Diet*. 2021;34(3):572–584.
57. Keaver L, Walsh L, Callaghan H, Houlihan C. Nutrition guidance for cancer patients and survivors—a review of websites of Irish healthcare and charitable organisations and cancer centres. *Eur J Cancer Care (Engl)*. 2020;29(2).
58. Funk C. Key findings about Americans' confidence in science and their views on scientists' role in society. *Pew Research Center*. 2020 Available at. www.pewresearch.org/fact-tank/2020/02/12/key-findings-about-americans-confidence-in-science-and-their-views-on-scientists-role-in-society.

CHAPTER 12

Nutrition in Immunology, Infection and Allergy

Kaninika Basu ■ Mary Feeney

LEARNING POINTS

- Define the burden of allergic disease
- Understand the role of the immune system and different cell populations involved in allergy
- Differentiate between different types of food hypersensitivity responses, recognise their presentation and understand their diagnosis and management
- Recognise how food allergy can impact on nutrition and diet

CASE STUDY 12.1 Allergy Case Example 1

ALLERGY CASE EXAMPLE: DELAYED COW'S MILK ALLERGY IN AN INFANT

A 10-week-old male infant presents with abdominal distension, painful flatus, vomiting, loose, mucous-containing stools, poor sleep and irritability. He was tracking growth centiles for age.

Consider Early Feeding History

He was exclusively breastfed from birth until 6 weeks of age. Infant formula was then introduced alongside breastfeeds; after 3 weeks the formula was switched to a 'comfort' formula due to poor feed tolerance and increased vomiting after bottle feeds. Formula feeds were stopped 2 days prior to presentation in the clinic and he recommenced exclusive breastfeeding.

Consider Individual and Family History of Atopic Disease

Infantile colic, dry skin and cradle cap reported.
Father has asthma and allergic rhinitis. No other family history of atopy.

Consider Medications

Colic relief drops (lactase drops) trialled between 2–4 weeks of age, and comfort infant formula (partially hydrolysed, prethickened formula) trialled for 1 week (9–10 weeks of age) with no improvement in symptoms.

Presentation considered suggestive of a diagnosis of non-immunoglobulin E (IgE)-mediated cow's milk allergy due to positive family history of atopy, presence of typical delayed-onset allergy symptoms involving more than one body system and worsening of symptoms concurrent with introduction of cow's milk (i.e., infant formula).

Investigations

Specific IgE/skin prick testing not indicated due to delayed symptom onset.

Maternal elimination of cow's milk for 2–4 weeks to be followed by home reintroduction to confirm a diagnosis of non-IgE-mediated cow's milk allergy.

Outcome/Follow-up

At 16 weeks of age, mother reports gastrointestinal symptoms significantly reduced following elimination of cow's milk. He was easier to settle and sleeping for longer periods at night. Symptoms worsened over the week of maternal reintroduction of cow's milk but had resettled a few days after cow's milk was eliminated again. Diagnosis of non-IgE-mediated cow's milk allergy was confirmed, continued dietary avoidance of cow's milk in maternal diet while breastfeeding and infant diet during complementary feeding was recommended. He should be reassessed in 6 months or at around 12 months of age.

CASE STUDY 12.2 Allergy Case Example 2

ALLERGY CASE EXAMPLE: ATOPIC ECZEMA, COW'S MILK AND EGG ALLERGY IN AN INFANT

An 18-week-old female infant presented to the clinic with early onset severe flexural and facial eczema. She developed dry skin at around 3 weeks of age. Mild eczema was diagnosed at 7 weeks of age and topical emollients were prescribed. Growth was following appropriate weight-for-age and height-for-age centiles.

Consider Feeding History

She is currently exclusively breastfeeding and is reported to be feeding well. When fed a small volume of an infant formula at 14 weeks of age, she developed hives and refused to finish the bottle.

Consider Individual and Family History of Atopic Disease

Parents report prior history of neonatal acne and ongoing cradle cap.

Father has seasonal rhinitis and asthma, and mother had childhood eczema. Older sibling has eczema and tree nut allergies.

Mother was concerned about food allergies, particularly cow's milk and nut allergies, due to siblings' allergy history.

Presentation and history suggestive of IgE-mediated cow's milk allergy. Early onset infantile eczema and atopic history increases risk for other food allergies, particularly egg and peanut.

Investigations

Allergy testing is indicated due to history of immediate-onset allergy symptoms.

Results

Skin prick test (SPT): cow's milk extract 2 mm; cow's milk fresh 6 mm; egg white 13 mm; raw egg 23 mm; peanut, almond, cashew, sesame, pine nut: 0 mm.

Specific IgE: total IgE 19; cow's milk 0.54; hen's egg 3.2; peanut 0.10; almond 0.07; cashew 0.06; walnut 0.01; hazelnut 0.01; sesame 0.01 kU/L

Allergic sensitisation is indicated by SPT wheal diameter ≥ 3 mm or a specific IgE level of ≥ 0.35 kU/L. Refer to Table 12.4: 'Diagnostic Values for Skin Prick and Specific IgE Testing' for reference ranges.

Outcome

Eczema management: Mild topical steroids for facial eczema to be applied twice daily for 7 days and moderate topical steroid applied to trunk and limbs twice daily for up to 14 days, or until eczema resolves and itching stops, and once control achieved to continue to apply at weekends.

Diet: Strict dietary avoidance of cow's milk and hen's egg recommended due to diagnosed cow's milk and hen's egg allergies, and proactive introduction of peanut recommended to prevent peanut allergy. Since mother planned to continue breastfeeding, no hypoallergenic formula was needed. Expressed breast milk or plant-based alternative milk drinks were recommended for use in food preparation. Maternal elimination of cow's milk and hen's egg was recommended for 2–4 weeks, followed by gradual reintroduction of cow's milk and then hen's egg, to establish impact on eczema exacerbations. Maternal diet was reviewed for nutritional adequacy, and maternal supplementation of vitamin D and calcium was recommended. Complementary feeding was discussed and introduction of peanut recommended once first foods had been introduced.

Questions to Consider at Follow-Up

Assess skin condition and discuss topical management.

Assess impact of maternal elimination of cow's milk and egg. Has there been any notable improvement in eczema during avoidance and/or worsening skin symptoms with reintroduction. Will ongoing dietary avoidance be necessary?

Assess infant feeding and growth. Is breastfeeding ongoing, does prescription of a hypoallergenic formula need to be considered, are there any concerns with complementary feeding (i.e., introduction of common allergen foods, introduction of peanut)? Is growth following age-appropriate centiles?

If ongoing dietary avoidance is recommended, consider onward referral for dietitian assessment and advice to ensure nutritional adequacy.

CASE STUDY 12.3 **Allergy Case Example 3**

ALLERGY CASE EXAMPLE: WHEAT-DEPENDENT EXERCISE-INDUCED ANAPHYLAXIS

A 19-year-old woman presented to the clinic following a number of episodes of collapse following exercise over a 2-year period. She reported four episodes occurring after moderate physical activity, three involving collapse after running as well as urticaria, angioedema and wheeze. One episode involved vomiting only.

History suggestive of food-dependent exercise-induced anaphylaxis (FDEIA).

INVESTIGATIONS

Wheat is the most common trigger of FDEIA, and omega-5 gliadin has high diagnostic sensitivity. Other common triggers for anaphylaxis should be tested to rule out an IgE-mediated allergy.

Results

Wheat 1.7 kU/L

Omega-5 gliadin 7.42 kU/L (≥ 0.35 kU/L has specificity >95% for wheat-dependent exercise-induced anaphylaxis (WDEIA))

Cow's milk, soy, cod, tree nuts—negative

Allergic sensitisation is indicated by SPT wheal diameter ≥ 3 mm or a specific IgE level of ≥ 0.35 kU/L. Refer to Table 12.4: 'Diagnostic Values for Skin Prick and Specific IgE Testing' for reference ranges.

Exercise challenge after eating wheat-containing bread: negative. A negative exercise challenge does not exclude a diagnosis of FDEIA.

Outcome

Diagnosis of WDEIA is made.

Advice to avoid wheat in combination with exercise. Supervised physical activity can continue. Antihistamines and an adrenaline autoinjector prescribed. Avoidance of alcohol and nonsteroidal anti-inflammatory drugs before exercise also emphasised as these cofactors may increase likelihood of a reaction.

CASE STUDY 12.4 **Allergy Case Example 4**

ALLERGY CASE EXAMPLE: EOSINOPHILIC OESOPHAGITIS IN AN ADULT

A 28-year-old man presented to the clinic with a 2-year history of dysphagia of increasing severity. At one point the dysphagia was severe enough to call an ambulance. He recently experienced immediate-onset symptoms after eating foods containing cow's milk such as chocolate and in a cereal and became concerned about a worsening allergy. He reported bananas cause mild oral irritation. He reported a previous medical history of childhood asthma and mild allergic rhinitis. He had horses and dogs as pets.

Investigations

SPTs: Negative to common inhalant allergens, including dog and horse; positive to cow's milk; specific IgE blood tests: positive to cow's milk and banana

Gastroscopy: 1- to 2-cm superficial-looking tear (muscle seen to be intact) was seen at the posterior wall about 1 cm from the stenosis.

Outcome

History and investigations suggestive of eosinophilic oesophagitis (EOE).

He was initially treated with 6 weeks of proton pump inhibitor followed by exclusion diet (cow's milk and banana). He is regularly followed up by gastroscopy and biopsy.

Introduction

In the late 19th and early 20th centuries, a notable group of scientists led by Louis Pasteur, Paul Ehrlich, Elie Metchnikoff, Jules Bordet and Emil A. von Behring described an immune system, the function of which was to defend the body from attacks by microorganisms. Literally, it meant a 'system that exempts' from disease. While the immune system ensured protection against a noxious agent, or at least the occurrence of some process strictly advantageous to the host, it is important to understand the consequences of its overstimulation. In the wave of industrialisation of Europe and North America, there was a reduction in infectious diseases due to new antitoxin parenteral treatments and vaccines; however, new diseases and strange reactions were rising which were difficult to explain. In 1859, Charles Harrison Blackley, a doctor in Manchester, England, reported that he suffered from what were called summer colds, with seasonal sneezing, watery eyes, and a runny nose. Viennese paediatrician Clemens von Pirquet Freiher first proposed that the immune system played a role in the pathogenesis of infectious diseases in addition to the role of microorganisms and their toxins.[1]

Burden of Disease

Allergy is the most common chronic disease in Europe with up to 20% of patients living with a severe debilitating disease.[1,2] The World Allergy Organisation estimate of allergy prevalence of the whole population by country ranges between 10% and 40%.[3] More than 150 million Europeans suffer from chronic allergic diseases, and the current prediction is that by 2025 half of the entire EU population will be affected. The avoidable indirect costs of failure to properly treat allergy in the EU is estimated to range between €55 and €151 billion per annum.[1] Around 11–26 million members of the European population are estimated to suffer from food allergy. This prevalence if projected onto the world's population translates into 240–550 million people with potential food allergy, a huge global health burden.[4]

The UK has one of the highest prevalence rates of allergic conditions in the world, with over 20% of the population affected by one or more allergic disorders.[5] Allergic disorders are a huge burden of cost on health care systems. In 2009, it was reported that allergic diseases across all ages costs the UK National Health Service an estimated £900 million a year, mostly through prescribed treatments in primary care, representing 10% of the general practitioner prescribing budget.[6] An estimated 1%–10% of adults and children have a diagnosed food hypersensitivity; however, about 20% of the population experience some reactions to foods, suggesting that they might have an undiagnosed food hypersensitivity.[5] From 1992 to 2012 there was a 615% increase in the rate of hospital admissions for anaphylaxis in the UK.[2] Between March 2013 and February 2014 there was a 7.7% increase in hospital admissions with a primary diagnosis of an allergy, compared with the previous year. In the same year, 19.2% of emergency admissions were due to anaphylactic reactions and 19.2% were for 'other' allergic reactions.[7] In addition to hospital admissions, patients suffering from allergy often have to significantly change their lifestyles to reduce their allergic reactions. Food allergies can be a particular concern in young children, where the incidence of food allergy, which may be life threatening, is estimated to be greater in toddlers (5%–8%) than in adults (1%–2%). Food allergy affects 3%–6% of children in the developed world. In the UK, it is estimated that the prevalence for food allergy is 7.1% in breastfed infants, with 1 in 40 developing peanut allergy and 1 in 20 developing egg allergies. However, over the last 20 years, while hospital admissions due to food anaphylaxis have continued to increase across all age groups, deaths have not. Furthermore, over the same time period, the case fatality rate has more than halved, from 0.7% in 1998 to 0.3% in 2018.[2]

Pathologic and Protective Cell Populations

Despite decades of research and detailed knowledge of the critical role of IgEs and mast cells in allergies, the physiological, beneficial function of the pathologic and protective cells in allergy are still not completely understood. However, some of the cell populations which participate in this process have been identified (Table 12.1).

TABLE 12.1 ■ **Pathologic and Protective Cell Population Attributed to Participation in Allergic Diseases**

Cell Type	Function
Eosinophil	Proinflammatory white blood cell
Antigen-presenting cell	Mediate cellular immune response
Basophil	Histamine-containing leukocytes derived from bone marrow
T helper 2 cells	Protective type II immune responses
Mast cells	Early interaction with environmental antigens and allergens, secretion of histamine
Regulatory T cells	Control immune response to self
Invariant TCR+CD1d-restricted natural killer T cells	Regulate development of asthma and allergy
Innate lymphoid cells	Functionally mirrors T helper cells
Commensal bacteria	Barrier protective response to prevent allergic sensitisation of food

Antibodies, also known as immunoglobulins, are glycosylated protein molecules which are present on the surface of B cells and either serve as antigen receptors or are secreted into the extracellular space where they bind and neutralise their target antigens. In the context of allergy, IgE is an important antibody. It is typically the least abundant antibody (0.05%) found in serum. Monomers of IgE consist of two heavy chains (ε chain) and two light chains, with the ε chain containing 4 immunoglobulin-like constant domains (Cε1–Cε4). IgE has an essential role in type I hypersensitivity reactions (i.e., allergic diseases, anaphylaxis) and providing immunity against parasites such as helminths and protozoa.

EOSINOPHILS

The eosinophil is a specialised cell of the immune system. This proinflammatory white blood cell has a bilobed nucleus and cytoplasm filled with approximately 200 large granules containing enzymes and proteins with different (known and unknown) functions. High eosinophil count in peripheral blood most often indicates a parasitic infection, an allergic reaction or cancer. Allergic conditions associated with high eosinophil count, either locally in tissue or in peripheral blood, include eosinophilic oesophagitis (EOE), gastro-oesophageal reflux disease (GORD), proton pump inhibitor-responsive oesophageal eosinophilia, drugs, infection, autoimmune conditions, and primary hypereosinophilic syndromes.

ANTIGEN-PRESENTING CELLS

Antigen-presenting cells (APCs) are a heterogeneous group of immune cells that mediate the cellular immune response by processing and presenting antigens for recognition by certain lymphocytes such as T cells. Classical APCs include dendritic cells, macrophages, Langerhans cells and B cells. APCs play a pivotal role in transferring information from the periphery of the organism to lymphoid organs to initiate the activation of naive T cells. Dendritic cells, Langerhans cells and macrophages are also critical in the induction of allergic inflammation by presenting allergens to T lymphocytes and by contributing to the local recruitment of effector cells.[6]

BASOPHILS

Basophils are bone marrow-derived circulating leukocytes. They are highly granular mononuclear cells. Basophils make up less than 1% of leukocytes in humans but they are the only circulating leukocytes that contain histamine, and they share many similarities with the mast cells. Like mast cells, basophils become activated by antigen cross-linking of FcεRI receptor-bound IgE to undergo rapid degranulation and release their cellular contents. In addition, basophils can be activated without IgE cross-linking by inflammatory mediators such as complement factors C5a and C3a, eosinophil major basic protein, platelet-activating factor and chemokines.[7–9]

T HELPER 2 CELLS

T helper (Th) H62 cells are involved in protective type II immune responses, which are important for eradication of extracellular parasites and bacterial infection and also contribute to chronic inflammatory diseases, such as asthma and allergy. They produce interleukin (IL)-4, IL-5, IL-10, and IL-13, which are important for the induction and development of humoral immune responses. IL-4 and IL-13 activate B-cell proliferation and antibody production. Th2 cell-mediated inflammation is characterised by the presence of eosinophils and basophils, as well as extensive mast cell degranulation, a process dependent on cross-linking surface-bound IgE.[10–14]

MAST CELLS

Mast cells are derived from haematopoietic stem cells. They are widely distributed throughout vascularised tissues, particularly near surfaces exposed to the external environment, such as skin, airways and gastrointestinal tract. They interact early with environmental antigens and allergens. They are long-lived cells which can reenter the cell cycle and proliferate after appropriate stimulation. Increases in numbers of mast cells, and changes in their tissue distribution and/or phenotypic characteristics, can occur during Th2-cell responses and other settings associated with persistent inflammation and/or tissue remodelling. Th2 responses are often also associated with increased numbers of circulating basophils, hematopoietic cells that are developmentally distinct from mast cells but that can secrete mediators, including histamine, also produced by mast cells. Mast cells, like basophils, constitutively express on their surface substantial numbers of FcεRI, the high-affinity receptor for IgE, and the number of surface FcεRI is positively regulated by ambient concentrations of IgE. Ag- and IgE-dependent activation of mast cells, via aggregation of FcεRI when bi- or multivalent Ag-antigen (Ag) is recognised by the cells' surface FcεRI-bound IgE, initiates a complex secretory response. This FcεRI-dependent mast cell activation response includes the rapid release (in minutes) of cytoplasmic granule-associated mediators such as histamine, heparin and other proteoglycans; several proteases and certain cytoplasmic-granule-associated cytokines; the secretion of de novo synthesised lipid mediators (including cysteinyl leukotrienes and prostaglandins) and the production, with a prolonged kinetics, of many cytokines, chemokines and growth factors. Aggregation of only a small fraction of the mast cell's FcεRI is sufficient to trigger mast cell activation and mediator secretion; as a result, individual mast cells can be simultaneously sensitised to respond to many different specific antigens. The extent to which mast cells secrete various types of mediators can vary according to the strength of the activation signal, with release of some cytokines occurring at lower antigen concentrations than the concentration required to induce substantial degranulation and release of stored mediators. The magnitude of mast cell activation in response to antigen and IgE can also be positively or negatively regulated by exposure to ligands for many other receptors expressed by this cell type.[15–22]

REGULATORY T CELLS

Regulatory T cells (also called Tregs) are T cells which have a role in regulating or suppressing other cells in the immune system. Tregs control the immune response to self and antigens and help prevent autoimmune and allergic disease. 'Natural' Tregs are produced by normal thymus; however, 'adaptive' Tregs are formed by differentiation of naïve T cells outside the thymus (e.g., periphery) or in cell culture.

INVARIANT TCR+ CD1D-RESTRICTED NATURAL KILLER T CELLS

Invariant T-cell receptor (TCR)+ CD1d-restricted natural killer T (iNKT) cells play an important role in regulating the development of asthma and allergy.[23] iNKT cells can function to skew adaptive immunity toward Th2 responses or can act directly as effector cells at mucosal surfaces in diseases such as ulcerative colitis and bronchial asthma. These cells have been found in lungs of patients with chronic asthma and oesophageal cells in patients with EOE, suggesting their relevance in atopic diseases.

INNATE LYMPHOID CELLS

Innate lymphoid cells (ILCs) are unique subsets of lymphocytes that do not express rearranged antigen receptors but transcriptionally and functionally mirror Th cells. ILCs can induce a type 2 inflammatory response and produce type 2 cytokines IL-4, IL-5, IL-9, and IL-13 as well as other effector molecules, e.g., vascular endothelial growth factor. A subset of IL-25-responsive ILC2s, in addition, produces IL-17 and is termed inflammatory ILC2 as, in murine models, ILC2 plays a role in food allergy.[24–29]

COMMENSAL BACTERIA

Human bodies contain 10 times more microbes than eukaryotic cells, which collectively encode 100–1000 times more genetic information and are referred to as the microbiome. Over the course of millions of years of coevolution, commensal bacteria have participated in and delivered many physiological functions essential to our health.

The commensal bacterial community composition varies by anatomic site. Enterobacteria and vaginally derived lactic acid-producing bacteria initially predominate; breast milk, which harbours its own microbiome, favours the emergence of Bifidobacteria, which extract nutrients from human milk glycans. Subsequent microbial successions eventually result in a diverse and unique microbiota. In the neonatal, the emerging microbiome is critically intertwined with the maturation of the immune system of its host and profoundly influenced by environmental factors.

Antibiotic use and the consumption of a high-fat, low-fibre diet have a major, and rapid, impact on gut bacterial populations with long-term consequences for both overall microbial community structure and the regulation of host immunity. Recent studies suggest the role of mucosa-associated commensal bacteria in eliciting a barrier protective response critical to preventing allergic sensitisation to food, and those colonise the intestine and other mucosal sites are now widely regarded as integral to promoting normal human physiology. Commensals are now known to influence broad aspects of the mammalian immune system and have been identified as key modifiers in multiple human disease states including allergy.[30–36]

Pathology

Epidemiologist Strachan observed an inverse correlation between hay fever and the number of older siblings in a study of more than 17,000 British children born in 1958.[37] His observations suggest that lifestyle changes in industralised countries have led to a decrease of the infectious burden while a rise of allergic and autoimmune diseases was observed. This is known as the 'hygiene hypothesis', which proposes that allergic reactions, in which the immune system misfires on innocuous environmental triggers like pollen or peanuts, are driven by a lack of exposure to parasites or other pathogens.[37]

In healthy individuals, when the immune system recognises a substance as foreign, B cells produce antibodies. This is known as sensitisation and is a normal immune response. In individuals with allergy, the immune system identifies a harmless substance as a threat. Thus, allergy is an immune response to an innocuous substance, also known as allergen. Allergens are proteins or antigens and can be found in a noninfectious substance such as peanut or pollen. Allergens trigger the immune system to respond in a detrimental way, causing tissue damage and serious illness. These deleterious immune responses are known as hypersensitivities and cause a range of undesirable reactions leading to diarrhoea, bloating, cough, wheeze, rash, inflammation or anaphylaxis. Food hypersensitivity reactions can be broadly classified into allergic and nonallergic hypersensitivity (Fig. 12.1). Nonallergic hypersensitivity includes food intolerance, and allergic hypersensitivity can be further classified into IgE-mediated and non-IgE-mediated allergies. IgE-mediated allergy is characterised as a type I hypersensitivity. Other hypersensitivity reactions (II, III and IV) are mediated by other antibody classes, immune cells or cellular components. Food allergy is a common IgE-mediated allergic hypersensitivity.

Some people may have an inherited tendency toward allergies, a condition known as atopy. Atopy refers to the genetic tendency to develop allergic diseases such as allergic rhinitis, asthma and atopic dermatitis (eczema). Atopy is typically associated with heightened immune responses to common allergens, especially inhaled allergens and food allergens.

Food intolerance is a nonallergic response that does not involve the immune system and takes place in the digestive system. It occurs when the body systems are unable to properly breakdown the food. This could be due to enzyme deficiencies, sensitivity to food additives or reactions to naturally occurring chemicals in foods. Often, people can eat small amounts of the food without causing problems.

A food allergy, however, involves the immune system. For instance, if a patient has an allergy to cow's milk, the patient's immune system identifies cow's milk as an invader or allergen. The immune system overreacts by producing IgE, which then travel to specific cells that release chemicals, causing an allergic reaction. Each type of IgE has specific 'sensors' for each type of allergen. IgE-mediated reactions typically occur immediately after ingestion whereas non-IgE-mediated are delayed and take up to 48 hours to develop, but still involve the immune

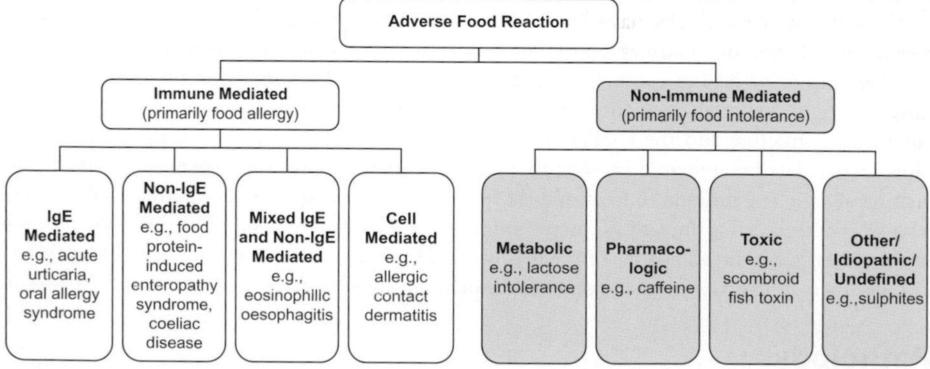

Fig. 12.1 Types of food hypersensitivity. *IgE*, Immunoglobulin E. (From Australian Society of Clinical Immunology and Allergy. Food intolerance. Available at: https://www.allergy.org.au/patients/food-other-adverse-reactions/food-intolerance.)

system. Non-IgE-mediated food allergies are caused by a reaction involving other components of the immune system apart from IgE antibodies, hence the name. The mechanism of non-IgE-mediated food allergy is not well understood, and although the immune system is presumed to be involved, 'non-IgE-mediated food allergy' is an umbrella term for a range of predominantly gastrointestinal food allergies that affect the full length of the gut and have also been implicated in atopic eczema.

Food allergies can occur to any food. The commonest triggers are cow's milk, peanut, tree nuts, egg, soya, wheat, fish and shellfish. Some food allergic reactions occur due to cross-reactivity, such as pollen food syndrome (PFS) or oral allergy syndrome in which the sensitising allergens are usually pollens and the immune system recognises homologous allergens in certain raw fruits or vegetables or some tree nuts. A newly recognised allergy is lipid transfer protein allergy which is more commonly found in the Mediterranean population but has recently also been reported in Northern European population. Meat allergy is relatively uncommon and can develop at any time in life. The mechanism is not very well understood yet, however, and has been attributed to additives in meat preparation or prior exposure to tick bite.

Pathogenesis

Encountering an allergen once is usually necessary to develop an allergy. When allergens enter the body, APCs at body surfaces capture and present them to immune cells, particularly T cells, initiating a cascade of immune responses. This response is similar to the response of the immune system to a microbe. Through a number of immune interactions between T cells and B cells, B cells produce allergen-specific IgE antibodies. Once released into the blood, IgE binds to mast cells, as well as other immune cells such as basophils.[13]

The immune system of patients with allergy develops sensitisation where specific IgE antibodies can recognise allergens. IgEs bind and interact with cells that express a specific receptor called FcεR1, as previously described. When reexposed to the allergen, mast cells (with IgE bound to their FcεR1 receptors) immediately react by rapidly releasing different mediators (e.g., histamine, proteases or cytokines) that cause the classic allergic symptoms (Fig. 12.2). These symptoms depend on the tissue where the contact with the allergen happens and can range from sneezing, allergic rhinitis, wheeze and acute asthma (respiratory tract) to diarrhoea, abdominal pain and oral-allergy syndrome (gastrointestinal tract) or itching, acute urticaria, angioedema, conjunctivitis (skin and mucous membrane). Systemic exposure to allergens can activate a large number of mast cells from different organs at the same time, causing anaphylaxis, a serious and life-threatening allergic reaction.

Basophils and mast cells have long been implicated in the pathogenesis of allergic disease as high levels of mediators common to both cell types are found in tissue locations relevant to allergic diseases. Basophils are also a source of the major Th2-driving cytokine, IL-4, early in immune responses. Basophils are rapidly recruited to the skin, lung or nose, following antigen challenge in humans, and are found in elevated numbers in asthma, allergic rhinitis, atopic dermatitis and nasal polyps. In these conditions, recruited basophils participate in late-phase reactions by the production and release of a number of mediators such as histamine, LTC4 and IL-4. Thus basophils may fulfil pathological roles in both the onset and chronicity of allergic disease.

Approach to a Patient With Food Allergy

Accurate diagnosis of food allergy is vital to prevent allergic reactions (Table 12.2) and to avoid unnecessary dietary restrictions which can significantly impact on nutrition and on quality of life.

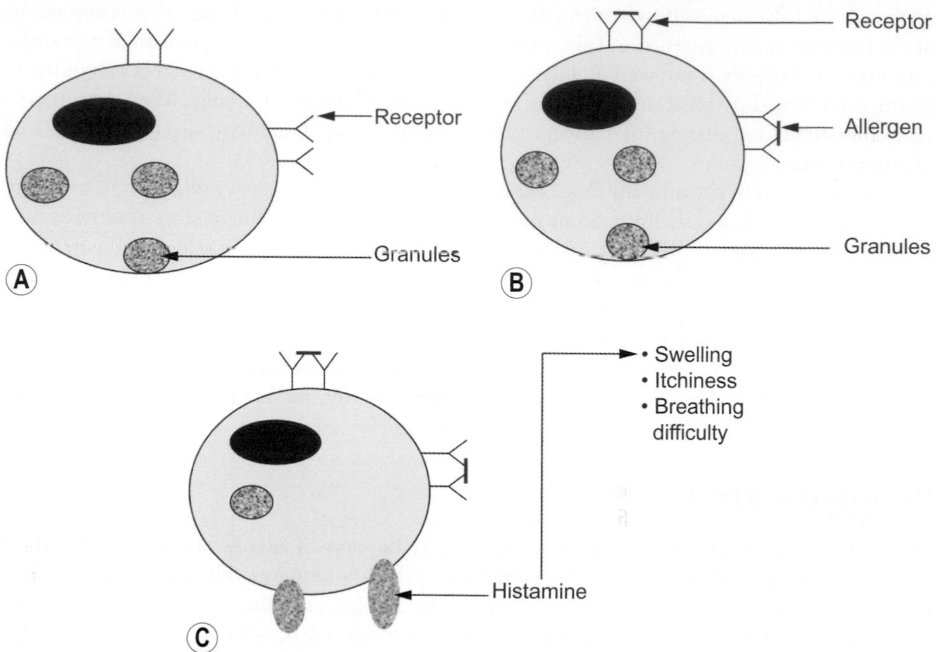

Fig. 12.2 Schematic representation of mast cell-mediated allergic reaction.

TABLE 12.2 ■ **Symptoms Associated With Allergic Reactions**

System	Symptoms
Skin	Flushing/erythema, pruritus, urticarial, angio-oedema, eczema
Oropharyngeal	Pruritus, oedema (lips, tongue, pharynx), vocal changes/hoarseness (laryngeal oedema), throat closure
Gastrointestinal	Dysphagia, acute abdominal pain, colicky abdominal pain, nausea, vomiting, diarrhoea/loose frequent stools, blood or mucous in the stool, constipation, gastro-oesophageal reflux disease, perianal redness, back arching
Upper and lower airway	Conjunctivitis, nasal itching, sneezing, rhinorrhoea, cough, chest tightness, wheeze, shortness of breath, stridor
Cardiovascular	Dizziness, hypotension, tachycardia, hypotonia (collapse)
Anaphylaxis	Multisystem involvement (e.g., skin symptoms plus respiratory or cardiovascular symptom) or two or more symptoms from different symptom categories
Other	Pallor, tiredness, faltering growth, malnutrition

Modified from Skypala IJ, Brown T, Meyer R, et al. The development of a standardised diet history tool to support the diagnosis of food allergy. *Clin Transl Allergy*. 2015;5:7.

ALLERGY-FOCUSSED HISTORY

The allergy-focussed history forms the cornerstone of diagnosis in food allergy (Fig. 12.3). The information that arises supports the clinician to establish the likelihood of an allergy diagnosis, to distinguish between IgE-mediated and non-IgE-mediated reactions and decide if any additional tests are needed to confirm the diagnosis (Table 12.3). It also guides appropriate selection of allergens to be tested.[38,39]

INVESTIGATIONS

IgE-Mediated Food Allergy

SPTs and specific IgE blood tests are used to detect IgE sensitisation in the skin or blood to a specific food.[40] The presence of food-specific IgE indicates that the individual is sensitised to the food but does not necessarily indicate a clinical allergy to the food, and so the results must be considered in the context of the allergy-focussed clinical history.[40,41]

Skin Prick Tests. Drops of commercial food allergen extracts are placed on the skin and a lancet or needle is used to prick the epidermis through the extract allowing the allergen to come into contact with mast cells in the skin. Modified SPT, known as prick-to-prick testing, may be carried out using fresh food samples where no commercial extract is available for the allergen in question or when there are concerns about the stability of the allergen in the commercial extract (e.g., fruits and vegetables). Positive and negative controls of histamine and saline, respectively, should always be included to account for skin reactivity and dermatographism ('writing on the skin': a benign, localised hive-like reaction to pressure on the skin). After 15–20 minutes, the wheal and flare for each prick test should be measured. While SPTs have high sensitivity, they have a low specificity such that a positive SPT result indicates with a 50% positive predictive accuracy that the patient has an IgE-mediated allergy to the food. This is why the clinical history is key; without it, false-positive results can lead to over-diagnosis of food allergy. A negative SPT (negative predictive value > 90%) is very useful to exclude IgE-mediated food allergy. Please see Fig. 12.4 for an example of the Skin Prick Test.[40,41]

Specific IgE Blood Testing. Serum-specific IgE tests detect the presence of circulating allergen-specific IgE using fluorescent-labelled antibody assays to a suspected food allergen. Levels are quantified as levels of kilounits of allergen per litre (kU/L); however, there are different laboratory methodologies available, and results may not be comparable.[40] This type of testing is useful where SPT is not available or is difficult due to severe eczema or dermatographism or if antihistamines cannot be discontinued. They are also useful to evaluate any discrepancies between SPT and clinical history or to confirm the diagnosis indicated by SPT. As for SPT, specific IgE testing should be guided by the clinical history and indiscriminate testing to multiple allergens avoided due to the risk of false-positive test results.[40,41]

Allergic sensitisation is typically defined as SPT wheal diameter ≥ 3 mm or a specific IgE level of ≥0.35 kU/L. Individuals can have allergic sensitisation without necessarily going on to have a clinical reaction if they eat the culprit food. Diagnostic values usually using a cutoff with a 95%–100% positive predictive value have been generated based on the probability of a clinical reaction during oral food challenges and use of these cutoff values can improve the specificity of SPT and specific IgE, helping to confirm the diagnosis of food allergy or to decide when to perform an oral food challenge. Of note, 95%–100% positive predictive values occur at lower SPT measurements in infants under 2 years of age (e.g., egg ≥ 3–5 mm) compared with older children and adults (e.g., egg ≥ 7 mm) (Table 12.4). Diagnostic cutoffs can be variable across populations and should be defined as per local patient population and allergy prevalence. While the likelihood of being allergic increases as SPT size increases and with higher specific IgE results, this does not predict the *severity* of an allergic reaction. Changes in SPT and/or specific IgE tests over time can be indicative that the individual may be outgrowing the allergy (decreasing) or that the allergy is

The iMAP Allergy-focused Clinical History

for Suspected Cow's Milk Allergy in Infancy

'The Cornerstone of the Diagnosis'

Ask about:

- A family history of atopic disease (atopic dermatitis,asthma, allergic rhinitis or food allergy) in parents or siblings

  - a reported history along with symptoms of suspected cow's milk allergy makes the diagnosis more likely; this applies to both IgE-mediatedand non-IgE-mediated

- Sources of cow's milk protein and how much is being or was ingested:

  Exclusive breast feeding - when cow's milk protein from maternal diet comes through in the breast milk (low risk of clinical allergy)

  Mixed feeding - when cow's milk protein is given to the breast feeding infant e.g., top-up formulas, on weaning with solids

  Formula-feeding infant - the commonest presentation, particularly in countries where there is poor adherence with the WHO guidance (14) of exclusive breastfeeding for 6 months

- Presenting symptoms, to include:

  - if more than one symptom, the sequence of clinical presentation of each one
  - age of first onset
  - timing of onset following ingestion (atopic dermatitis-such 'timing' can be very variable)

    IgE-mediated - usually within minutes, but can be up to 2 hours

    Non-IgE-mediated - usually after $\geq$ 2 hours or even days

  - duration, severity and frequency
  - reproducibility on repeated exposure
  - amount and form of milk protein that may be causing symptoms

- Details of any concern with feeding difficulties and/or poor growth
- Details of any changes in diet and any apparent response to such changes
- Details of any other previous management, including medication, for the presenting symptoms and any apparent response to this

Fig. 12.3 Allergy-focused clinical history for the diagnosis of cow's milk allergy. (Reproduced from Venter C, Brown T, Meyer R, et al. Better recognition, diagnosis and management of non-IgE-mediated cow's milk allergy in infancy: iMAP-an international interpretation of the MAP (Milk Allergy in Primary Care) guideline. *Clin Transl Allergy*. 2017;7:26.)

TABLE 12.3 ■ **Type of Allergy and Relevant Diagnostic Tests**

Diagnosis	Diagnostic Tests
IgE-mediated food allergy	Allergy-focussed history Skin prick test Specific IgE blood test Component-resolved diagnostic tests Oral food challenge
Non-IgE-mediated food allergy	Allergy-focussed history Single food exclusion followed by reintroduction Multiple food exclusions followed by sequential reintroduction Elemental or protein hydrolysate formula diets

IgE, Immunoglobulin E.

persistent (no change or increasing) and unlikely to be outgrown. There is no lower age limit for performing SPT or specific IgE blood tests.[40]

The results of SPT and/or specific IgE can sometimes be discordant with the clinical history and with each other; in this scenario specific IgE component testing or an oral food challenge is recommended.[40]

Specific IgE Component Testing. Specific IgE to allergen components can refine the diagnosis of allergy, e.g., to differentiate between a peach allergy which may induce a potentially severe reaction (sensitisation to lipid transfer protein, PruP3) or mild oral symptoms of pollen food syndrome (sensitisation to Bet v1 homologue, Pru P1).[40]

Oral Food Challenges. Oral food challenges, in particular double-blind, placebo-controlled food challenges, are considered the 'gold standard' assessment for the diagnosis of food allergy.[42] Essentially, they involve an individual eating the allergen food under clinical supervision while observed for allergic symptoms. The procedure is resource intensive and involves a risk of potentially severe allergic reactions. They may be used where use of other diagnostic tests has not been able to confirm allergy or tolerance to a food, to determine complete or partial resolution of allergy to a food previously avoided or to identify reaction thresholds or the role of suspected allergy cofactors in reactions. In clinical practice, the procedure can be individualised to the patient's needs. Different dosing schedules may be used, starting with low doses to identify reaction thresholds and ensuring a typical portion of the food is eaten without symptoms to confirm tolerance. Different food preparations may be used such as baked or fresh (uncooked) milk, similarly baked or cooked egg or with the food blinded in a recipe (e.g., due to anxiety about eating the food making it difficult to distinguish between subjective symptoms due to fear and those due to allergy). In research settings, use of standardised protocols such as those developed by the American Academy of Allergy, Asthma and Clinical Immunology together with the European Academy of Allergy and Clinical Immunology are recommended.[43]

MANAGEMENT OF FOOD ALLERGY

The mainstay of food allergy management is avoidance of the culprit food(s) to prevent acute and/or chronic symptoms. Individuals are provided with emergency rescue medications and action plans to treat allergic symptoms in the event of accidental ingestion. Allergen avoidance advice should be individualised as not all individuals need to completely avoid the allergen (e.g., some individuals with cow's milk or egg allergies can tolerate them in baked forms, and some individuals diagnosed with an allergy to one tree nut, e.g., cashew, may be tolerant to other nuts and benefit from including them in their diet).[44] Such flexibility can be important to improve nutrition and to support inclusion of

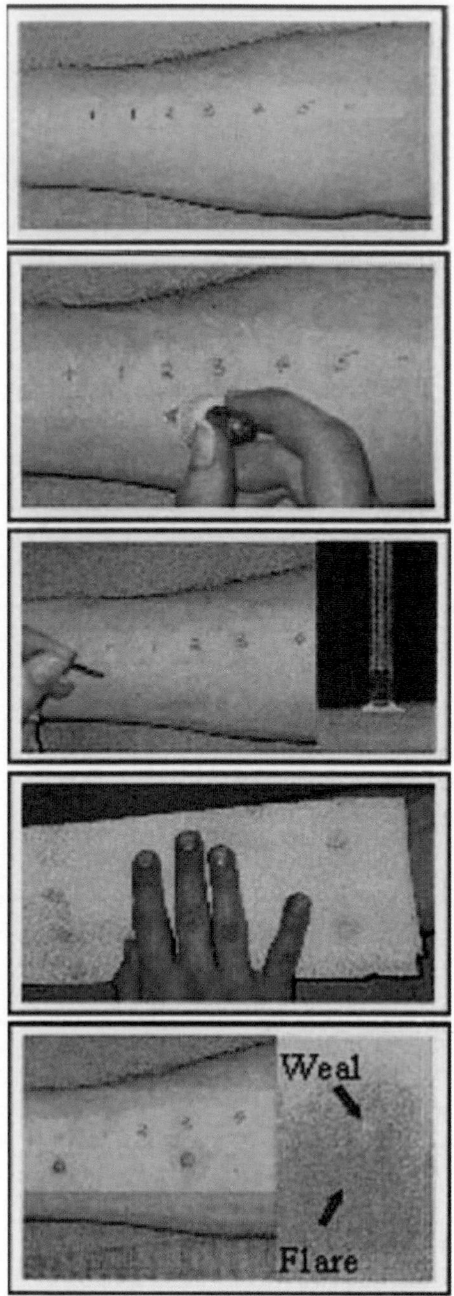

Fig. 12.4 Skin prick testing. (Adapted from patient information leaflet used at the Paediatric Allergy clinic, Ninewells Hospital, Dundee, UK.)

TABLE 12.4 ■ **Diagnostic Values for Skin Prick and Specific IgE Testing**

Foods	Skin Prick Test 95% PPV	Specific IgE 95% PPV	Specific IgE 50% NPV
Cow's milk[a]	≥8 mm Infants ≤ 2 years: 6 mm	15 kU/L Infants ≤ 2 years: 5 kU/L	2 kU/L
Egg[a]	≥7 mm Infants ≤ 2 years: 4–5 mm	7 kU/L Infants ≤ 2 years: 2 kU/L	2 kU/L
Peanut	≥8 mm Infants ≤ 2 years: 4 mm	15–34 kU/L	2 kU/L with history of reaction; 5 kU/L with no history of reaction
Fish		20 kU/L	
Tree nuts	≥8 mm walnut ≥12 mm cashew	20 kU/L	
Sesame	≥8 mm	50 kU/L (86% PPV)	
Wheat		≥100	

[a]Note values do not apply to baked milk or baked egg.
IgE, Immunoglobulin E; NPV, negative predictive value; PPV, positive predictive value.
Modified from Foong RX, Santos AF. Biomarkers of diagnosis and resolution of food allergy. *Pediatr Allergy Immunol*. 2021;32:223–233. https://doi.org/10.1111/pai.13389.

foods that may be culturally important. Allergy management can become more complex for health care practitioners but for families, the improvements to health and quality of life can be significant.[45]

Non-IgE-Mediated Food Allergy

The immune response which drives allergic manifestations of non-IgE-mediated food allergy does not involve food-specific IgE antibodies and therefore SPT and specific IgE tests are not useful in the diagnosis of this type of allergy.[38,40] If the allergy-focussed history is suggestive of a non-IgE-mediated food allergy, a trialled elimination of the suspected allergen(s) followed by controlled reintroduction with monitoring for any allergic symptoms is used to confirm the diagnosis. Usually the recommended exclusion period is 2–4 weeks; however, in some cases a longer exclusion period up to 6 weeks is appropriate. If symptoms resolve or significantly improve during the elimination period and worsen or reoccur during the reintroduction, this confirms the diagnosis, and the allergen food(s) should be avoided for a longer period. The reintroduction phase may not be appropriate for individuals who have experienced severe delayed reactions; they should be evaluated in a specialist clinic.

Single Food Exclusion Diet. All sources of a single food (e.g., cow's milk) are excluded from the individual's diet. In the case of breastfeeding infants, maternal exclusion of the food may also be recommended.[46]

Multiple Food Exclusion Diet. Sometimes it is easier to identify a culprit food through eliminating more than one food during the diagnostic exclusion diet, or multiple food allergies are suspected. The foods to exclude are chosen based on the allergy-focussed clinical history and the foods most commonly associated with the presenting condition (e.g., cow's milk and egg (and soya) for eczema, cow's milk, egg and wheat for EOE).

Elemental or Protein Hydrolysate Formula Diets. In cases of severe symptoms or when multiple food exclusion diets have been unsuccessful in identifying culprit foods but allergy is still suspected, a diet solely using elemental sip feeds (for teenagers and adults) or amino acid formula feeds (for infants and children) may be used.

The diagnostic accuracy of such diets relies on careful adherence during the elimination period. It is important that individuals are well informed about which food(s) to avoid, labelling reading, eating out, informing child care settings, provide suitable alternatives both for nutrition and ease following the diet.

Reintroduction. The exclusion diet should be followed by reintroduction of the food(s) to confirm or exclude the diagnosis of food allergy. In breastfed infants, reintroduction may be phased with the mother reintroducing the food(s) in her own diet prior to introducing to her infant. It is important that the reintroduction plan is formulated at the beginning of the diagnostic diet, as it can be difficult to motivate individuals to reintroduce a food if their symptoms have significantly improved. However, this step is vital to avoid unnecessary ongoing dietary restrictions as symptoms may not reoccur following reintroduction. Dietary restrictions can be challenging to adhere to and may be expensive and may affect growth and nutrition, particularly in children.[38,45]

Assessing Acquisition of Tolerance/Partial Tolerance: Use of 'Ladders'

While allergies to peanut, tree nuts, sesame, fish and shellfish tend to be lifelong, other allergies including cow's milk, egg, soya and wheat are usually outgrown in early childhood, and monitoring for the development of tolerance is a key part of food allergy management.[45]

For IgE-mediated allergy, repeat allergy testing is used to decide whether it is safe to introduce the food. A significant reduction (e.g., 50% decrease specific IgE over a 12-month period) would indicate increasing likelihood that the food would be tolerated. An oral food challenge under clinical supervision may be recommended and if negative, continued consumption of the allergen food at home advised.

Individuals with mild to moderate non-IgE-mediated allergy are usually recommended to trial introduction of the allergen at home using a ladder approach, generally after around 6 months of avoidance and when asymptomatic. The first foods to be introduced are those where the allergen (e.g., cow's milk or egg) is present in small amounts and in a food which has undergone extensive heating (e.g., baked in a biscuit, cake or savoury muffin). The rationale is based on the fact that extensive heating changes the structure of heat labile allergens, making them more likely to be tolerated by the individual.[47,48]

Impact of Allergy on Nutrition

Common allergen foods provide essential nutrients and their avoidance can affect nutritional adequacy, particularly when the food in question is a key source for important macro and micronutrients (e.g., cow's milk or wheat, legumes in the case of vegan/vegetarians, and in those with additional nutritional needs such as young children).[38,49,50]

Concurrent allergic disease such as atopic eczema or gut inflammation can increase nutritional requirements; this has been associated with growth faltering (weight and height stunting) in many studies of infants and children with food allergy, particularly cow' milk allergy, multiple food allergies and atopic eczema.[49,50] Studies have shown increased risk of nutritional compromise with increasing numbers of foods avoided. Increased gut permeability can also increase nutrient needs

TABLE 12.5 ■ **Common Food Allergens and Their Nutrient Content**

Allergen	Nutrients
Cow's milk	Protein, carbohydrate, fats, vitamin A, vitamin D, riboflavin, pantothenic acid, vitamin B12, calcium, magnesium, phosphate
Egg	Protein, riboflavin, biotin, vitamin A, vitamin B12, vitamin D, vitamin E, pantothenic acid, selenium, iodine, folate
Wheat	Carbohydrate, fibre, protein, thiamine, riboflavin, niacin, calcium, iron, folate if fortified
Fish	All fish: Protein, iodine. Fish bones: calcium, phosphorus, fluoride. Fatty fish: Protein, fat, vitamins A and D, omega-3 fatty acids
Soya	Protein, thiamine, riboflavin, pyridoxine, folate, calcium, phosphorus, magnesium, Iron, zinc, fibre
Peanut	Protein, fats, vitamin E, niacin, magnesium

Modified from Skypala IJ, Venter C, Meyer R, et al. The development of a standardised diet history tool to support the diagnosis of food allergy. *Clin Transl Allergy*. 2015;5:7. https://doi.org/10.1186/s13601-015-0050-2.

and may be associated with micronutrient deficiencies and may impact negatively on growth and catch-up growth.[50]

It has been difficult to estimate the impact of dietary restrictions on micronutrient intakes due to limitations of dietary intake assessment methods and biomarkers of nutritional status. Children on an elimination diet (of various foods) have shown a lower intake of some key micronutrients, including vitamin D, folic acid, calcium, zinc, iron and B vitamins. There is limited data to indicate risk for nutritional deficiencies when intakes are inadequate and whether such impacts are reversed with reintroduction of the food(s), though cases of nutritional rickets, iodine and iron deficiency due to restricted diets in allergic patients have been published.[50]

Nutritional status should be reviewed prior to and regularly during ongoing dietary avoidance to ensure nutritional adequacy. Dietary advice should be individualised to ensure access to suitable safe (allergen free) and nutritious alternatives while addressing needs for growth/catch-up growth or weight gain, identifying nutrients at risk of inadequate intakes (Table 12.5) and advising on alternative food sources or using supplements if required.

Feeding Difficulties and Restricted Diets

Individuals with food allergy are often reported to experience additional challenges with feeding and eating such as fussy or picky eating, food aversion or refusal, feeding difficulties, dietary over-restriction or anxiety, all of which affect nutrition additional to restrictions necessitated by the diagnosed allergy.[49–51]

Food allergies most commonly occur during the first 2 years of life, overlapping with feeding development. Acquisition of feeding skills can be interrupted due to delayed or limited exposure to textures or flavours during complementary feeding.[50,51] This may be due to uncertainty of the diagnosis, parental anxiety to progress with introducing new foods due to fear of a reaction. An infant or child with persistent symptoms such as vomiting, gastro-oesophageal reflux, abdominal pain or constipation may develop negative associations with new foods and feeding aversions. This may delay attainment of oro-motor and/or sensory feeding skills. Where faltering growth occurs, parental anxiety may increase and feeding style may involve ignoring of hunger and satiety cues to increase dietary intake.[51] Although many improve with support, some feeding difficulties may persist after food allergies have resolved (e.g., 11.5-year-old children with previous cow's milk allergy on unrestricted diets had higher scores for avoidant eating behaviour than control group children without previous allergy).

For many, constant vigilance around food and fear of reactions affects quality of life. Children may learn caution through parental modelling as they get older. For both children and adults, feelings of anxiety can cause symptoms that mimic allergy, leading to uncertainty about food choices and limiting of foods to those considered 'safe' and excluding tolerated foods. Avoidance diets entail a heightened awareness of food and diet and some association with eating disorders (e.g., avoidant restrictive food intake disorder has been reported).[52–54]

These challenges are often well managed by families once the allergy diagnosis has been established and symptoms improve as they learn to navigate allergy management. Peer support can be a fundamental part of this. Additional multidisciplinary care or referral to feeding or psychological support services may be needed.

Allergy Treatment

Promising advances have been made in immunotherapy and desensitisation for the treatment of food allergy, in particular for peanut allergy. These approaches are not yet widely available outside of research programmes; however, their use in clinical settings is likely to increase as they gain regulatory approval.[55]

Allergy Prevention

A number of dietary approaches have been investigated for allergy prevention. Most promising have been findings that proactive introduction of peanut and cooked egg during complementary feeding and continued consumption are effective to prevent development of these allergies in infants from both high-risk and general populations.[56–58] This has led to changes in infant feeding guidelines in a many countries, particularly those with high prevalence of these allergies (Table 12.6). It is not yet known whether a similar effect would occur for other common allergen foods and further research is ongoing.

Vitamin D insufficiency has been found to be associated with challenge-proven food allergy in infants, and the rise in food allergy has occurred in conjunction with increasing prevalence of vitamin D deficiency. However, vitamin D supplementation during pregnancy, during breastfeeding and in infants has not been shown to reduce prevalence of food allergy. While fish oil supplementation during pregnancy has been found to protect against development of asthma, its supplementation during pregnancy and breastfeeding and in infancy has not been shown to reduce prevalence of food allergy.[59]

Although breastfeeding confers many important benefits to infants, studies to date show no benefit of breastfeeding over cow's milk formulae to prevent development of allergy to foods such as cow's milk, soya and egg. Studies have also investigated the role of avoiding potential food allergens during pregnancy, when breastfeeding and in infancy. This alone and in combination with environmental interventions (such as house dust mite elimination) have been found to have little to no effect on food allergy in early childhood.[59]

Management of Food Allergy Summary

- Avoidance of culprit food(s) to prevent acute and/or chronic symptoms is the mainstay of food allergy management.
- Allergen avoidance advice should be individualised as avoidance of an allergen food in all forms is not necessary for many individuals with food allergies, and nutritional status should be regularly assessed.

TABLE 12.6 ■ **Comparing Recommendations for Peanut and Egg Introduction for Allergy Prevention**

Region/ Country	Allergen Foods Included	Recommended Age for Introduction	Allergy Screening Prior to Introduction
USA (NIAID)	Peanut	Introduce at 4–6 months in infants with severe eczema, egg allergy or both. Introduce at around 6 months in accordance with family preferences and cultural practices in infants with mild to moderate eczema. Freely introduce together with other solid foods and in accordance with family preferences and cultural practices for infants without any eczema or food allergy.	Precautionary specific IgE testing is recommended prior to peanut introduction for infants with severe eczema, egg allergy or both.
Australia (ASCIA)	All common allergen foods	At around 6 months but not before 4 months, start to introduce a variety of foods, continue breastfeeding All infants should be given allergenic solid foods including peanut butter, cooked egg, dairy and wheat products in the first year of life. This includes infants at high risk of allergy.	No specific screening is recommended prior to introduction of specific allergen foods.
UK (COT)	Cooked egg, Peanut	Peanut and egg do not need to be differentiated from other complementary foods. Introduce at around 6 months alongside continued breastfeeding. Deliberate exclusion of peanut or hen's egg beyond age 6–12 months may increase the risk of allergy. Families of infants with history of early onset eczema or suspected food allergy may wish to seek medical advice before introducing these foods.	No specific screening is recommended prior to introduction.
UK (BSACI) Infants at higher risk of allergy	Cooked egg, peanut	Infants at higher risk of developing a food allergy may benefit from the introduction of foods containing egg and peanut from 4 months alongside other complementary foods.	Routine screening prior to introduction is not recommended. If allergy testing is undertaken, it is recommended that it should only be done by someone with the experience and competence to interpret the results. Testing should not be performed where there is not rapid access to a service that can promptly undertake a supervised food challenge.

Continued

TABLE 12.6 ■ **Comparing Recommendations for Peanut and Egg Introduction for Allergy Prevention—cont'd**

Region/ Country	Allergen Foods Included	Recommended Age for Introduction	Allergy Screening Prior to Introduction
Europe (EAACI)	Cooked egg, peanut	In countries where prevalence of the allergies is high, peanut and well-cooked egg should be introduced as part of complementary feeding. According to the studies, it appears that the best age to introduce egg and peanut is from 4–6 months of life. Professionals should advocate introducing egg and peanut alongside continued breastfeeding.	Screening is not specified.

ASCIA, Australasian Society of Clinical Immunology and Allergy; *BSACI*, British Society for Allergy & Clinical Immunology; *COT*, Committee on Toxicity of Chemicals in Food, Consumer Products and the Environment; *EAACI*, European Academy of Allergy and Clinical Immunology; *IgE*, Immunoglobulin E; *NIAID*, National Institute of Allergy and Infectious Diseases.

Modified from:

Togias A, Cooper SF, Acebal ML, et al. Addendum guidelines for the prevention of peanut allergy in the United States: Report of the National Institute of Allergy and Infectious Diseases-sponsored expert panel. *J Allergy Clin Immunol*. 2017;139:29–44;

Netting MJ, Campbell DE, Koplin JJ, et al. An Australian consensus on infant feeding guidelines to prevent food allergy: Outcomes from the Australian Infant Feeding Summit. *J Allergy Clin Immunol Pract*. 2017;5:1617–1624;

Scientific Advisory Committee on Nutrition. Assessing the health benefits and risks of the introduction of peanut and hen's egg into the infant diet before six months of age in the UK. A Joint Statement from the Scientific Advisory Committee on Nutrition and the Committee on Toxicity of Chemicals in food, Consumer products and the Environment. Available at: https://cot.food.gov.uk/sites/default/files/jointsacncotallergystatement-april2018.pdf;

Turner PJ, Feeney M, Meyer R, Perkin MR, Fox AT. Implementing primary prevention of food allergy in infants: New BSACI guidance published. *Clin Exp Allergy*. 2018;48:912–915;

and

Halken S, Muraro A, de Silva D, et al. EAACI guideline: Preventing the development of food allergy in infants and young children (2020 update). *Pediatr Allergy Immunol*. 2021;32:843–858.

- Some allergies such as cow's milk or egg allergy are commonly outgrown in early childhood; monitoring for acquisition of tolerance is a key part of food allergy management.
- Food immunotherapy and desensitation are promising treatment approaches shown in research settings to increase the amount of allergen exposure an allergic individual can tolerate without symptoms and to reduce the risk of severe allergic reactions. Some treatments have achieved regulatory approval in some countries (e.g., peanut immunotherapy).

Proactive introduction of peanut and cooked egg during complementary feeding and continued consumption have been found to prevent development of these allergies in infants from both high-risk and general populations. Further research for other food allergies is ongoing as well as for combination approaches (e.g., proactive eczema prevention in combination with food allergen introduction in infancy).

Common Food Allergy Disorders

Please see Table 12.7 for an overview of Food Induced Allergic Disorders.

TABLE 12.7 ■ **Food Induced Allergic Disorders**

Disorder	Clinical Features	Typical Age Group	Common Foods Involved
IgE-mediated			
Pollen food syndrome	Pruritus, mild oedema confined to oral cavity	Onset after pollen allergy established (i.e., older children, adult)	Raw fruits, raw vegetables, tree nuts, peanut, soya Cooked forms typically tolerated
Urticaria/angioedema	Triggered by ingestion or direct contact	More common in children than adults	Primarily major allergens
Rhinoconjunctivitis/ asthma	Accompanies food-induced allergic reaction but rarely occur as isolated symptoms; may be triggered by inhalation of aerosolised food protein	More common in children than adults; associated with occupational allergy in adults	General: major allergens; occupational: wheat, egg, seafood
Gastrointestinal symptoms	Nausea, emesis, abdominal pain and diarrhoea triggered by food ingestion	Any age	
Anaphylaxis	Rapidly progressive, multiple organ system reaction	Any age	More commonly: peanut, tree nuts, shellfish, fish, cow's milk, egg
Food dependent, exercise-induced anaphylaxis	Food triggers anaphylaxis only if ingestion followed temporally by exercise; cofactors may be involved	Onset late childhood/ adulthood	Most commonly described: wheat (most common), shellfish, celery, nuts
Mixed IgE- and non-IgE-mediated			
Atopic eczema/ dermatitis	Associated with food in 30%–40% of children with moderate to severe eczema	Most common in infancy or early childhood	Major allergens, particularly egg and cow's milk
Eosinophilic gastrointestinal disorders	Symptoms vary on site(s) of intestinal tract affected and degree of eosinophilic inflammation	Any age	Multiple
Non-IgE-mediated			
Dietary protein-induced proctitis/proctocolitis	Mucus and bloody stools in infants	Infancy	Cow's milk (through breastfeeding)

Continued

TABLE 12.7 ■ **Food Induced Allergic Disorders—cont'd**

Disorder	Clinical Features	Typical Age Group	Common Foods Involved
Food protein-induced enterocolitis syndrome	Chronic exposure: emesis, diarrhoea, poor growth, lethargy; Reexposure after restriction: emesis, diarrhoea, hypotension ~2 hours after ingestion	Infancy	Cow's milk, soy, rice, oat

IgE, Immunoglobulin E.
Modified from Sicherer SH, Sampson HA. Food allergy. *J Allergy Clin Immunol*. 2010;125(2 Suppl 2):S116–S125. https://doi.org/10.1016/j.jaci.2009.08.028, and Muraro A, Werfel T, Hoffmann-Sommergruber K, et al. EAACI Food Allergy and Anaphylaxis Guidelines Group. EAACI food allergy and anaphylaxis guidelines: diagnosis and management of food allergy. *Allergy*. 2014;69(8):1008–1025. https://doi.org/10.1111/all.12429.

TABLE 12.8 ■ **Common Symptoms of IgE- and non-IgE-Mediated Cow's Milk Allergy**

Body System	IgE-Mediated	Non-IgE-Mediated
Gastrointestinal	Vomiting, diarrhoea, abdominal pain/colic	Irritability, colic, vomiting, reflux, food refusal or aversion, diarrhoea-like stools (loose and/or more frequent), constipation, soft stools with excessive straining, blood and/or mucus in stools, abdominal discomfort or pain, painful flatus
Skin	Acute pruritus, erythema, urticaria (hives), angioedema Acute 'flaring' of persisting atopic dermatitis	Pruritus (itching), erythema (flushing) Nonspecific rashes Persistent atopic dermatitis Faltering growth
Respiratory	Acute rhinitis and/or conjunctivitis	

IgE, Immunoglobulin E.
Modified from Fox A, Brown T, Walsh J, et al. An update to the Milk Allergy in Primary Care guideline. *Clin Transl Allergy*. 2019;9:40. https://doi.org/10.1186/s13601-019-0281-8.

COW'S MILK ALLERGY

Aetiopathology

Cow's milk allergy can present at any time in infancy, including soon after birth in breastfed infants, when formula milk is introduced, or when foods containing cow's milk are given during complementary feeding.[39] It is the most common cause of food allergy in early life, with prevalence ranging between 1.9% and 4.9% worldwide. It can induce acute, IgE-mediated reactions with allergic symptoms occurring within 2 hours of exposure or delayed, non-IgE-mediated reactions with symptoms occurring more than 2 hours and up to 72 hours after exposure.[60] Infants can also present with mixed, IgE- and non-IgE mediated cow's milk allergy (Table 12.8).

IgE-mediated reactions are usually easily identified and managed through total dietary elimination of cow's milk. Non-IgE-mediated cow's milk allergy is more difficult to diagnose, in part due to overlap of symptoms with other common conditions of infancy such as colic, constipation, gastro-oesophageal reflux and/or atopic eczema.[39] Of note, altered bowel habit, reflux, constipation and colic may occur in more than half of otherwise healthy infants. It can also be confused with lactose intolerance, a nonallergic food hypersensitivity reaction which typically occurs due to secondary lactase deficiency following an acute gastrointestinal infection, often resulting in inappropriate management with low lactose infant formula.[39]

Clinical Features

Diagnosis. A diagnosis of cow's milk allergy begins with the allergy focussed history (see Fig.12.3). A family history of atopy, presence of typical symptoms particularly involving more than one body system, worsening of symptoms concurrent with introduction of cow's milk (e.g., infant formula) are supportive of a diagnosis of non-IgE-mediated cow's milk allergy.[39,60,61] SPT and specific IgE testing are not indicated in the absence of immediate-onset symptoms. The diagnosis should be confirmed by a 2- to 4-week elimination of cow's milk showing symptom improvement or resolution, followed by home reintroduction with reoccurrence of symptoms. In exclusively breastfed children, cow's milk products should be eliminated in the maternal diet then reintroduced in the mother's diet in previously consumed amounts and over a 1-week period.[61,62] Follow-up consultation is essential to assess the outcome and to ensure rechallenge has occurred.

Treatment. The mainstay of management is ongoing dietary avoidance of cow's milk, usually for a minimum of 6 months from diagnosis. Cow's milk does not need to be avoided by the breastfeeding mother for a majority of infants, unless symptomatic while exclusively breastfeeding or suspected to react to cow's milk in the maternal diet, in which case a trial period of maternal elimination is recommended.[62] Dietary advice to support ongoing cow's milk avoidance by the mother (if required) and during complementary feeding should be provided. Breastfeeding should be supported, including discussion of any concerns about safety of breastfeeding and nutritional adequacy of infant and mother. Maternal supplementation of 1000 mg calcium, 10 μg vitamin D is recommended to avoid nutritional deficiencies. A hypoallergenic infant formula may be unnecessary if full breastfeeding continues to 12 months of age or beyond. Should a hypoallergenic infant formula be required, extensively hydrolysed infant formula milks are generally tolerated by over 90% of infants with a cow's milk allergy.[39] An amino acid formula is usually reserved for infants with one or more of the following: anaphylaxis to cow's milk, severe growth faltering (weight loss >2 centiles), severe early onset eczema unresponsive to standard topical treatments, confirmed food protein-induced enterocolitis syndrome (FPIES), confirmed EOE.[39]

Prognosis. In a majority of infants with cow's milk allergy, the allergy is outgrown by primary school age, with many becoming partially tolerant to baked cow's milk at an earlier age.[60] For IgE-mediated cow's milk allergy, repeat allergy testing guides the timing of introduction and a clinically supervised challenge may be recommended prior to introducing cow's milk at home. When cow's milk allergy persists into later childhood and/or adulthood, this tends to be associated with more severe allergy and risk for anaphylaxis.

In non-IgE-mediated cow's milk allergy, reintroduction is usually at home. A ladder approach is usually followed starting with foods containing small amounts of extensively heated cow's milk, progressing to foods containing higher amounts of milk protein and less heating with pasteurised fresh milk the last step of the ladder.[39] The duration at each stage varies and should be guided by a dietician.

ATOPIC ECZEMA

Aetiopathology

Atopic dermatitis or eczema is a chronic inflammatory disorder of the skin, characterised by an impaired skin barrier.[63–65] Early onset eczema is strongly associated with the development of food allergy, particularly egg and peanut allergy. Risks for sensitisation are increased with longer duration and severity of the eczema. Skin barrier integrity is impaired (loss of function gene mutations have been found) and sensitisation to food allergens occurs via the skin.[65,66]

Routine specific IgE and/or skin prick testing (Fig. 12.4) for food allergy is not recommended, as a high proportion of children with atopic eczema demonstrate asymptomatic allergic sensitisation. False-positive testing can lead to unnecessary dietary restrictions.[63–65] Testing is only recommended when the individual has a history suggestive of food allergy or moderate to severe eczema which is unresponsive to optimised topical treatments. Where food allergy is a factor in atopic eczema, it is more commonly non-IgE-mediated or mixed IgE and non-IgE-mediated and usually in children under 1 year of age rather than older children. Allergy prevention trials in recent years have found that earlier introduction of egg and peanut and ongoing consumption is effective to prevent those allergies.[56,57] Many international organisations have changed feeding guidelines (see Table 12.6).

Investigations

Specific IgE or skin prick testing should be guided by the history (e.g., suspected immediate reaction to cow's milk or egg). A trial elimination and reintroduction guided by an allergy-focussed history may be useful therapeutically when there are other symptoms suggestive of non-IgE-mediated allergy, particularly when growth is faltering (see Table 12.8).[63,64] The most common foods implicated in atopic eczema are cow's milk and/or egg.[65]

Advice on precautionary testing prior to introduction of peanut varies across countries (see Table 12.6). For infants with a history of severe eczema and or an egg allergy, the National Institute of Allergy and Infectious Diseases expert panel recommends that evaluation with peanut-specific IgE, skin prick testing or both be strongly considered before introduction of peanut to determine if peanut should be introduced, and if so, the preferred method of introduction.[66] The rationale is due to early onset and longer duration of eczema associated with increased risk of egg and also peanut allergy. Positive allergy testing does not necessarily indicate clinical allergy, and oral food challenge testing may be indicated to confirm sensitisation or allergy.[65,67] A list of useful guidelines and website for more information is seen in Table 12.10.

Treatment

Topical therapy involves moisturisers to restore the skin barrier and antiinflammatories to manage inflammation. In moderate to severe eczema, mild topical steroids may be used for facial eczema with application twice daily for 7 days or until eczema resolves and itching stops. Moderate topical steroid to be applied on trunk and limbs twice daily for up to 14 days or until eczema resolves and itching stops. Once control achieved, continue to apply at weekends.[64]

Elimination, guided by the allergy-focussed history, should be for 2–4 weeks followed by sequential reintroduction to identify whether eczema is triggered. Maternal elimination may be recommended during breastfeeding during the diagnostic elimination diet with trialled reintroduction at a later stage to establish whether ongoing avoidance is warranted.[38]

Suitable foods for introducing cooked egg include scrambled egg, omelette, or mashed hard-boiled egg and for introducing peanut include smooth peanut butter, puffed peanut snacks, peanut flour or ground peanut. Once established, egg and peanut should continue to be regularly eaten. Additional resources have been published.[66,68–70]

POLLEN FOOD SYNDROME

Aetiopathology

'Pollen food syndrome' and 'oral allergy syndrome' are umbrella terms for reactions to foods which occur due to allergy to pollen or less commonly to latex.[71] PFS is more prevalent in older children and young adults. PFS occurs in 40%–70% of individuals sensitised to pollens and around 2% of the general population. The main allergens involved are the pathogenesis-related 10 proteins and profilins. The most common sensitising allergen is Bet V1, from Silver Birch which cross reacts with pathogenesis-related 10 allergens such as those found in stone fruits, carrot, celery, coriander, almond, hazelnut, soybean or peanut. Profilin allergens in grass, mugwort and ragweed pollen can also trigger reactions (e.g., to banana, melon, tomato or peanut).[71] Affected individuals typically experience transient, mild, localised oral or oropharyngeal symptoms such as pruritis, paraesthesia and/or angioedema. Abdominal symptoms including nausea and vomiting may also occur. Occasionally symptoms can be severe, especially where high concentrations of the allergen are eaten (e.g., fresh fruit smoothie, soy protein shake).[71,72]

Diagnosis

A positive clinical history may be enough to diagnose the condition, for example, if only raw fruits or vegetables are involved and symptoms are typical. Skin prick testing to pollens and prick-to-prick testing to foods identified from the allergy-focussed history such as specific fresh fruits, vegetables or soy milk are helpful to confirm diagnosis; whole foods contain all of the allergens involved in PFS whereas commercial test solutions do not.[72] Component-resolved diagnosis can be helpful to distinguish between PFS and primary allergy to peanut, tree nuts, seeds, legumes or lipid transfer protein allergens.

Treatment

Affected individuals should avoid trigger foods in raw form; they typically are able to eat the same fruits or vegetables cooked or canned due to the denaturation of the protein by heat. Peeling, pureeing or microwaving for 60 seconds or less can be adequate to allow the individual to tolerate the food. Overrestriction is not uncommon due to uncertainty of the diagnosis and lack of specific dietary advice. There is no need to avoid any cross-reacting foods unless they cause symptoms. When peanut or tree nuts are implicated, roasted nuts may be tolerated and support from an experienced dietitian can be helpful especially when multiple foods are avoided.[72] While immunotherapy treatments are effective for allergic rhinitis symptoms, they do not usually prevent PFS.

FOOD-DEPENDENT EXERCISE-INDUCED ANAPHYLAXIS

Aetiopathology

Exercise-induced anaphylaxis is a rare condition in which anaphylaxis can occur during or after physical activity.[73] In around 30%–50% of cases it is food dependent, occurring after the individual has eaten a specific food before physical activity, or occasionally after physical activity. Wheat is the most common trigger food, known as WDEIA (or omega-5 gliadin allergy).[74] Additional cofactors such as nonsteroidal antiinflammatory drugs and/or alcohol can also be associated. The physical activity which triggers the response does not need to be strenuous, particularly in the context of other cofactors; in some cases walking, climbing stairs or dancing can cause a reaction. Other food triggers include prawns, tomato, celery, lettuce, apple, peach, peanut, tree nuts, soya, maize and cow's milk. It should be noted that the trigger food does not always cause symptoms every time it is eaten and exercising without having eaten the trigger food usually causes no symptoms.

Diagnosis

Diagnosis is made from the clinical history and understanding the combination of food triggers and cofactors in exercise-induced anaphylaxis. The individual may not suspect a food trigger, especially as they may be eating it regularly without any symptoms. Specific IgE to omega-5 gliadin (Tri a 19), a wheat allergen component, has been shown to have a sensitivity of up to 80% and a specificity of above 95% in WDEIA and has a higher sensitivity than specific IgE to wheat or gluten for diagnosing WDEIA. A negative omega-5-gliadin has a high negative predictive value.[74] An exercise challenge (eating the trigger food and exercising under clinical supervision) may be useful in some cases but often they are negative, even where the food trigger is known and consumed at the time of the exercise challenge. Accuracy of diagnostic challenge for WDEIA may be improved by using concentrated gluten flour as the wheat source for the challenge.[75]

Treatment

Avoidance of food triggers in combination with exercise significantly reduces the risk of future reactions. Some individuals can consume the trigger food when resting (e.g., in the evening), while others must avoid it completely. Physical activity with supervision can continue. It is important to avoid alcohol and taking nonsteroidal antiinflammatory drugs before exercise. Antihistamines (to treat early onset symptoms) and an adrenaline autoinjector must always be prescribed because one-third of patients continue to have allergic reactions despite dietary advice.[73]

EOSINOPHILIC OESOPHAGITIS

Aetiopathology

EOE is a chronic disorder of the digestive system in which large numbers of eosinophils are present in the oesophagus. This condition is characterised by vomiting, stomach or chest pain, failure to thrive (particularly in children), difficulty swallowing and food getting stuck in the throat. The frequency of EOE has been estimated to be approximately 1 in 2000 individuals. This condition has been reported in multiple North continents including Europe, Australia, and America.[76]

The symptoms of EOE may be variable, more so in people of different ages. Common symptoms include dysphagia, food impaction, nausea, vomiting, poor growth, weight loss, abdominal pain, poor appetite and malnutrition.[77–79] These symptoms often overlap with symptoms of GORD and may often lead to diagnostic dilemma. EOE patients do not typically respond to anti-GORD therapy. Some patients with pronounced oesophageal eosinophilia may have complete responses to proton pump inhibitor therapy, thus making it the first-line therapy used for the treatment of GORD. However, these patients do not typically have GORD but rather a disease variant similar to EOE.[80–83]

EOE is caused by the presence of a large number of eosinophils in the oesophagus. The production and accumulation of eosinophils may be caused by many factors such as immune hypersensitivity responses to particular foods or environmental proteins (allergens) in some affected individuals. Some individuals with this condition have been found to have an unusually high expression of a particular gene called *eotaxin-3*. This gene codes for a protein that is important in controlling the accumulation of eosinophils. EOE can run in families but the risk for additional family members is <5% unless they are twins with the EOE patient. Several genes have been identified to contribute to EOE including *CAPN14* and *TSLP*. A fundamental step in the development of EOE is loss of oesophageal barrier function which is mediated by loss of antiproteases such as SPINK7 and desmosomal proteins such as desmoglein-1 and dysregulated expression of the *CAPN14* gene product (calpain-14).[84]

EOE often presents with symptoms similar to several other gastrointestinal conditions including:

1. GORD, characterised by reflux of the contents of the stomach or small intestines into the oesophagus
2. Ulcerative colitis, characterised by chronic inflammation and ulceration of the lining of the colon
3. Crohn disease, an inflammatory bowel disease characterised by severe, chronic inflammation of the intestinal wall or any portion of the gastrointestinal tract

Management[85–88]

Diagnosis. The diagnosis of EOE is often delayed because of a lack of awareness of this condition. Upper gastrointestinal endoscopy and small tissue biopsy is required to count eosinophils and to look for tissue injury and thickening of tissue.

Elevated expression of eotaxin-3 is part of a whole panel of dysregulated genes expressed by the oesophagus of patients with EOE, termed the 'EOE transcriptome' which divides patients into different subgroups, referred to as endotypes.[78]

Treatment. Many children and adults with EOE show improvement with proton pump inhibitor therapy. The proton pump inhibitors exert their effects by direct action rather than blockade of stomach acid alone. Individuals with EOE often have other atopic conditions such as asthma or eczema.

The main approaches to dietary management of EOE are elemental diet (amino acid or elemental sip feed) or empiric food elimination based on the most common food triggers (i.e., cow's milk, egg, wheat, soy, nuts, fish). Dietary eliminations based on positive allergy SPT, specific IgE or patch testing have not been found to be more successful than elimination of one or more of the common trigger foods. Detection of sensitisation may also be indicative of concomitant food allergy. While elemental diets are very effective in achieving remission, they are generally unpalatable and difficult to sustain for long periods. Nasogastric or gastrostomy tube feedings may be necessary to achieve adequate volumes of the formula to meet nutritional needs. Empiric food eliminations may follow a 'step-down' approach in which six foods are eliminated followed by sequential reintroduction and monitoring, or a 'step-up' approach eliminating one food (most commonly cow's milk) and eliminating additional common trigger foods only if remission is not achieved. The goal is to find an approach with the fewest dietary restrictions that maintains remission of symptoms.

Steroids are often used to control inflammation if dietary changes alone are not sufficient. Regular endoscopies and biopsies are performed to monitor the effectiveness of treatment.

Complications. EOE is a chronic disease limited to the oesophagus and has a persistent or spontaneously fluctuating course. So far it does not seem to limit life expectancy, but it often substantially impairs the quality of life. To date, there has been no association with malignant conditions, but there is concern that the chronic, uncontrolled inflammation will evoke irreversible structural alterations of the oesophagus, leading to tissue fibrosis, stricture formation and impaired function. This oesophageal remodelling may result in several disease-inherent and procedure-related complications (Table 12.9).[89–93]

TABLE 12.9 ■ **Complications Associated With EOE**

Conditions	Clinical Features
Inflammatory conditions	Furrows, exudates, oedema, oesophageal rings, stenosis
Perforation	Boerhaave syndrome, fibrostenotic condition, oesophageal dilatation
Gas in hepatic portal venous system	Intraluminal gas enters the portal venous circulation due to oesophageal dilation for strictures associated with EOE
Intramucosal dissection of the oesophagus	Separation of mucosa or submucosa leading to false lumen creation
Oesophageal dysmotility	Mucosal infiltration by eosinophils and their interaction with the microenvironment and inflammatory cytokines
Achalasia-like changes	Abnormal buildup of eosinophils in muscularis propria leading to myoactive, neuroactive and cytotoxic secretory products from the eosinophils
Adrenal insufficiency	Low morning cortisol levels

EOE, Eosinophilic oesophagitis.

TABLE 12.10 ■ **Useful Guidelines and Websites**

Food allergy prevention	Addendum guidelines for the prevention of peanut allergy in the United States, 2017 https://www.niaid.nih.gov/sites/default/files/addendum-peanut-allergy-prevention-guidelines.pdf ASCIA guidelines for infant feeding and allergy prevention, 2017 https://www.allergy.org.au/hp/papers/infant-feeding-and-allergy-prevention BSACI early feeding guidance, 2018 https://www.bsaci.org/professional-resources/resources/early-feeding-guidelines/ EAACI food allergy prevention, 2021 https://onlinelibrary.wiley.com/doi/10.1111/pai.13496
CMPA	The Milk Allergy in Primary Care Guideline https://gpifn.org.uk/imap/
GORD	NICE GORD 2015 Pediatric Gastroesophageal Reflux Clinical Practice Guidelines: Joint Recommendations of the North American Society for Pediatric Gastroenterology, Hepatology, and Nutrition (NASPGHAN) and the European Society for Pediatric Gastroenterology, Hepatology, and Nutrition (ESPGHAN)

ASCIA, Australasian Society of Clinical Immunology and Allergy; *BSACI*, British Society for Allergy & Clinical Immunology; *CMPA*, Cow's milk protein allergy; *EAACI*, European Academy of Allergy and Clinical Immunology; *GORD*, gastro-oesophageal reflux disease; *NICE*, National Institute for Health and Care Excellence.

References

1. Akdis CA, Agache I, eds. Global Atlas of Allergy. Munich, Germany: European Academy of Allergy and Clinical Immunology; 2014.
2. Conrado AB, Ierodiakonou D, Gowland MH, Boyle RJ, Turner PJ. Food anaphylaxis in the United Kingdom: Analysis of national data, 1998–2018. *BMJ*. 2021;372:n251.
3. Igea JM. The history of the idea of allergy. *Allergy*. 2013;68(8):966–973. https://doi.org/10.1111/all.12174.
4. World Allergy Organization. *WAO White Book on Allergy*. Available at: https://www.worldallergy.org/UserFiles/file/WhiteBook2-2013-v8.pdf.
5. Levy ML, Price D, Zheng X, Simpson C, Hannaford P, Sheikh A. Inadequacies in UK primary care allergy services: national survey of current provisions and perceptions of need. *Clinical and experimental allergy: journal of the British Society for Allergy and Clinical Immunology*. 2004;34(4):518–519. https://doi.org/10.1111/j.1365-2222.2004.1945.x.
6. Bubnoff DV, Geiger E, Bieber T. Antigen presenting cells in allergy. *J Allergy Clin Immunol*. 2001;108:329–339.
7. GOV.UK. Corporate report. HSCIC annual report and accounts 2014 to 2015. Available at: https://www.gov.uk/government/publications/hscic-annual-report-and-accounts-2014-to-2015.
8. Patil SU, Bunyavanich S, Berin MC. Emerging food allergy biomarkers. *J Allergy Clin Immunol Pract*. 2020;8:2516–2524.
9. Min B. Basophils: What they 'can do' versus what they 'actually do'. *Nat Immunol*. 2008;9:1333–1339.
10. Moro K, Yamada T, Tanabe M, et al. Innate production of T(H)2 cytokines by adipose tissue-associated c-Kit(+)Sca-1(+) lymphoid cells. *Nature*. 2010;463:540–544.
11. Pelly VS, Kannan Y, Coomes SM, et al. IL-4-producing ILC2s are required for the differentiation of TH2 cells following Heligmosomoides polygyrus infection. *Mucosal Immunol*. 2016;9:1407–1417.
12. Lee JB, Chen CY, Liu B, et al. IL-25 and CD4(+) TH2 cells enhance type 2 innate lymphoid cell-derived IL-13 production, which promotes IgE-mediated experimental food allergy. *J Allergy Clin Immunol*. 2016;137(4):1216–1225.e5. https://doi.org/10.1016/j.jaci.2015.09.019.

13. Galli SJ, Tsai M. IgE and mast cells in allergic disease. *Nat med.* 2012;18(5):693–704. https://doi.org/10.1038/nm.2755.
14. Ezzat MH, Hasan ZE, Shaheen KY. Serum measurement of interleukin-31 (IL-31) in paediatric atopic dermatitis: Elevated levels correlate with severity scoring. *J Eur Acad Dermatol Venereol.* 2011;25:334–339.
15. Enerback L, Pipkorn U, Granerus G. Intraepithelial migration of nasal mucosal mast cells in hay fever. *Int Arch Allergy Appl Immunol.* 1986;80:44–51.
16. Galli SJ, Kalesnikoff J, Grimbaldeston MA, Piliponsky AM, Williams CM, Tsai M. Mast cells as "tunable" effector and immunoregulatory cells: Recent advances. *Annu Rev Immunol.* 2005;23:749–786.
17. Kalesnikoff J, Galli SJ. New developments in mast cell biology. *Nat Immunol.* 2008;9:1215–1223.
18. Kawakami T, Galli SJ. Regulation of mast-cell and basophil function and survival by IgE. *Nat Rev Immunol.* 2002;2:773–786.
19. Kitamura Y. Heterogeneity of mast cells and phenotypic change between subpopulations. *Annu Rev Immunol.* 1989;7:59–76.
20. Metcalfe DD, Baram D, Mekori YA. Mast cells. *Physiol Rev.* 1997;77:1033–1079.
21. Rivera J, Gilfillan AM. Molecular regulation of mast cell activation. *J Allergy Clin Immunol.* 2006;117:1214–1225.
22. Ryan JJ, Kashyap M, Bailey D, et al. Mast cell homeostasis: A fundamental aspect of allergic disease. *Crit Rev Immunol.* 2007;27:15–32.
23. Meyer EH, DeKruyff RH, Umetsu DT. iNKT cells in allergic disease. *Curr Top Microbiol Immunol.* 2007;314:269–291.
24. Mjösberg JM, Trifari S, Crellin NK, et al. Human IL-25- and IL-33-responsive type 2 innate lymphoid cells are defined by expression of CRTH2 and CD161. *Nat Immunol.* 2011;12:1055–1062.
25. Mjösberg J, Bernink J, Golebski K, et al. The transcription factor GATA3 is essential for the function of human type 2 innate lymphoid cells. *Immunity.* 2012;37:649–659.
26. Karta MR, Broide D, Doherty TA. Insights into group 2 innate lymphoid cells in human airway disease. *Curr Allergy Asthma Rep.* 2016;16.8.
27. von Moltke J, O'Leary CE, Barrett NA, Kanaoka Y, Austen KF, Locksley RM. Leukotrienes provide an NFAT-dependent signal that synergizes with IL-33 to activate ILC2s. *J Exp Med.* 2017;214:27–37.
28. Price AE, Liang HE, Sullivan BM, et al. Systemically dispersed innate IL-13-expressing cells in type 2 immunity. *Proc Natl Acad Sci U S A.* 2010;107:11489–11494.
29. Chu DK, Llop-Guevara A, Walker TD, et al. IL-33, but not thymic stromal lymphopoietin or IL-25, is central to mite and peanut allergic sensitization. *J Allergy Clin Immunol.* 2013;131(1):187–200.e2008. https://doi.org/10.1016/j.jaci.2015.09.019.
30. Cho I, Blaser MJ. The human microbiome: At the interface of health and disease. *Nat Rev Genet.* 2012;13:260–270.
31. Dominguez-Bello MG, Costello EK, Contreras M, et al. Delivery mode shapes the acquisition and structure of the initial microbiota across multiple body habitats in newborns. *Proc Natl Acad Sci U S A.* 2010;107:11971–11975.
32. Feehley T, Stefka AT, Cao S, Nagler CR. Microbial regulation of allergic responses to food. *Semin Immunopathol.* 2012;34:671–688.
33. Olle B. Medicines from microbiota. *Nat Biotechnol.* 2013;31:309–315.
34. Sela DA, Chapman J, Adeuya A, et al. The genome sequence of Bifidobacterium longum subsp. infantis reveals adaptations for milk utilization within the infant microbiome. *Proc Natl Acad Sci U S A.* 2008;105:18964–18969.
35. The Human Microbiome Project Consortium. Structure, function and diversity of the healthy human microbiome. *Nature.* 2012;486:207–214.
36. Turnbaugh PJ, Ley RE, Hamady M, et al. The human microbiome project. *Nature.* 2007;449:804–810.
37. Strachan DP. Hay fever, hygiene, and household size. *BMJ.* 1989;299(6710):1259–1260. https://doi.org/10.1136/bmj.299.6710.1259.
38. Skypala IJ, Venter C, Meyer R, et al. The development of a standardised diet history tool to support the diagnosis of food allergy. *Clin Transl Allergy.* 2015;5:7. https://doi.org/10.1186/s13601-015-0050-2.
39. Venter C, Brown T, Meyer R, et al. Better recognition, diagnosis and management of non-IgE-mediated cow's milk allergy in infancy: iMAP-an international interpretation of the MAP (Milk Allergy in Primary Care) guideline. *Clin Transl Allergy.* 2017;7:26. https://doi.org/10.1186/s13601-017-0162-y.

40. Gomes-Belo J, Hannachi F, Swan K, Santos AF. Advances in Food Allergy Diagnosis. *Curr Pediatr Rev.* 2018;14(3):139–149. https://doi.org/10.2174/1573396314666180423105842.
41. Foong R, Giovannini M, Du Toit G. Improving diagnostic accuracy in food allergy. *Curr Opin Allergy Clin Immunol.* 2019;19:224–228.
42. Feeney M, Marrs T, Lack G, et al. Oral food challenges: The design must reflect the clinical question. *Curr Allergy Asthma Rep.* 2015;15(8):51.
43. Consensus report of American Academy of Allergy, Asthma and Clinical Immunology and the European Academy of Allergy and Clinical Immunology standardizing double blind, placebo controlled oral food challenges. Available at: https://www.jacionline.org/article/S0091-6749(12)01663-6/pdf.
44. Cox AL, Nowak-Wegrzyn A. Innovation in Food Challenge Tests for Food Allergy. *Curr Allergy Asthma Rep.* 2018;18(12):74. https://doi.org/10.1007/s11882-018-0825-3.
45. Anagnostou K, Stiefel G, Brough H, du Toit G, Lack G, Fox A. Active management of food allergy: An emerging concept. *Arch Dis Child.* 2014;100(4):386–390.
46. Rajani PS, Martin H, Groetch M, Järvinen KM. Presentation and Management of Food Allergy in Breastfed Infants and Risks of Maternal Elimination Diets. *J Allergy clin immunol Pract.* 2020;8(1):52–67. https://doi.org/10.1016/j.jaip.2019.11.007.
47. Leonard SA, Caubet JC, Kim JS, Groetch M, Nowak-Węgrzyn A. Baked milk- and egg-containing diet in the management of milk and egg allergy. *J Allergy clin immunol Pract.* 2015;3(1):13–24. https://doi.org/10.1016/j.jaip.2014.10.001.
48. Lambert R, Grimshaw KEC, Ellis B, Jaitly J, Roberts G. Evidence that eating baked egg or milk influences egg or milk allergy resolution: a systematic review. *Clinical and experimental allergy : journal of the British Society for Allergy and Clinical Immunology.* 2017;47(6):829–837. https://doi.org/10.1111/cea.12940.
49. Mehta H, Groetch M, Wang J. Growth and nutritional concerns in children with food allergy. *Curr Opin Allergy Clin Immunol.* 2013;13(3):275–279.
50. Meyer R. Nutritional disorders resulting from food allergy in children. *Pediatr Allergy Immunol.* 2018;29:689–704.
51. Chehade M, Meyer R, Beauregard A. Feeding difficulties in children with nonIgE-mediated food allergic gastrointestinal disorders. *Ann Allergy Asthma Immunol.* 2019;122:603–609.
52. Fitzgerald M, Frankum B. Food avoidance and restriction in adults: a cross-sectional pilot study comparing patients from an immunology clinic to a general practice. *J Eat Disord.* 2017;5:30. https://doi.org/10.1186/s40337-017-0160-4.
53. Jafri S, Frykas TL, Bingemann T, Phipatanakul W, Bartnikas LM, Protudjer JLP. Food Allergy, Eating Disorders and Body Image. *J Affect Disord Rep.* 2021;6:100197. https://doi.org/10.1016/j.jadr.2021.100197.
54. Patrawala MM, Vickery BP, Proctor KB, Scahill L, Stubbs KH, Sharp WG. Avoidant-restrictive food intake disorder (ARFID): A treatable complication of food allergy. *J Allergy Clin Immunol Pract.* 2022;10(1):326–328.e2. https://doi.org/10.1016/j.jaip.2021.07.052.
55. Wood RA, Sampson HA. Oral immunotherapy for the treatment of peanut allergy: Is it ready for prime time? *J Allergy Clin Immunol Pract.* 2014;2:97–98.
56. Du Toit G, Roberts G, Sayre PH, et al. Randomized trial of peanut consumption in infants at risk for peanut allergy. *N Engl J Med.* 2015;372(9):803–813.
57. Perkin MR, Logan K, Tseng A, et al. Randomized Trial of Introduction of Allergenic Foods in Breast-Fed Infants. *N Engl J Med.* 2016;374(18):1733–1743. https://doi.org/10.1056/NEJMoa1514210.
58. Feeney M, Du Toit G, Roberts G, et al. Impact of peanut consumption in the LEAP Study: Feasibility, growth and nutrition. *J Allergy Clin Immunol.* 2016;138(4):1108–1118.
59. Mazzocchi A, Venter C, Maslin K, Agostoni C. The Role of Nutritional Aspects in Food Allergy: Prevention and Management. *Nutrients.* 2017;9(8):850. https://doi.org/10.3390/nu9080850.
60. Fox A, Brown T, Walsh J, et al. An update to the Milk Allergy in Primary Care guideline. *Clin Transl Allergy.* 2019;9:40. https://doi.org/10.1186/s13601-019-0281-8.
61. Koletzko S, Niggemann B, Arato A, et al. Diagnostic approach and management of cow's-milk protein allergy in infants and children: ESPGHAN GI Committee practical guidelines. *J Pediatr Gastroenterol Nutr.* 2012;55(2):221–229. https://doi.org/10.1097/MPG.0b013e31825c9482.
62. Høst A, Husby S, Østerballe O. A prospective study of cow's milk allergy in exclusively breast-fed infants. *Acta Paediatr.* 1988;77:663–670.

63. Muraro A, Werfel T, Hoffmann-Sommergruber K, et al. EAACI food allergy and anaphylaxis guidelines: diagnosis and management of food allergy. *Allergy*. 2014;69(8):1008–1025. https://doi.org/10.1111/all.12429.
64. NICE. *Atopic Eczema in Children*. National Institute for Health and Clinical Excellence; 2007. Available at https://www.nice.org.uk/guidance/cg57.
65. Eichenfield LF, Tom WL, Berger TG, et al. Guidelines of care for the management of atopic dermatitis: section 2. Management and treatment of atopic dermatitis with topical therapies. *J Am Acad Dermatol*. 2014;71(1):116–132. https://doi.org/10.1016/j.jaad.2014.03.023.
66. Togias A, Cooper SF, Acebal ML, et al. Addendum guidelines for the prevention of peanut allergy in the United States: Report of the National Institute of Allergy and Infectious Diseases-sponsored expert panel. *J Allergy Clin Immunol*. 2017;139:29–44.
67. Sweeney A, Sampath V, Nadeau KC. Early intervention of atopic dermatitis as a preventive strategy for progression of food allergy. *Allergy Asthma Clin Immunol*. 2021;17:30.
68. Turner PJ, Feeney M, Meyer R, Perkin MR, Fox AT. Implementing primary prevention of food allergy in infants: New BSACI guidance published. *Clin Exp Allergy*. 2018;48:912–915.
69. Netting MJ, Campbell DE, Koplin JJ, et al. An Australian consensus on infant feeding guidelines to prevent food allergy: Outcomes from the Australian Infant Feeding Summit. *J Allergy Clin Immunol Pract*. 2017;5:1617–1624.
70. Bird JA, Groetch M, Allen KJ, et al. Conducting an Oral Food Challenge to Peanut in an Infant. *J Allergy clin immunol Pract*. 2017;5(2):301–311.e1. https://doi.org/10.1016/j.jaip.2016.07.019.
71. Muluk NB, Cingi C. Oral allergy syndrome. *Am J Rhinol Allergy*. 2018;32:27–30.
72. Gunawardana MA, Rey-Garcia H, Skypala IJ. Nutritional management of patients with pollen food syndrome: Is there a need? *Curr Treat Options Allergy*. 2018;5:500–514.
73. Minty B. Food-dependent exercise-induced anaphylaxis. *Can Fam Physician*. 2017;63(1):42–43.
74. Matsuo H, Dahlstrom J, Tanaka A, et al. Sensitivity and specificity of recombinant omega-5 gliadin-specific IgE measurement for the diagnosis of wheat dependent exercise-induced anaphylaxis. *Allergy*. 2008;63:233–236.
75. Brockow K, Kneissl D, Valentini L, et al. Using a gluten oral food challenge protocol to improve diagnosis of wheat-dependent exercise-induced anaphylaxis. *J Allergy Clin Immunol*. 2015;135 977.e4–984.e4.
76. Eosinophilic Esophagitis. Rare Disease Database. Avaibile at https://rarediseases.org/rare-diseases/eosinophilic-esophagitis/.
77. Truskaite K, Dlugosz A. Prevalence of eosinophilic esophagitis and lymphocytic esophagitis in adults with esophageal food bolus impaction. *Gastroenterol Res Pract*. 2016;2016:1–6.
78. Nguyen N, Furuta GT, Menard-Katcher C. Recognition and assessment of eosinophilic esophagitis: The development of new clinical outcome metrics. *Gastroenterol Hepatol*. 2015;11(10):670–674.
79. Lucendo AJ, Friginal-Ruiz AB, Rodriguez B. Boerhaave's syndrome as the primary manifestation of adult eosinophilic esophagitis. *Two case reports and a review of the literature. Dis Esophagus*. 2011;24(2):E11–E15.
80. Issa D, Alwatari Y, Smallfield GB, Shah RD. Spontaneous transmural perforation in eosinophilic esophagitis: Rare case presentation and role of esophageal stenting. *J Surg Case Rep*. 2019;2019(6):rjz190.
81. Jon Spechler S, Konda V, Souza R. Can eosinophilic esophagitis cause achalasia and other esophageal motility disorders? *Am J Gastroenterol*. 2018;113:1594–1599.
82. Martin L, Santander C, Lopez Martin MC, et al. Esophageal motor abnormalities in eosinophilic esophagitis identified by high-resolution manometry. *J Gastroenterol Hepatol*. 2011;26(9):1447–1450.
83. Nurko S, Rosen R. Esophageal dysmotility in patients who have eosinophilic esophagitis. *Gastrointest Endosc Clin N Am*. 2008;18(1):73–89.
84. Blanchard C, Wang N, Stringer KF, et al. Eotaxin-3 and a uniquely conserved gene-expression profile in eosinophilic esophagitis. *J Clin Invest*. 2006;116(2):536–547. https://doi.org/10.1172/JCI26679.
85. Hirano I, Chan ES, Rank MA. GA Institute and the Joint Task Force on Allergy-Immunology Practice Parameters clinical guidelines for the management of eosinophilic esophagitis. *Gastroenterology*. 2020;158:1776–1786.
86. Lucendo AJ, Molina-Infante J, Arias A, et al. Guidelines on eosinophilic esophagitis: Evidence-based statements and recommendations for diagnosis and management in children and adults. *United European Gastroenterol J*. 2017;5(3):335–358.

87. Groetch M, Venter C, Skypala I, et al. Dietary therapy and nutrition management of eosinophilic esophagitis: A work group report of the American Academy of Allergy, Asthma, and Immunology. *J Allergy Clin Immunol Pract.* 2017;5(2):312–324.e29.
88. Kliewer KL, Cassin AM, Venter C. Dietary therapy for eosinophilic esophagitis: Elimination and reintroduction. *Clin Rev Allergy Immunol.* 2018;55(1):70–87.
89. Straumann A. The natural history and complications of eosinophilic esophagitis. *Gastrointest Endosc Clin N Am.* 2008;18(1):99–118; ix. https://doi.org/10.1016/j.giec.2007.09.009. ix.
90. Bose P, Kumar S, Nebesio TD, et al. Adrenal insufficiency in children with eosinophilic esophagitis treated with topical corticosteroids. *J Pediatr Gastroenterol Nutr.* 2019;70:324–329.
91. Fianchi F, De Matteis G, Cianci R, et al. Acute intramucosal dissection in eosinophilic esophagitis. *Clin J Gastroenterol.* 2019;12:525–529.
92. Okada S, Azuma T, Kawashita Y, Matsuo S, Eguchi S. Clinical evaluation of hepatic portal venous gas after abdominal surgery. *Case Rep Gastroenterol.* 2016;10(1):103–112.
93. Sgro A, Betalli P, Battaglia G, et al. An unusual complication of eosinophilic esophagitis in an adolescent: Intramural esophageal dissection. *Endoscopy.* 2012;44(Suppl 2). E419–4E20.

SECTION C

Nutrition and Population Health

SECTION OUTLINE

CHAPTER 13

Nutrition and Mental Health

Sabrina Mörkl ■ Sonja Lackner ■ Kirsty Alderton ■ Sandra Holasek

LEARNING POINTS

By the end of this chapter, you should be able to:

- Define psychobiotics and compare and contrast prebiotics, probiotics and postbiotics
- Describe how psychobiotic approaches could be integrated into future psychiatric care
- Understand nutrition in the context of the most common psychiatric disorders (depression, anxiety, psychosis) and describe the state-of-the-art dietary interventions for psychiatric disorders
- Demonstrate the basics of giving dietary advice with the technique of motivational interviewing
- Describe the steps required for mindful eating

Disclaimer: Dietary interventions (psychobiotics) should be used alongside psychotherapy and psychopharmacological interventions as an important pillar in the biopsychosocial treatment model for mental disorders.

CASE STUDY 13.1 Vitamin B1 Deficiency

[Reported from elsewhere.[1–3]]

Mr. L. is a 45-year-old man with a history of alcohol use disorder and bariatric surgery. Further investigation revealed symptoms of confusion, slowed response, general weakness, problems with memory and language. On neurological examination he revealed horizontal and vertical nystagmus and ptosis as well as diminished tendon reflexes.

Laboratory Tests

The patients showed elevated mean corpuscular volume (MCV) as well as elevated liver parameters. Serum thiamine levels were reduced.

Nutritional Anamnesis

The wife of Mr. L. reported that he was not eating regularly after he had bariatric surgery 6 months before. He had been consuming high amounts of alcohol for several years (>6 glasses of wine and beer per day).

Diagnosis

A magnetic resonance tomography (MRT) revealed white matter hyperintensities in the periaqueductal grey, mammillary body, thalamus and cortex.

Treatment

Mr. L. was immediately treated with thiamine intravenously. Neurological symptoms were alleviated in the consecutive days.

Conclusion

Wernicke encephalopathy, first described in 1881 by Carl Wernicke, is an acute disorder of the central nervous system caused by thiamine deficiency. It is characterised as a clinical triad of acute mental confusion, ataxia and ophthalmoparesis, but also other symptoms such as gastrointestinal symptoms,

CASE STUDY 13.1 Vitamin B1 Deficiency—(Continued)

cerebellar signs, seizures, frontal lobe dysfunction, amnesia and altered mental state can occur. Only 8.2% of patients exhibit the classical diagnostic triad.[3]

The disease is most typically observed in patients with chronic alcohol abuse, but it can also follow an unbalanced diet, bariatric surgery, vomiting and anorexia nervosa. In this case report, thiamine deficiency resulted in a combination effect of alcoholism and malnutrition due to bariatric surgery. It is of utmost importance to treat thiamine deficiency immediately as delays in treatment can result in irreversible dementia and death.

Thiamine (also called vitamin B1) is essential for cell growth and development. The active form of thiamine is called thiamine pyrophosphate. It is a coenzyme necessary for the metabolism processes of lipids, glucose and amino acids. Deficiency of B1 results in metabolic disturbances leading to oxidative stress, excitotoxicity of neurons, inflammation, impaired neurogenesis, impairment of blood-brain-barrier, lactic acidosis and decreased astrocyte function.[4,5] These metabolic changes lead to damages of distinctive, vulnerable parts of the brain such as the thalamus, the mammillary bodies and the periaqueductal areas.[6]

Usually, thiamine levels are low in patients with Wernicke encephalopathy, but they can also be normal in a few cases. As Wernicke encephalopathy is considered a medical emergency, it needs to be treated immediately as neurological damage can be serious.

CASE STUDY 13.2 Vitamin B12 Deficiency, Depression, and Psychosis

[Reported from elsewhere.[7]]

Mr. M., a 23-year-old man, presented at the psychiatry department with a several months' history of persistent depressed mood. Further anamnesis revealed anhedonia, fatigability, distracted concentration, altered psychomotor ability, disturbances of sleep, feelings of guilt and death wishes, low self-esteem, loss of appetite and mood-congruent third-person acoustic hallucinations. He reported similar episodes over the past years. Hamilton Depression Rating Scale test resulted in a score of 22, indicating moderate depressive symptoms. Physically, the patient presented striking pallor, knuckle hyperpigmentation and a beefy tongue. He had altered perception and coordination and reflexes of the limbs and spasticity.

Laboratory Tests

Blood analysis revealed reduced haemoglobin, packed cell volume and mean corpuscular haemoglobin concentration (haemoglobin of 11.9 g/dL, reference range, 13–17; packed cell volume of 32.9 L/L, reference range, 40–50; mean corpuscular haemoglobin concentration of 36.2 g/L, reference range, 315–345) whereas mean corpuscular haemoglobin and MCV were increased (mean corpuscular haemoglobin of 43.9 pg, reference range, 27–32; MCV of 121.1 fL, reference range, 80–101).

Vitamin B12 level was reduced (155 pg/mL, reference range, 175–885), and folic acid level was within the normal range (7.2 ng/mL, reference range, 3–17).

Nutritional Anamnesis

Mr. M. reported adhering to a lifelong vegetarian diet. A few months before his presentation at the clinic, he stopped consuming animal-based food such as eggs and dairy products completely. Due to the current anorexic episode, he additionally reduced the total amount of food and skipped meals.

Diagnosis

According to *Diagnostic and Statistical Manual of Mental Disorders, Fifth Edition* criteria,[8] Mr. M. was diagnosed with major depressive disorder (MDD). The MDD was recurrent and currently presented as a severe depressive episode accompanied by psychotic symptoms. Additionally, a megaloblastic anaemia due to vitamin B12 deficiency was diagnosed.

Treatment

Functional cobalamin deficiency can be treated with high dosages of vitamin B12. Thus, intramuscular vitamin B12 was administered to capture nutritional deficiencies as well as potential digestive disturbances. Furthermore, he received cobalamin 1000 mcg/d for 10 days. Afterward, this dose was given every second day for a week and was then further reduced to weekly supplementation.

To treat the MDD and the psychotic symptoms, escitalopram 20 mg/d and olanzapine 20 mg/d were prescribed, respectively.

Continued

CASE STUDY 13.2 Vitamin B12 Deficiency, Depression, and Psychosis—(Continued)

Shortly after treatment onset, significant improvements of psychiatric and neurologic symptoms were observed including remarkably improved Hamilton Depression Rating Scale (HAM-D) scores. Premorbid levels were achieved after 5 months.[7]

Long-Term Recommendation

Nutritional counselling to avoid insufficient supply with vitamin B12 was recommended. For vegan diets the regular supplementation of vitamin B12 is mandatory to counteract a vitamin B12 deficiency.[9]

Conclusion

Vitamin deficiencies may present in various neuropsychiatric disorders. The nutritional status should be taken into consideration in treatment, and nutritive inequalities should be resolved as a part of treatment. The efficacy of whole-diet intervention as well as nutrient-based interventions on the improvement of psychotic symptoms need to be tested further in clinical trials. However, both appear to be promising in the treatment of psychiatric diseases and, based on the current research status, an implication for dietary interventions given.[10] It is important to emphasise further that the consumption of a high-quality diet containing sufficient amounts of nutrients is essential and nutritional counselling should be included in regular treatment settings.[11]

CASE STUDY 13.3 Iron and Depression

[Adapted from elsewhere.[12–14]]

A 44-year-old woman, Miss R., presented to psychiatry outpatient services to treat her recurrent depressive disorder (moderate depression without psychotic symptoms). The patient's history showed that she had been suffering from a depressive disorder since the age of 33. There was no history of obsessive-compulsive disorders, impulse control disorders, substance use or eating disorders. Over the previous 5 years, she had started consuming ice cubes to cope with life stressors. According to the patient, whenever she was feeling tense or low, she would have an intense desire to eat ice cubes. She would only feel better after the consumption of ice cubes and iced drinks, independent of seasons. Initially, she consumed about 250–500 g of ice cubes per day. Progressively, the quantity of ice cube consumption increased to about 10–12 kg of ice cubes per day. She spent hours preparing ice cubes, which led to significant psychosocial dysfunction and interpersonal problems. Because of problems with heartburn, she took omeprazole.

Physical Exam and Laboratory Tests

Physical examination did not reveal any pathologies. Lab tests show microcytic, hypochromic anaemia, and low MCV, mean corpuscular haemoglobin and mean corpuscular haemoglobin concentration, haemoglobin, serum iron, serum ferritin (<10 mg/dL).

Nutritional Anamnesis

Miss R. has a body mass index of 22.5 kg/m^2. She eats infrequently. Due to her work as a leading secretary of a company, she often eats in canteens. In the evening she usually eats ready-made meals from the microwave. She loves bread, spaghetti and pastry and frequently drinks coffee, black tea and milk. Miss R. became a vegetarian 4 months ago. Emotional eating is problematic.

Diagnosis

Major depression

Iron deficiency due to low iron absorption (pagophagia, treatment with proton pump-inhibitor omeprazole), low iron intake (vegetarian diet) and low iron absorption (frequent coffee and tea consumption with meals (polyphenols and tannins))

Treatment

Laboratory tests point to a remarkable iron deficiency. The patient was referred to a dietitian. Iron was substituted intravenously to fill up iron stores. Further, dietary advice was given to achieve a proper iron intake with a vegetarian diet (legumes, nuts and seeds, leafy greens, dark chocolate, and vitamin C rich fruit for iron absorption). It was recommended to avoid coffee and tea with meals as polyphenols lower iron absorption. When the patient reduced coffee consumption, heartburn stopped, and omeprazole was discontinued. Additionally, she received venlafaxine and cognitive behavioural psychotherapy.

CASE STUDY 13.3 Iron and Depression—(Continued)

Conclusion

When patients present with typical somatic symptoms and depression, they should be asked about dietary intake, bowel movements, restless legs symptoms[15] and medication[16] to rule out iron deficiency. Possible differential diagnosis such as coeliac disease should be checked.[17]

Pagophagia has been shown to be associated with iron deficiency.[14,18] Accordingly, it has been shown to respond to the treatment of underlying deficiency without any other intervention.

Additional Information

Iron deficiencies show typical signs comparable with symptoms of depression and are often overlooked in psychiatry.

Iron is essential for oxygen supply, electron transport in the mitochondria's respiratory chain, the proper function of enzymes (catalase, peroxidase), and gene expression. Further, iron is required for the myelination of brain white matter and the spinal cord. It is a cofactor for several neurotransmitter synthesis enzymes such as serotonin (tryptophan-hydroxylase) and dopamine-synthesis (tyrosine hydroxylase). Iron is also involved in monoamine metabolism and monoamine transporters. Further, brain iron status modulates gamma-aminobutyric acid and glutamate homeostasis.

It is long known that iron deficiency can result in decreased productivity, decreased performance, immune disorders and neural dysfunction. Patients suffering from depression often exhibit symptoms similarly found in iron deficiency such as fatigability and tiredness. Many depressive symptoms (low mood, irritability, fatigue, sleepiness) in patients with deficient iron levels can be resolved with iron supplements before improvements in red blood cell count occur. This could be due to improved levels of neurotransmitters and iron-dependent enzymes that are not related to the concentration of haemoglobin. A recent study published in *Psychiatry and Clinical Neuroscience* report data of 11876 Japanese individuals and found that the rate of self-reported lifetime history of iron deficiency was higher in the depression group for both men and women. Likewise, iron supplementation seems to lead to a significant improvement of postpartum depression.

CASE STUDY 13.4 Low Microbiome Diversity and Malnutrition/Anorexia Nervosa

Miss V., a 24-year-old woman diagnosed with anorexia nervosa according to *International Statistical Classification of Diseases and Related Health Problems, 10th Revision* criteria,[19] was treated at a local psychiatric clinic. She weighed 38.5 kg and her body mass index was 13.3 kg/m^2; however, she had already gained 1.5 kg in the 18 days she was hospitalised. Besides the psychotherapy, the patient received nutritional therapy including standarised portions of the regular hospital menu and energy-dense sip food three times a day. The patient scored 26 for the Beck's Depression Inventory,[20] and 46 for the HAMD[21] psychiatric questionnaires, indicating moderate to severe depressive mood, respectively, although she had been treated with Seroquel (quetiapine) 50 mg + 25 mg as an antidepressant.

Clinical History

Her disease history revealed reoccurring severe episodes of extremely restrictive eating behaviour with a documented onset 3 years before and several hospitals stays lasting from some days up to several months. However, her first documented hospital stay was 7 years before due to a severe episode of MDD.

Laboratory Tests

The patient was enrolled for a cross-sectional study investigating energy-sensing differences in female subjects of diverse energy status. Therefore, a stool sample of the patient was collected and a microbiome analysis by 16s-RNA-sequencing—a method to gain genetic information of the microbes present in the sample—was performed. Her microbiome diversity was clearly reduced in comparison with the other study participants[22] (Chao-1 index: 884, range within the study population 689–2267, median 1286; Shannon index: 5.95, range: 4.88–7.29, median 6.39).

Dietary Assessment

Based on the results of an interviewer-guided, twice-repeated 24-hour recalls, the average daily energy intake of the patient was 1882 kcal (7882 kJ). She consumed around 179 g of carbohydrates (39% of

Continued

CASE STUDY 13.4 Low Microbiome Diversity and Malnutrition/Anorexia Nervosa—(Continued)

total energy), 88 g of fat (41% of total energy) and 92 g of protein (20% of total energy). Her dietary fibre intake amounted to 5.78 g/d, which is far too low (recommended daily intake above 30 g[23]).

The assessment of the food diversity revealed that she had chosen food from 11 different food groups of a total of 22 food groups and her diet was composed of 19 different food items. She consumed only 26.5 g of fruits and 88 g of vegetables a day which is below the nutritional recommendations.[24]

Anthropometry

The patient's height of 1.7 m was measured by a stadiometer. Her weight of 38.5 kg was measured in fasting condition in the morning, and the circumferences of her waist (52 cm), hip (77 cm) and upper arm (19 cm) were taken by a nonflexible measuring tape. The triceps skinfold of 7 mm was assessed by a Harpenden caliper. All anthropometric measures were taken in accordance with the guidelines of the International Society for the Advancement of Kinanthropometry.[25] The patient's body fat was assessed by measuring her subcutaneous adipose tissue thickness at defined body sites by ultrasound.[26,27] The sum of subcutaneous adipose tissue at the measurement sites was 24.42 mm (reference: <28 mm, medical surveillance recommended; 35–80 mm, desirable range[28]). In total, the anthropometric measures indicated severe malnutrition.

Clinical Management

Anorexia nervosa, as one of the most common diseases in adolescence with the highest mortality of all psychiatric diseases, is characterised by nutritional restriction, immune response and severe behavioural symptoms. The role of the gut microbiome is therefore crucial.

Hospital food, sip food and nutritional therapy may have enhanced diversity within the duration of hospitalisation.

Influence of Medication on Microbiome Diversity

Antidepressants have known antibiotic effects and may have altered the intestinal microbial composition of the patient. Additionally, poor dietary choices and extreme restrictive eating behaviour/low amounts of food might have contributed to reduced microbial diversity in Veronica's stool sample.

There is a brief window of treatment opportunity in the course of anorexia nervosa with a starvation process often becoming self-perpetuating. The gut microbiota might be a possible indicator for predicting and monitoring this disorder. The low microbiome diversity of our patient might be a consequence of a 7-year disease history.[29,30]

Conclusion

Significant differences in the microbiome between the restrictive and binge-purging subtypes of anorexia nervosa have been observed. This could help explain why restrictive subtype patients need dramatically more calories to gain weight compared with patients with the binge-purging subtype.[31] Because of the strong restrictive subtype of our patient, the altered microbiome leads to a high need of energy.

Overview and Introduction

HOW CAN FOOD AND NUTRITION AFFECT MENTAL HEALTH?

Both over- and undernutrition, low dietary quality and nutritional deficiencies are linked to psychiatric disorders. According to the World Health Organization, 'Health is a state of complete physical, mental and social well-being', a state which seems unreachable. More than 450 million people worldwide suffer from mental disorders,[32] despite intensive efforts to improve mental health care. Psychiatric treatment encompasses a whole array of approaches, from psychotherapy to psychopharmacology and electroconvulsive therapy. However, patients do not satisfactorily respond to the current state of the art therapies. Only one-third of patients with depression reach complete remission,[33] which reflects our incomplete understanding of the aetiology and pathophysiology of psychiatric disorders. Indeed, all psychopharmacological approaches in psychiatry are symptom based (i.e., most of them work by inhibiting the reuptake of neurotransmitters, while not at the same time addressing other pathways such as neurotransmitter synthesis/availability by food, inflammation, brain plasticity, feeding time and circadian rhythms). A balanced diet, as part of a healthy lifestyle, is a key factor for the health of an individual, not only physically but also in terms of mental health.

Nutritional modifications could, besides having a positive influence on patients' overall health, target psychiatric disorders in a multifactorial approach. To improve both the prevention and treatment of psychiatric disorders, it is of utmost importance to expand our understanding of the underlying mechanisms and the therapeutic management of the disorders by recognising their multifactorial nature and apply a multisystemic treatment.

The field of nutritional psychiatry has evolved with rapidity over the past several years, with an increasing amount of dietary or nutrient-based (nutraceutical) intervention studies being initiated and more preclinical and epidemiological data being available. Nutritional psychiatry involves prescriptive dietary modification/improvement and/or the use of nutrient-based supplementation to prevent or treat psychiatric disorders. Several studies have shown the relationships between diet and mental disorders.[34,35] In a study by Jacka et al., participants with better diet quality were less likely to be depressed, while a high intake of processed foods was associated with increased levels of anxiety.[34] Micronutrients are vital to the proper functioning of the nervous and the immune system and several of these are often lacking in nonbalanced eating behaviour. In particular, low intakes of selenium, zinc, iron, magnesium, vitamin B12 and folic acid were found to be associated with increased depression risk.[36–40]

Studies point out that certain dietary types, such as the Mediterranean diet, are associated with a lower incidence of mental illness.[41–43] The consumption of fruit, vegetables, lean meat, fish, nuts and whole grain along with a low intake of processed and sugary foods was inversely associated with depression and depressive symptoms.

Diet represents a significant factor in shaping the gut microbiome and its metabolites. At the same time, studies have shown profound alterations of gut microbiota in patients with psychiatric disorders and symptoms of depression and anxiety.[44–46] In fact, dietary modification can change the complex assembly of bacteria which inhabit the human gastrointestinal tract (GIT) within days,[47] thereby changing the complex communication system between the GIT, the micro-organisms which inhabit it and the peripheral and central nervous systems. This is termed the microbiota–gut–brain axis (MGBA). All interventions that modify the MGBA (such as dietary modification, specific prebiotics (i.e., nondigestible fibre), probiotics (living bacteria), antibiotics, synbiotics (combinations of pre- and probiotics), postbiotics (bacterial fermentation products such as short chain fatty acids) and faecal microbiota transplantation) could be regarded as psychobiotics, as they are suggested to improve mental health through their microbiota-modifying properties.[48,49]

At the completion of this section, the reader will have learned about the definition and use of 'psychobiotics', have an overview of current dietary approaches for mental disorders, including depression, anxiety disorders, psychosis spectrum disorders and attention deficit hyperactivity disorder (ADHD) and be able to give dietary advice to patients.

WHAT IS A PSYCHOBIOTIC?

Bacteria, viruses, protozoa, archaea and fungi belong to the complex environment which resides in the GIT termed the 'gut microbiota', while the genetic information these bacteria carry is termed the 'gut microbiome'. Bacteria outnumber the number of body cells slightly and are essential for a range of physiological processes. Interestingly, cellular organelles such as mitochondria, the adenosine-triphosphate-producing power plants of the cells, are also of bacterial origin and seem to be related to Proteobacteria,[50] underlining the central role of bacteria for life, health and disease.

Every human being has a fingerprint-like individuality of microbial communities, and despite this the terms of 'dysbiosis' and 'healthy gut microbiome' are controversial.[51] The gut microbiome produces neurotransmitters such as serotonin, gamma-aminobutyric-acid, noradrenaline and dopamine[52] and has a role in synthesising micronutrients such as vitamin K and B-group vitamins including biotin, cobalamin, folates, nicotinic acid, pantothenic acid, pyridoxine, riboflavin and thiamine.[53]

The MGBA involves neural (vagus nerve and enteric nervous system), endocrine (cortisol and hypothalamic-pituitary-adrenal axis) and immune (cytokine) pathways, which are altered in psychiatric disorders. Notably, the MGBA could be targeted and modified with 'psychobiotics'. But what is a psychobiotic?

Originally, psychobiotics were defined as health-promoting bacteria, which, when ingested in adequate amounts, have a positive effect on mental health.[48,49] According to this prior definition, psychobiotics included only living bacteria. Recently, this definition was changed: the term 'psychobiotic' now also contains all microbiota-targeted interventions such as plant fibres (prebiotics), which enhance the growth of beneficial bacteria, enabling them to build butyrate, and propionate (postbiotics), which also have psychobiotic properties[49,54,55] (Fig. 13.1).

DIETARY PATTERNS AND DIETARY QUALITY: THE MEDITERRANEAN VERSUS WESTERN DIET

The Mediterranean diet (also often called a Cretan diet) is a form of diet inspired by the Mediterranean countries in the 1960s. It is by far the dietary pattern with the most substantial evidence base for mental health benefits. Studies showed that a Mediterranean diet not only leads to a lower incidence of cardiovascular disorders but also to better mental health status.[56] A

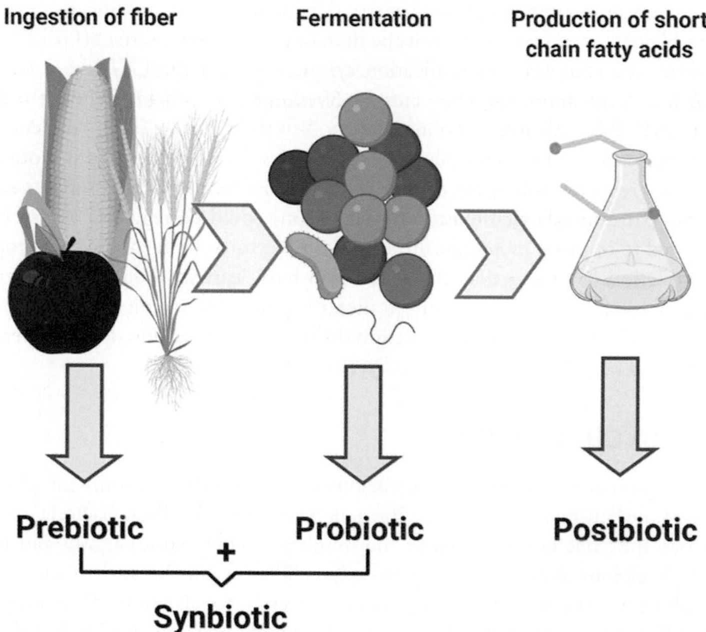

Fig. 13.1 Psychobiotics. (Created with BioRender.com.)

Mediterranean diet with nuts has a reduced risk for the development of depression.[42] The following key components define a Mediterranean diet: vegetables, fruit, nuts, legumes, fish and unsaturated fats.[57] Many components of a Mediterranean diet have been catalogued in a list of foods high in antidepressant nutrients. The highest-scoring foods were bivalves such as oysters and mussels, various seafoods, and plant foods such as leafy greens, lettuces, peppers, and cruciferous vegetables.[58] Both low intake of healthy food and high intakes of processed foods seem problematic for mental health.

Adherence to a Mediterranean diet was connected to a lower risk for depression with a linear dose–response relationship.[59] For example, the large European PREDIMED study demonstrated a reduced risk for incident depression in people with type 2 diabetes who were randomised to a Mediterranean diet with nuts, compared with a low-fat diet control group.[60] A Mediterranean diet ensures an adequate nutritional intake,[61] combines the effects of single nutrients and targets various mechanisms, including antiinflammatory, antioxidant, neurogenesis and microbiome- and immune-modifying activities.[62] Nevertheless, if a Mediterranean style diet is disassembled into its individual components, there is no single ingredient which accounts for its positive effects alone. It appears as though the complex characteristics of the nutritional composition are the basis for its efficacy.[63] This multifactorial perspective implies that such a prescriptive approach may potentially improve people's responses beyond an effect garnered from isolated nutrients.[64] However, a Mediterranean diet only reduces measurable symptoms of depression when a clinical diagnosis of depression is present.[65] The Supporting the Modification of Lifestyle in Lowered Emotional States trial included only patients with clinical depression. A modified Mediterranean diet intervention was associated with improvement in depression as measured with the Montgomery Asberg Depression Rating Scale compared with a social support intervention.[66] Stahl and colleagues showed that dietary coaching could prevent elderly persons from developing symptoms of depression.[67] Importantly, this nutritional intervention was as effective as a psychotherapeutic treatment. This study's participants, who received dietary coaching for 6 weeks, experienced a 40%–50% reduction of depressive symptoms and higher quality of life. These effects even persisted long term for 2 further years.[67] The time for dietary coaching was similar to short-time psychotherapy: Stahl et al. employed six to eight sessions of dietary advice over a 6- to 12-week period with semiannual booster sessions (3, 9, and 15 months after the treatment phase). While the first session lasted 1 hour, the following sessions took 30 minutes each.[67] In the study of Jacka et al., participants took part in seven individual dietary support sessions of roughly 60 minutes (four sessions weekly and three sessions every 2 weeks).[66] The dietary coaching study of Bersani et al. involved five weekly group sessions (in groups of eight patients) which took 90 minutes each.[68] Likewise, an Italian study showed effects of nutritional psychoeducation in patients with affective disorders and psychosis. In comparison with state-of-the-art psychoeducation, the dietary intervention group showed significant improvements of symptom severity, sleep quality and Mediterranean diet adherence.[68] Firth et al. summarised the results of 16 randomised controlled trials with a total of 45826 participants and could show that dietary interventions significantly reduce depressive symptoms.

Therefore, dietary advice to improve mental health seems to be a cost-effective, practical, nonpharmacological add-on intervention for patients suffering from depression.

THE ROLE OF MICRONUTRIENTS IN MENTAL HEALTH

Micronutrients are vital to the proper functioning of the nervous and the immune system, and a number of micronutrients such as selenium, zinc, iron, magnesium, vitamin B12 and folic acid are found to be inversely associated with increased depression risk.[36–40] Zinc, folate and other nutrients are lowered as a result when the immune system is activated and may be the consequence of mental illness itself. Further, qualitative and quantitative nutritional deficiencies, malabsorption, stress, age and genetic polymorphisms could demand a higher intake of nutrients to maintain the function of the central nervous system.[69] Micronutrients such as vitamins and minerals play an important role in the appropriate physiology and maintenance of health. Deficiencies of minerals and vitamins result in various disorders including neuropsychiatric diseases due to their essential contribution to neurological structures and signalling.

Besides the minerals that will be discussed in the following section, several vitamins, especially those belonging to the group of B vitamins, vitamin C and the fat-soluble vitamin D[70] and other antioxidant vitamins such as vitamin A and E, have been adversely associated with the occurrence of neuropathologies and may result in delirium, dementia, cognitive impairments or depression,[70] as well as psychosis and schizophrenia.[10]

A putative mechanism for vitamin D and the occurrence of autism, a neurodevelopmental disease, are primarily based on vitamin D's crucial role in neuroprotection in brain development, its function in cell proliferation and differentiation, immunomodulation as well as steroidogenesis and regulation of neurotransmission. Thus, it has been suggested that prenatal vitamin D deficiency may alter brain development.[71]

The neuropsychiatric effects of vitamin C result in adverse mood, depression and cognitive impairment long before symptoms of scurvy manifest. These can mechanistically be explained by vitamin C's substantial role in neurotransmitter synthesis and release in the brain. Vitamin C is involved in the conversation of dopamine to noradrenaline, the modulation of dopaminergic and glutamatergic neurotransmission, and the release of catecholamine and acetylcholine from synaptic vesicles and prevents neuronal damage in the brain due to its antioxidant properties.[72] Low vitamin C is attributed to poor dietary choices and low fruit and vegetable intake[10] which can often be observed in patients suffering from psychiatric diseases.[73]

Severe thiamine (vitamin B1) deficiency is often connected to chronic alcohol abuse and may result in Korsakoff syndrome as a consequence of inadequately treated Wernicke encephalopathy. Symptoms are global amnesia and major neurocognitive disorders.[74]

Recently, the correlation of nutritional deficiencies and first-episode psychosis have been described. Striking results have been observed for reduced levels of folate, vitamin D and vitamin C in the early onset of schizophrenia,[10] whereas in long-term schizophrenia, additional deficiencies of vitamins B12 and E were identified.

As an example of the effect of nutrient deficiency on mental health, vitamin B12 deficiency will be discussed in more depth. Vitamin B12 deficiency is reported to be a commonly overlooked cause of psychiatric morbidity.[7] A considerable number of people report on adhering to a vegan diet which appears to be an ongoing trend that has been established over the past decades. However, vegans are at risk of vitamin B12 deficiency since the main food sources of this nutrient are animal products.[10,75]

Mechanistically, the psychogenic and neurological effects of vitamin B12 deficiency can be explained by the vitamin's role in homocysteine cleavage in methionine metabolism. In brief, homocysteine is metabolised through demethylation of dietary methionine and can be remethylated to methionine via two pathways: besides the enzymatic and vitamin B6-dependent metabolisation to cysteine, homocysteine is remethylated by a vitamin B12 and folate-dependent mechanism[76] (Fig. 13.2).

Additionally, high levels of homocysteine in plasma are associated with oxidative stress leading to damage of dopaminergic neurons and interrupted dopamine biosynthesis, and the homocysteine's neurotoxicity (by induction of DNA strand breakage, DNA hypomethylation, oxidative stress and apoptosis) may lead to brain damage, which in turn may be a molecular mechanism for cognitive impairment and depression.[76]

For the synthesis of neurotransmitters such as dopamine, noradrenaline, adrenaline, melatonin and serotonin, intermediates of the methionine-homocysteine pathway (S-adenosylmethionine and A-adenosylhomocysteine) donate the required methyl groups. Thereby, vitamin B12 and

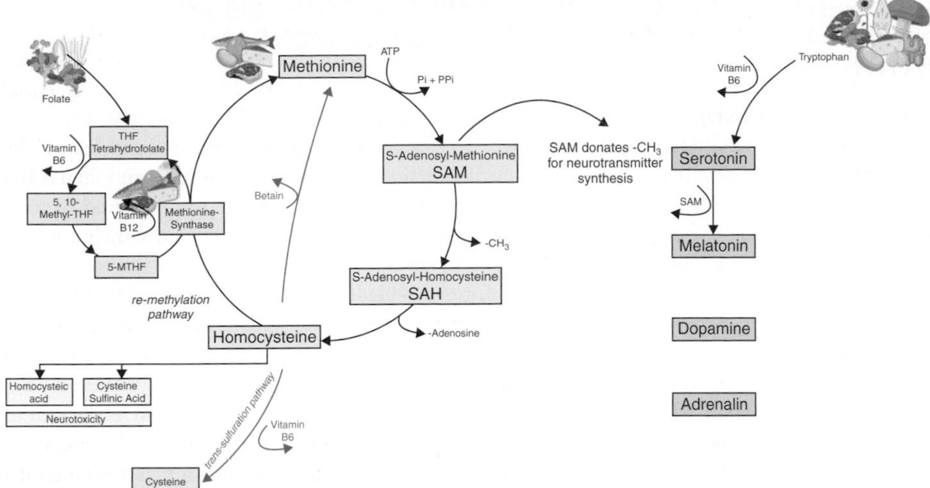

Fig. 13.2 The role of B vitamins in mental health. *MTHF*, Methyl-THF. (Created with BioRender.com.) (Modified from Bhatia P, Singh N. Homocysteine excess: delineating the possible mechanism of neurotoxicity and depression. *Fundam Clin Pharmacol*. 2015;29(38):522–528.

folate are required for converting homocysteine into S-adenosylmethionine, which exhibits an antidepressant function and plays a role in reducing oxidative stress via elevated production of glutathione[76] (see Fig. 13.2).

Thus, vitamin B12 deficiency and, to a lesser extent, folate deficiency are associated with depressive disorders,[76] as well as the aetiology of psychosis and schizophrenia.[10] Interestingly, it has already long been known that neuropsychiatric symptoms can precede anaemia and may occur with normal blood count.[77] However, it is reported that in clinical practice vitamin B12 deficiency without manifestation of anaemia often remains unconsidered and therefore untreated.[7] Thus, the evaluation of vitamin B12 status is warranted to ensure an adequate treatment of psychiatric symptoms.

Pathophysiological Theories of Mental Disorders

INFLAMMATORY THEORIES OF MENTAL DISORDERS

Apart from vulnerability and psychosocial factors, nutrition and inflammation are crucial circumstances relevant to the pathogenesis of depression. The inflammatory hypothesis of depression states that inflammatory processes influence the brain and cause symptoms such as anxiety and low mood. Persons with mental health issues predominantly show an inflammatory, unhealthy lifestyle, including poor dietary choices and nutritional deficiencies.[78,79] A poor diet has been shown to precede mental disorders and to be a risk factor for illness onset.[80] Commonly, patients with mood disorders consume a Western-style diet with less nutrient-dense foods, high amounts of fat and sugar and excess dietary energy compared with the general population.[81,82] Red and processed meat intake may be an additional risk factor for depression.[82] This may be due to proinflammatory arachidonic acid found in animal products, which increases suicide risk.[83] A Western-style diet alters gut microbiota composition and increases inflammatory pathways, leading to depressive symptoms.[38] Indeed, patients with depression show severely altered gut microbial composition.[84,85]

BIOCHEMISTRY OF MOOD: MONOAMINE HYPOTHESIS AND NECESSARY NUTRITIONAL COFACTORS FOR MONOAMINE SYNTHESIS

Schildkraut postulated that one of the reasons for depression could be a lack of neurotransmitters such as serotonin, noradrenaline or dopamine.[86] In this context, it is important to know about the necessary steps of serotonin synthesis and their interactions with inflammation. Tryptophan is the precursor of serotonin. If someone consumes tryptophan-rich food, for example, found in tofu, fish or soybeans, this tryptophan is either turned into serotonin and subsequently melatonin or follows another branch, where it is converted to kynurenine, kynurenic acid and quinolinic acid (Fig. 13.3). Kynurenine can be converted to various metabolites; some of these are considered neuroprotective (e.g., kynurenic acid), while others are neurotoxic (e.g., 3-hydroxykynurenine and quinolinic acid).

Indoleamine 2,3-dioxygenase is responsible for converting tryptophan to kynurenine and is triggered by inflammation. Therefore, indoleamine 2,3-dioxygenase activation is linked to increases in kynurenine and reductions in serotonin associated with depression.[87] While serotonin is antidepressant, quinolinic acid is neuroinflammatory, stimulates the brain excessing glutamate activity and inhibiting N-methyl-D-aspartate (NMDA) receptors and as a result promotes depression.[88,89] Kynurenine pathway metabolites have immune- and neuromodulatory properties. A number of factors determine whether tryptophan is broken down to serotonin or follows the neurotoxic branch to quinolinic acid. These include dietary choices, the presence of nutritional deficiencies, levels of stress and physical activity.[90]

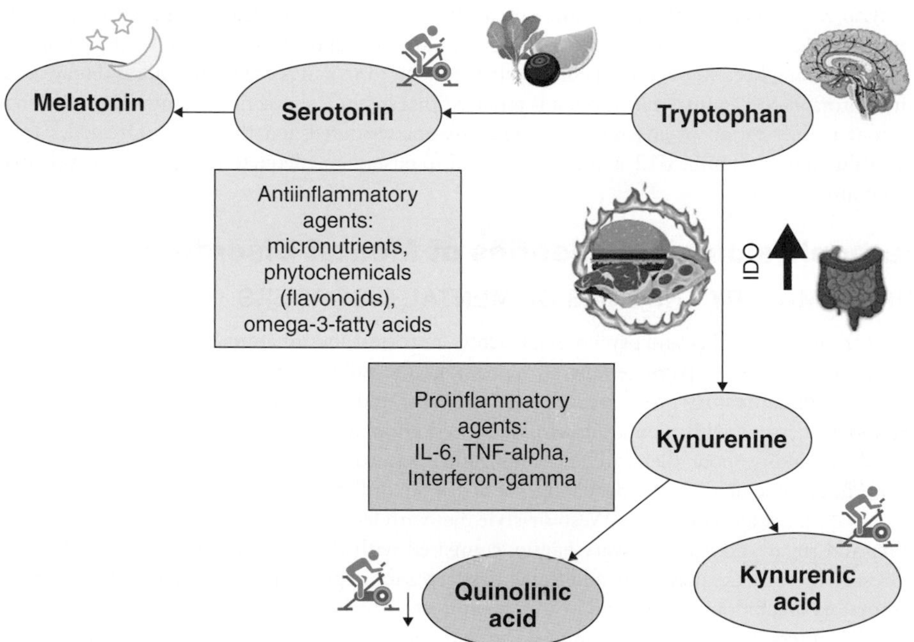

Fig. 13.3 **Tryptophan-kynurenine pathway in the context of nutrition and physical exercise.** *IDO*, Indoleamine 2,3-dioxygenase; *IL*, interleukin; *TNF*, tumour necrosis factor.

Nutritional Therapy for Psychiatric Disorders

NUTRITIONAL THERAPY FOR DEPRESSION

Being one of the most prevalent and severe mood disorders, major depression is deleterious to the patients' quality of life and of enormous socioeconomic impact. According to the World Health Organization, depression is the second most frequent cause of disability-adjusted life years in the age category of 15 to 44 years for both genders, with the number of patients continuing to grow. Depression is prevalent in the general population and presents with significant disability, as well as increased morbidity and premature mortality.[91]

Interestingly, many patients with depression crave sugars and carbohydrates, which could be attributed to a central deficiency in tryptophan, a serotonin precursor. Through insulin, glucose ingestion facilitates the entry of tryptophan into the brain.[92] Therefore, subjects eating high-carbohydrate diets experience less depressive symptoms and mood disturbances than people with low-carbohydrate diets.[93,94] Fig. 13.4 shows the synthesis of neurotransmitters involved in psychiatric disorders (serotonin, melatonin, dopamine, noradrenaline) along with dietary cofactors.[95–100] Monoamine oxidase (MAO) is responsible for the breakdown of neurotransmitters. Therefore, MAO blockers are used as second-line antidepressants as they cause a range of side effects.

Phytochemicals (i.e., found in berries, green tea, apples, grapes) and spices (turmeric, oregano, cinnamon, cloves) naturally inhibit MAO and lead to higher neurotransmitter availability.[101] One micronutrient has a range of physiological effects: for example, copper, which is found in legumes, nuts and cocoa, is a cofactor for the respiratory chain, antioxidative defence and synthesis of noradrenaline from dopamine and directs iron metabolism.[102]

Supplements used for treating depression are vitamin D, folic acid, vitamin B12, S-adenosyl-L-methionine, omega-3 polyunsaturated fatty acids, and zinc. Some micronutrients are important for synthesis of neurotransmitters, and others are responsible for neuronal differentiation and

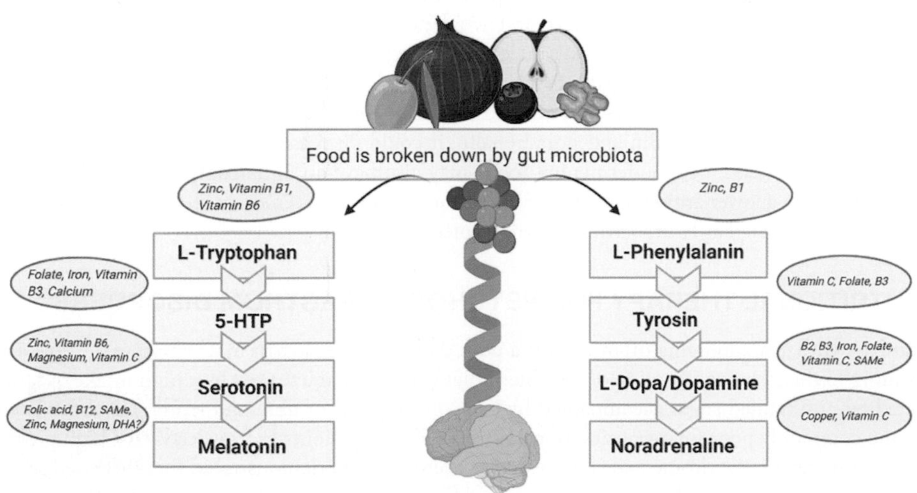

Fig. 13.4 Synthesis of neurotransmitters and necessary cofactors. *DHA*, Docosahexaenoic acid; *5-HTP*, 5-hydroxytryptophan; *SAMe*, S-adenosyl-L-methionine. (Figure created with Biorender.com.)

receptor expression. For example, vitamin D is important for dopamine signal transduction and enhances dopamine release and a higher vitamin D level is associated with a reduced depression risk.

However, for most of the micronutrients alone, the available data are not yet sufficient or inconclusive. Moreover, the form and delivery of micronutrients seem to be crucial to ensure effects. As for antioxidants and folate, they were found to work only when consumed from food sources and not from dietary supplements.[103,104] Another critical point are the possible interactions of micronutrients with antidepressants (i.e., some antidepressants may lower B vitamins[105,106]). To date, randomised controlled trials support the role of omega 3 fatty acids and zinc in the treatment of depression,[107] which will now be described in detail.

Depressed patients show a lower eicosapentaenoic acid and docosahexaenoic acid status,[108] and supplementation with omega-3 fatty acids improves symptoms of depressed patients, especially in those with high inflammatory markers.[109] Omega-3 fatty acid consumption (containing 1.5 to 2 g of eicosapentaenoic acid per day) has mood-stimulating effects in depressed patients.[110,111] Omega-3-supplements are currently in many treatment guidelines for major depression, for instance, in the guideline of the International Society for Nutritional Psychiatry Research.[112]

Zinc is involved in cellular immune response, hormone regulation and regulation of the hypothalamic-pituitary-adrenal axis. Therefore, a zinc deficiency could lead to depressive symptoms via activation of inflammatory processes[113] (and modification of the NMDA receptor[114]). Interestingly, zinc levels are lower in people with depression regardless of diet and increase in depressed patients after recovering from the depressive episode (without having taken any supplements). Studies show the beneficial effect of zinc as an add-on therapy to antidepressants.[107,115]

NUTRITIONAL THERAPY FOR ANXIETY

For anxiety, nutritional treatment options are not well researched. In addition to healthy guidelines such as eating a balanced diet, staying hydrated and avoiding excessive caffeine and alcohol intake, some additional considerations can help with anxiety. For example, complex carbohydrates are metabolised more slowly and, therefore, help maintain stable blood sugar levels, which prevents anxiety. Further, a regular eating pattern and avoidance of meal skipping result in constant blood sugar levels and may relieve feelings of anxiety. A dietary pattern rich in vegetables was shown to increase the tone of the parasympathetic nervous system.[116] A 2010 review found magnesium (for example, in grains, dairy, legumes, liver) could be a nutrient relevant for anxiety treatment.[117] As magnesium impedes adrenalin and noradrenalin, it could decrease anxiety symptoms due to its sympatholytic effect.[118] Some fermented foods may also have an antianxiety effect.[119] Anxiety is correlated with a lower antioxidant state.[120] Therefore, it stands to reason to recommend foods rich in antioxidants, such as fruit, berries, nuts and spices.[121]

NUTRITIONAL THERAPY FOR PSYCHOSIS-SPECTRUM DISORDERS

Patients with schizophrenia often exhibit a poor diet, especially when in a symptomatic episode. Adding to this, the consumption of a Western diet (mainly characterised by a high intake of saturated fat and refined sugar accompanied by low consumption of fibre and fruit[122]) is also related to the commonly poor financial situation of schizophrenic patients.[123] This leads to a high prevalence of metabolic syndrome and cardiovascular events.[124] Peet demonstrated that increased sugar consumption results in a decreased state of mind for schizophrenic patients with poor social functioning and a higher number of days spent in hospital.[125] In schizophrenia, fatty acid supplementation,[126] vitamin D and probiotic supplementation[127] showed positive results, while vitamin B supplementation did not improve symptoms.[128] However, data are limited by small sample sizes, short study duration and insufficient characterisation of patients. There is also some evidence that people with psychosis show increased antibodies to gliadin, a protein from grains that forms a part of gluten.[129] A specific subset of patients with schizophrenia may benefit from a gluten-free diet. However, more extensive clinical trials are needed to confirm this association.[130]

A diet recommended since the 1920s is the ketogenic diet, a controlled high-fat, low-protein, and low-carbohydrate diet.[131] In animal models, a ketogenic diet improved anxiety-related behaviours, depression-like behaviour and autism-spectrum disorder-related and schizophrenia-related behaviour, which may be partly attributable to changes in the gut microbiota.[132,133] However, these studies have limited generalisability to human conditions. To date, studies in patients are lacking and inconclusive. Therefore, there is no sufficient evidence for the use of a ketogenic diet in mental disorders such as schizophrenia.[134] However, to date, according to a Cochrane review on dietary advice for patients with schizophrenia, interventional studies are sparse and more research is needed to determine whether dietary intervention has an effect.[135]

NUTRITIONAL THERAPY FOR ADHD

ADHD in adulthood is a frequent disorder with a prevalence of 2.5%, which can successfully be treated by pharmacotherapy in 50%–70% of cases. Commonly, patients with ADHD show unhealthy dietary patterns. Current evidence is not strong enough to recommend specific dietary interventions for ADHD. A subgroup of children and adolescents may benefit from elimination diets (i.e., removal of particular food from the diet to eliminate potential allergens such as eggs, wheat, dairy, soy or artificial additives such as colours, flavours, sweeteners, monosodium glutamate and preservatives), but studies are scarce.[136] Further, there is still a lack of evidence for nutrient supplementation such as omega-3s and vitamin supplementation.[137]

SUPPLEMENTS/NUTRACEUTICALS AND PSYCHIATRY

Nutritional supplements or nutraceuticals were initially defined as 'a food or part of a food that has medical or health benefits, including the prevention and treatment of disease'.[138] As mentioned previously, there is some rationale for using nutraceuticals to treat psychiatric disorders, but still more evidence from randomised controlled trials is needed.

Most interventional studies with nutrients to date use a shotgun approach without sufficient biomarkers and checking for individual deficiencies of patients with psychiatric disorders. Therefore, they are often found to be not more effective than placebo. For example, the most extensive study to date on vitamin D supplementation for depression did not show a preventive effect on the incidence or recurrence of depression,[139] and a combination nutraceutical product did not outperform placebo in the treatment of depression.[140] This underlines the importance of testing baseline nutrient levels and inflammatory markers and adapting the nutritional intake according to baseline deficiencies, that is, by supplementing vitamins only when the patient demonstrates a deficiency (personalised nutrition); however, studies on these subjects are currently lacking.

Some recent approaches include the use of herbs and spices in psychiatry, such as saffron (*Crocus sativus*)[141] or turmeric (curcumin). A meta-analysis of randomised controlled trials for saffron supports its use for major depression as it is significantly more effective than a placebo.[142] Saffron's antidepressant effects are due to its serotonergic, antioxidant, antiinflammatory, neuroendocrine and neuroprotective effects.[143] The same is true for turmeric with its active compound curcumin[144]: neurochemically, curcumin could inhibit the MAO which subsequently regulates serotonin and dopamine levels, reduces inflammatory response, enhances neurogenesis and improves activities of antioxidant enzymes.[145]

Of course, a patient does not just live on individual nutrients alone or singular food items but eats a whole diet with several components interacting with each other and influencing brain function. Therefore, a whole-food, whole-diet approach may be more beneficial than the recommendation of a single nutrient supplement, a single probiotic or a particular type of food.

Giving Dietary Advice and Motivational Interviewing

Many people make efforts to improve their mental health through their diet; however, lasting dietary change remains difficult for many patients.

To change dietary behaviour, a technique called Motivational Interviewing (MI) may be useful. This technique was developed by the clinical psychologists William Miller and Stephen Rollnick and is an evidence-based, goal-directed and focused form of counselling. MI is a method to influence clients in the direction of behavioural change (i.e., a dietary change). Changes are often accompanied by ambivalence—a part of a person wants to stick to the old behaviour, while another part wants to change. This ambivalence causes anxiety, which frequently leads to procrastination and inhibition of a decision to change behaviour. MI helps in resolving ambivalence and helps elicit a motivation to change.[146]

To do MI, four core skills are necessary: open questions, affirmations, reflection and summaries. An open question is a question that cannot be answered by either yes or no and is used to gather information. Affirmations set a positive stimulus to confirm the decision of the patient (i.e., give a neutral observation of a person's strengths, resources, efforts, values) while reflections recapitulate the contents of the patient's statements in other words, which communicates attention and understanding. Table 13.1 gives an example of core skills in the nutritional context. Table 13.2 gives an overview on the processes of motivational interviewing, which are not linear but continuously run alongside a therapeutic process.[146]

MI aims to enhance personal control and self-efficacy and is useful for changing current health behaviors.[147] Therefore, it should be known and used by clinicians in the mental health sector to motivate for dietary change.

TABLE 13.1 ■ **Core Skills of Motivational Interviewing**

Open questions	**Tell me about your diet!** **What does your typical lunch look like?** **What do you have for breakfast?**
Affirmations	I really appreciate that you are willing to change your diet! Wow, you took your time to have breakfast for 3 days this week—how did you manage that? I really enjoyed talking with you today.
Reflections	It sounds like you… Maybe you are wondering if…am I right? So you feel…
Summary	Let me see if I understand so far… This is what I got so far…Please tell me if I missed anything.

Modified from Miller WR, Rollnick S. *Motivierende Gesprächsführung: Motivational Interviewing: 3. Auflage des Standardwerks in Deutsch*. Fribourg: Lambertus-Verlag; 2015.

TABLE 13.2 ■ **Overview on the Processes of Motivational Interviewing**

Processes	**Description**
Engaging	Every process starts with engaging, because without active engagement a goal cannot be reached.
Focusing	Motivational interview sets a trajectory toward a common goal.
Evoking	A goal (i.e., dietary change) is identified and agreed on; a 'change' talk is started to enhance the motivation for change.
Planning	Key strategies are planned to mobilise change.

Modified from Miller WR, Rollnick S. *Motivierende Gesprächsführung: Motivational Interviewing: 3. Auflage des Standardwerks in Deutsch*. Fribourg: Lambertus-Verlag; 2015.

Mindful Eating

There has been convincing evidence for a positive effect of mindfulness-based interventions concerning individual well-being and physical health in recent years. Mindfulness-based meditation and eating become more and more important in the prevention and treatment of chronic diseases.[148]

Mindfulness is the individual observation of direct experience using an open and nonjudgmental strategy. The Mindfulness-Based Stress Reduction program by Jon Kabat Zinn is used internationally, mainly to manage depression. There is also evidence for mindfulness in the management of pain and psychological well-being. As regards eating disorders and eating behaviour, there has been a focus on binge eating since the 1990s, with the development of using mindful eating in obese and overweight people. Mindful eating is defined as developing an awareness of physical versus psychological hunger and satiety. There is a strong focus on training the individual to notice distressing thoughts and emotions early, being able to tolerate distress and not to let it make the person eat more. The activity of several brain regions is altered in individuals practicing mindfulness. The findings show an overall calming of brain regions associated with subjective and cognitive appraisal of emotions. Mindfulness increases grey matter concentration in the left hippocampus and posterior cingulated cortex, temporo-parietal junction and cerebellum, as well as in areas associated with learning, emotional and self-referential processing. Self-monitoring of food intake is often disturbed by environmental cues, like packaging size and colouring. Mindfulness training can interrupt these automatic, nonconscious external influences.

Consequently, it is possible to reduce food intake in overweight conditions. Potential associated mechanisms in overweight people are increased awareness of and increased responsiveness to (1) internal physical cues, (2) internal emotional cues, (3) external cues.[149]

Mindfulness-based interventions are increasingly used to alter eating behaviours, reduce food cravings and promote weight regulation. The underlying mechanisms are hard to identify because a range of different components are used in complex intervention sets. Decentering based strategies are potential and investigated in more detail. This helps to understand the elective parts of mindfulness interventions.

Decentering, referring to seeing thoughts and feelings as temporary events, separated from oneself, has been found to change food intake and reduce chocolate consumption. Additionally, decentering can improve the ability to exercise self-control. Mechanisms that interact have been identified here: there is evidence that snacking on high-calorie food is often habitual and may occur as an automatic response to certain cues such as internal events like thoughts or memories. By decentering from these thoughts, more controlled decision-making is possible.[150]

Acceptance-based behavioural therapy focuses on awareness of internal experiences and emotions to accept those as temporary and not fixed character traits. A key component of this concept are mindfulness strategies.[151]

Mindfulness meditation was intensively studied by Mantzios and colleagues,[152] showing potential effects on weight loss and maintenance. They included sitting breath awareness practice to cultivate attention, nonreactivity and nonjudgment. Mindfulness walking meditation has its focus on body awareness. Mindful hunger awareness and eating meditation by taking a deep breath before eating, for example, resulted in changed eating quality.

Daubenmier and colleagues[153] conducted a weight calorie-restricted study with a 5.5-month diet and exercise intervention. They assessed the effectiveness of adding a mindfulness-based stress reduction and eating awareness training. The authors reported some significant clinical differences between the groups, but no difference in weight loss. Mason and colleagues followed a similar protocol to Daubenmier and included the Reward-based Eating Drive scale, wherein they could report on differences in the treatment groups.[153]

The inclusion of mindful eating as a prominent component of weight management programs has a high potential to improve long-term outcomes.[154]

Restraint and emotional eating, as maladaptive eating behaviour, are common in eating disorders. Lower levels of direct engagement with the eating experience are seen in patients with eating disorders. Compared with people with obesity, patients with anorexia nervosa and binge eating show lower access to direct experience while eating. Mindfulness is referring to self-regulation of attention to focus on the present-moment experience with an attitude of openness, acceptance of bodily sensations and emotions. Mindful eating is inversely correlated to the severity of eating disorders and seems to increase positive mood and healthy food choices. Mindful eating training could therefore be helpful in decreasing the anxiety response to food cues and confront the fear of eating in patients with eating disorders. In obese individuals, mindful eating may be useful only as a savouring tool but not to change eating behavior.[155]

PRACTISE MINDFUL EATING. THE RAISIN MEDITATION, MINDFUL EATING EXERCISE BY JON KABAT-ZINN[156]

Holding, seeing, and touching: Examine a raisin as if you had never seen it before. What does it look like? How does it fit in your hand, and how do the ridges feel on the pads of your fingers?

Smelling: Smell its aroma and get a sense of it. Does the smell arouse your senses? Does your mouth or stomach react?

Placing: Place the raisin on your tongue and hold it there. Turn the raisin around in your mouth, without chewing. How are you reacting? How does this raisin feel?

Tasting: Place the raisin between your teeth and bite. When you bite, notice the texture. Note the flavours as they release. Pause after a few bites and experience the flavour and texture in your mouth. Continue chewing and noticing—does its taste change?

Swallowing: Note the intention to ingest and the position your mouth takes. Finally, swallow the raisin and end up with a smile.

The Raisin Meditation, a mindful eating exercise by Jon Kabat-Zinn, is a wonderful example of what mindful eating can be. This intense sensual experience leads to full awareness of food in the moment.

Dietary Recommendations for General and Mental Health

As far as we are concerned, we should recommend a simple, plant-based diet for patients with psychiatric disorders. Evidence to date indicates that a Mediterranean-style diet is advisable.[66,68] Recommendations based on plates seem useful for teaching the patients what an ideal main-meal plate should look like: half the plate should be filled with a diverse range of vegetables and salads, a quarter with unprocessed protein (like fish, red meat, tofu, legume, cheese) and the final quarter with whole grains such as whole-grain pasta, quinoa, barley, or brown rice. Further, easily memorable concepts to increase vegetable and fruit intake (such as 'eat the rainbow',[157] thus advising the patient to add different-coloured fruits and vegetables to every meal) could be used within this concept. Future human studies will show whether an additional intake of fermented foods such as kefir is helpful to influence the symptoms of psychiatric disorders.[158] Of course, diet is no substitute for adequate psychopharmacological therapy but should be one of the pillars of psychiatric treatment. Psychiatric disorders are multifactorial, and therefore need to be treated in a systemic, biopsychosocial fashion.[159]

Conclusion

As research methodology improves and understanding of the gut health's relation to not only inflammation but also to psychiatry grows, practitioners can incorporate measurable lifestyle interventions to guide patients toward sustainable improvements in both their physical and mental health. By working with the patient to improve gut health (in addition to ongoing therapy), there is potential to improve the individual's quality of life while also treating the symptoms of psychiatric disorders. Nutritional psychiatry is a young field, and future studies will show whether approaches of personal nutrition should be integrated in standard care. Of course, psychiatric disorders cause patients to eat a less healthy diet which alters the gut microbiome and inflammatory pathways, but conversely, an altered gut microbiome could influence dietary behaviour and could subsequently be a risk factor for the development of mental disorders. Nevertheless, it may not be important to know which of these factors was there first to escape this vicious circle. It may be more important for clinicians to be aware that psychiatric disorders are multifactorial diseases that need to be treated in a multifactorial way. While acute diseases can be seen mechanistically, most chronic and psychiatric diseases need to be seen systemically. So, when one part of the system (for example, diet) is changed, it automatically influences other parts of the system (gut microbiome, cognition, mood, appetite). Therefore, the mental health clinician should be aware of interventions targeting mental health and the microbiota–gut–brain axis.

References

Note: This chapter contains an extended reference list due to the novel and emerging nature of this field.

1. Boulanger AS, Paquette I, Létourneau G, Richard-Devantoy S. Thiamine et encéphalopathie de Gayet-Wernicke: quelles règles de prescription? [Wernicke encephalopathy: Guiding thiamine prescription]. *L'Encephale*. 2017;43(3):259–267. https://doi.org/10.1016/j.encep.2016.04.011.
2. Liang H, Wu L, Liu LL, Han J, Zhu J, Jin T. A case report: Non-alcoholic Wernicke encephalopathy associated with polyneuropathy. *J Int Med Res*. 2017;45(6):1794–1801.
3. Galvin R, Bråthen G, Ivashynka A, et al. EFNS guidelines for diagnosis, therapy and prevention of Wernicke encephalopathy. *Eur J Neurol*. 2010;17(12):1408–1418. https://doi.org/10.1111/j.1468-1331.2010.03153.x.
4. Abdou E, Hazell AS. Thiamine deficiency: an update of pathophysiologic mechanisms and future therapeutic considerations. *Neurochem Res*. 2015;40(2):353–361. https://doi.org/10.1007/s11064-014-1430-z.

5. Alcaide ML, Jayaweera D, Espinoza L, Kolber M. Wernicke's encephalopathy in AIDS: a preventable cause of fatal neurological deficit. *Int J STD AIDS*. 2003;14(10):712–713. https://doi.org/10.1258/095646203322387992.
6. Sechi G, Serra A. Wernicke's encephalopathy: new clinical settings and recent advances in diagnosis and management. *Lancet Neurol*. 2007;6(5):442–455. https://doi.org/10.1016/S1474-4422(07)70104-7.
7. Rao NP, Kumar NC, Raman BR, Sivakumar PT, Pandey RS. Role of vitamin B12 in depressive disorder—a case report. *Gen Hosp Psychiatry*. 2008;30(2):185–186.
8. American Psychiatric Association *Diagnostic and Statistical Manual of Mental Health Disorders: DSM-5*. 5th ed. Washington DC: American Psychiatric Publishing; 2013.
9. Weikert C, Trefflich I, Menzel J, et al. Vitamin and mineral status in a vegan diet. *Dtsch Arztebl Int*. 2020;117(35-36):575–582. https://doi.org/10.3238/arztebl.2020.0575.
10. Firth J, Carney R, Stubbs B, et al. Nutritional deficiencies and clinical correlates in first-episode psychosis: A systematic review and meta-analysis. *Schizophr Bull*. 2018;44(6):1275–1292.
11. Khosravi M, Sotoudeh G, Amini M, et al. The relationship between dietary patterns and depression mediated by serum levels of Folate and vitamin B12. *BMC Psychiatry*. 2020;20:63. https://doi.org/10.1186/s12888-020-2455-2.
12. Mehra A, Sharma N, Grover S. Tekrarlayan Majör Depresif Bozukluğu Olan Bir Kadın HastadaPagofaji: Bir Olgu Sunumu ve Literatür Derlemesi [Pagophagia in a Female with Recurrent Depressive Disorder: A Case Report with Review of Literature]. *Turk Psikiyatri Derg*. 2018;29(2):143–145.
13. Khatib MA, Rahim O, Kania R, Molloy P. Case report: Iron deficiency anemia: Induced by long-term ingestion of omeprazole. *Dig Dis Sci*. 2002;47(11):2596–2597.
14. Barton JC, Barton JC, Bertoli LF. Pagophagia in men with iron-deficiency anemia. *Blood Cells Mol Dis*. 2019;77:72–75.
15. Seeman MV. Why are women prone to restless legs syndrome? *Int J Environ Res Public Health*. 2020;17(1):368. https://doi.org/10.3390/ijerph17010368.
16. Hamano H, Niimura T, Horinouchi Y, et al. Proton pump inhibitors block iron absorption through direct regulation of hepcidin via the aryl hydrocarbon receptor-mediated pathway. *Toxicol Lett*. 2020;318:86–91.
17. Dahlerup JF, Eivindson M, Jacobsen BA, et al. Diagnosis and treatment of unexplained anemia with iron deficiency without overt bleeding. *Dan Med J*. 2015;62(4):C5072.
18. Parry-Jones B. Pagophagia, or compulsive ice consumption: A historical perspective. *Psychol Med*. 1992;22(3):561–571.
19. World Health Organization *International Statistical Classification of Diseases and Related Health Problems: 10th Revision (ICD-10)*. 5th ed. Geneva: WHO Library Cataloguing-in-Publication Data; 2016.
20. Beck AT, Ward CH, Mendelson M, Mock J, Erbaugh J. An inventory for measuring depression. *Arch Gen Psychiatry*. 1961;4:561–571.
21. Hamilton M. A rating scale for depression. *J Neurol Neurosurg Psychiatry*. 1960;23:56–62.
22. Mörkl S, Lackner S, Müller W, et al. Gut microbiota and body composition in inpatients with anorexia nervosa in comparison to athletes, overweight, obese and normal weight controls. *Int J Eat Dis*. 2017;50(12):1421–1431.
23. Deutsche Gesellschaft für Ernährung (DGE), Österreichische Gesellschaft für Ernährung (ÖGE), Schweizerische Gesellschaft für Ernährung (SGE), *D-A-CH-Referenzwerte für die Nährstoffzufuhr*. 2 (4) ed. Bonn: Neuer Umschau Buchverlag; 2018.
24. Federal Ministry Republic of Austria. Social Affairs, Health, Care and Consumer Protection. The Austrian Food Pyramid. 2022. Available at: https://broschuerenservice.sozialministerium.at/Home/Download?publicationId=617. Accessed 10.05, 2020.
25. Stewart A, Marfell-Jones M, Olds T, De Ridder J. International Standards for Anthropometric Assessment. Lower Hut, New Zealand: International Society for the Advancement of Kinanthropometry; 2011. ISBN: 0-620-36207-3.
26. Lackner S, Mörkl S, Müller W, et al. Novel approaches for the assessment of relative body weight and body fat in diagnosis and treatment of anorexia nervosa: A cross-sectional study. *Clin nutr*. 2019;38(6):2913–2921. https://doi.org/10.1016/j.clnu.2018.12.031.
27. Müller W, Lohman TG, Stewart AD, et al. Subcutaneous fat patterning in athletes: Selection of appropriate sites and standardisation of a novel ultrasound measurement technique: Ad hoc working group on body composition, health and performance, under the auspices of the IOC Medical Commission. *Br J Sports Med*. 2016;50(1):45–54.

28. Ackland TR, Müller W. Imaging method: Ultrasound. In: Hume PA, Kerr DA, Ackland TR, eds. *Best Practice Protocols for Physique Assessment in Sport*. 1st ed. Singapore: Springer; 2018:131–141.
29. Treasure J, Zipfel S, Micali N, et al. Anorexia nervosa. *Nat Rev Dis Primers*. 2015;1:15074.
30. Treasure J, Stein D, Maguire S. Has the time come for a staging model to map the course of eating disorders from high risk to severe enduring illness? An examination of the evidence. *Early Interv Psychiatry*. 2015;9(3):173–184.
31. Mack I, Cuntz U, Grämer C, et al. Weight gain in anorexia nervosa does not ameliorate the faecal microbiota, branched chain fatty acid profiles, and gastrointestinal complaints. *Sci Rep*. 2016;6:26752.
32. Saraceno B. The WHO World Health Report 2001 on mental health. *Epidemiol Psichiatr Soc*. 2011;11:83–87.
33. Tranter R, O'Donovan C, Chandarana P, Kennedy S. Prevalence and outcome of partial remission in depression. *J Psychiatry Neurosci*. 2002;27(4):241.
34. Jacka FN, Mykletun A, Berk M, Bjelland I, Tell GS. The association between habitual diet quality and the common mental disorders in community-dwelling adults: the Hordaland Health study. *Psychosom med*. 2011;73(6):483–490. https://doi.org/10.1097/PSY.0b013e318222831a.
35. Godos J, Currenti W, Angelino D, et al. Diet and mental health: Review of the recent updates on molecular mechanisms. *Antioxidants*. 2020;9(4):346. https://doi.org/10.3390/antiox9040346.
36. Quirk SE, Williams LJ, O'Neil A, et al. The association between diet quality, dietary patterns and depression in adults: a systematic review. *BMC psychiatry*. 2013;13:175. https://doi.org/10.1186/1471-244X-13-175.
37. Murakami K, Mizoue T, Sasaki S, et al. Dietary intake of folate, other B vitamins, and omega-3 polyunsaturated fatty acids in relation to depressive symptoms in Japanese adults. *Nutrition*. 2008;24(2):140–147. https://doi.org/10.1016/j.nut.2007.10.013.
38. Sandhu KV, Sherwin E, Schellekens H, Stanton C, Dinan TG, Cryan JF. Feeding the microbiota-gut-brain axis: diet, microbiome, and neuropsychiatry. *Transl Res*. 2017;179:223–244. https://doi.org/10.1016/j.trsl.2016.10.002.
39. Briguglio M, Dell'Osso B, Panzica G, et al. Dietary neurotransmitters: A narrative review on current knowledge. *Nutrients*. 2018;10(5):591. https://doi.org/10.3390/nu10050591.
40. Wei P, Keller C, Li L. Neuropeptides in gut-brain axis and their influence on host immunity and stress. *Comput Struct Biotechnol J*. 2020;18:843–851. https://doi.org/10.1016/j.csbj.2020.02.018.
41. Mantzorou M, Vadikolias K, Pavlidou E, et al. Mediterranean diet adherence is associated with better cognitive status and less depressive symptoms in a Greek elderly population. *Aging Clin Exp Res*. 2021;33(4):1033–1040. https://doi.org/10.1007/s40520-020-01608-x.
42. Sánchez-Villegas A, Delgado-Rodríguez M, Alonso A, et al. Association of the Mediterranean dietary pattern with the incidence of depression: the Seguimiento Universidad de Navarra/University of Navarra follow-up (SUN) cohort. *Arch. Gen. Psychiatry*. 2009;66(10):1090–1098. https://doi.org/10.1001/archgenpsychiatry.2009.129.
43. Vicinanza R, Bersani FS, D'Ottavio E, et al. Adherence to Mediterranean diet moderates the association between multimorbidity and depressive symptoms in older adults. *Arch. Gerontol. Geriatr*. 2020;88:104022. https://doi.org/10.1016/j.archger.2020.104022.
44. Bastiaanssen TFS, Cowan CSM, Claesson MJ, Dinan TG, Cryan JF. Making sense of… the microbiome in psychiatry. *Int J Neuropsychopharmacol*. 2019;22(1):37–52. https://doi.org/10.1093/ijnp/pyy067.
45. Mörkl S, Wagner-Skacel J, Lahousen T, et al. The role of nutrition and the gut-brain axis in psychiatry: A review of the literature. *Neuropsychobiology*. 2018:1–9. Advance online publication. https://doi.org/10.1159/000492834.
46. Painold A, Mörkl S, Kashofer K, et al. A step ahead: Exploring the gut microbiota in inpatients with bipolar disorder during a depressive episode. *Bipolar Disord*. 2019;21(1):40–49. https://doi.org/10.1111/bdi.12682.
47. David L, Maurice C, Carmody R, et al. Diet rapidly and reproducibly alters the human gut microbiome. *Nature*. 2014;505:559–563. https://doi.org/10.1038/nature12820.
48. Dinan TG, Stanton C, Cryan JF. Psychobiotics: a novel class of psychotropic. *Biol. Psychiatry*. 2013;74(10):720–726. https://doi.org/10.1016/j.biopsych.2013.05.001.
49. Sarkar A, Lehto SM, Harty S, Dinan TG, Cryan JF, Burnet PWJ. Psychobiotics and the manipulation of bacteria-gut-brain signals. *Trends Neurosci*. 2016;39(11):763–781.
50. Roger AJ, Muñoz-Gómez SA, Kamikawa R. The origin and diversification of mitochondria. *Current Biol*. 2017;27(21):R1177–R1192.

51. Moloney RD, Desbonnet L, Clarke G, Dinan TG, Cryan JF. The microbiome: Stress, health and disease. *Mamm Genome*. 2014;25(1–2):49–74.
52. Cheung SG, Goldenthal AR, Uhlemann A, Mann JJ, Miller JM, Sublette ME. Systematic review of gut microbiota and major depression. *Front Psychiatry*. 2019;10:34.
53. Hill MJ. Intestinal flora and endogenous vitamin synthesis. *Eur J Cancer Prev*. 1997;6(Suppl 1):S43–S45. https://doi.org/10.1097/00008469-199703001-00009.
54. Gibson GR, Roberfroid MB. Dietary modulation of the human colonic microbiota: Introducing the concept of prebiotics. *J Nutr*. 1995;125(6):1401–1412.
55. Liu RT, Walsh RFL, Sheehan AE. Prebiotics and probiotics for depression and anxiety: A systematic review and meta-analysis of controlled clinical trials. *Neurosci Biobehav Rev*. 2019
56. Muñoz MA, Fíto M, Marrugat J, Covas MI, Schröder H, REGICOR and HERMES investigators. Adherence to the Mediterranean diet is associated with better mental and physical health. *Br J Nutr*. 2009;101(12):1821–1827. https://doi.org/10.1017/S0007114508143598.
57. Trichopoulou A, Kouris-Blazos A, Wahlqvist ML, et al. Diet and overall survival in elderly people. *BMJ*. 1995;311(7018):1457–1460.
58. LaChance LR, Ramsey D. Antidepressant foods: An evidence-based nutrient profiling system for depression. *World J Psychiatr*. 2018;8(3):97–104. https://doi.org/10.5498/wjp.v8.i3.97.
59. Molendijk M, Molero P, Sánchez-Pedreño FO, Van der Does W, Martínez-González MA. Diet quality and depression risk: A systematic review and dose-response meta-analysis of prospective studies. *J Affect Disord*. 2018;226:346–354.
60. Sánchez-Villegas A, Martínez-González MA, Estruch R, et al. Mediterranean dietary pattern and depression: the PREDIMED randomized trial. *BMC Med*. 2013;11:208. https://doi.org/10.1186/1741-7015-11-208.
61. Milaneschi Y, Bandinelli S, Penninx BW, et al. Depressive symptoms and inflammation increase in a prospective study of older adults: a protective effect of a healthy (Mediterranean-style) diet. *Mol Psychiatry*. 2011;16(6):589–590. https://doi.org/10.1038/mp.2010.113.
62. Marx W, Moseley G, Berk M, Jacka F. Nutritional psychiatry: the present state of the evidence. *Proc Nutr Soc*. 2017;76(4):427–436. https://doi.org/10.1017/S0029665117002026.
63. Schwingshackl L, Hoffmann G. Does a Mediterranean-type diet reduce cancer risk? *Curr Nutr Rep*. 2016;5(1):9–17.
64. Sarris J, Logan AC, Akbaraly TN, et al. Nutritional medicine as mainstream in psychiatry. *Lancet Psychiatry*. 2015;2(3):271–274.
65. Wardle J, Rogers P, Judd P, et al. Randomized trial of the effects of cholesterol-lowering dietary treatment on psychological function. *Am J Med*. 2000;108(7):547–553. https://doi.org/10.1016/s0002-9343(00)00330-2.
66. Jacka FN, O'Neil A, Opie R, et al. A randomised controlled trial of dietary improvement for adults with major depression (the 'SMILES' trial). *BMC Med*. 2017;15(1):23.
67. Stahl ST, Albert SM, Dew MA, Lockovich MH, Reynolds III CF. Coaching in healthy dietary practices in at-risk older adults: A case of indicated depression prevention. *Am J Psychiatry*. 2014;171(5): 499–505.
68. Bersani FS, Biondi M, Coviello M, et al. Psychoeducational intervention focused on healthy living improves psychopathological severity and lifestyle quality in psychiatric patients: Preliminary findings from a controlled study. *J Ment Health*. 2017;26(3):271–275.
69. Akhondzadeh S, Gerbarg PL, Brown RP. Nutrients for prevention and treatment of mental health disorders. *Psychiatr Clin North Am*. 2013;36(1):25–36.
70. Maxwell 4th PJ, Montgomery SC, Cavallazzi R, Martindale RG. What micronutrient deficiencies should be considered in distinct neurological disorders? *Curr Gastroenterol Rep*. 2013;15(7):331–337.
71. Ali A, Cui X, Eyles D. Developmental vitamin D deficiency and autism: Putative pathogenic mechanisms. *J Steroid Biochem Mol Biol*. 2018;175:108–118.
72. Plevin D, Galletly C. The neuropsychiatric effects of vitamin C deficiency: a systematic review. *BMC Psychiatry*. 2020;20:315. https://doi.org/10.1186/s12888-020-02730-w.
73. Aucoin M, LaChance L, Cooley K, Kidd S. Diet and psychosis: A scoping review. *Neuropsychobiology*. 2020;79(1):20–42.
74. Arts NJ, Walvoort SJ, Kessels RP. Korsakoff's syndrome: A critical review. *Neuropsychiatr Dis Treat*. 2017;13:2875–2890.

75. Oh R, Brown DL. Vitamin B12 deficiency. *Am Fam Physician*. 2003;67(5):979–986.
76. Bhatia P, Singh N. Homocysteine excess: Delineating the possible mechanism of neurotoxicity and depression. *Fundam Clin Pharmacol*. 2015;29(6):522–528.
77. Lindenbaum J, Healton EB, Savage DG, et al. Neuropsychiatric disorders caused by cobalamin deficiency in the absence of anemia or macrocytosis. *N Engl J Med*. 1988;318(26):1720–1728.
78. Scott D, Happell B. The high prevalence of poor physical health and unhealthy lifestyle behaviours in individuals with severe mental illness. *Issues Ment Health Nurs*. 2011;32(9):589–597. https://doi.org/10.3109/01612840.2011.569846.
79. Teasdale SB, Ward PB, Samaras K, et al. Dietary intake of people with severe mental illness: systematic review and meta-analysis. *Br J Psychiatry*. 2019;214(5):251–259. https://doi.org/10.1192/bjp.2019.20.
80. Lassale C, Batty GD, Baghdadli A, et al. Healthy dietary indices and risk of depressive outcomes: a systematic review and meta-analysis of observational studies. *Mol Psychiatry*. 2019;24:965–986. https://doi.org/10.1038/s41380-018-0237-8.
81. Lopresti AL, Jacka FN. Diet and bipolar disorder: A review of its relationship and potential therapeutic mechanisms of action. *J Altern Complement Med*. 2015;21(12):733–739. https://doi.org/10.1089/acm.2015.0125.
82. Nucci D, Fatigoni C, Amerio A, Odone A, Gianfredi V. Red and processed meat consumption and risk of depression: A systematic review and meta-analysis. *Int J Environ Res Public Health*. 2020;17(18):6686. https://doi.org/10.3390/ijerph17186686.
83. Vaz JS, Kac G, Nardi AE, Hibbeln JR. Omega-6 fatty acids and greater likelihood of suicide risk and major depression in early pregnancy. *J Affect Disord*. 2014;152–154,76–82. https://doi.org/10.1016/j.jad.2013.04.045.
84. Valles-Colomer M, Falony G, Darzi Y, et al. The neuroactive potential of the human gut microbiota in quality of life and depression. *Nat Microbiol*. 2019;4:623–632. https://doi.org/10.1038/s41564-018-0337-x.
85. Sanada K, Nakajima S, Kurokawa S, et al. Gut microbiota and major depressive disorder: A systematic review and meta-analysis. *J Affect Disord*. 2020;266:1–13. https://doi.org/10.1016/j.jad.2020.01.102.
86. Schildkraut JJ. The catecholamine hypothesis of affective disorders: A review of supporting evidence. *Am J Psychiatry*. 1965;122(5):509–522.
87. Miura H, Ozaki N, Sawada M, Isobe K, Ohta T, Nagatsu T. A link between stress and depression: Shifts in the balance between the kynurenine and serotonin pathways of tryptophan metabolism and the etiology and pathophysiology of depression. *Stress*. 2008;11(3):198–209.
88. Guillemin GJ. Quinolinic acid, the inescapable neurotoxin. *FEBS J*. 2012;279(8):1356–1365.
89. Myint AM, Kim Y, Verkerk R, et al. Tryptophan breakdown pathway in bipolar mania. *J Affect Disord*. 2007;102(1–3):65–72.
90. Joisten N, Kummerhoff F, Koliamitra C, et al. Exercise and the Kynurenine pathway: Current state of knowledge and results from a randomized cross-over study comparing acute effects of endurance and resistance training. *Exerc Immunol Rev*. 2020;26:24–42.
91. Walker ER, McGee RE, Druss BG. Mortality in mental disorders and global disease burden implications: a systematic review and meta-analysis. *JAMA Psychiatry*. 2015;72(4):334–341. https://doi.org/10.1001/jamapsychiatry.2014.2502.
92. Berlin I, Vorspan F, Warot D, Manéglier B, Spreux-Varoquaux O. Effect of glucose on tobacco craving. Is it mediated by tryptophan and serotonin? *Psychopharmacology*. 2005;178(1):27–34. https://doi.org/10.1007/s00213-004-1980-x.
93. Brinkworth GD, Luscombe-Marsh ND, Thompson CH, et al. Long-term effects of very low-carbohydrate and high-carbohydrate weight-loss diets on psychological health in obese adults with type 2 diabetes: randomized controlled trial. *J Intern Med*. 2016;280(4):388–397. https://doi.org/10.1111/joim.12501.
94. Wurtman JJ, Brzezinski A, Wurtman RJ, Laferrere B. Effect of nutrient intake on premenstrual depression. *Am J Obstet Gynecol*. 1989;161(5):1228–1234. https://doi.org/10.1016/0002-9378(89)90671-6.
95. Peuhkuri K, Sihvola N, Korpela R. Dietary factors and fluctuating levels of melatonin. *Food & Nutrition Research*. 2012;56:17252. https://doi.org/10.3402/fnr.v56i0.17252.
96. Morton DJ. Possible mechanisms of inhibition and activation of rat N-acetyltransferase (EC 2.3.1.5.) by cations. *J Neural Transm*. 1989;75(1):51–64. https://doi.org/10.1007/BF01250643.

97. Zaouali-Ajina M, Gharib A, Durand G, et al. Dietary docosahexaenoic acid-enriched phospholipids normalize urinary melatonin excretion in adult (n-3) polyunsaturated fatty acid-deficient rats. *J Nutr.* 1999;129(11):2074–2080. https://doi.org/10.1093/jn/129.11.2074.
98. Maximino C. *Serotonin and Anxiety: Neuroanatomical, Pharmacological, and Functional Aspects.* New York: Springer; 2012.
99. Gropper SS, Smith JL. *Advanced Nutrition and Human Metabolism.* Boston, USA: Cengage Learning; 2012. ISBN 9781133104056.
100. Duff J. Chapter Fourteen - Nutrition for ADHD and Autism. In: Cantor DS, Evans JR, eds. *Clinical Neurotherapy.* Boston: Academic Press; 2014:357–381.
101. Dixon Clarke SE, Ramsay RR. Dietary inhibitors of monoamine oxidase A. *J Neural Transm.* 2011;118(7):1031–1041. https://doi.org/10.1007/s00702-010-0537-x.
102. Widhalm K. *Ernährungsmedizin: mit 219 Tabellen.* Deutscher Ärzte-Verlag, Köln; 2009.
103. Payne ME, Steck SE, George RR, Steffens DC. Fruit, vegetable, and antioxidant intakes are lower in older adults with depression. *J Acad Nutr Diet.* 2012;112(12):2022–2027. https://doi.org/10.1016/j.jand.2012.08.026.
104. Sharpley AL, Hockney R, McPeake L, Geddes JR, Cowen PJ. Folic acid supplementation for prevention of mood disorders in young people at familial risk: a randomised, double blind, placebo controlled trial. *J Affect Disord.* 2014;167:306–311. https://doi.org/10.1016/j.jad.2014.06.011.
105. Pinto J, Huang YP, Rivlin RS. Inhibition of riboflavin metabolism in rat tissues by chlorpromazine, imipramine, and amitriptyline. *J Clin Invest.* 1981;67(5):1500–1506. https://doi.org/10.1172/jci110180.
106. Viljoen M, Swanepoel A, Bipath P. Antidepressants may lead to a decrease in niacin and NAD in patients with poor dietary intake. *Med Hypotheses.* 2015;84(3):178–182. https://doi.org/10.1016/j.mehy.2014.12.017.
107. Schefft C, Kilarski LL, Bschor T, Köhler S. Efficacy of adding nutritional supplements in unipolar depression: A systematic review and meta-analysis. *Eur Neuropsychopharmacol.* 2017;27(11):1090–1109. https://doi.org/10.1016/j.euroneuro.2017.07.004.
108. Lin PY, Huang SY, Su KP. A meta-analytic review of polyunsaturated fatty acid compositions in patients with depression. *Biol Psychiatry.* 2010;68(2):140–147.
109. Rapaport MH, Nierenberg AA, Schettler PJ, et al. Inflammation as a predictive biomarker for response to omega-3 fatty acids in major depressive disorder: A proof-of-concept study. *Mol Psychiatry.* 2016;21(1):71–79.
110. Adams PB, Lawson S, Sanigorski A, Sinclair AJ. Arachidonic acid to eicosapentaenoic acid ratio in blood correlates positively with clinical symptoms of depression. *Lipids.* 1996;31(Suppl):157.
111. Bae JH, Kim G. Systematic review and meta-analysis of omega-3-fatty acids in elderly patients with depression. *Nutr Res.* 2018;50:1–9.
112. Guu TW, Mischoulon D, Sarris J, et al. A multi-national, multi-disciplinary Delphi consensus study on using omega-3 polyunsaturated fatty acids (n-3 PUFAs) for the treatment of major depressive disorder. *J Affect Disord.* 2020;265:233–238.
113. Martínez-Cengotitabengoa M, Carrascón L, O'Brien JT, et al. Peripheral inflammatory parameters in late-life depression: A systematic review. *Int J Mol Sci.* 2016;17(12):2022. https://doi.org/10.3390/ijms17122022.
114. Pittenger C, Sanacora G, Krystal JH. The NMDA receptor as a therapeutic target in major depressive disorder. *CNS Neurol Disord Drug Targets.* 2007;6(2):101–115.
115. Lai J, Moxey A, Nowak G, Vashum K, Bailey K, McEvoy M. The efficacy of zinc supplementation in depression: Systematic review of randomised controlled trials. *J Affect Disord.* 2012;136(1–2):e31–e39.
116. Young HA, Benton D. Heart-rate variability: a biomarker to study the influence of nutrition on physiological and psychological health. *Behav Pharmacol.* 2018;29(2 and 3-Spec Issue):140–151. https://doi.org/10.1097/FBP.0000000000000383.
117. Lakhan SE, Vieira Karen F%J. Nutritional and herbal supplements for anxiety and anxiety-related disorders: Systematic review. *Nutr J.* 2010;9(1):42.
118. Shimosawa T, Takano K, Ando K, Fujita T. Magnesium inhibits norepinephrine release by blocking N-type calcium channels at peripheral sympathetic nerve endings. *Hypertension.* 2004;44(6):897–902. https://doi.org/10.1161/01.HYP.0000146536.68208.84.
119. Hilimire MR, DeVylder JE, Forestell Catherine A%J. Fermented foods, neuroticism, and social anxiety: An interaction model. *Psychiatry Res.* 2015;228(2):203–208.

120. Xu Y, Wang C, Klabnik J, M O'Donnell J. Novel therapeutic targets in depression and anxiety: Antioxidants as a candidate treatment. *Curr Neuropharmacol.* 2014;12(2):108–119.
121. Wu A, Noble EE, Tyagi E, Ying Z, Zhuang Y, Gomez-Pinilla F. Curcumin boosts DHA in the brain: Implications for the prevention of anxiety disorders. *Biochimica et Biophysica Acta.* 2015;1852(5): 951–961. https://doi.org/10.1016/j.bbadis.2014.12.005.
122. Dipasquale S, Pariante CM, Dazzan P, Aguglia E, McGuire P, Mondelli V. The dietary pattern of patients with schizophrenia: A systematic review. *J Psychiatr Res.* 2013;47(2):197–207.
123. Royal B. Schizophrenia: Nutrition and alternative treatment approaches. *Schizophr Bull.* 2015;42(5):1083–1085.
124. Andrade C. Cardiometabolic risks in schizophrenia and directions for intervention, 2: nonpharmacological interventions. *J Clin Psychiatry.* 2016;77(8):964.
125. Peet M. International variations in the outcome of schizophrenia and the prevalence of depression in relation to national dietary practices: An ecological analysis. *Br J Psychiatry.* 2004;184(5):404–408.
126. Chia SC, Henry J, Mok YM, Honer WG, Sim K. Fatty acid and vitamin interventions in adults with schizophrenia: A systematic review of the current evidence. *J Neural Transm.* 2015;122(12):1721–1732.
127. Ghaderi A, Banafshe HR, Mirhosseini N, et al. Clinical and metabolic response to vitamin D plus probiotic in schizophrenia patients. *BMC Psychiatry.* 2019;19(1):77. https://doi.org/10.1186/s12888-019-2059-x.
128. Allott K, McGorry PD, Yuen HP, et al. The Vitamins in Psychosis study: A randomized, double-blind, placebo-controlled trial of the effects of vitamins B12, B6, and folic acid on symptoms and neurocognition in first-episode psychosis. *Biol Psychiatry.* 2019;86(1):35–44. https://doi.org/10.1016/j.biopsych.2018.12.018.
129. Okusaga O, Yolken RH, Langenberg P, et al. Elevated gliadin antibody levels in individuals with schizophrenia. *World J Biol Psychiatry.* 2013;14(7):509–515. https://doi.org/10.3109/15622975.2012.747699.
130. Kalaydjian AE, Eaton W, Cascella N, Fasano A. The gluten connection: the association between schizophrenia and celiac disease. *Acta Psychiatr Scand.* 2006;113(2):82–90. https://doi.org/10.1111/j.1600-0447.2005.00687.x.
131. Hee Seo J, Mock Lee Y, Soo Lee J, Chul Kang H, Dong Kim H. Efficacy and tolerability of the ketogenic diet according to lipid: nonlipid ratios—comparison of 3: 1 with 4: 1 diet. *Epilepsia.* 2007;48(4):801–805.
132. Newell C, Bomhof MR, Reimer RA, Hittel DS, Rho JM, Shearer J. Ketogenic diet modifies the gut microbiota in a murine model of autism spectrum disorder. *Mol Autism.* 2016;7(1):37.
133. Ma D, Wang AC, Parikh I, et al. Ketogenic diet enhances neurovascular function with altered gut microbiome in young healthy mice. *Sci Rep.* 2018;8(1):6670. https://doi.org/10.1038/s41598-018-25190-5.
134. Bostock E, Kirkby KC, Taylor BVM. The current status of the ketogenic diet in psychiatry. *Front Psychiatry.* 2017;8:43.
135. Pearsall R, Thyarappa Praveen K, Pelosi A, Geddes J. Dietary advice for people with schizophrenia. *Cochrane Database Syst Rev.* 2016;3(3):CD009547. https://doi.org/10.1002/14651858.CD009547.pub2.
136. Nigg JT, Holton K. Restriction and elimination diets in ADHD treatment. *Child Adolesc Psychiatr Clin N Am.* 2014;23(4):937–953. https://doi.org/10.1016/j.chc.2014.05.010.
137. Gan J, Galer P, Ma D, Chen C, Xiong T. The effect of vitamin D supplementation on attention-deficit/hyperactivity disorder: A systematic review and meta-analysis of randomized controlled trials. *J Child A Psychopharmacol.* 2019;29(9):670–687. https://doi.org/10.1089/cap.2019.0059.
138. Kalra EK. Nutraceutical--definition and introduction. *AAPS PharmSci.* 2003;5(3):E25. https://doi.org/10.1208/ps050325.
139. Okereke OI, Reynolds CF 3rd, Mischoulon D, et al. Effect of long-term vitamin D3 supplementation vs placebo on risk of depression or clinically relevant depressive symptoms and on change in mood scores: A randomized clinical trial. *JAMA.* 2020;324(5):471–480. https://doi.org/10.1001/jama.2020.10224.
140. Sarris J, Byrne GJ, Stough C, et al. Nutraceuticals for major depressive disorder-more is not merrier: An 8-week double-blind, randomised, controlled trial. *J Affect Disord.* 2019;245:1007–1015. https://doi.org/10.1016/j.jad.2018.11.092.
141. Gohari AR, Saeidnia S, Mahmoodabadi MK. An overview on saffron, phytochemicals, and medicinal properties. *Pharmacogn Rev.* 2013;7(13):61.
142. Tóth B, Hegyi P, Lantos T, et al. The Efficacy of Saffron in the Treatment of Mild to Moderate Depression: A Meta-analysis. *Planta Medica.* 2019;85(1):24–31. https://doi.org/10.1055/a-0660-9565.

143. Lopresti AL, Drummond PD. Saffron (Crocus sativus) for depression: A systematic review of clinical studies and examination of underlying antidepressant mechanisms of action. *Hum Psychopharmacol.* 2014;29(6):517–527.
144. Fusar-Poli L, Vozza L, Gabbiadini A, et al. Curcumin for depression: a meta-analysis. *Crit Rev Food Sci Nutr.* 2020;60(15):2643–2653. https://doi.org/10.1080/10408398.2019.1653260.
145. Zhang Y, Li L, Zhang J. Curcumin in antidepressant treatments: An overview of potential mechanisms, pre-clinical/clinical trials and ongoing challenges. *Basic Clin Pharmacol Toxicol.* 2020;127(4):243–253. https://doi.org/10.1111/bcpt.13455.
146. Miller WR, Rollnick S. *Motivierende Gesprächsführung: Motivational Interviewing: 3. Auflage des Standardwerks in Deutsch.* Freiburg im Breisgau: Lambertus-Verlag; 2015.
147. Martins RK, McNeil DW. Review of motivational interviewing in promoting health behaviors. *Clin Psychol Rev.* 2009;29(4):283–293.
148. Gaiswinkler L, Kaufmann P, Pollheimer E, et al. Mindfulness and self-compassion in clinical psychiatric rehabilitation: A clinical trial. *Mindfulness.* 2020;11(2):374–383.
149. Warren JM, Smith N, Ashwell M. A structured literature review on the role of mindfulness, mindful eating and intuitive eating in changing eating behaviours: Effectiveness and associated potential mechanisms. *Nutr Res Rev.* 2017;30(2):272–283.
150. Tapper K, Ahmed Z. A mindfulness-based decentering technique increases the cognitive accessibility of health and weight loss related goals. *Front Psychol.* 2018;24(9):587.
151. Forman EM, Butryn ML, Juarascio AS, et al. The mind your health project: A randomized controlled trial of an innovative behavioral treatment for obesity. *Obesity (Silver Spring).* 2013;21(6):1119–1126.
152. Mantzios M, Wilson JC. Mindfulness, eating behaviours, and obesity: A review and reflection on current findings. *Curr Obes Rep.* 2015;4(1):141–146.
153. Daubenmier J, Moran PJ, Kristeller J, et al. Effects of a mindfulness-based weight loss intervention in adults with obesity: A randomized clinical trial. *Obesity (Silver Spring, Md.).* 2016;24(4):794–804. https://doi.org/10.1002/oby.21396.
154. Dunn C, Haubenreiser M, Johnson M, et al. Mindfulness approaches and weight loss, weight maintenance, and weight regain. *Curr Obes Rep.* 2018;7(1):37–49.
155. Soler J, Cebolla A, Elices M, et al. Direct experience while eating in a sample with eating disorders and obesity. *Front Psychol.* 2018;9:1373.
156. Kabat-Zinn J. *Full Catastrophe Living.* New York: Dell-Publishing; 1991.
157. Graham TG, Ramsey D. *The Happiness Diet: A Nutritional Prescription for a Sharp Brain, Balanced Mood, and Lean, Energized Body.* Potter/Ten Speed/Harmony/Rodale; 2012.
158. Aslam H, Green J, Jacka FN, et al. Fermented foods, the gut and mental health: A mechanistic overview with implications for depression and anxiety. *Nutr Neurosci.* 2020;23(9):659–671.
159. Egger JW. *Integrative Verhaltenstherapie und psychotherapeutische Medizin: ein biopsychosoziales Modell.* Wiesbaden: Springer-Verlag; 2015.

CHAPTER 14

Nutrition in Public Health, Policy, Prevention and Implementation

Celia Laur ■ Lauren Ball ■ Jørgen Torgerstuen Johnsen ■
Mercedes Zorrilla Tejeda

LEARNING POINTS

By the end of this chapter, you should be able to:

- Describe the purpose of public health nutrition approaches at local, national and international levels, including how each of these approaches can be interconnected
- Explain how changes at the individual and population levels need appropriate implementation of a policy or programme, building on quality improvement methodology and implementation science to encourage sustainable change
- Understand that public health policies and programmes need adequate implementation to be effective and how the extent of the impact can be monitored using outcome and process measures
- Understand the overall purpose of the health-related sustainable development goals and provide examples of how the goals have been used to inform public health nutrition strategies at the national and international level
- Describe how competencies for improving nutrition care at any level go beyond clinical skills to include collaborative work, leadership and advocacy to drive improvement and impact

Note: In lieu of case studies this chapter uses case examples within the conceptual and explanatory text

Introduction

Previous chapters have focused on topics related to clinical nutrition care to meet patients' individual needs. This chapter takes a wider view on nutrition-related prevention and policy implementation and its impact at local, national and international levels. Public health nutrition policies at each of these levels have potential for improving the nutritional health of populations. However, such improvements will not occur without a focus on implementation, process and impact.

Introduction to Implementation Science and Behaviour Change

There is a lot to consider when thinking about developing, sustaining and/or spreading a public health nutrition initiative and a lot can be learned from other fields. Quality improvement methodology is one area, for example, by using the Model for Improvement:

Plan-Do-Study-Act cycles, to work through small changes that make sense in a local context.[1] Implementation science can also inform how to change practice, and has been defined as 'the scientific study of methods to promote the systematic uptake of research findings and other evidence-based practices into routine practice, and, hence, to improve the quality and effectiveness of health services'.[2] Applying principles from implementation science builds off work that is more generalisable, facilitating use of theories, models and frameworks that can help guide progress.

Considering behaviour change theory can also be useful, such as thinking through capability, opportunity and motivation for changing behaviour.[3] For example, when supporting a target population in cooking healthy meals, participants may have high levels of *motivation* to cook; however, they may not have the appropriate cooking skills (*capability*) or be able to afford the healthier options (*opportunity*). The Consolidated Framework for Implementation Research (CFIR) can also be useful to help think through the context that may be impacting a proposed change. The CFIR constructs include intervention characteristics (i.e., evidence strength, cost, adaptability), outer setting (i.e., external policy and incentives), inner setting (i.e., structural characteristics, culture, compatibility, readiness, resources), characteristics of individuals (i.e., knowledge and beliefs about the intervention, self-efficacy) and process (i.e., planning, engaging, opinion leaders, champions).[4] The CFIR website includes details about the constructs and tools to use in practice.[5]

A key component to effective implementation is to work directly with those most impacted by the change, making sure that the work meets a real need, in a way that makes sense and is appropriate to those most impacted. There are many opportunities to learn more about how to put evidence into practice, including online training modules about implementation science.[6]

MONITORING PROGRESS

When implementing any initiative, it is important to understand the starting point (i.e., what is the nature and prevalence of the problem in that setting) and to monitor progress (i.e., if the change is making a difference). Monitoring can include outcome measures (i.e., weight change, decreased hospitalisations) and process measures (i.e., how many sessions were delivered, and how many people attended each session) to understand if the initiative is being implemented as intended and is having the desired impact. If outcome measures indicate a programme or policy is not having an impact on the target audience, process measures can help explain why. For example, if rates of diabetes did not change in a diabetes prevention programme, process measures can show if it was being delivered as intended. It is important to recognise the difference between a programme or policy that is not working because of the original design or because it was not implemented as intended.

For ongoing monitoring of progress, there is growing interest in Learning Health Systems as a way to work toward high-value health care. Learning Health Systems are 'dynamic health ecosystems where scientific, social, technological, policy, legal and ethical dimensions are synergistically aligned to enable cycles of continuous learning and improvement to be routinised and embedded across the system, thus enhancing value through an optimised balance of impacts on patient and provider experience, population health and health system costs'.[7] To achieve sustained, population-level impact, Learning Health Systems encourage change processes that adapt to system need and are continuous over time.[7,8] All of these factors that affect implementation can be considered at the local, national and international levels and all are impacted by policy.

POLICY IMPLEMENTATION

Policy refers to 'law, regulation, procedure, admirative action, incentive, or voluntary practice of governments and other institutions'.[9,10] More specifically, food policy focuses on challenges with the food systems and the nutritional, health and environmental outcomes. Food policy influences the food system and what people eat through agricultural, fishing, farming industries/land, animal welfare, food trade and social and labour policies. Thus, food policy shapes who eats what, when, where and at what cost, giving it immense impact on our nutrition, health, livelihoods, communities, nature, climate, cities, and countryside. For example, a food policy can require fortification of salt with iodine, can mandate how food products are labelled or can involve adding a tax on sugar. Policy can also impact what types of food are grown and produced, which then impacts the physical environment and thus may impact the climate (e.g., increased soy or palm oil production which leads to drastic land losses in our rainforest). With the crosscutting nature of food and nutrition, policies can be wide ranging, such as ways to encourage breastfeeding or changing the food environment by limiting the development of fast-food venues near schools. Given this wide spectrum, food and nutrition policy can be influenced and driven by the global momentum to tackle the malnutrition issues we face today.[11]

GLOBAL MOMENTUM

To prevent and manage malnutrition in all its forms, the World Health Organization held a World Health Assembly in 2012 which endorsed a comprehensive implementation plan on maternal, infant and young child nutrition. Six global nutrition targets were specified with an aim to achieve them by 2025 including[12]:

- Achievement of a 40% reduction in the number of children under 5 who are stunted
- Achievement of a 50% reduction in anaemia among women of reproductive age
- Achievement of a 30% reduction in low birth weight
- Ensuring that there is no increase in childhood overweight
- Increasing the rate of exclusive breastfeeding in the first 6 months up to at least 50%
- Reducing or maintaining childhood wasting at less than 5%

In 2015, the 2030 Agenda for Sustainable Development was adopted by all United Nations Member States, focused on peace and prosperity for people and the planet.[13] Central to this agenda were the 17 Sustainable Development Goals (SDGs), which recognised that 'ending poverty and other deprivations must go hand-in-hand with strategies that improve health and education, reduce inequality, and spur economic growth—all while tackling climate change and working to preserve our oceans and forests.'[13] Of the recommended 17 SDGs, SDG2: 'End hunger, achieve food security and improved nutrition, and promote suitable agriculture' contains clear goals for improved nutrition. Target 2.2 of SDG2 focuses directly on malnutrition: 'By 2030 end all forms of malnutrition, including achieving by 2025 the internationally agreed targets on stunting and wasting in children under five years of age, and address the nutritional needs of adolescent girls, pregnant and lactating women, and older persons.' SDG3: 'Ensure healthy lives and promote well-being for all at all ages,' focuses on access to essential health care services for all and highlights how important nutrition is to the 2030 agenda.[14]

The World Health Assembly and the SDG targets are closely monitored to demonstrate global progress toward these goals. Reports such as the Global Nutrition Report and the World Health Organization (WHO) Global Nutrition Policy Report and databases such as the Global Database on the Implementation of Nutrition Action provide valuable information on the countries progress and food/nutrition policy implementation toward these global targets. Reports and databases like these are a vital asset for our understanding of the issues and how well the different countries are meeting these goals, and thus aim to keep governments to their commitments.[11]

Achieving these global goals cannot be done in silos and will take multiple approaches at the local, national and international levels. To further explore these approaches, case examples are used to demonstrate the role of food policy and effective implementation at each level.

Nutrition Care Strategies at a Local Level

Local governments are in a unique position to support the health and well-being of the populations in which they serve. In most countries, government health services are responsible for identifying the health care needs of their local populations and shaping services to meet these needs. Similarly, nongovernment or private health services indirectly support population health by aligning their services with the needs of the region.

Most of the time, the health care needs of a local area overlap with the health care needs of a country or region of the world. Such overlap provides opportunity for local initiatives to be developed that also support national and global health priorities. For example, the Baby-Friendly Hospital Initiative (BFHI) is a global, evidence-based public health initiative that is primarily implemented at local levels to support new mothers to breastfeed.[15]

CASE EXAMPLE: INITIATIVES TO SUPPORT BREASTFEEDING IN AUSTRALIA

Rationale

One of the most effective measures a mother can take to protect the health of her infant and herself is to breastfeed.[16] Exclusive breastfeeding (i.e., no other oral intake) has been shown to at least modestly protect against excessive infant weight gain and later obesity.[17] This effect may be a result from differences in weight gain that occurs between breastfed and formula-fed infants.[17] Most women understand the importance of breastfeeding and want to breastfeed, but they need high-quality, accessible support to overcome barriers that are commonly experienced. For example, although most mothers can physically lactate, mothers who do not receive adequate breastfeeding education and lactation support may produce insufficient milk to nourish the infant or may experience pain when feeding.

Alignment With National and Global Priorities

WHO recommends that infants start breastfeeding within the first hour after birth and are exclusively breastfed for the first 6 months of life.[18] The WHO/United Nations Children's Fund BFHI (Baby-Friendly Hospital Initiative) was introduced in Australia in 1993 and its governance was passed to the Australian College of Midwives. In 2006, the initiative was renamed to the Baby Friendly Health Initiative to reflect its expansion into community health facilities.[19] In 2008, the Australian College of Midwives adopted a 7-point plan based on plans from Canada and the United Kingdom, which awarded the first community health service accreditation.

Components of the Initiative

For a local health facility to be awarded accreditation with the programme, all 7 points need to be addressed[20]:

- Point 1: Have a written breastfeeding policy that is routinely communicated to all staff and volunteers.
- Point 2: Educate all staff in the knowledge and skills necessary to implement the breastfeeding policy.
- Point 3: Inform women and their families about breastfeeding being the biologically normal way to feed a baby and about the risks associated with not breastfeeding.
- Point 4: Support mothers to establish and maintain exclusive breastfeeding for 6 months.

- Point 5: Encourage sustained breastfeeding beyond 6 months with appropriate introduction of complementary foods.
- Point 6: Provide a supportive atmosphere for breastfeeding families and for all users of the child health service.
- Point 7: Promote collaboration between staff and volunteers, breastfeeding support groups and the local community to protect, promote and support breastfeeding.

Evaluation of the Initiative

For hospitals which implemented the BFHI, exclusive breastfeeding rates during the first 6-months modestly improved.[21] However, the uptake of the BFHI has been suboptimal due to barriers within health systems. In 2017, only 22% of maternity hospitals had been accredited as Baby Friendly. Process measures regarding the programme are not routinely collected (i.e., number of practices that are continuously implemented, proportion of total newborns in an accredited unit that are being breastfed), which makes it challenging to identify the best use of resources to continue with the programme.[21] Development of Learning Health Systems may facilitate this monitoring, increasing the understanding of if, and highlighting when the intervention is being implemented effectively and having the desired impact on the target population.

This case example demonstrates that even when local initiatives align with national and global priorities, lack of monitoring and evaluation can make it difficult to understand the impact and the benefits of the programme on the target population.

Nutrition Care Strategies at a National Level

National governments are well placed to implement health initiatives that have the potential to positively affect their entire population and therefore support other economic and population priorities. National strategies can influence local implementation and be informed by international strategies. For example, the World Cancer Research Fund International designed the NOURISHING policy framework and policy database in 2013 with the aim to promote healthy diets and reduce noncommunicable diseases and obesity.[22] Each letter of the acronym, NOURISHING, stands for 1 of the 10 evidence-based policy areas where national governments should focus and take action (Box 14.1). Three key domains include the food environment, food systems and behaviour change communication, with each domain having the potential to influence how and what people eat. This tool provides information to policy makers, researchers and local communities about what other countries are doing around the world and thus can be used to inform local and national strategies.

To demonstrate the integration of international and national strategies, a series of case examples are provided, focused on food labelling, industry collaboration and public awareness campaigns.

BOX 14.1 ■ Nourishing Framework Policy Areas[22]

- Nutrition label standards and regulation on the use of claims and implied claims on food
- Offer healthy food and set standards in public institutions and other specific settings
- Use economic tools to address food affordability and purchase initiatives
- Restrict food advertising and other forms of commercial promotion
- Improve nutritional quality of the whole food supply
- Set incentives and rules to create a healthy retail and food service environment
- Harness food supply chain and actions across sectors to ensure coherence with health
- Inform people about food and nutrition through public awareness
- Nutrition advice and counselling in health care settings
- Give nutrition education and skills

CASE STUDY 14.1 Applying International Strategies at a National Level for Salt Reduction

Rationale. According to WHO, cardiovascular diseases (CVDs) are the main cause of death around the world, contributing to approximately 18 million deaths per year.[23] The majority of CVDs can be prevented by modifying diet and lifestyle behaviours.[24] It is well documented that diets that are high in salt can increase blood pressure, and therefore the risk of developing heart failure, heart attacks, stroke and kidney diseases.[25] Reduction of salt intake is recognised by WHO as having the potential to save many lives and money.

International Alignment. To support national initiatives in meeting this international priority, WHO designed SHAKE, a technical package for salt reduction with the objective to help governments to decrease salt consumption of their population. The five components of the SHAKE tool are[26] *Surveillance*: Measure and monitor salt use; *Harness Industry*: Promote the reformulation of foods and meals to contain less salt; *Adopt standards for labelling and marketing*: Implement standards for effective and accurate labelling and marketing of food; *Knowledge*: Educate and empower individuals to eat less salt; *Environment*: Support settings to promote healthy eating. Key steps to support implementation of the SHAKE tool are in Box 14.2.

National Implementation of International Recommendations (UK). In 2003, the Scientific Advisory Committee on Nutrition published an evidence report that highlighted the risks of high salt intake and blood pressure. After this, the Food Standard Agency and the Consensus Action on Salt and Health started collaborating with the food industry in the United Kingdom to (1) create a voluntary salt reduction programme and (2) develop public awareness campaigns to educate the population about the risks of eating too much salt.[27] The key to promote the reformulation of foods in this programme was working closely with all sectors of the food industry to meet the targets. This approach aligns with the SHAKE recommendations, specifically *Harness industry*, and increase *Knowledge*.

Evaluation. This collaborative programme resulted in a decrease of salt intake in the UK population, and many products contain 55% less sodium than before this initiative.[28] Between 2003 and 2011, the UK salt reduction programme resulted in a salt intake reduction of 15%. Since then, Australia, Canada, the United States and other countries have followed their example.[27]

BOX 14.2 ■ To Support Implementation, the SHAKE Tool Highlights the Following Key Steps of a National Salt Reduction Programme Development[26]

1. Advocate for salt reduction
2. Form a small leadership team
3. Identify, survey and consult with stakeholders
4. Establish a broader advisory group and hold regular meetings
5. Set national target for population salt intake
6. Identify and agree on specific programme objectives
7. Develop the specific activities and the implementation programme
8. Develop a monitoring and evaluation plan
9. Review of the overall salt reduction programme plan by stakeholders and advisory group
10. Sign off by the senior government leader responsible for the programme

CASE STUDY 14.2 A Sample of National Front-of-Pack Food Labelling Strategies

Rationale. A strong example of a national, system-level, approach is food labelling, which aims to encourage industry to improve and reformulate foods that are high in salt, sugar and *trans*-fats. The implementation of front-of-package labelling is also thought to help consumers to make informed food purchases and to easily identify healthier options when purchasing food, aiming to make the healthy

CASE STUDY 14.2 Sample of National Front-of-Pack Food Labelling Strategies—(Continued)

choice the easy choice.[29] These labels can be described in either graphical forms, symbols, wording or numbers depending on country-specific regulations.[30] The support of governments, scientific organisations, academia, the food industry and consumers is essential for a successful implementation of food labelling.[31]

The Nutritional Warning Approach. In 1993, Finland made it compulsory to include the warning 'high salt content' on the label of foods that were above specific percentages for salt. This strategy resulted in reformulation of different foods. Between 1979 and 2007 there was a 25%–30% salt intake reduction resulting from this systematic action on salt that included public awareness campaigns that empowered people to identify healthy options.[32] In Latin America, Chile was the first country to adopt the nutritional warning approach in food labelling.[33] Their approach requires customers to be informed on the package when the food contains an excess amount of a critical nutrients that are directly linked to noncommunicable diseases. Example warnings included: high in sugar; high in calories; high in saturated fats; and high in sodium. Mexico, Peru and Uruguay have followed Chile's example and this labelling is mandatory.[34–36] Brazil and Canada are considering the adaptation of this approach.[37–40]

Consumer-Friendly Systems. France has taken a different approach to food labelling, using a consumer-friendly system, the NutriScore Label.[41] This system classifies foods and beverages into five categories, using a colour scale that goes from dark green to dark red, and each colour contains a letter A–E as the ranking score. Positive nutrients include fibre, protein, fruits and vegetables. Negative nutrients include energy, saturated fatty acids, sugars and salt.[42] The Nordic keyhole labelling is another example of a positive labelling approach. This labelling approach aims to make healthy choices easy through labelling food products that contain less fat, sugar, salt and more dietary fibre and whole grain. This approach is thought to make it easier for the consumer to find products filling the requirement and allows food producers to stand out with healthier products.[43]

Evaluation. Labelling can be an easier option for the consumer to navigate through aisles of food products. However, as shown previously, there is no one size fits all solution, and countries need to evaluate what would be the best option in their context. Labelling is also facing challenges as businesses try to reduce the regulation and implementation of labelling that can be damaging to their products' reputation and sale. For example, the design of the Chile and Mexican labels are often seen as less friendly and direct than the traffic light or Nordic keyhole labelling schemes. A recent study from Chile found that after the labelling scheme was introduced, they experienced a significant decline in beverages sold high in sugar, saturated fat, sodium or calories.[44] As labelling is dealt with differently across the globe, an action network, established by France and Australia under the United Nations Decade of Action on Nutrition (2016–2025), was set up to create space for discussing, sharing knowledge, and supporting the development, implementation and advocacy for nutrition labelling.[45]

Nutrition Care Strategies at an International Level. International collaboration, policy development, and implementation are key to meeting the SDGs to improve health at a global scale. Just as national strategies can be informed by international strategies, international strategies can also be informed by learning from national experience. A strong example of national experience leading to international strategies, which, in turn, strengthen other national strategies, is in the reduction of *trans*-fatty acids (TFAs).

CASE STUDY 14.3 Global Action to Reduce Trans-Fatty Acids

Rationale. TFA and its increased health risk is discussed in Chapter 1, 'Basic Principles of Nutrition'. Several studies have shown a relationship between TFA consumption and increased risk of CVD. Thus, as part of a healthy diet, WHO recommends that total TFA intake be limited to less than 1% of total energy intake. Given a 2000-calorie diet, it is less than 2.2 g/day.[46]

National Strategies. In 2004, Denmark became to first country to restrict industrially produced TFA in all food products. Although it is difficult to infer causality, in the 3-year period after the introduction of these restrictions, the CVD rates decreased by 3.2% compared with similar countries who did not implement restrictions.[47] In the United States, between 2007 and 2013, counties in New York State that

Continued

CASE STUDY 14.3 Global Action to Reduce Trans-Fatty Acids—(Continued)

implemented TFA restrictions had 7.8% fewer hospital admissions for heart attacks after implementing restrictions, compared with counties without TFA restrictions.[48]

In Argentina, between 2004 and 2014, an estimated 1.3% to 6.7% annual reduction in CVD was associated with a near elimination of industrially produced TFA.[49] However, the road was long between 2004 and 2014, and Argentina worked hard on implementing several policies to reduce industry-produced TFA. The first approach was to ask industry to voluntarily reformulate their food by replacing approximately 40% of industry produced TFA from cooking oils like vegetable oils. The voluntary approach was achieved mainly with *trans* fat free sunflower oil.[50] Therefore, regulations enforcing mandatory labelling of industry produced TFA were needed as voluntary approaches did not work, and the enforcement was introduced in 2006. However, introduction of TFA labelling also had challenges, but with support from the Pan American Health Organization, the Argentine Ministry of Health negotiated with industry to eliminate industry-produced TFA. Thus, the country's food code was amended and by the end of 2014, industry produced TFAs in foods were not allowed to exceed 2% of total fats in vegetable oils and margarines and 5% of total fats in other foods.[50]

TFA elimination is challenging. Lack of regulatory capacities, laboratory capacities and accurate and reliable TFA data are common challenges countries face while eliminating TFAs.[51] Nevertheless, identifying the barriers such as limited human and financial resource, food sampling and testing for assessing TFAs in food brings opportunities and incentives for prioritization to confront the obstacles and challenges countries face. Understanding the barriers and other lessons learned from the countries that initially attempted regulation of TFAs led to the development of the international strategy, called the REPLACE framework.

The International Framework. The REPLACE framework (Box 14.3), a globally aimed action package to eliminate industrially produced TFAs from the global food supply, was brought forth by WHO and Resolve to Save Lives in 2018. The REPLACE road map objective is to make the world *trans*-fat free by 2023 by providing countries with tools to help eliminate industrially produced TFAs from its food supplies.[52] REPLACE is a significant example of impactful policy action at a global scale and is renowned as the first global initiative to eliminate a risk factor for CVD. It is estimated that 500,000 lives could be saved per year with this approach.[52]

Evaluation and Impact. After that launch of the REPLACE framework in 2018, and up until end of 2020, 2.4 billion people in 32 countries are thought to have experienced the benefit of mandatory TFA policies. Sixteen countries (covering over 768 million people) had these best practices implemented by the end of 2020, and the number of countries is projected to increase to at least 40 by 2022. 'Best practices' refers to 'legislative or regulatory measures that limit industrially produced TFA in foods in all settings and are in line with the recommended approach. The two best-practice policies for TFA elimination are: 1) Mandatory national limit of 2g industrially produced TFA per 100g of total fat in all foods; and 2) Mandatory national ban on the production or use of partially hydrogenated oils as an ingredient in all foods'.[51,53] While 67 countries (in 2020) have national policy commitment to eliminated TFAs in their national policies, strategies, or action plans, 27 countries have other complementary measures in place, and 18 countries have adapted less restrictive legislative or regulatory measures.[53] The WHO is also providing technical support to achieve their aim to be *trans*-fat free by 2023. Successful and influential policies and frameworks, like REPLACE, are needed to combat malnutrition in all its forms as we are living an increasingly global world.

REPLACE in Action

The work to eliminate TFAs in Nigeria is a recent example of a country who took on the REPLACE framework and its best practices.[51] The implementation of the best practice was expected by the end of 2020, and Nigeria owes its success to the political will within the government, the National Agency for Food and Drug Administration and Control, Federal Ministry of Health and civil society who provided advocacy, legal support and convening stakeholders throughout the policy process. The prioritization and implementation were achieved with guidance from the technical working group on best practices for TFA elimination and strong campaigning by civil society advocates to raise public knowledge of the health harms of TFAs and to build its support for regulations. Due to the hard work of the Nigerian Government, the WHO, and civil society to advance and implement regulations, industry also began activating its awareness and issues around TFA elimination. A workshop on reformulation of products high in TFAs was thus conducted for small and medium-sized companies. Seeing the increase of interest from industry reinforced the government's interest and commitment to implementing the REPLACE action package.[53]

CASE STUDY 14.3 Global Action to Reduce Trans-Fatty Acids—(Continued)

BOX 14.3 ■ The Six Actions Areas of the REPLACE Framework[52]

- REview dietary sources of industrially produced *trans*-fat and the landscape for required policy change.
- Promote the replacement of industrially produced *trans*-fat with healthier fats and oils.
- Legislate or enact regulatory actions to eliminate industrially produced *trans*-fat.
- Assess and monitor *trans*-fat content in the food supply and changes in *trans*-fat consumption in the population.
- Create awareness of the negative health impact of *trans*-fat among policy makers, producers, suppliers and the public.

Capacity Building

This chapter demonstrates that improving nutrition care in individuals goes well beyond clinical care to include prevention, implementation, and policy at the local, national and international levels. Each of these levels interact with local, national, and international strategies, each informing the other. Clearly, achieving population impact cannot be done in silos, requiring a multidisciplinary team effort that brings together a variety of expertise and experience to drive change.

Having a solid foundation of nutrition education is an important place to start to develop the knowledge and skills to understand and advocate for change. Programmes such as the summer school in Applied Human Nutrition, delivered by the NNEdPro Global Centre for Nutrition and Health, provide one option for brief yet intensive training to build this foundation.[54] Dietitians and nutrition professionals are the experts in nutrition, yet having members within a multidisciplinary team with a basic understanding of nutrition, and the ability to critically appraise nutrition evidence, will help to widen reach.

Leadership and advocacy skills are also important to drive change, using an evidence-based approach along with clear communication to present a strong and actionable message. Implementation, change management and systems thinking skills can help you to think though how to make a change, considering the individual involved and the positioning within the local, national, and international contexts. All these skills, when applied within a multidisciplinary team, help to drive improvements in nutrition at all levels.

Conclusion

Having a population-level impact involves the integration of local, national and international strategies, each building on the other. A solid foundation in nutrition knowledge and critical appraisal as well as an overview of implementation strategies and the role of leadership within this are an important start-up toolkit toward achieving population level impact.

References

1. Langley G, Moen R, Nola K, Noal T, Norman C, Provost L. *The Improvement Guide*. 2nd ed. San Francisco, CA: Jossey- Bass; 2009.
2. Eccles MP, Mittman BS. Welcome to implementation science. *Implement Sci*. 2006;1(1):1.
3. Michie S, van Stralen M, West R. The behaviour change wheel: A new method for characterising and designing behaviour change interventions. *Implement Sci*. 2011;6(42).

4. Damschroder LJ, Aron DC, Keith RE, Kirsh SR, Alexander JA, Lowery JC. Fostering implementation of health services research findings into practice: A consolidated framework for advancing implementation science. *Implement Sci*. 2009;4(50).
5. CFIR Research Team-Center for Clinical Management Research. Consolidated framework for implementation research. 2021. Available at: https://cfirguide.org/constructs/. Accessed February 15, 2021.
6. The Centre for Implementation. Courses and events. 2020. Available at: https://thecenterforimplementation.com/courses. Accessed November 12, 2020.
7. Menear M, Blanchette M-A, Demers-Payette O, Roy D. A framework for value-creating learning health systems. *Health Res Policy Syst*. 2019;17(79).
8. Friedman CP, Rubin JC, Sullivan KJ. Toward an information infrastructure for global health improvement. *Yearb Med Inform*. 2017;26(1):16–23.
9. Centers for Disease Control and Prevention. Definition of Policy. Office of the Associate Director for Policy and Strategy. 2015. Available at: https://www.cdc.gov/policy/analysis/process/definition.html. Accessed March 22, 2021.
10. Observatory of Public Sector Innovation. Public Policy. 2015. Available at: https://oecd-opsi.org/guide/public-policy/. Accessed March 22, 2021.
11. Hawkes C, Parsons K. *Brief 1: Tackling Food Systems Challenges: The Role of Food Policy*. London, UK: Centre for Food Policy; 2019.
12. World Health Organization. Global nutrition targets 2025: policy brief series. 2014. World Health Organization. https://www.who.int/publications/i/item/WHO-NMH-NHD-14.2.
13. United Nations. Department of Economic and Social Affairs. Sustainable development. Do you know all 17 SDGs? 2021. Available at: https://sdgs.un.org/goals. Accessed February 15, 2021.
14. United Nations. Department of Economic and Social Affairs. Sustainable development. Make the SDGs a reality. 2021. Available at: https://sdgs.un.org/. Accessed February 15, 2021.
15. Abrahams SW, Labbok MH. Exploring the impact of the Baby-Friendly Hospital Initiative on trends in exclusive breastfeeding. *Int Breastfeed J*. 2009;4:11.
16. U.S. Department of Health and Human Services. *Executive Summary: The Surgeon General's Call to Action to Support Breastfeeding*. Washington, DC; 2011. Centers for Disease Control and Prevention. https://www.cdc.gov/breastfeeding/resources/calltoaction.htm.
17. Moore T, Arefadib N, Deery A, West S. The First Thousand Days: An Evidence Paper. 2017. The Royal Children's Hospital Melbourne. https://www.rch.org.au/ccch/.
18. World Health Organization. *Indicators for Assessing Infant and Young Child Feeding Practices*. World Health Organization; 2008.
19. BFHI Australia. Baby Friendly Health Initiative. 2021. Available at: https://bfhi.org.au/. Accessed February 15, 2021.
20. The Global Criteria for Baby Friendly Community Health Services in Australia. 2013. World Health Organization. https://www.who.int/publications/who-guidelines.
21. Atchan M, Davis D, Foureur M. Applying a knowledge translation model to the uptake of the Baby Friendly Health Initiative in the Australian health care system. *Women Birth*. 2014;27(2):79–85.
22. World Cancer Research Fund International. NOURISHING framework. 2013. Available at: https://www.wcrf.org/int/policy/policy-databases/nourishing-framework. Accessed February 15, 2021.
23. World Health Organization. Accelerating salt reduction in Europe: A country support package to reduce population salt intake in the WHO European Region. 2020. World Health Organization. https://apps.who.int/iris/handle/10665/340028.
24. World Health Organization. Noncommunicable diseases. Fact Sheets. 2015. Available at: https://www.who.int/news-room/fact-sheets/detail/noncommunicable-diseases. Accessed March 22, 2021.
25. Stanner S, Coe S. *Cardiovascular Disease: Diet, Nutrition and Emerging Risk Factors*. 2nd Edition. 2019. Wiley Blackwell - Oxford UK.
26. World Health Organization. *The SHAKE Technical Package for Salt Reduction*. Geneva, Switzerland; 2016. World Health Organization. https://apps.who.int/iris/handle/10665/250135.
27. He FJ, Brinsden HC, Macgregor GA. Salt reduction in the United Kingdom: A successful experiment in public health. *J Hum Hypertens*. 2014;28(6):345–352.
28. Ni Mhurchu C, Capelin C, Dunford EK, Webster JL, Neal BC, Jebb SA. Sodium content of processed foods in the United Kingdom: Analysis of 44,000 foods purchased by 21,000 households. *Am J Clin Nutr*. 2011;93(3):594–600.

29. Hawkes C, Smith TG, Jewell J, et al. Smart food policies for obesity prevention. *Lancet*. 2015; 385(9985):2410–2421.
30. World Health Organization. *Guiding Principles and Framework Manual for Front-of-Pack Labelling for Promoting Healthy Diets*. WHO; 2019. World Health Organization. https://www.who.int/publications/m/item/guidingprinciples-labelling-promoting-healthydiet.
31. Food and Agriculture Organization of the United Nations. *Handbook on Food Labelling to Protect Consumers*. Rome; 2016. Food and Agriculture Organization of the United Nations. https://www.fao.org/publications/card/en/c/fc5f4bc2-650a-4704-9162-9eb9b3a1fdd0/.
32. Trieu K, Neal B, Hawkes C, et al. Salt reduction initiatives around the world—A systematic review of progress towards the global target. *PLoS One*. 2015;10(7).
33. Reyes M, Garmendia ML, Olivares S, Aqueveque C, Zacarías I, Corvalán C. Development of the Chilean front-of-package food warning label. *BMC Public Health*. 2019;19(1):906.
34. Diario Oficial de la Federación. Diario Oficial de la Federación. 2020. Available at: https://www.dof.gob.mx/nota_detalle.php?codigo=5597654&fecha=31/07/2020. Accessed March 22, 2021.
35. Decreto Supremo. Aprueban Manual de Advertencias Publicitarias en el marco de lo establecido en la Ley N° 30021, Ley de promoción de la alimentación saludable para niños, niñas y adolescentes, y su Reglamento aprobado por Decreto Supremo N° 017-2017-SA. El Peruano. 2017. Available at: https://busquedas.elperuano.pe/normaslegales/aprueban-manual-de-advertencias-publicitarias-en-el-marco-de-decreto-supremo-n-012-2018-sa-1660606-1/. Accessed March 22, 2021.
36. Normative y Avisos Legales del Uruguay. Decreto N° 272/018. Normative y Avisos Legales del Uruguay. 2018. Available at: https://www.impo.com.uy/bases/decretos/272-2018/1. Accessed March 22, 2021.
37. Agência Nacional de Vigilância Sanitária—Anvisa. Publicado relatório de AIR sobre rotulagem nutricional—Português (Brasil). Ministerio da Saude. 2019. Available at: https://www.gov.br/anvisa/pt-br/assuntos/noticias-anvisa/2019/publicado-relatorio-de-air-sobre-rotulagem-nutricional. Accessed March 22, 2021.
38. Agencia Nacional de Vigilancia Sanitaria. Painel de Processos Regulatorio. 2020. Available at: https://app.powerbi.com/view?r=eyJrIjoiODQwZWIxMjAtYTAwYi00ZWZlLTg0NzQtMjQ1NGFiMDVkOGUyIiwidCI6ImI2N2FmMjNmLWMzZjMtNGQzNS04MGM3LWI3MDg1ZjVlZGQ4MSJ9. Accessed March 22, 2021.
39. Government of Canada. Regulations Amending Certain Regulations Made Under the Food and Drugs Act (Nutrition Symbols, Other Labelling Provisions, Partially Hydrogenated Oils and Vitamin D). 2018. Gov of Canada. https://www.canada.ca/en/health-canada/corporate/about-health-canada/legislation-guidelines/acts-regulations/forward-regulatory-plan/plan/healthy-eating-provisions-front-pack-labelling-other-labelling-provisions-industrially-produced-trans-fats-vitamin-d.html.
40. Prime Minister of Canada JT. Minister of Health mandate letter. Government of Canada. 2019. Available at: https://pm.gc.ca/en/mandate-letters/2019/12/13/minister-health-mandate-letter. Accessed March 22, 2021.
41. Development of a new front-of-pack nutrition label in France: the five-colour Nutri-Score. Julia C and Hercberg S. Public Health Panorama. Volume 3, 357–820. https://www.euro.who.int/__data/assets/pdf_file/0008/357308/PHP-1122-NutriScore-eng.pdf.
42. World Cancer Research Fund. NOURISHING and MOVING policy database. 2020. Available at: https://policydatabase.wcrf.org/level_one?page=nourishing-level-one#step2=0#step3=309. Accessed March 22, 2021.
43. New guidelines make the Keyhole even greener. Nordic Co-operation. 2021. https://www.norden.org/en/news/new-guidelines-make-keyhole-even-greener.
44. Taillie LS, Reyes M, Colchero MA, Popkin B, Corvalán C. An evaluation of Chile's Law of Food Labeling and Advertising on sugar-sweetened beverage purchases from 2015 to 2017: A before-and-after study. *PLoS Med*. 2020;17(2):e1003015.
45. United Nations Decade of Action on Nutrition. France and Australia announced the establishment of the Global Action Network on Nutrition Labelling. United Nations. 2019. Available at: https://www.un.org/nutrition/news/france-australia-announced-establishment-global-action-network-nutrition-labelling. Accessed March 22, 2021.
46. World Health Organization. Healthy diet. Fact Sheet No. 394. 2018. Available at: https://www.who.int/publications/m/item/healthy-diet-factsheet394. Accessed March 22, 2021.

47. Restrepo BJ, Rieger M. Denmark's policy on artificial trans fat and cardiovascular disease. *Am J Prev Med.* 2016;50(1):69–76.
48. Brandt EJ, Myerson R, Perraillon MC, Polonsky TS. Hospital admissions for myocardial infarction and stroke before and after the trans-fatty acid restrictions in New York. *JAMA Cardiol.* 2017;2(6):627–634.
49. Rubinstein A, Elorriaga N, Garay OU, et al. Eliminating artificial trans fatty acids in Argentina: estimated effects on the burden of coronary heart disease and costs. *Bull World Health Organ.* 2015;93:614–622.
50. Boushey CJ, Kerr DA, Wright J, Lutes KD, Ebert DS, Delp EJ. Use of technology in children's dietary assessment. *Eur J Clin Nutr.* 2009;63(Suppl 1):S50–S57.
51. World Health Organization. Countdown to 2023: WHO report on global trans-fat elimination 2020. 2020. World Health Organization. https://apps.who.int/iris/handle/10665/334170.
52. WHO plan to eliminate industrially-produced trans-fatty acids from global food supply. May 2019. World Health Organization. https://www.who.int/news/item/14-05-2018-who-plan-to-eliminate-industrially-produced-trans-fatty-acids-from-global-food-supply.
53. World Health Organization. TFA Country Score Card. Global database on the Implementation of Nutrition Action (GINA). 2021. Available at: https://extranet.who.int/nutrition/gina/en/scorecard/TFA. Accessed February 15, 2021.
54. NNEdPro Global Centre for Nutrition and Health. 7th NNEdPro Foundation certificate and summer school in applied human nutrition. 2021. Available at: https://www.nnedpro.org.uk/summer-school. Accessed February 15, 2021.

SECTION D

Appendix of Nutrition Toolkits

SECTION OUTLINE

APPENDIX 1

Nutrition and Clinical Science: Toolkit for Further Reading

Duane Mellor

Introduction

The nature of medical course design, structure and delivery varies between countries as well as between medical schools within the same country, as different medical schools will have different approaches to education. However, there is a common basis in all medical programmes of a core theme of what are often called the basic or biomedical sciences. These may be taught as discrete science topics such as physiology, biochemistry or anatomy, within system-based blocks of teaching (e.g., cardiovascular system) or a combination of both. Whereas each of these approaches highlight the importance of various scientific disciplines, especially anatomy, nutrition can at times be covered only fleetingly or worse, completely absent. This toolkit will consider how nutrition and principles of nutritional science are implicitly included in the curriculum despite not always being explicitly covered as a stand-alone topic. The toolkit will then delve into how nutritional principles might be applied, not only in the basic sciences but also in a clinical setting.

Although rare, in some countries, regulatory organisations governing the teaching and licensing of medicine request the inclusion of nutrition as a specific topic within the components of biomedical science. Others may include it as part of clinical skills acquisition. If not specifically placed in the curriculum, nutrition may appear within clinical specialities such as endocrinology and gastrointestinal (GI) medicine, or as part of public health teaching under epidemiology. Despite its presence, nutrition may not always be overtly obvious to students early in their medical career journeys. Some doctors report that they have received only 3 hours of nutrition teaching during their degree, perhaps only recognising the explicit nutritional management of disease (e.g., artificial feeding via parenteral and enteral routes). This is only the very tip of the iceberg which exists in any medical curriculum, as there are clear aspects of nutritional science deeply imbedded in the underpinning of medical sciences. Bearing in mind that medical curricula are already packed full of content, more explicit nutrition teaching may not be the answer, but rather, better highlighting and signposting by medical educators could be effective. This may help medical trainees to connect the scientific principles with the application of nutrition and even application with respect to food-based recommendations and counselling.

With this view, then, overall, the core principles of nutritional science are implicitly embedded across the biomedical sciences from metabolism and biochemistry through to cell biology and physiology. As this book focuses on the essential principles of nutrition in medicine and health care, there may be underlying aspects of human biology, especially biochemistry and physiology, which might be useful to help with the interpretation and application of the other chapters. This toolkit aims to highlight these connections and suggest links to other key medical textbooks to further your understanding of nutrition, while also deepening your knowledge of the underpinning of biomedical principles and science of nutrition.

SECTION 1: NUTRITION WITHIN THE BASIC SCIENCE UNDERPINNING MEDICINE

Cell Biology

The different cell types with differing metabolic demands interact together to determine our overall metabolic requirements, which ultimately informs our nutritional requirements as a whole organism. This key principle is useful when considering metabolic processes, organisation and transport systems within cells, tissues and organs.

Perhaps one of the most challenging aspects of cell and molecular biology for medical students is the number of transporters and channels in cell membranes. Students must decipher not only which are key to memorise, but also how they can be clinically relevant, especially with respect to disease as these transporters and channels are targets for therapeutic agents. With respect to digestion, which is covered in Chapter 2.1 in this toolkit, there are several transporters which explain what substrates can appear in circulation, as well as those which cannot. In some tissues, sodium transport is vital, not only with respect to maintaining membrane potentials, but also fluid in the intra- and extracellular compartment, which in turn influences blood pressure and disease risk. Therefore, linking how molecules are transported from the GI tract lumen into the enterocyte as well as into and out of cells within the body is inherently related to nutrition. These are the only ways of maintaining the internal environment in response to either dietary inputs or losses from the body which have not been replaced.

To revisit related core aspects of cell biology, it is worth reading:

- Ritter JM, et al. How drugs act: Cellular aspects—excitation, contraction and secretion. In *Rang and Dale's Pharmacology*. 9th ed. Elsevier; 2020:52–68.
- Caplan MJ. Functional organisation of the cell. In: Boron W, Boulpaep E, eds. *Medical Physiology*. 3rd ed. Elsevier; 2016:8–46.

Genetics Including Epigenetics

The area of genetics and molecular nutrition has grown exponentially over the past few decades with the advent of polymerase chain reaction technology and the Human Genome project.

Genetics has increased our understanding of a range of diseases in which there is direct inheritance. For example, phenylketonuria which, in its classic form, is an autosomal recessive disorder caused by mutations in both alleles of the gene that is responsible for the enzyme phenylalanine hydroxylase. This gene is located on chromosome 12, and in phenylketonuria, the inability to metabolise phenylalanine to tyrosine results in high levels of this amino acid with potential complications of learning difficulties, organ damage and altered posture and gait. This can be managed using a low-phenylalanine diet (it cannot be completely removed from the diet as it is an essential amino acid and cannot be synthesised de novo).

Genetics can also interact with nutrition where single nucleotide polymorphisms occur. These are single base mutations which subtly alter the transcription of proteins. They can occur at varying rates for different single nucleotide polymorphisms within populations, leading to interactions with the diet. They tend to be associated with an increased risk of disease which might be moderated by dietary factors or lifestyle. An example is the presence of apolipoprotein A1 which influences high-density lipoprotein cholesterol levels and therefore may influence the risk of cardiovascular disease (CVD) or type 2 diabetes mellitus (T2DM), or the link between neural tube defects in children of mothers with the G allele of phosphatidylethanolamine-N-methyltransferase which alters choline metabolism, a substance not normally essential in the diet but may become so in periods of increased requirements, as in the case in pregnancy.

Epigenetics is an emerging area which investigates how environmental factors can influence the expression of genes. This has been hypothesised to be the mechanism by how the thrifty phenotype (the concept that disease later in life has its origins in utero, based on Barker's developmental origins of health and disease) may occur. This supposes that a challenging metabolic environment during intrauterine development and infancy may predispose an individual to increased risk of T2DM and CVD. Similar outcomes have been seen in studies of infants whose parents have had bariatric surgery prior to conception, in which gene expression seems to be altered by the alteration of the metabolic environment.

A final consideration of genetics with respect to diet is that many of the long-term conditions which are significantly influenced by diet and lifestyle, such as T2DM and CVD, appear to be influenced by several genes across several chromosomes. This means that using genetics to influence dietary choice can be very challenging, and although interesting associations are being shown from genome-wide association studies, there is currently limited clinical application of this practice.

To revisit related core aspects of genetics including epigenetics, it is worth reading:

- Stephenson J, Heslehurst N, Hall J, et al. Before the beginning: nutrition and lifestyle in the preconception period and its importance for future health. *Lancet* 2018; 391(10132):1830–1841.

Biochemistry and Metabolism

For many students, biochemical pathways can be a chore to be absorbed and regurgitated for exams only on a need to recall basis. However, an understanding of biochemistry from a nutritional perspective could help with understanding pathways and metabolism in a way that might help to embed the principles within a live and often clinical context. This may lead to practical applications later in careers.

With respect to intermediary metabolism, the substrates are those derived from the macronutrients (carbohydrates, fats, and proteins). However, the pathways of glycolysis, the Krebs cycle and beta-oxidation tend to omit where the deaminated keto acids and other monosaccharides enter these metabolic pathways.

Beyond macronutrients, normal metabolism requires several cofactors and enzymes which are dependent on micronutrients for normal reactions. These include riboflavin (vitamin B2) and niacin (vitamin B3), which are essential for the synthesis of the high-energy electron carriers flavin adenine dinucleotide and nicotinamide adenine dinucleotide, required for the synthesis of adenosine triphosphate in the electron transport chain. Similarly, hexokinase, phosphofructokinase, aldolase, phosphoglycerate kinase and pyruvate kinase are regulated by magnesium ions. This may explain why organs with high metabolic demands such as the liver are also an excellent source of these vitamins and minerals when eaten, as in the case of lamb's liver.

To revisit related core aspects of metabolism and biochemistry, it is worth reading:

- Shulman GI, Petersen KF. Metabolism. In: Boron W, Boulpaep E, eds. *Medical Physiology*. 3rd ed. Elsevier; 2016:1170–1192.

Physiology and Pathology

In Section B, physiology will be considered in more depth, relative to the body's organ systems. In principle, understanding of function in the normal condition (physiology) and the abnormal condition (pathology) is a central tenet of medical teaching.

To revisit the principles and core aspects of physiology, there are number of excellent textbooks; some are more in-depth than others. As suggested texts as starting points or for revision of principles, it is worth reading:

- Costanzo LS. *Physiology*. 6th ed. Elsevier; 2018.
- Susan Mulroney, Adam Myers. *Netter's Essential Physiology*. 2nd ed. Elsevier; 2016.

For more a more in-depth understanding of physiological principles relevant to medicine, see:

- Bruce M. Koeppen, Bruce A. Stanton. *Berne and Levy Physiology*. 7th ed. Elsevier; 2017.
- Boron W, Boulpaep E. *Boron and Boulpaep Medical Physiology*. 3rd ed. Elsevier; 2018.

Pharmacology

For some, the metabolic principles of pharmacology are considered to be a more important science than nutrition. However, the principles of metabolism of an ingested chemical substance and that of a drug or medication have several similarities. These are perhaps more obvious for bioactive compounds in foods which are not typically considered as nutrients (e.g., polyphenols). However, the principles of ADME (absorption, distribution, metabolism and excretion) used in pharmacokinetics can also be applied to nutrition.

An emerging area of research is drug–nutrient interactions, especially considering we have an ageing population and, as a consequence, the challenge of managing individuals treated with multiple pharmacological agents.

For an overview of food-drug interaction, see:

- Boullata JI, Hudson LM. Drug-nutrient interactions: a broad view with implications for practice. *J Acad Nutr Diet* 2012;112(4):506–517.
- Jeffrey K. Aronson, ed. *Meyler's Side Effects of Drugs*. 16th ed. Elsevier; 2016.

For a more general overview of pharmacology, which has some links to nutrition:

- James M. Ritter, Rod J. Flower, Graeme Henderson, Yoon Kong Loke, David MacEwan, Humphrey P. Rang. *Rang & Dale's Pharmacology*. 9th ed. Elsevier.

Immunology and Infection

Often, improving nutritional intake and status is thought to enhance or even boost immune function. Current evidence does not support these claims in relation to foods or specific nutrients, however, and the only existing health claims are in relation to foods and nutrients supporting normal function/health rather than enhancing it. This has been covered elsewhere in this textbook.

For an overview of immunology, including response to infection, see:

- David Male, Stokes Peebles, Victoria Male. *Immunology*. 9th ed. Elsevier; 2020.

Genomics and Personalised Medicine

Like many aspects of life in the 21st century, people are now seeking a more personalised approach to health care. Personalised medicine and personalised nutrition are emerging areas of research, which aims to make use of large amounts of data in order to individualise care. This can be a challenging area with respect to nutrition as the focus on the data may not always give due respect to the personal and cultural preferences of individuals. This may subsequently lead to poor engagement with and adherence to any nutritional management plans formulated using such data-driven approaches.

- Kelsell DP, Linton KJ. Molecular cell biology and human genetics. In: Parveen Kumar, Michael L Clark, eds. *Kumar and Clark's Clinical Medicine*. Elsevier; 2016.

SECTION 2: NUTRITION WITHIN THE SYSTEMS TEACHING WITH MEDICINE

Overview of Gastrointestinal Tract

There are several key functional principles of the GI tract which ultimately impact on nutritional status and health. Understanding the role and function of the different secretions in the different segments of the GI tract is an important foundation of these principles. These broadly can be categorised into the following areas:

- Lubrication
- Protection of the GI mucosa
- Adjustment of the pH of the contents within the GI lumen
- Protection against infection
- Hydrolysing (digestive) enzymes

Ingestion

It is important to consider how such an everyday afterthought like swallowing is controlled, and how it can be impeded in many scenarios such as neurological conditions, including cerebrovascular events.

Saliva performs a key role in lubricating the ingested food to form a bolus that can be swallowed. This may need special consideration in conditions where the function of the salivary glands is impeded (e.g., Sjogren's syndrome and mumps). Saliva has further functions including that of digestion, which largely occurs via the amylase it contains. These digestive functions are numerous and varied, such as the early digestion of carbohydrates, as well as the inhibition of bacteria and the production of bicarbonate to buffer acid produced by oral bacteria. Through the chewing of food, a lubricated bolus is formed that can, under normal physiological conditions, be swallowed. Under altered physiological conditions, like in the case of a cerebral vascular accident, the interaction between the texture and consistency of foods and fluids and swallow function becomes a key consideration. Such dysphagia may require use of thickened fluids and texture-modified foods to assist with the control of the bolus which is inhibited by the neurological insult. On the other hand, in the case of oesophageal tumours, oral control of the bolus is not the issue, as normal fluids can be controlled through the oral and pharyngeal phase and pass any blockages in the oesophagus. In this case the trouble arises when solid foods become stuck above the stricture caused by the tumour despite bolus formation after chewing. This may lead to undernutrition and associated weight loss.

Digestion

Digestion occurs at several locations throughout the GI system and is linked to adaptations which increase surface area and blood supply to different parts of the system. The main functions of the stomach are storage, bacterial management, secretion of protective mucus and acid secretion into the stomach lumen (with bicarbonate in the mucus and mucosa to minimise risk of tissue injury), along with intrinsic factor, which is required to facilitate vitamin B12 absorption. The function of the acid is to reduce pH, which facilitates chemical digestion of food particles, along with physical digestion from the churning of the powerful muscular contractions, reducing bacterial load and activation of pepsin (a protein digesting enzyme). This results in the bolus that enters the stomach and is converted into chyme which is released periodically into the duodenum. During these processes the stomach secretes a similar amount of fluid as is ingested per day (approximately 2 L per day).

The initial part of the duodenum receives the acidic chyme from the stomach, and it is quickly neutralised to a weak alkali. To achieve this chemical change, the epithelium of the duodenum is protected by mucus containing bicarbonate, which acts alongside pancreatic juices and bile, which, along with the bile's acids and salts, is rich in bicarbonate. Both the exocrine pancreas (via its acini) and the biliary system are adapted to secrete concentrated bicarbonate-rich secretions. The duodenum along with the stomach and oesophagus completes the anatomical foregut. The duodenum continues into the jejunum (and then ileum) to form the small intestine. As well as being a site of absorption, it is important to note that the duodenum contains chemical sensing cells (akin to taste receptors) which have a role in controlling hormonal release to help maintain the internal environment following a meal. This can influence appetite.

The role of digestion, which includes secretion of enzymes, mucus and water balances, facilitates absorption. Fig.A 1.1 shows the sodium and water secretion into the GI tract and the primary mechanisms of water absorption.

Absorption

The role of the stomach with respect to absorption is limited. Fluid is secreted into the stomach so the hypertonic food bolus is diluted, and further dilution occurs in the duodenum, so that ultimately it can reach the jejunum in an isotonic state. The absorptive capacity of the GI tract is

Section of GI Tract	Oral intake	Saliva	Stomach	Pancreas/ Bile	Jejunum	Ileum	Caecum	Proximal colon	Distal colon
Sodium (mmol/l)	150	50	60–100	150/150	100–150				3
Fluid volume (ml)	2000	1000	2000	2000/1000	1000				
GI Lumen									
Residue									
Fluid Volume (ml)							1500		100
Volume Fluid Absorbed (ml)					4000–5000	3000–4000		1400	
Mucosal resistance					Leaky	Mod-leaky	Mod-Tight	Tight	Tight
Absorptive Mechanism					Na – nutrient* Na-H	Na-Cl Na – nutrient* Na	Na SCFA	NaCl SCFA	Na

*nutrient include glucose and amino acids

Fig. A.1.1 Schematic showing sodium and fluid movement in the gastrointestinal (GI) tract. *SCFA*, Short chain fatty acid.

relative to the surface area, and so because the stomach has rugae folds to facilitate expansion after a meal, absorption is usually restricted to some drugs and alcohol.

Most of the absorption in the GI tract occurs in the small intestine. However, it is important to consider net absorption and secretion of fluid and electrolytes as this can prove to be significant in diarrheal disease as well as following bowel surgery, particularly following the formation of stoma (e.g., ileostomies and colostomies). In the duodenum and proximal jejunum, there is net secretion of water, while most of absorption of macronutrients occurs in the jejunum. Water-soluble nutrients are transported from the intestine via portal circulation to the liver. This is essential to buffer the variation in substrate supply from meals, so that the systemic circulation is not exposed to extremes of substrate levels. Lipid-soluble material (triglycerides, cholesterol and fat-soluble vitamins—vitamins A, D, E and K) are absorbed into the lymph which drains into the vena cava.

In the terminal ileum, bile acids are reabsorbed along with vitamin B12; therefore, having an intact terminal ileum (which can be damaged or resected due to inflammatory bowel disease) is essential to prevent deficiency and megaloblastic anaemia. The colon is primarily a site for short-chain fatty acid (SCFA) absorption and some water and electrolytes. The role of SCFAs in human health includes acting as an energy substrate for enterocytes, as well as influencing plasma glucose and lipids, depending on the composition of SCFA which are produced by the fermentative action of the colonic microflora can ultimately. Additionally, there is increasing evidence that they may also influence mental health.

Transportation

Following absorption, either via portal circulation or the lymphatic system, nutrients can circulate freely, bind to serum proteins (e.g., albumen), or form part of larger lipid structures such as lipoproteins. For many nutrients, including glucose and amino acids, circulating levels are highly regulated by hormonal and neurological mechanisms. The role of transport proteins, which are steadily released in the fasted state, can help regulate circulating levels, as can the effect of tissues in uptake of any postprandial peaks, such as those that could occur with potassium.

Excretion

The purpose of this toolkit is not to summarise how nutrition can be used to manage disease of the colon. However, normal function of the colon and regular bowel habit is linked to an adequate fibre intake, adequate fluid intakes and regular physical activity. When reviewing the concepts linked to constipation, diarrhoea, and faecal continence, it is worth spending time reviewing the neurological control of defaecation. This should include the general principles that the parasympathetic nervous system is linked to defaecation, the sympathetic nervous system is linked to retaining and somatic nervous control gives voluntary control. This can be useful when considering the effects of spinal injury (e.g., cauda equine syndrome) on bowel control, as this provides an opportunity to work through the control pathways in health and disease.

For more information, see

- Johns JS. "Neurogenic Bowel." In: Walter Frontera, Julie Silver, Thomas Rizzo, eds. *Essentials of Physical Medicine and Rehabilitation: Musculoskeletal Disorders, Pain, and Rehabilitation*. 4th ed. Philadelphia: Elsevier, 2019:786–791.

For a review of the general principles of GI physiology, it is worth reviewing the following resources.

GI system:

- Binder HJ. Organisation of gastrointestinal system. In: Boron W, Boulpaep E, eds. *Medical Physiology*. 3rd ed. Elsevier; 2016:852–862.
- Lindsay J, Langmead L, Preston SL. Gastrointestinal disease. In: Parveen Kumar, Michael L Clark, eds. *Kumar and Clark's Clinical Medicine*. 9th ed. 2016:357–436.

Stomach:

- Binder HJ. Gastric function. In: Boron W, Boulpaep E, eds. *Medical Physiology*. 3rd ed. Elsevier; 2016:863–878.

Small intestine:

- Binder HJ. Intestinal fluid and electrolyte movement. In: Boron W, Boulpaep E, eds. *Medical Physiology*. 3rd ed. Elsevier; 2016:889–913.
- Binder HJ, Mansbach CM. Nutrient digestion and absorption. In: Boron W, Boulpaep E, eds. *Medical Physiology*. 3rd ed. Elsevier; 2016:914–943.

Renal and Urinary Systems

Nutrition often focuses on food intake, whereas the physiological role of the renal system (especially the kidneys) is essential for reabsorption from the filtrate in the nephron. With pathology related to this (e.g., renal failure and nephrotic syndrome), numerous nutritional and medical management challenges are presented.

The role of the kidneys extends further than just one of resorption when you consider their role in maintenance of haemostasis, iron and vitamin D metabolism, which also have nutritional implications.

For more information on renal physiology see the following, and reflect how this can link to nutrition:

- Gienisch G, Windhager EE, Aronson PS. Organization of the urinary system. In: Boron W, Boulpaep E, eds. *Medical Physiology*. 3rd ed. Elsevier; 2016:722–738.
- Yaqoob MM, Ashman N. Kidney and urinary tract disease. In: *Kumar and Clark's Clinical Medicine*. 9th ed. 721–793.

Cardiovascular and Respiratory Systems

The relationship between nutrition and the cardiovascular and respiratory systems is covered in Chapters 5 and 6, and their roles are inextricably linked to nutrition, both in terms of organ function and nutrient metabolism. Examples of these relationships include how oxygen availability may influence substrate use in energy metabolism or the role of electrolytes and calcium on cardiomyocyte function.

To review cardiovascular physiology, see:

- Boulpaep EL. Organization of the cardiovascular system. In: Boron W, Boulpaep E, eds. *Medical Physiology*. 3rd ed. Elsevier; 2016:410–428.
- Bunce NH, Ray R. Cardiovascular disease. In: Parveen Kumar, Michael L Clark, eds. *Kumar and Clark's Clinical Medicine*. 9th ed. 2016:931–1056.

To review respiratory physiology, see:

- Boron WF. Organization of the respiratory system. In: Boron W, Boulpaep E, eds. *Medical Physiology*. 3rd ed. Elsevier; 2016:590–605.
- Frew AJ, et al. Respiratory disease. In: Parveen Kumar, Michael L Clark, eds. *Kumar and Clark's Clinical Medicine*. 9th ed. 2016:1057–1137.

Reproductive System

The role of nutrition in the reproductive system is covered in Chapter 7. For more details on the physiological principles linked to reproductive health, see the resources below.

To review physiology and endocrine principles underpinning reproductive function, see:

- Nelson-Piercy C, Mullins EWS, Regan L. Women's health. In: Parveen Kumar, Michael L Clark, eds. *Kumar and Clark's Clinical Medicine*. 9th ed. 2016:1291–1310.

Musculoskeletal System

The role of muscle is manyfold, but two of the most well known are that of physical activity, with an obvious link to weight management, and its role in glucose regulation with respect to diabetes. The key principles of physiology that have clear relationships with nutrition are:

1. The role of GLUT-4 transporters and how they respond to insulin.
   Typically, muscles require the action of insulin to express GLUT-4 transporters on their cell membranes. Therefore, in the absence of insulin (e.g., in undiagnosed type 1 diabetes mellitus), muscles become deficient in glucose, leading to amino acid fluxes out of muscle. This in part explains the muscle wasting seen in those newly diagnosed with type 1 diabetes mellitus.
2. The role of exercise in maintaining GLUT-4 transporters in the cell membranes of the myocytes and decreasing the rate degradation.
   This in part explains the insulin and glucose-sensitising effects of exercise, which is at its greatest with respect to glucose in the first 1–2 hours postexercise and can last up to 24 hours with respect to insulin.
3. How different muscles contain different amounts of glycogen.
   This is related to the size of the muscle (capacity) and how it is trained and then replenished with glycogen following exercise/work depending on glucose supply from the diet. An additional consideration is the variation between different muscle types—fast-twitch (type 1) muscle, which preferentially use glucose, or slower twitch (type 2) muscle fibres which preferentially oxidise fatty acids. These different types of muscle fibre, which are partly influenced by genetics, can be modulated by training and may then influence success at different types of sporting activity (e.g., sprints compared with marathon running).
4. That glucose released from glycogen cannot be directly released into circulation.
   This glucose is unable to help maintain plasma glucose due to the lack of glucose 6 phosphatase in muscle.
5. That the release of lactate from muscle enters the Cori cycle in the liver.
   This lactate has undergone anaerobic respiration and can be released into circulation during exercise when insulin levels are reduced, and counterregulatory hormones (glucagon and catecholamines) are increased. This may occur even in athletes without diabetes, resulting in hyperglycaemia.

To review the physiological principles at a cellular level, see:

- Moczydlowski EG. Cellular physiology of skeletal, cardiac, and smooth muscle. In: Boron W, Boulpaep E, eds. *Medical Physiology*. 3rd ed. Elsevier; 2016:228–251.

Nervous System

There are a number of primary biomedical points with respect to neurological anatomy and nutrition, which are interrelated with function in health and disease.

1. The first of these underpin the principles of the chemical gradients with respect to sodium and potassium ions which set up the resting action potential. This relates back to the chemistry of these group 1 metals and also helps to account for the pharmacological action of lithium treatments.
2. The second is how other mineral ions can influence neurological function, including calcium and the role of fatty acids, especially the long-chain fatty acids (including omega 3 fatty acids which are essential for the myelination of longer neurones) and the distinct role of cyanocobalamin (vitamin B12) with respect to myelination.
3. Finally, from a basic biological perspective, it is important to note how a number of B vitamins, especially thiamine, riboflavin and niacin, are essential as part of cofactors in intermediary metabolism and electron transfer chains in the mitochondria. This in part explains the neurological symptoms seen with deficiency disease. In part these deficiency diseases are a reflection of the high energy demands of the nervous system, which typically accounts for around 25% of resting energy expenditure.

The fuel substrates for the nervous system have an influence on wider health and disease. Neurones cannot metabolise fatty acids; in the fed state they preferably metabolise glucose, and in the fasted (both starvation and nutritional ketosis) state, they metabolise ketones which need to be synthesised from acetyl acetyl coenzyme A in the liver (produced from beta oxidation of fatty acids). The relevance of this is related to the use of and interest in low-carbohydrate diets, which have become of increasing interest in both people with diabetes (mainly T2DM) and also those with epilepsy, especially where the epilepsy may be linked to the deficiency of rate-limiting steps in glycolysis (e.g., phosphofructokinase or pyruvate dehydrogenase) where a ketogenic (very-low-carbohydrate) diet can be an effective treatment option. There is increasing interest in the potential effects of diet in relation to this, linked to cognitive decline and dementia. This area does not advocate very-low-carbohydrate diets, but perhaps more moderate intakes and restrictions of free sugars and ultraprocessed foods sources of carbohydrate which are rapidly absorbed.

To review neurological physiology, see:

- Ransom BR. Organization of the nervous system. In: Boron W, Boulpaep E, eds. *Medical Physiology*. 3rd ed. Elsevier; 2016:254–274.

Summary of Toolkit

The purpose and principle of this toolkit is to encourage exploration of the interrelationship between the principles underpinning biomedical sciences (which are essential to form a comprehensive understanding of medicine) and the science and application of nutrition. This may be through using your understanding of nutrition to apply some of the more abstract principles of biology and physiology, or vice versa, but the overall goal is to both facilitate your understanding of nutrition and help improve your understanding of the medical sciences and, ultimately, enhance your practice.

APPENDIX 2

Weight Stigma – A Practical Guide for Clinicians

Ally Jaffee ■ Hala El-Agib El-Shafie ■ Iain Broadley

The weight stigma that some patients experience, as detailed below, should have no place in health care.

Examples of lived patient experience:

> *Had a doctor's appointment to discuss suspected endometriosis, as I was being examined on the table, stripped naked from the waist down…the doctor grabbed a handful of my belly fat, jiggled it about, and announced to the nurse, 'She needs to get rid of THIS first.'*
>
> *Visiting my GP [general practitioner] with chest pains, to be told to 'go home and look in the mirror, as that was what was wrong with me', to later that evening being rushed into hospital because I couldn't breathe. I was diagnosed with bronchitis.*
>
> —LANGUAGE MATTERS (OBESITY UK)[1]

Many UK medical schools require graduates to say a variation of the Hippocratic oath.[2] In each of these there is a variation of 'do no harm'. Similarly, the general medical council produces a booklet on good medical practice.[3] It is a legal stipulation and part of the code of ethics that all doctors must treat every single patient with respect and without discrimination.

The general medical council outlines this in 'Domain 4: Maintaining Trust', encompassing treat patients and colleagues fairly and without discrimination[3], which states the following:

'You must give priority to patients on the basis of their clinical need if these decisions are within your power. If inadequate resources, policies or systems prevent you from doing this, and patient safety, dignity or comfort may be seriously compromised, you must raise your concern in line with our guidance and your workplace policy. You should also make a record of the steps you have taken'.[4]

'The investigations or treatment you provide or arrange must be based on the assessment you and your patient make of their needs and priorities, and on your clinical judgement about the likely effectiveness of the treatment options.[5] You must not refuse or delay treatment to patients because you believe that a patient's actions or lifestyle have contributed to their condition'.[5]

What Is Weight Stigma?

'Weight stigma' refers to societal devaluation on the basis of body weight that can lead to people of higher weight being subject to prejudice and discrimination.[6]

Weight stigma is present in all aspects of society including education, health care, and the media.[7,8] Compared with other forms of discrimination, weight discrimination is most often reported by adults.[9] Research shows that 80% of British adults believe that people with obesity are viewed differently because of their weight, and 62% believe that people are more likely to discriminate against people who are overweight compared with people of different ethnic background (60%), sexual orientation (56%), or gender (40%).[10]

A weight stigma investigation showed that doctors are the second most common source of stigma out of a possible 20 sources,[11] with 53% of obese individuals reporting inappropriate comments made by their doctors,[12] and 40% of health care students witnessed senior colleagues making negative comments and jokes about obese patients.[13] A review of surveys that included individuals with overweight and obesity showed that 55% of patients with obesity have reported cancelling an appointment because they were anxious about being weighed.[14] Experiences of weight stigma in young adults is linked to concerns of increased depression, anxiety, poor body image, and unhealthy eating behaviours.[15]

Reluctance to engage with the health care system for fear of judgement may be reduced with greater education on weight stigma for health care professionals (HCPs). Appropriately addressing the multifactorial causes of obesity, while training HCPs to communicate effectively, will create a nonstigmatising practice in which patients with obesity can be treated equally.

Concept of Bias: Conscious and Unconscious Bias

Whether implicit (unconscious) or explicit (conscious), physicians may have negative attitudes toward people with excess body weight. Implicit weight bias is defined as unconscious negative attitudes toward people with excess weight.[16] This negative attitude may affect the treatment provided to those being negatively biased, while those providing the treatment may not even acknowledge that they hold these beliefs. A recent study of a large cohort of medical students found that 74% of physicians exhibited implicit weight bias and 67% endorsed explicit weight bias.[15] The first step to reducing weight bias and stigma in health care is to become aware of one's own bias.

Scan the QR code in Fig. A 2.1 to test yourself.

Biases can result in less time spent rapport building, resulting in reduced empathy and reassurance when dealing with overweight or obese patients.[17] Indirect weight stigma is also common and easily overlooked. A 2012 study found physical barriers to be one of the most stigmatising situations reported by participants.[11] Physical barriers in health care settings include:

Fig. A.2.1 Touch screen test. Weight IAT by project implicit, Harvard University.

narrow chairs,
chairs with arm rests,
narrow walkways, and
lack of appropriate weighing equipment, surgical gowns, and suitable blood pressure cuffs.[18]

HCPs have a critical role in beginning the discussion around obesity.[18] If done effectively, it can improve a patient's experience by reducing anxiety and other negative effects of experienced stigma and therefore reduce health care avoidance in the long term.

Fig. A 2.2 demonstrates examples, effects and enforcers of weight stigma, and who weight stigma affects.

Barriers Associated with Treating Obesity

HCPs aim to provide their patients with the highest quality of care. However, the presence of weight stigma can lower this quality of care for patients with excess weight.[19] Many HCPs view obesity as an avoidable risk factor that makes their ability to prevent or treat a disease more difficult.[19,20] This is an oversimplification which results in continued weight stigma.[19] As well as the multifactorial causes of obesity, there are numerous other barriers to treating obesity mentioned herein.[21]

Outcomes/Behaviour Changes as a Result of Weight Stigma

The existence of weight stigma and bias in health care may have a range of potential negative outcomes for patients including[22] see Fig. 2.4:

- changes in eating and activity (binge eating, lower motivation to exercise);
- increased blood pressure, blood sugar, and cortisol;
- reduced engagement with health care services;
- weight gain;
- depression, anxiety, suicidal tendencies;
- more advanced, poorly controlled chronic disease; and
- lower health-related quality of life.[23]

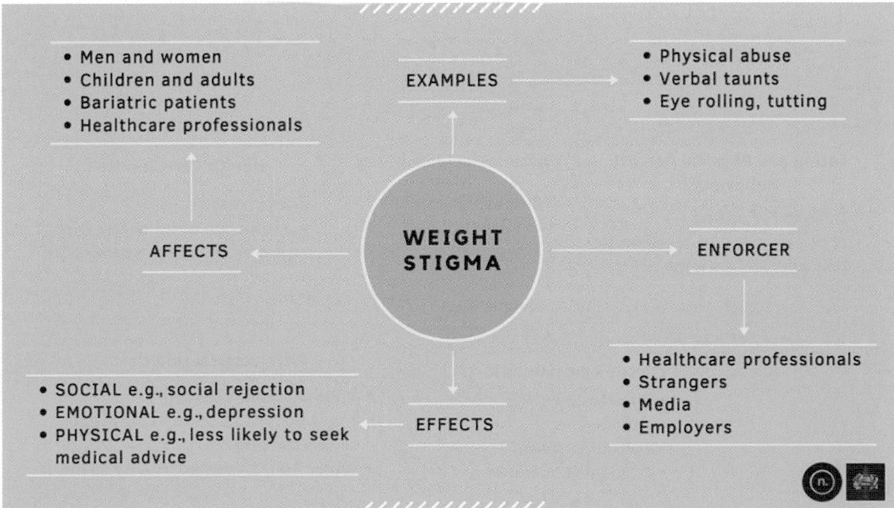

Fig. A.2.2 Weight stigma through affects, examples, enforcers and effect. (Modified from Puhl et al. 2016.)

Research has shown that people who had reported experiencing weight discrimination had a 60% greater risk of dying independent of body mass index.[24,25] Numerous studies have shown a higher prevalence of health care avoidance in people with higher body mass indexes, often as a result of body weight stigma.[26] This avoidance of health care can eventually lead to untreated or undiagnosed medical conditions associated with patients with obesity.[22] This is explained in Fig. A 2.3.

The Weight Set-Point Theory and Weight Stigma

The set point theory states that our bodies have a preset weight baseline hardwired into our DNA and that our weight and how much it changes from that set-point might be limited. The theory suggests that some individuals have higher weight set-points than others and that our bodies fight to stay within these ranges.[27] It is important for health care professionals to diffuse the blame that

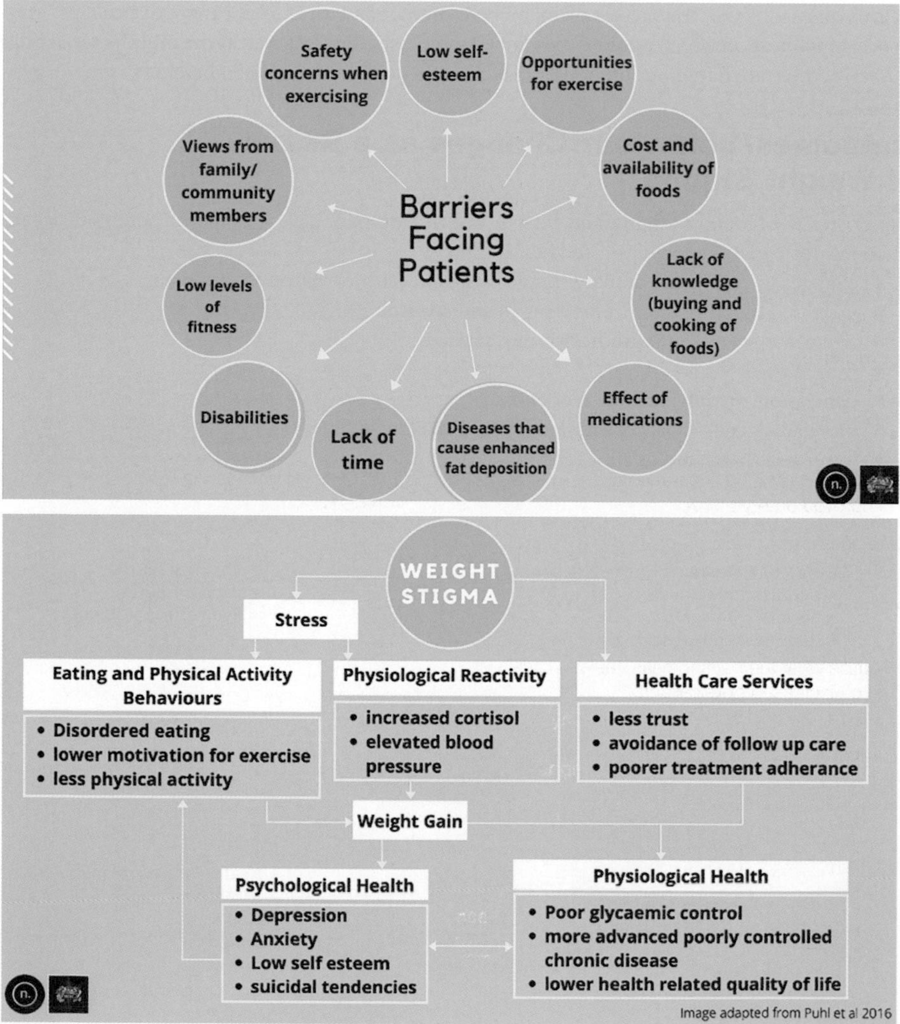

Fig. A.2.3 The barriers patients face that may lead to untreated or undiagnosed medical conditions associated with obesity (*Top*). Weight stigma and health related factors (*Bottom*). (Modified from Puhl et al. 2016.)

patients cast upon themselves during their weight loss journey, and this can be done by educating the patients on the physiological adaptations associated with dieting (e.g., homeostasis regulating hormonal changes).[27] Therefore, understanding the idea behind the set-point theory and how it provides evidence of the body's adaptive responses to energy changes is significant.

Nonverbal and Verbal Communication—Dos and Don'ts

It is necessary to implement an appropriate, nonjudgemental approach from all HCPs to minimise the prevalence of weight stigma in the primary care setting. Nonverbal communication is essential in providing effective patient care. Nonverbal communication includes:

facial expressions,
body language,
eye contact and gestures.[28]

Research has shown that in situations where verbal and nonverbal communication is contradictory, nonverbal communication often outweighs the verbal.[29] This highlights the importance of both forms of communication supporting and complementing each other.

The dos	The don'ts
Seek permission to discuss weight with patient.	Assume patient is ready or willing to discuss their weight.
Address the concern that brought the patient to you before discussing their weight.	Focus solely on the patient's weight particularly when it is not the reason for the visit.
Ask patient and use words chosen by the patient to describe excess weight – can be different for each patient.	Use terms that are judgemental or disrespectful to patient.
Acknowledge the patient is not his or her symptoms—'the patient has obesity'.	Refer to patient as his or her symptoms—'the patient is obese'.
Consider the patient's life—what works for one may not work for another.	Use language that generalises or stereotypes.
Focus on positives (achievements, potential for improved quality of life).	Threaten patient with long-term consequences of obesity.
Use questions that encourage a more open discussion.	Use closed questions—yes-or-no answering.
Acknowledge that obesity is a multifactorial complex condition.	Simplify the intervention for obesity—'Eat less, move more'.
Prioritise what the patient measures as success (e.g., increased physical activity irrespective of weight loss).	Focus on biomedical markers as a measure of success.
Collaborate with the patient to set out achievable goals and suggest useful support.	Use prescriptive language when talking about diet and lifestyle changes.

Public Health Messages

Public health campaigners should aim to generate positivity around health messaging by promoting healthy relationships with food and body image. However, at this time, there is limited evidence to suggest that these public health campaigns (e.g., Change4Life) are effective in reducing the rates of obesity.[30] Currently, there are concerns about the negative impact these public health messages may have by focusing on body shape and size. Despite evidence of biological and genetic factors contributing to weight regulation, obesity campaigns and policies frame it as personal choice.[15] The weight-loss competition TV show *The Biggest Loser*, aired in America, Asia,

Australia, and the Arab world, focuses on weight status and weight loss, which augments weight stigma and unhealthy weight-control behaviours.[31]

Instead, a more positive weight-neutral approach may provide lasting benefits (e.g., 'health at every size' approach).[32]

The World Health Organisation has set out some tactics to improve action on the message being communicated to the public in relation to behaviour change.

These include:

- involve partners early in the campaign and
- use trusted messengers such as registered dietitians who can remove barriers and stigma around making the change.

Ensure the target population has access to resources. For example, liaising with GP practices to ensure appropriate referrals. Additionally, some principles for effective communication have been set out. These include:

- Accessible—Identify effective communication channels such as making all information available online.
- Relevant—Know, listen, tailor, and motivate the audience.
- Timely—Communicate early and at the right time.
- Understandable—Use simple language, use real stories, and make it visual.

At a national level, the health development agency, alongside the National Health Service in the UK, has set out characteristics which evidence suggests are key elements for success in behaviour change. These include:

- When appropriate, intervene at multiple levels.
- Tailor messages in terms of age, gender, and culture.
- Ensure information is basic but accurate.
- Collaborate with services in the community, for example, providing transport links from community centres to clinics.
- Address peer norms and social pressures.

Recognition of Weight Stigma Among Medical Practitioners

Recently, the Royal College of Physicians in the UK, along with over 100 other medical and scientific organisations, signed a global pledge to end obesity stigma.[33]

This statement and accompanying recommendations highlighted the prevalence of weight stigma in society and the need for education around weight stigma to change the current public narrative of obesity. This acknowledgement of weight stigma as an issue is an encouraging step in the right direction.

How to Improve Practice

In the UK, the percentage of the adult population with obesity has increased from 26% in 2016 to 29% in 2017–2018.[34] Current models do not appear to be working on a population level, which must be reconsidered. Next we suggest some actions that may help clinicians to improve in practice.

1. **Appropriate communication with patients**
   - Refer to the dos and don'ts.
   - Practice appropriate verbal and nonverbal communication (e.g., eye contact).
   - Use a patient-centred approach.[30]

- Tailor health interventions based on the patient's circumstances (i.e., health status, perceived barriers). Some examples of this may include a patient affected by type 2 diabetes[35] or a patient taking certain/specific medications that contribute to weight gain.

2. **Appropriate referrals**
   - Presently, it is common for primary care practices to issue referrals to commercial weight loss programmes free of charge to the patient. Such services include Slimming World, Weight Watchers, Noom, and more.
   - It is not always the best option for GPs to refer their patients to such services, as these organisations offer programmes that are contradictory to the evidence we know regarding intentional weight loss and its outcomes.
   - As a GP, it is important to educate and contemplate appropriate referrals for patients with obesity to protect them from stigmatising and fat-phobic environments.
   - GPs and health care professionals with reliable nutrition qualifications should work simultaneously to provide patients with group support services that encompass a non-stigmatising, patient health, and well-being ethos.
3. **Inclusive physical environment**
   - Examples include:
     - appropriately sized furniture in waiting areas (e.g., chairs/ sofas);
     - appropriately sized furniture and equipment within consultation rooms (e.g., scales, blood pressure cuffs, chairs/sofas);
     - appropriate messaging on posters/information sheets; and
     - recording a patient's weight only when necessary and giving each patient the option of not knowing the recorded result).
   - Nonstigmatising images can be sourced from World Obesity's image bank.[36]
4. **Gaining patient feedback and auditing**
   - The Royal College of General Practitioners provide recommendations for gaining patient feedback for GPs.[37] This includes patient participation groups[38] and the national patient survey.
   - Patient feedback can help practices discover areas requiring improvement as well as what is being done well. This is also a way to audit and monitor the progress of anything new that has been implemented.[37]
5. **Checking your area for what services/support are available (e.g., support groups)**
   - Referrals: including HCPs (e.g., registered dietitian, weight management services)
   - BEAT Charity HelpFinder[39]—a search engine for finding eating disorder support (e.g., registered dietitians, support groups, National Health Service community centres)
   - Support groups, including:
     - Online support groups
     - BEAT Charity Nightingale[40] (binge-eating disorder online support group)
     - Obesity UK support groups (online and some face-to-face)
     - HOOP UK[41]
   - Local cooking and teaching classes, including:
     - Hackney[42]—London, UK
     - Cakebread Cellars[43]—Rutherford, California, USA
     - The Homeland Cooking School[44]—Auckland City, New Zealand
     - Kitchen Lab[45]—Beirut, Lebanon
6. **Appropriate approach to obesity treatment**
   - Propose a weight-neutral, healthy eating approach for obesity treatment. By improving health and fitness, mortality risk is reduced, regardless of an individual's weight.[46]

- Focus on improving fitness and overall health rather than the number on the scale.[13] This approach incorporates health benefits instead of intentional weight loss.[47]

7. **Continual professional development and further reading**
   - Training of current and new staff in GP practice
   - Examples of training: World Obesity SCOPE[48] obesity management training and eating disorder training by Anorexia and Bulimia Care[49]
   - More detailed recommendations for weight management covered by National Institute for Health and Clinical Excellence guidelines[50]

Weight stigma is concerningly prevalent in health care along with other aspects of life. There are decades of research showing us that the diets and weight loss programmes and campaigns are short-term fixes and are not tackling the obesity issue; if anything, they are making it worse. Without a systematic and attitude change, we risk a continuous increase in obesity and weight stigma.

References

1. The European Association for the Study of Obesity. Talking about obesity. Language matters guide. (2020). Obesity UK. Available at https://easo.org/talking-about-obesity-obesityuk-language-matters-guide/
2. Patient. The Hippocratic Oath and Good Medical Practice. Available at https://patient.info/doctor/ideals-and-the-hippocratic-oath.
3. General Medical Council. Home. Available at https://www.gmc-uk.org/.
4. General Medical Council. Domain 2: Safety and quality. 2022. Available at https://www.gmc-uk.org/ethical-guidance/ethical-guidance-for-doctors/good-medical-practice/domain-2----safety-and-quality.
5. General Medical Council. Domain 4: Maintaining trust. Available at https://www.gmc-uk.org/ethical-guidance/ethical-guidance-for-doctors/good-medical-practice/domain-4---maintaining-trust
6. Puhl RM. Obesity stigma: Important considerations for public health. *Am J Public Health*. 2010;100(6):1019–1028. https://doi.org/10.2105/AJPH.2009.159491.
7. Obesity Action California. Understanding obesity stigma brochure—Obesity Action Coalition. Available at https://www.obesityaction.org/our-community/discover-the-oacs-community/?gclid=CjwKCAjwxr2iBhBJEiwAdXECw73n1bZT19vKhfXKQGp21csjnNP2LhFkXpbR0dIRPowPXFBvXfj_ThoCFrsQAvD_BwE.
8. University of Connecticut. Weight bias & stigma. UConn Rudd Center for Food Policy & Health. Available at https://uconnruddcenter.org/research/weight-bias-stigma/.
9. Latner JD, O'Brien KS, Durso LE, Brinkman LA, MacDonald T. Weighing obesity stigma: The relative strength of different forms of bias. *Int J Obes*. 2008;32(7):1145–1152. https://doi.org/10.1038/ijo.2008.53.
10. Hazell C. Weight revealed as the UK's most common form of discrimination. Available at https://britishlivertrust.org.uk/weight-uks-most-common-discrimination/#:~:text=Weight%20revealed%20as%20the%20UK's%20most%20common%20form%20of%20discrimination,-Posted%20on%3A%2-011th&text=New%20research%20reveals%20that%20more,against%20someone%20who%20is%20overweight.
11. Puhl RM, Brownell KD. Confronting and coping with weight stigma: an investigation of overweight and obese adults. *Obesity (Silver Spring, Md.)*. 2006;14(10):1802–1815. https://doi.org/10.1038/oby.2006.208.
12. Puhl RM, Brownell KD. Psychosocial origins of obesity stigma: toward changing a powerful and pervasive bias. *Obesity Reviews*. 2003;4:213–227. https://doi.org/10.1046/j.1467-789X.2003.00122.x.
13. Chakravorty T. Fat shaming is stopping doctors from helping overweight patients-here's what medical students can do about it. *BMJ (Clinical research ed.)*. 2021;375:n2830. https://doi.org/10.1136/bmj.n2830.
14. Alberga AS, Forhan M, Russell-Mayhew S. Weight bias and health care utilization: a scoping review. 2019;20:e116. https://doi:10.1017/S1463423619000227
15. Brown A, Flint SW, Batterham RL. Pervasiveness, impact and implications of weight stigma. *eClinicalMedicine*. 2022:47.

16. Kirk SFL, Ramos Salas X, Alberga AS, Russell-Mayhew S. Canadian Adult Obesity Clinical Practice Guidelines: Reducing Weight Bias, Stigma and Discrimination in Obesity Management, Practice and Policy. Available from: https://obesitycanada.ca/guidelines/weightbias.
17. Durkin M. Doctor, your weight bias is showing. Available at https://acpinternist.org/archives/2017/02/weight.htm.
18. McGowan BM. A practical guide to engaging individuals with obesity. *Obes Facts*. 2016;9(3):182–192. https://doi.org/10.1159/000445193.
19. Phelan SM, Burgess D, Yeazel MW, Hellerstedt WL, Griffin JM, van Ryn M. Impact of weight bias and stigma on quality of care and outcomes for patients with obesity. *Obes Rev*. 2015;16(4):319–326. https://doi.org/10.1111/obr.12266.
20. Foster GD, Wadden TA, Makris AP, et al. Primary Care Physicians' Attitudes about Obesity and Its Treatment. *Obesity Research*. 2003;11:1168–1177. https://doi.org/10.1038/oby.2003.161.
21. National Institute for Health and Clinical Excellence. Working with people to prevent and manage overweight and obesity: the issues. Obesity prevention. Guidance. NICE. Available at https://www.nice.org.uk/guidance/cg43/chapter/working-with-people-to-prevent-and-manage-overweight-and-obesity-the-issues.
22. Stanford FC. Addressing weight bias in medicine. Harvard Health. 2019. Available at https://www.health.harvard.edu/blog/addressing-weight-bias-in-medicine-2019040316319.
23. Puhl R, Suh Y. Health consequences of weight stigma: Implications for obesity prevention and treatment. *Curr Obes Rep*. 2015;4(2):182–190. https://doi.org/10.1007/s13679-015-0153-z.
24. Tomiyama AJ, Carr D, Granberg EM, et al. How and why weight stigma drives the obesity 'epidemic' and harms health. *BMC Med*. 2018;16(1):1–6. https://doi.org/10.1186/s12916-018-1116-5.
25. Sutin ARP, Stephan Y, Terracciano A. Weight discrimination and risk of mortality. *Psychol Sci*. 2015;26(11):1803–1811. https://doi.org/10.1177/0956797615601103.
26. Mensinger JL, Tylka TL, Calamari ME. Mechanisms underlying weight status and healthcare avoidance in women: A study of weight stigma, body-related shame and guilt, and healthcare stress. *Body Image*. 2018;25:139–147.
27. What you need to know about Set Point Theory. Healthline. Available at https://www.healthline.com/health/set-point-theory.
28. Nonverbal communication skill list and examples. The Balance. Available at https://www.thebalancemoney.com/nonverbal-communication-skills-2059693.
29. Inui TS, Carter WB. A Guide to the Research Literature on Doctor/Patient Communication. In: Lipkin M, Putnam SM, Lazare A, Carroll JG, Frankel RM, eds. *The Medical Interview. Frontiers of Primary Care*. New York, NY: Springer; 1995. https://doi.org/10.1007/978-1-4612-2488-4_41.
30. Walls HL, Peeters A, Proietto J, et al. Public health campaigns and obesity – a critique. *BMC Public Health*. 2011;11:136. https://doi.org/10.1186/1471-2458-11-136.
31. Kenney EL, Wintner S, Lee RM, Austin SB. Obesity Prevention Interventions in US Public Schools: Are Schools Using Programs That Promote Weight Stigma. *Preventing chronic disease*. 2017;14:E142. https://doi.org/10.5888/pcd14.160605.
32. Health at every size. Nutritional Sciences. 2021. Available at https://nutrisci.wisc.edu/2021/01/14/health-at-every-size/
33. Royal College of Physicians signs global pledge to end obesity stigma. Royal College of Physicians. 2020. Available at https://www.rcplondon.ac.uk/news/royal-college-physicians-signs-global-pledge-end-obesity-stigma
34. Statistics on Obesity, Physical Activity and Diet. National Health Service. 2019. Available at https://digital.nhs.uk/data-and-information/publications/statistical/statistics-on-obesity-physical-activity-and-diet
35. Leitner DR, Frühbeck G, Yumuk V, et al. Obesity and type 2 diabetes: Two diseases with a need for combined treatment strategies—EASO can lead the way. *Obes Facts*. 2017;10(5):483–492. https://doi.org/10.1159/000480525.
36. Weight stigma. World Obesity Federation. Available at https://www.worldobesity.org/what-we-do/our-policy-priorities/weight-stigma
37. Guidance on supporting information for appraisal and revalidation. General Medical Council. 2021. Available at https://www.gmc-uk.org/registration-and-licensing/managing-your-registration/revalidation/guidance-on-supporting-information-for-appraisal-and-revalidation
38. Welcome to the National Association for Patient Participation. National Association for Patient Participation. N.D. Available at https://napp.org.uk/

39. Welcome to Helpfinder. Beat Eating disorders. n.d. Avaible at https://helpfinder.beateatingdisorders.org.uk/
40. Nightingale - Online Support Group. Beat Eating disorders. n.d. Available at https://www.beateatingdisorders.org.uk/get-information-and-support/get-help-for-myself/i-need-support-now/online-support-groups/nightingale-online-support-group/
41. Hoop (UK). Hoop: Helping Overcome Obesity Problems. n.d. Available at https://www.talkhealthpartnership.com/charities/hoop
42. Cooking classes in Hackney. Hackney. n.d. Available at https://hackney.gov.uk/cooking-classes
43. Private Cooking Classes. Cakebread Cellars. n.d. Available at https://www.cakebread.com/cooking-classes.html
44. Learn to cook in our state of the art space. Homeland Cooking School. n.d. Available at https://homelandnz.com/cooking-school/
45. Cook with Friends. Kitchen lab. n.d. Available at https://kitchenlabo.com/
46. Angadi SGAGS. Obesity treatment: Weight loss versus increasing fitness and physical activity for reducing health risks. *iScience*. 2021:24. https://doi.org/10.1016/j.isci.2021.102995.
47. Gaesser GA, Angadi SS. Obesity treatment: Weight loss versus increasing fitness and physical activity for reducing health risks. *iScience*. 2021;24(10):102995. https://doi.org/10.1016/j.isci.2021.102995.
48. SCOPE. World Obesity Federation. n.d. Available at https://www.worldobesity.org/training-and-events/scope
49. Anorexia and Bulimia Care. Anorexia & Bulimia Care ABC. n.d. Available at https://amhp.org.uk/member/anorexia-and-bulimia-care/
50. NICE guidelines. National Institute for Health and Care Excellence. n.d. Available at https://www.nice.org.uk/about/what-we-do/our-programmes/nice-guidance/nice-guidelines

APPENDIX 3

Nutrition and COVID-19: Toolkit of Emerging Evidence

Shane McAuliffe ■ James Bradfield ■ Taskforce

Introduction

The coronavirus disease (COVID-19) pandemic of 2019, which fully came to global attention in 2020, was an outbreak like few have ever experienced before. The pandemic affected almost all industries and workplaces, with a near complete stagnation of international travel, closure of workplaces and practices like social distancing and face mask wearing becoming the norm in many countries around the world. However, few workforces were affected like those working in hospitals and health services around the world as they dealt with the initial wave of cases, the fallout from the disease and subsequent surges in cases since. All aspects of patient care were examined to see how outcomes could be improved for those who contracted severe acute respiratory syndrome coronavirus 2 (SARS-CoV-2), including nutrition. This appendix presents some of the evidence for the role and importance of nutrition in the development, management and recovery from COVID-19.

Origin of the Disease and Declaration of a Pandemic

Coronaviruses are a large family of viruses, named for their appearance which imitates the spikes on a crown. There have been coronavirus outbreaks in the past, perhaps most notably the severe acute respiratory syndrome coronavirus (SARS-CoV-1) outbreak in 2002, more commonly referred to as SARS. Though this outbreak was classified as an epidemic rather than a pandemic, it had a higher case fatality rate than COVID-19.

The first cases of COVID-19 were reported in the Chinese city of Wuhan on December 31, 2019, when a cluster of pneumonia cases of unknown aetiology were detected. Shortly afterward, the virus thought to be causing these conditions was identified via genetic sequencing and referred to as a novel coronavirus. China reported their first deaths from the disease while cases began to appear in other countries around the world. Authorities quickly identified Huanan Seafood Market as a common exposure point for many of the first cases and it was subsequently closed; however, the origin of disease remains a topic of debate. Wuhan entered a strict lockdown with restrictions on movement in and out of the city, while it became clear that the virus is spread by droplets (i.e., by coughing, sneezing or touching your face) and to a lesser extent surface contact. More recently it has been acknowledged that aerosol is also a primary route of spread.

From January 22 to 23, the World Health Organisation (WHO) convened a meeting to determine if this outbreak warranted declaration as a Public Health Emergency of International Concern. Initially not determined to be so, the WHO reversed their decision on January 30 following identification of cases in countries around the world including in America and Europe. In February, the virus was renamed as SARS-CoV-2 and on March 11, the WHO declared the outbreak as a pandemic.

By the end of February, several countries, including Italy and Iran, emerged as major outbreak centres where health care systems struggled to deal with an influx of cases. In subsequent weeks, in many countries around the world, rules were enforced to prevent large gatherings of people, many events were cancelled, and lockdowns and travel bans became common methods that governments used to try and curtail rising cases.

For current updates on nutrition and COVID-19 please refer to the online resources of the NNEdPro Nutrition and COVID-19 Taskforce: www.nnedpro.org.uk/covid-19nutrition-resources

COVID-19

COVID-19 is the disease that develops after infection with SARS-CoV-2. Though many signs and symptoms have been identified as hallmarks of the disease, the following are considered the most typical:

- High temperature
- A new continuous cough
- Loss of taste and/or smell

Most patients who develop COVID-19 have mild disease and are able to manage their condition at home with rest and simple supportive measures. Patients should isolate themselves from friends or family to prevent onward transmission. Recommended isolation periods vary between countries but generally range between 10 and 14 days from the onset of symptoms. Public health tracking and tracing systems for identifying patients and their recent contacts have been developed all over the world, usually based on mobile phone technology, with varying levels of success.

Some patients will develop symptoms serious enough to require hospitalisation. Typically, these include breathlessness, chest pain, fever, fatigue, and gastrointestinal symptoms. The most common indication for hospital admission is to treat hypoxia with supplemental oxygen. Delivery mechanisms range from simple noninvasive devices (nasal cannula, simple face mask) to advanced noninvasive respiratory support (continuous positive airway pressure), to invasive mechanical ventilation (tracheal intubation and ventilation), as required. If a patient requires a level of care which cannot be achieved safely on a regular ward, they will be moved to an intensive care unit (ICU). Over the course of the pandemic, several other treatments were developed such as giving patients the antiinflammatory glucocorticoid dexamethasone; however, at present, there is still no specific cure for COVID-19. At the time of writing, there have been almost 120 million confirmed cases of COVID-19 around the world with almost 2.6 million deaths. Risk factors, treatments and challenges related to nutrition will be discussed later in this appendix.

VACCINES

From early in the pandemic, it became clear that there would be a great need for a reliable vaccine given the presence of the virus in almost every country worldwide. Despite this, in February 2020, the WHO announced that it did not expect a vaccine to be available for at least 18 months. In June and August, Chinese and Russian authorities, respectively, announced that they had developed vaccines though they did not become widely available at the time. The UK authorised the use of vaccines in December 2020 and a national vaccination programme was rolled out. Since then, others have been authorised in countries around the world with vaccination programmes designed to vaccinate as many people as possible, beginning with those most vulnerable.

THE ROLE OF NUTRITION IN COVID-19

Given the sustained global impact of the COVID-19 pandemic, almost all areas of health and lifestyle have been called into question and examined in relation to the disease. Observational research into COVID-19 outcomes has shown that people with nutrition-related noncommunicable conditions such as the metabolic syndrome, obesity[1] and diabetes mellitus[2] are at greater risk of mortality and morbidity. In addition, much has been written about the importance of nutrition in COVID-19 prevention and clinical management.[3] Specific attention has been given to the role of nutrition in immune health in the context of COVID-19,[4] and dietary micronutrients in infectious disease,[5] with particular interest in vitamin D and COVID-19.[6]

As with all aspects of COVID-19, ongoing research yields more new information each day, and it is difficult to keep pace with novel findings. Nonetheless, the following core topics are worthy of further discussion in the context of nutrition in health care. It is important to note that, to date, there is no evidence that any specific food or diet can prevent or treat COVID-19, and a balanced dietary pattern that supports overall health remains the core principle of dietary advice.

Nutrition of the Primary Prevention of COVID-19

NUTRITION AND INFECTION

Infection increases the metabolic demand for energy-yielding substrates, to facilitate the production of immune system cells and mediators.[2] These are primarily glucose, amino acids and fatty acids. Vitamins and minerals are required as cofactors. This means that good nutritional status is an essential requirement for the body to respond to the challenge of infection effectively. Conversely, malnutrition in all its forms has the potential to dampen the body's immune system and impair its function. Poor nutritional status can therefore result in a blunted response, which is made clear by conditions of nutritional deficiencies.[2,3] Groups at higher risk of COVID-19 also tend to be at higher risk of micronutrient deficiencies and poorer overall nutritional status.[3,7]

Malnutrition is characterised by chronic inflammation and higher susceptibility to infection. Through rapid changes in food environments and living conditions, a global nutrition transition is generating a new double burden of malnutrition in which undernutrition and overweight coexist within populations, and often within individuals. Both states have the potential to impair adequate functioning of the immune system.[8]

DESPITE TWO DISTINCT CLINICAL PRESENTATIONS, WE OBSERVE COMMON AETIOLOGICAL CHARACTERISTICS AND PATHWAYS IN UNDERNUTRITION AND OVERNUTRITION:[8]

- Early life undernutrition increases the risk of obesity in later life
- Altered metabolism
- Chronic underlying inflammation
- Gut dysfunction (enteropathy)
- Excess energy and macronutrient intake often coincides with micronutrient deficiencies in overweight individuals

UNDERNUTRITION

Mortality from COVID-19 has been highest among older people and those with comorbidities, who are also often most at risk of undernutrition in society. Malnutrition in these groups is often community acquired and associated with poor clinical outcomes in secondary care. It is estimated that 23% of European older adults are at high risk of malnutrition.[9] In the UK, this figure is about 29% of adult patients who are admitted to hospitals.[10]

Admission to hospital with poor nutritional reserve is predictive of poorer clinical outcomes.[11] Compounding this, COVID-19 is associated with a huge metabolic cost, particularly in patients requiring intensive care, where severe depletion of lean and functional mass has been observed.[12] This is likely to be significant in the recovery phase of disease.

MALNUTRITION IS ASSOCIATED WITH WORSE CLINICAL OUTCOMES IN THOSE ADMITTED TO SECONDARY CARE,[11] INCLUDING:

- Impaired immune response to infection
- Increased muscle depletion
- Increased frequency of complications
- Increased length of stay
- Increased morbidity and mortality

OVERNUTRITION

There has been significant interest in the role of poor metabolic health predicting susceptibility to and worse outcomes from COVID-19. This patient group generally comprises those with obesity, insulin resistance and clinical features of the metabolic syndrome.[13] It is well recognised that patients with obesity who develop acute respiratory distress syndrome tend to have worse outcomes. Explanatory physiological mechanisms underlying this include diminished recruitment of lung tissue and lower ventilatory pressures even without well-established lung injury.[14] Another potentially important factor is the increased concentration of circulating proinflammatory cytokines in these patients during critical illness.[2] Observations from the influenza H1N1 epidemic suggest poorer vaccine response and overall recovery in those living with obesity.[14]

Many of these factors exist across metabolic conditions including obesity, type 2 diabetes and cardiovascular disease, which have been associated with higher rates of severe COVID-19 infection and mortality. While the rate of infection appears similar, global data suggest that patients with diabetes have up to threefold higher mortality rate compared with the rates seen in COVID-19 patients overall (7.3% versus 2.3%).[15] Poorer glycaemic control appears to be a key factor in this relationship, as demonstrated from large data sets in both the UK and China.[16,17] Higher rates of mortality have also been observed in patients with hypertension.[18]

MICRONUTRIENTS

Micronutrients are required for normal immune functions through a number of mechanisms,[2,3] from external physical barriers to the production of immune proteins, cells and inflammatory mediators. Therefore, optimal nutritional status is required for an optimal immune response.

MICRONUTRIENTS FUNCTION IN MULTILEVEL IMMUNE SYSTEM RESPONSE[2]

- Development and maintenance of physical barriers, skin and mucous membranes
- Production of antimicrobial proteins
- Activity of immune cells
- Mediation of inflammatory processes

Micronutrient deficiencies impair the function of the immune system, increasing susceptibility to infection. Infection causes inflammation, resulting in higher metabolic demands and increased nutritional requirements.[2] Specific micronutrient deficiencies have been associated with the risk of respiratory tract infections (RTIs) and disease outcomes.[3] Some of the pathophysiological effects of, and immune responses to, COVID-19 share characteristics with those observed in other well-described acute respiratory infections, suggesting potential roles of specific micronutrients in the prevention and treatment of COVID-19.

A SELECTION OF KEY MICRONUTRIENTS WHICH HAVE LONGSTANDING ASSOCIATIONS WITH RTIs[3]

- Vitamin A: Infectious disease in children
- Vitamin C: RTIs in older adults and common cold
- Vitamin D: RTI, tuberculosis, chronic obstructive pulmonary disease, asthma
- Vitamin E: RTI in the institutionalised elderly
- Selenium: Enhanced antiviral immunity
- Zinc: Common cold, pneumonia in elderly populations

Higher rates of micronutrient deficiency are seen in certain population groups. Analysis from the latest UK National Diet and Nutrition Survey highlighted associations between inadequacy of certain micronutrients (A, E, C and D) and respiratory complaints in the UK population, which remained after adjustment for age and sex, body mass index, household income and smoking status.[19]

Age is the number one predictor of mortality from COVID-19,[17] and there is a general deterioration of immune function associated with ageing. This process is known as immunosenescence, and it affects both innate and adaptive immune systems.[3,7] A further mismatch exists between reduced dietary intakes and impaired nutrient absorption, as well as increased requirements to compensate for deficits in cellular function and the inflammatory response associated with ageing.[20] These factors lead to increased susceptibility to infections, poorer response to vaccination and higher levels of micronutrient deficiencies in older adults.[20]

The potential role of vitamin D in the prevention and treatment of COVID-19 has been discussed in a range of peer-reviewed publications. There is a strong association between contracting COVID-19 and its severity, including mortality, and vitamin D insufficiency and deficiency.[21] However, vitamin D is also a negative acute phase reactant so the presence, and direction, of causality in this association is unclear from the observational studies reporting it. Robust interventional trials proving a benefit from vitamin D supplementation in COVID-19 prevention and treatment are lacking. Vitamin D supplementation is already widely recommended for the general population to reduce the risk of deficiency and associated disease, specifically musculoskeletal disease.[22] This is recommended for all people during autumn and winter, when insufficient sunlight is available to meet requirements, and all year in groups at highest risk of deficiency, including older housebound individuals, those with darker skin tones and those living at higher latitudes.[4,23] During the COVID-19 pandemic, the UK expanded provision of vitamin D supplements to vulnerable groups at highest risk during winter months.[24]

KEY POINTS IN RELATION TO VITAMIN D AND COVID-19

- Currently, there is not sufficient peer-reviewed and published evidence to support a specific role for vitamin D supplementation for the prevention or treatment of COVID-19.
- Avoiding vitamin D deficiency is important for health. For this reason, measures to prevent deficiency should be supported at all times.
- This is possible through obtaining sufficient vitamin D from natural sunlight, some food products (particularly those fortified with vitamin D) and moderately dosed vitamin D supplements if required, particularly for those who are at higher risk of deficiency.
- Appropriate recommendations for vitamin D supplementation are available globally, including by the National Institute for Health and Care Excellence, European Food Safety Authority and the American Institute of Medicine.
- Clinically proven insufficiency and deficiency require treatment with higher doses of supplementation. Individuals at highest risk of deficiency (based on demographics, skin tone, comorbidities, and cultural and lifestyle factors) may require supplementation at

higher doses than those recommended by national population guidelines, and this should be done under appropriate clinical supervision.
- Further research continues to be undertaken to discover a potential therapeutic role for vitamin specific to COVID-19 infection.

CONCLUSION

Importantly, unlike age, nutritional status can be considered a modifiable risk factor in the prevention and treatment of COVID-19. Nutrition support provided as part of routine clinical practice has been shown to improve outcomes (including from infectious complications of illness) of those at nutritional risk in large randomised clinical trials, with benefits demonstrated in both older patients and those with comorbidities.[25,26]

Improvements in metabolic health are also possible through nutritional intervention, which may prove protective against COVID-19 infection. The COVID-19 pandemic provides a platform for the promotion of healthy diet and lifestyle choices to the population at large. Additional emphasis on public health messaging can be used as an opportunity to facilitate discussions around nutrition-related behaviour change at a population level and promote the inclusion of nutrition into routine health care practice.[27]

In other respiratory infections, correction of micronutrient deficiencies has been effective in promoting improved immune responsiveness, granted the key observation of effect in these cases has been in those with deficient status.[2,3] This emphasises the importance of robust systems for testing and treating nutritional insufficiencies and deficiencies, in cases of COVID-19 infection and more widely. Advances in our understanding of the importance of nutritional status in COVID-19 can provide a catalyst for all health care professionals to embed nutritional care into routine practice.

KEY RECOMMENDATIONS TO PROMOTE HEALTHY DIETARY PATTERNS AND NUTRITIONAL ADEQUACY IN THE POPULATION[28]

- Eating foods from a variety of food groups will typically be sufficient to meet energy, protein and micronutrient requirements in the general population. Aiming to improve overall dietary diversity while maintaining dietary quality should be a primary focus.
- Global food-based dietary guidelines make recommendations for a variety and diversity of whole vegetables, fruits, berries, nuts, seeds, grains and pulses, along with some meat, eggs, dairy products and fish.
- Common to these recommendations is to reduce food items associated with poorer health outcomes, such as refined grains, free sugars and processed meat products.
- In higher-risk groups where dietary intakes are unlikely to be sufficient to meet nutritional requirements, supplementation should be considered as an addition to good overall dietary practices.
- In those with preexisting malnutrition or at risk of malnutrition, nutrient- and calorie-dense foods and beverages can help to improve energy intake.
- Vitamin D is found in only a handful of foods, and many population groups have inadequate status, especially during the winter months. To ensure adequate vitamin D, supplementation guidelines should be followed while taking into account special conditions and common risk factors such as age, skin colour and obesity.
- These recommendations must be considered in the context of the COVID-19 pandemic, during which concerns related to food access and affordability have impacted common dietary practices.

COVID-19 and Nutrition in Primary Care: Social Inequalities

People's diets and therefore nutritional status are affected by much more than just their knowledge and preferences around food. Though previously nutrition research has been heavily weighted toward a reductionist approach,[29] there is now a greater appreciation for the social determinants of health which influence food choices and eating behaviour.

The social determinants of health are commonly described as those conditions in which people are born, grow, live, work and age.[30] These too have been examined in the context of the COVID-19 pandemic, and unsurprisingly, reports have suggested that those from more socioeconomically disadvantaged backgrounds tend to suffer disproportionally from COVID-19.[31,32] Socioeconomic factors that may increase an individual's likelihood of contracting COVID-19 include living conditions (such as multigenerational households, inability to socially distance), working in manual jobs where working from home is not possible and relying on public transport to get to and from work. Nutritional status is also strongly correlated with socioeconomic status and local food environment and may influence outcomes in COVID-19.

There is a further relationship between those with poor health and COVID-19, mediated by higher levels of nutrition-related noncommunicable diseases. Socioeconomic status is inversely correlated with conditions like cardiovascular disease, diabetes and cancer, all of which are related to greater odds of severe disease and mortality in COVID-19.[33] Of course, health inequalities reflect social inequalities at large, and addressing them requires systemic changes that are unlikely to occur in the short term.

Structural change requires time, investment, multisector buy-in and the will of those in positions of power. In the UK, health inequalities have been formally in the public consciousness since at least 1980 with the publishing of the Black Report[34], however, COVID-19 has once again forced this issue under the microscope and into everyday discourse. It remains to be seen what effect this will have on improving health care accessibility in the future.

NUTRITION IN THE TREATMENT AND MANAGEMENT OF COVID-19

The relevance of nutritional status in COVID-19 infection is made clear by the important role it plays in the functioning of the immune system and consequently, viral immunity.[2] Therefore, malnutrition is associated with immune dysfunction that confers poorer outcome from infection. It is also true that individuals from groups most likely to be hospitalised with COVID-19 are also likely to have malnutrition at admission.

Useful resources designed to support optimising nutritional status during and after COVID-19 illness include appropriate pathways for the use of oral nutritional supplements.[35] These first-line principles can be applied to patients with COVID-19 in all settings, be that home, primary care facility, hospital ward or ICU. Regular monitoring of nutritional status is then key to identify patients who require escalation of nutrition support.

NUTRITION SCREENING

Given unprecedented service pressures during the COVID-19 pandemic, standard procedure and practice has been difficult to maintain. Accordingly, nutrition screening and assessment will have been impacted.[27] Perhaps understandably, the focus of hospital teams has been on urgent medical issues such as respiratory failure, meaning nutrition care has been a lower priority.[27] The challenge of accurate nutrition screening is further complicated by staff shortages, increased workload, and added personal protective equipment requirements.[36] All these factors impact on a medical and nursing team's ability to obtain height and weight measurements, complete nutrition screening assessments and ultimately reflect the strain efficiently and accurately on services to ensure best practice has been maintained.[36]

These issues have been particularly stark in the intensive care setting, where anthropometric measures are imperative to help guide feed provision and dietetic management of nutrition support. In many cases weight was based on proxy measures and estimated at admission without subsequent repeat measurement until discharge from the unit. The lack of continuous measurement of anthropometric data makes monitoring the effectiveness of nutritional interventions extremely difficult.

Despite this, the importance of nutrition screening should not be overlooked and can still be incorporated into routine practice, even if using simplified tools. There are several validated screening tools which can be implemented with ease and identify those at nutritional risk, such as the Nutrition Risk Screening (2002), Malnutrition Universal Screening Tool and Mini Nutritional Assessment, all of which have been able to identify patients with COVID-19 at nutritional risk.[37] Importantly, this screening should be applied to all patients, as even those in normal and overweight categories remain at risk of malnutrition in acute illness, where the risk of sarcopenia is particularly high. Furthermore, sarcopenia has the potential to double mortality risk in critically ill patients.[1] Shared access to electronic health care records in the community can also be a source of recently recorded data where this has not been immediately available.

WARD-BASED NUTRITION CARE

Several barriers to ensuring adequate nutrition support to inpatients on hospital wards have existed during the COVID-19 pandemic. These issues stem from staffing pressures, side effects of illness and challenges placed on catering services in terms of food provision.[1,30]

BARRIERS TO OPTIMISING NUTRITION SUPPORT ON COVID-19 WARDS

Staff pressures
- Incomplete food record charts
- Insufficient support at mealtimes
- Redeployment of staff unfamiliar with ward-based nutrition care
- Less recognition of patient's struggling to eat

Effects of illness
- Difficulty breathing and requirement for supplemental oxygen
- Loss of appetite, taste and/or smell
- Frailty
- Gastrointestinal symptoms
- Cognitive disturbances, including low mood and delirium
- Dysphagia following ICU stay

Difficulties with food provision
- Staff sickness
- Requirement for personal protective equipment and safe working environments
- Disruption to supply chain and logistics

In terms of nutritional strategies, 'Food First' principles, with additional oral nutritional supplements if required, should always be employed as first-line therapy to meet nutritional requirements. Continuous assessment of dietary adequacy should be carried out by a registered dietitian (RD), with consideration of an escalation in nutrition support (via enteral and in some cases parenteral routes) based on individual ability to meet nutritional requirements and maintain both weight and physical function. In some instances, this importance has been recognised and nutrition support has been prioritised through oral, enteral and parenteral means where indicated, ultimately contributing toward improved outcomes in this patient population.[38]

NUTRITION IN THE INTENSIVE CARE UNIT: THE IMPORTANCE OF FEEDING

Critically ill patients provide significant cause for concern when nutrition screening is suboptimal, due to existing malnutrition in this patient group, multiple contributing sequelae of disease and, ultimately, a missed opportunity to contribute toward improved clinical outcomes.[39] Acute respiratory complications leading to ICU admission are a major contributor to morbidity and mortality in patients with COVID-19. These admissions may last days to weeks and even months, depending upon the severity of disease and recovery. During long stays in the ICU, prolonged immobilization and ventilatory support contribute to muscle mass losses, resulting in increasing difficulty in terms of functional recovery.[40] This is exacerbated further by the severe metabolic cost associated with the 'cytokine storm' characteristic of COVID-19, meaning nutritional depletion is a major risk.[12] Many ICU patients, especially those mechanically ventilated, will require enteral nutrition or parenteral nutrition facilitated by an RD to reduce the impact on morbidity and mortality.[37]

CHALLENGES ASSOCIATED WITH FEEDING

In the early stages of the pandemic, professional bodies published clinical guidelines for nutritional management strategies specifically for patients with COVID-19 in the ICU, including the British Dietetic Association[41] and European Society of Clinical Nutrition and Metabolism,[42] among others. These recommendations were provided to combat significant challenges and ensure best practice when providing nutrition support to critically ill COVID-19 patients. Common across these guidelines were specific recommendations to reflect some of the recurring challenges faced when providing nutrition in the ICU setting.

NOTABLE INTERRUPTIONS TO FEEDING OCCUR SECONDARY TO:

- Proning (turning the patient to the prone position to improve ventilation)
- Radiographic imaging to confirm tube placement/replacement
- High levels of sedative and analgesic medications causing
  - Gastrointestinal symptoms
  - High gastric aspirates

Common nutritional strategies employed in patients critically ill with COVID-19:

- Promotion of early enteral nutrition
- Use of prokinetic medications
- Manipulation of feeding rate/concentration during times of proning
- Consideration of postpyloric or supplementary parenteral nutrition if nasogastric feeding is poorly tolerated

Such complexity means feed composition and delivery requires regular review throughout the clinical course and should be altered depending on factors such as fluid restrictions and gastrointestinal tolerance, necessitating regular dietetic and specialist nursing support.[37]

The challenges of nutrition support extend beyond just mechanically ventilated patients with COVID-19, but also those requiring noninvasive ventilatory support. It is well documented that the patients in this group often struggle to meet their nutritional requirements orally.[43] Poor nutritional status is associated with poorer clinical course, higher rates of invasive ventilation and increased mortality in patients undergoing noninvasive ventilation.[44] Due to difficulty meeting nutritional requirements, early artificial nutrition support via nasogastric feeding is often indicated.[45] Nasogastric feeding for patients requiring noninvasive ventilation/continuous positive airway pressure has traditionally[46] and more recently[1] been considered unsafe due to possible risks, including air leakage, with gastrointestinal disturbance further exacerbating respiratory compromise. Similar to the ICU setting, rapidly synthesised consensus guidelines developed early in the pandemic set out measures to minimise risk in these patients, including the use of silicone dressing to secure tube to face, fine bore (8Fr) feeding tubes, early use of prokinetics (metoclopramide, erythromycin) and measurement of gastric aspirates to indicate feed tolerance.[45] In cases of poor tolerance, consideration of postpyloric feeding or parenteral nutrition is advised.[45] A key aspect of optimising nutrition care across these settings is through a focus on multidisciplinary working.

NUTRITION AS AN ADJUNCTIVE TREATMENT—THE ROLE OF MICRONUTRIENTS

Micronutrients play an indispensable role in supporting immune function during times of illness,[2] which has been reflected by recent clinical guidelines from the European Society for Clinical Nutrition and Metabolism on the nutritional management of patients with COVID-19.[42] Much focus has been directed toward the potential of micronutrients as an adjunct to current treatments in mediating the inflammatory response observed with severe Covid-19 infection in the ICU setting. This has been prominent in the ICU setting, where specific micronutrients are thought to play a role in balancing the production of inflammatory cytokines to deal with the overreactive host response to infection and associated cytokine storm.[2] Accordingly, a number of clinical trials are underway to examine the benefit of vitamin and mineral supplementation in patients with COVID-19.

A range of micronutrients have been studied in the ICU setting more widely, many of which have demonstrated poorer outcomes in cases of deficient status and consequently have the potential to contribute to improved outcomes when status is corrected.[2] This comes with the caveat that plasma micronutrient concentrations must be interpreted with caution, given there is consistent evidence that most common measured micronutrients in the plasma are significantly lowered as part of the systemic inflammatory response irrespective of acute or chronic injury.[47] Raised C-reactive protein may provide an indication of this effect.

For example, vitamin D has been studied in ICU patients in the past, and severe deficiency in critical illness has been associated with poorer outcomes.[48] Interest in a potential therapeutic role for vitamin D in this patient group has accelerated during the COVID-19 pandemic.[49,50] An increasing depth of observational data on this relationship has prompted the initiation of clinical trial protocols in a bid to determine cause and effect.[51] Data from these studies have so far been mixed, and close attention must be paid to factors such as baseline status, optimal target ranges, clinical assays and measurable metabolites. Given that avoiding vitamin D deficiency is already an accepted target in this patient group, a pragmatic approach would be to routinely screen for and treat suboptimal status in all patients with COVID-19. This same logic can be applied to the many other micronutrients of interest, further details of which have been explored in a number of scoping reviews.[2,3]

In some instances, additional supplementation may be warranted based on mitigating factors. For example, provision of a vitamin preparation supplementing vitamins B and C (Pabrinex) is commonly provided for new patients considered at risk of refeeding syndrome on admission for an initial 10 days. This functions to prevent further electrolyte disturbances while also factoring in temporary deficits, particularly from inadequate enteral feed provision.

CONCLUSION

In the absence of robust interventional data, extrapolations based on existing knowledge of the relationship between nutrition, immunity and infection have informed the nutritional management of most patients with COVID-19. First-line principles include routine screening for malnutrition, screening and supplementation for insufficiency and deficiency, a food-first approach (in some cases supplemented by oral nutritional supplementation) and escalation to enteral and/or parenteral nutrition when appropriate. Optimising nutrition care requires a multidisciplinary approaching involving medical, nursing, dietetic and other allied health professional teams.

COVID-19 Recovery in the Community: Post Hospitalisation

Much of the discussion regarding COVID-19 and its impacts have focused on the impact on hospitals, critical care units and strained health care workforces. From the outset of the pandemic, there have been daily updates on the number of cases, the number of critical care beds occupied by patients with COVID-19 and the number of daily deaths. While clearly these figures have resonated with many and have been used as justification for governmental action, the fact remains that most patients who contact COVID-19 recover and most do not require hospitalisation.

There are now millions of people around the world living in the community after acute COVID-19. Many of these will have had a period where their appetite was poorer than usual, they faced difficulties feeding as described earlier or they were less physically active than they usually would be. A deterioration in physical and nutritional status is likely, takes time to recover and may require additional support. Bearing in mind the preexisting burden of malnutrition around the world, the effect of COVID-19 on nutritional status should be a cause for concern for all stakeholders. Here we describe some of the challenges likely to be faced in the years to come.

LONG COVID

Patients who suffer from COVID-19 are typically advised to isolate for 14 days from the onset of symptoms or the date of a positive test. During this period, the most common symptoms are a continuous cough, loss of smell and taste and a high temperature. However, other symptoms have also been reported, such as headache, shortness of breath, nausea, vomiting, diarrhoea and fatigue. For the majority of patients, these symptoms resolve themselves upon recovery but for some they persist for weeks to months, a phenomenon that has become known as 'long COVID'.

Loss of appetite, or anorexia, has also been reported as a symptom of long COVID that many have experienced. While this will likely directly affect diet and therefore nutritional status, other long-term symptoms may have similar consequences. Fatigue may make people less able to prepare meals, breathlessness can make eating both difficult and extremely tiring, while patients experiencing nausea and vomiting are likely to have reduced appetite. These symptoms often occur in combination with each other and therefore exert a synergistic effect on each other.

Undernutrition has been estimated to affect over 3 million people in the UK while 25%–34% of patients are estimated to be malnourished on admission to hospital.[52] Several reports have described clinically significant weight loss in COVID-19 patients,[53–55] and considering that older age is a significant risk factor for both COVID-19 and malnutrition, there may well be a silent increase in the prevalence or severity of malnutrition in the community. The British Dietetic Association has issued a policy statement on nutrition and the COVID-19 discharge pathway,[41] in which they advise that patients being discharged after treatment for COVID-19 are screened for malnutrition and that they have access to nutrition support from an RD if required. They highlight that good nutrition is essential in disease recovery and that not addressing nutrition is likely to result in a greater burden for many patients, plus primary and secondary care services.

Over the course of the pandemic, health services have been under strain to make beds available to patients who need them most. As a result, patients may have been discharged back into the community before their nutritional intakes and status were optimised, leading to an increased malnutrition burden. Like many issues in nutrition, this is not likely an issue which can be addressed in the short term but may require a shift in thinking about the importance of nutrition upon discharge and the effect that it may have on subsequent admissions.

Despite the obvious role and importance of nutrition in both the acute care of patients with COVID-19 and in those suffering from long COVID, the rapid guideline produced by the National Institute for Health and Care Excellence in the UK made no comments on diet or nutrition,[56] other than to mention that the expertise of dietetics may be required.

MANAGING MALNUTRITION IN THE COMMUNITY

The first step in managing malnutrition is to identify it. Numerous screening tools have been discussed throughout this book and it is worth revising Chapter 2 on the basic principles of screening and assessment. The British Dietetic Association advised that all patients who have suffered from COVID-19 should be screened upon discharge from hospital[41]; however, those patients who may be overweight or obese may not be considered at risk of malnutrition and therefore clinically significant weight loss, and indeed muscle loss, may go unnoticed.

Though COVID-19 has undoubtedly caused hardship on many fronts, it may also serve as an opportunity to improve the state of nutrition screening and further assessment in the community. We must also consider that in most cases, this screening will not be carried out by nutrition professionals like RDs, given that these services are usually accessed by onward referral. Therefore, the responsibility will likely fall on primary care practitioners to identify and appropriately triage patients.

Once malnutrition or risk thereof has been identified, it can be managed appropriately based on local guidelines and malnutrition pathways. Often screening tools provide information and guidance around when rescreening should occur. Generally, a high-energy, high-protein diet will be recommended for these patients, with a focus on selection of foods naturally high in energy and protein. Practices like food fortification may also be advised such as adding cream, cheese, and butter where possible to existing meals. Some patients may also benefit from the prescription of oral nutrition supplements,[35] especially considering some of the symptoms of long COVID discussed previously.

Like many nutrition interventions, the importance of monitoring and reviewing such patients is paramount. For many, symptoms will resolve in due course, and patients will likely then go back to eating as they had done previously. However, given time which has elapsed since the onset of both the COVID-19 pandemic and subsequent nutrition issues have become apparent, it is difficult to assess just what impact it will have in the long term.

NUTRITION: EVERYONE'S RESPONSIBILITY

As should now be clear, nutrition is not just the responsibility of nutrition professionals per se but rather the responsibility of all members of the multidisciplinary team in acute care and in the community. Nutrition and deterioration in nutritional status are important considerations in the development, disease course, recovery and rehabilitation from COVID-19, and there are many opportunities to influence outcomes in this pathway. As previously mentioned, dietetic services are generally accessed by onward referral and therefore only patients deemed to be at high enough risk will benefit from their expertise. Accordingly, doctors, nurses, allied health professionals, social workers, carers, friends and family members all have a role to play in maintaining good nutrition among those vulnerable patients, and either referring or requesting referral to experts as required.

Many guidelines and pathways exist for professionals and members of the public alike, where they can access good, reliable information to improve nutrition-related outcomes. COVID-19 will be remembered for many reasons and will leave a legacy on health care; however, one positive which could come about from its impact would be an increased acknowledgement of the role of nutrition. To address malnutrition in the community and reduce the risk of further infection from COVID-19 or any infectious disease which follows, there must be an appreciation that we all have a role in nutrition, no matter how small.

References

1. Wu Z, McGoogan JM. Characteristics of and important lessons from the coronavirus disease 2019 (COVID-19) outbreak in China: Summary of a report of 72 314 cases from the Chinese Center for Disease Control and Prevention. *JAMA*. 2020;323(13):1239–1242. https://doi.org/10.1001/jama.2020.2648.
2. Gupta R, Hussain A, Misra A. Diabetes and COVID-19: Evidence, current status and unanswered research questions. *Eur J Clin Nutr*. 2020;74(6):864–870. https://doi.org/10.1038/s41430-020-0652-1.
3. Fernández-Quintela A, Milton-Laskibar I, Trepiana J, et al. Key aspects in nutritional management of COVID-19 patients. *J Clin Med*. 2020;9(8):2589. https://doi.org/10.3390/jcm9082589.
4. Calder PC. Nutrition, immunity and COVID-19. *BMJ Nutr Prev Health*. 2020;3(1):74–92. https://doi.org/10.1136/bmjnph-2020-000085.
5. McAuliffe S, Ray S, Fallon E, Bradfield J, Eden T, Kohlmeier M. Dietary micronutrients in the wake of COVID-19: An appraisal of evidence with a focus on high-risk groups and preventative healthcare. *BMJ Nutr Prev Health*. 2020;3(1):93–99. https://doi.org/10.1136/bmjnph-2020-000100.
6. Lanham-New SA, Webb AR, Cashman KD, et al. Vitamin D and SARS-CoV-2 virus/COVID-19 disease. *BMJ Nutr Prev Health*. 2020;3(1):106–110. https://doi.org/10.1136/bmjnph-2020-000089.
7. Derbyshire E, Delange J. Covid 19: Is there a role for immunonutrition, particularly in the over 65s? *BMJ Nutr Prev Health*. 2020;3(1):100–105. https://doi.org/10.1136/bmjnph-2020-000071.
8. Barker LA, Gout BS, Crowe TC. Hospital malnutrition: Prevalence, identification and impact on patients and the healthcare system. *Int J Environ Res Public Health*. 2011;8(2):514–527. https://doi.org/10.3390/ijerph8020514.
9. Leij-Halfwerk S, Verwijs MH, van Houdt S, et al. Prevalence of protein-energy malnutrition risk in European older adults in community, residential and hospital settings, according to 22 malnutrition screening tools validated for use in adults ≥65 years: A systematic review and meta-analysis. *Maturitas*. 2019;126:80–89.
10. British Association for Parenteral and Enteral Nutrition (BAPEN). BAPEN publishes results of biggest malnutrition survey ever undertaken (Scotland). 2019. Available at: https://www.bapen.org.uk/media-centre/press-releases/377-bapen-publishes-results-of-biggest-malnutrition-survey-ever-undertaken-scotland.
11. Whittle J, Molinger J, MacLeod D, et al. Persistent hypermetabolism and longitudinal energy expenditure in critically ill patients with COVID-19. *Crit Care*. 2020;24:581. https://doi.org/10.1186/s13054-020-03286-7.
12. Bourke CD, Berkley JA, Prendergast AJ. Immune dysfunction as a cause and consequence of malnutrition. *Trends Immunol*. 2016;37(6):386–398. https://doi.org/10.1016/j.it.2016.04.003.
13. Steele RM, Finucane FM, Griffin SJ, Wareham NJ, Ekelund U. Obesity is associated with altered lung function independently of physical activity and fitness. *Obesity*. 2009;17(3):578–584. Available at. http://doi.wiley.com/10.1038/oby.2008.584.
14. Honce R, Schultz-Cherry S. Impact of obesity on influenza A virus pathogenesis, immune response, and evolution. *Front Immunol*. 2019;10:1071. https://doi.org/10.3389/fimmu.2019.01071.
15. Wu Z, McGoogan JM. Characteristics of and important lessons from the coronavirus disease 2019 (COVID-19) outbreak in China: Summary of a report of 72 314 cases from the Chinese Center for Disease Control and Prevention. *JAMA*. 2020;323(13):1239–1242. https://doi.org/10.1001/jama.2020.2648.
16. Barron E, Bakhai C, Kar P, et al. Associations of type 1 and type 2 diabetes with COVID-19-related mortality in England: A whole-population study. *Lancet Diabetes Endocrinol*. 2020;8(10):813–822. https://doi.org/10.1016/S2213-8587(20)30272-2.
17. Zhu N, Zhang D, Wang W, et al. A novel coronavirus from patients with pneumonia in China, 2019. *N Engl J Med*. 2020;382(8):727–733.

18. Gao C, Cai Y, Zhang K, et al. Association of hypertension and antihypertensive treatment with COVID-19 mortality: A retrospective observational study. *Eur Heart J.* 2020;41(22):2058–2066. https://doi.org/10.1093/eurheartj/ehaa433.
19. Almoosawi S, Palla L. Association between vitamin intake and respiratory complaints in adults from the UK national diet and nutrition survey years 1–8. *BMJ Nutr Prev Health.* 2020;3(2):403–408. https://doi.org/10.1136/bmjnph-2020-000150.
20. Wu D, Lewis ED, Pae M, Meydani SN. Nutritional modulation of immune function: Analysis of evidence, mechanisms, and clinical relevance. *Fron Immunol.* 2019;9. https://doi.org/10.3389/fimmu.2018.03160.
21. Carpagnano GE, Di Lecce V, Quaranta VN, et al. Vitamin D deficiency as a predictor of poor prognosis in patients with acute respiratory failure due to COVID-19. *J Endocrinol Invest.* 2020 Available at: https://pubmed.ncbi.nlm.nih.gov/32772324. Accessed October 31, 2020.
22. Public Health England. SACN vitamin D and health report. GOV.UK. https://www.gov.uk/government/publications/sacn-vitamin-d-and-health-report. Published July 20, 2016. Accessed December 21, 2022.
23. The Irish Longitudinal Study on Ageing. Vitamin D deficiency in Ireland – implications for COVID-19. Results from the Irish Longitudinal Study on Ageing (TILDA). Trinity College Dublin. Published April 2020. Accessed December 21, 2022.
24. UK Gov. At-risk groups to receive free winter supply of vitamin D. 2020. Available at: https://www.gov.uk/government/news/at-risk-groups-to-receive-free-winter-supply-of-vitamin-d.
25. Jie B, Jiang Z-M, Nolan MT, et al. Impact of nutritional support on clinical outcome in patients at nutritional risk: A multicenter, prospective cohort study in Baltimore and Beijing teaching hospitals. *Nutrition.* 2010;26:1088–1093.
26. Starke J, Schneider H, Alteheld B, Stehle P, Meier R. Short-term individual nutritional care as part of routine clinical setting improves outcome and quality of life in malnourished medical patients. *Clin Nutr.* 2011;30:194–201.
27. Mehta S. Nutritional status and COVID-19: An opportunity for lasting change. *Clin Med (Lond).* 2020;20(3):270–273. https://doi.org/10.7861/clinmed.2020-0187.
28. Birgisdottir BE. Nutrition is key to global pandemic resilience. *BMJ Nutr Prev Health.* 2020;3(2):129-132. https://doi.org/10.1136/bmjnph-2020-000160.
29. Shao A, Drewnowski A, Willcox DC, et al. Optimal nutrition and the ever-changing dietary landscape: A conference report. *Eur J Nutr.* 2017;56(Suppl 1):1–21. https://doi.org/10.1007/s00394-017-1460-9.
30. Who.int. 2021. Social determinants of health. Available at: https://www.who.int/teams/social-determinants-of-health. Accessed March 12, 2021.
31. Riley M. Health inequality and COVID-19: The culmination of two centuries of social murder. *Br J Gen Pract.* 2020;70(697):397. https://doi.org/10.3399/bjgp20X711965.
32. Dorn AV, Cooney RE, Sabin ML. COVID-19 exacerbating inequalities in the US. *Lancet.* 2020;395(10232):1243–1244. https://doi.org/10.1016/S0140-6736(20)30893-X.
33. Burström B, Tao W. Social determinants of health and inequalities in COVID-19. *Eur J Public Health.* 2020;30(4):617–618. https://doi.org/10.1093/eurpub/ckaa095.
34. Department of Health and Social Security. *Inequalities in Health: Report of a Research Working Group.* London, UK: Department of Health and Social Security; 1980.
35. Managing Adult Malnutrition. COVID-19 & good nutrition. 2020. Available at: https://www.malnutritionpathway.co.uk/covid19.
36. Minnelli N, Gibbs L, Larrivee J, Sahu KK. Challenges of maintaining optimal nutrition status in COVID-19 patients in intensive care settings. *JPEN J Parenter Enteral Nutr.* 2020;44(8):1439–1446. https://doi.org/10.1002/jpen.1996.
37. Liu G, Zhang S, Mao Z, Wang W, Hu H. Clinical significance of nutritional risk screening for older adult patients with COVID-19. *Eur J Clin Nutr.* 2020;74:876–883. https://doi.org/10.1038/s41430-020-0659-7.
38. Cintoni M, Rinninella E, Annetta MG, Mele MC. Nutritional management in hospital setting during SARS-CoV-2 pandemic: A real-life experience. *Eur J Clin Nutr.* 2020;74(5):846–847. https://doi.org/10.1038/s41430-020-0625-4.
39. Caccialanza R, Laviano A, Lobascio F, et al. Early nutritional supplementation in non-critically ill patients hospitalized for the 2019 novel coronavirus disease (COVID-19): Rationale and feasibility of a shared pragmatic protocol. *Nutrition.* 2020;74:110835. https://doi.org/10.1016/j.nut.2020.110835.

40. Wischmeyer P. Are we creating survivors… or victims in critical care? Delivering targeted nutrition to improve outcomes. *Curr Opin Crit Care*. 2016;22(4):279–284.
41. BDA. Covid-19/Coronavirus Clinical guidance. British Dietetic Association (BDA). https://www.bda.uk.com/practice-and-education/covid-19-coronavirus-clinical-guidance.html. Accessed December 21, 2022.
42. Barazzoni R, Bischoff SC, Breda J, et al. Espen expert statements and practical guidance for nutritional management of individuals with SARS-COV-2 infection. *Clin Nutr*. 2020;39(6):1631–1638. https://doi.org/10.1016/j.clnu.2020.03.022.
43. Reeves A, White H, Sosnowski K, Tran K, Jones M, Palmer M. Energy and protein intakes of hospitalised patients with acute respiratory failure receiving non-invasive ventilation. *Clin Nutr*. 2014;33(6):1068–1073. https://doi.org/10.1016/j.clnu.2013.11.012.
44. Terzi N, Darmon M, Reignier J, et al. Initial nutritional management during noninvasive ventilation and outcomes: A retrospective cohort study. *Crit Care*. 2017;21(1):293. https://doi.org/10.1186/s13054-017-1867-.
45. BAPEN. Route of Nutrition Support in Patients Requiring NIV & CPAP During the COVID-19 Response. BAPEN. https://www.bapen.org.uk/pdfs/covid-19/nutrition-in-niv-21-04-20.pdf. Accessed December 21, 2022.
46. Singer P, Rattanachaiwong S. To eat or to breathe? The answer is both! Nutritional management during noninvasive ventilation. *Crit Care*. 2018;22(1):27. https://doi.org/10.1186/s13054-018-1947-7.
47. McMillan DC, Maguire D, Talwar D. Relationship between nutritional status and the systemic inflammatory response: Micronutrients. *Proc Nutr Soc*. 2019;78(1):56–67. https://doi.org/10.1017/S0029665118002501.
48. Amrein K, Schnedl C, Holl A, et al. Effect of high-dose vitamin D_3 on hospital length of stay in critically ill patients with vitamin D deficiency: The VITdAL-ICU Randomized Clinical Trial. *JAMA*. 2014;312(15):1520–1530. https://doi.org/10.1001/jama.2014.13204.
49. Prevention and Treatment With Calcifediol of COVID-19 Induced Acute Respiratory Syndrome (COVIDIOL). ClinicalTrials.gov Identifier: NCT04366908. https://clinicaltrials.gov/ct2/show/NCT04366908.
50. Kohlmeier M. Avoidance of vitamin D deficiency to slow the COVID-19 pandemic. *BMJ Nutr Prev Health*. 2020;3(1):67–73. https://doi.org/10.1136/bmjnph-2020 000096.
51. Vimaleswaran KS, Forouhi NG, Khunti K. Vitamin D and COVID 19. *BMJ*. 2021;372:n544. https://doi.org/10.1136/bmj.n544.
52. BAPEN. 2021. Introduction to Malnutrition. Available at: https://www.bapen.org.uk/malnutrition-undernutrition/introduction-to-malnutrition?start=4. Accessed March 12, 2021.
53. Di Filippo L, De Lorenzo R, D'Amico M, et al. COVID-19 is associated with clinically significant weight loss and risk of malnutrition, independent of hospitalisation: A post-hoc analysis of a prospective cohort study. *Clin Nutr*. 2021;40(4):2420–2426. https://doi.org/10.1016/j.clnu.2020.10.043.
54. Li T, Zhang Y, Gong C, et al. Prevalence of malnutrition and analysis of related factors in elderly patients with COVID-19 in Wuhan, China. *Eur J Clin Nutr*. 2020;74(6):871–875. https://doi.org/10.1038/s41430-020-0642-3.
55. Bedock D, Bel Lassen P, Mathian A, et al. Prevalence and severity of malnutrition in hospitalized COVID-19 patients. *Clin Nutr ESPEN*. 2020;40:214–219. https://doi.org/10.1016/j.clnesp.2020.09.018.
56. National Institute for Health and Care Excellence. COVID-19 rapid guideline: Managing the long-term effects of COVID-19. NICE guideline [NG188]. 2020. Available at: https://www.nice.org.uk/guidance/ng188. Accessed March 12, 2021.

INDEX

Note: Page numbers followed by *f* indicate figures, *t* indicate tables, and *b* indicate boxes.

M

O

R

S

W

Z